6th edition

Phlebotomy
Exam Review

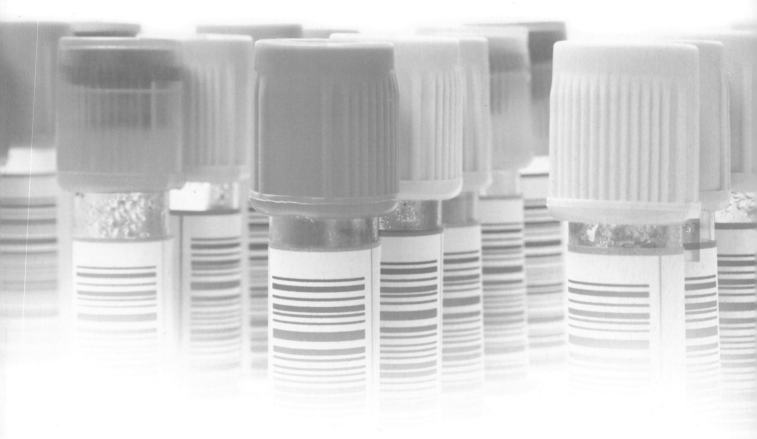

Ruth E. McCall, BS, MT (ASCP)
Retired Director of Phlebotomy and Clinical
   Laboratory Assistant Programs
Central New Mexico (CNM) Community College
Albuquerque, New Mexico

Cathee M. Tankersley, BS, MT (ASCP)
President, NuHealth Educators, LLC
Faculty Emeritus
Phoenix College
Phoenix, Arizona

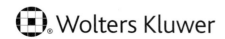
. Wolters Kluwer

Philadelphia • Baltimore • New York • London
Buenos Aires • Hong Kong • Sydney • Tokyo

Acquisitions Editor: Jonathan Joyce
Product Development Editor: Paula Williams
Editorial Assistant: Tish Rogers
Marketing Manager: Shauna Kelley
Production Project Manager: Marian Bellus
Design Coordinator: Terry Mallon
Artist/Illustrator: Jen Clements
Manufacturing Coordinator: Margie Orzech
Prepress Vendor: Aptara, Inc.

6th edition

9 8 7 6 5 4 3 2 1

Printed in the United States of America

978-1-4511-9454-8
Library of Congress Cataloging-in-Publication Data
available upon request

To all of the phlebotomy students who believe in quality education and national recognition for their profession. Thank you.

Ruth E. McCall
Cathee M. Tankersley

Reviewers

Justin Abeyta, AS
Sr. Clinical Laboratory Science Instructor
Lab Sciences
Arizona Medical Training Institute
Mesa, Arizona

Diana Alagna, RN
Medical Assistant Program Director
Medical Assisting
Stone Academy
Waterbury, Connecticut

Rhonda Anderson, PBT(ASCP)cm
Program Manager/Phlebotomy Instructor
Corporate and Career Development, Direct Care
Phlebotomy Program
Greenville Technical College
Greenville, South Carolina

**Belinda Beeman, CMA (AAMA),
PBT(ASCP), MEd**
Professor and Curriculum Coordinator
Medical Assisting
Goodwin College
East Hartford, Connecticut

Judith Blaney, MCLS
Phlebotomy Internship Coordinator
Allied Health
Manchester Community College
Manchester, New Hampshire

Kathy Bode, RN, BS, MS
Professor of Nursing Program
Allied Health Program Coordinator
Nursing and Allied Health
Flint Hills Technical College
Emporia, Kansas

Diane Butera, ASCP
CPT Instructor
Phlebotomy
Fortis Institute
Wayne, New Jersey

Marie Chouest, LPN
LPN Instructor
Health Sciences
Northshore Technical Community College
Bogalusa, Louisiana

Becky M. Clark, MEd, MT(ASCP)
Professor
Medical Laboratory Technology
J. Sargeant Reynolds Community College
Richmond, Virginia

Kelly Collins, MA, CPT1
Teacher
Allied Health
Tulare Adult School
Tulare, California

Silvia de la Fuente, MA, AHI
Phlebotomy Instructor
Allied Health Institute
Medical Programs and Phlebotomy
Estrella Mountain Community College
Avondale, Arizona

Desiree DeLeon, ASCP(PBT)cm, RN
RN Phlebotomy Instructor
Medical Lab Sciences
Central New Mexico Community College
Albuquerque, New Mexico

Mary Doshi, MA, MLS(ASCP)
Associate Professor/MLT Program Director
Medical Technology
San Juan College
Farmington, New Mexico

Amy Eady, MT(ASCP), MS(CTE), RMA
Director of Allied Health
Allied Health
Montcalm Community College
Sidney, Michigan

Kathleen Fowle, CPT
Certified Phlebotomist and Instructor
Pinellas Technical College
St. Joseph's Hospital
Clearwater, Florida

Tammy Gallagher, MT(ASCP)
Lead Phlebotomy Instructor
Emergency Medical Services
Butler County Community College
Butler, Pennsylvania

Faye Hamrac, MT, MS, BS
Phlebotomy Instructor
Health Sciences/Phlebotomy
Reid State Technical College
Evergreen, Alabama

Jacqueline Harris, CMA (AAMA), AHI (AMT)
Allied Health Program Chair
Medical Assisting, HCA, Medical Lab Tech
Wright Career College
Wichita, Kansas

Ronald Hedger, DO
Associate Professor of Primary Care
Clinical Education
Touro University Nevada
Henderson, Nevada

Eleanor Hooley, MT (ASCP)
Educator
Allied Health Department
Vancouver Community College
Vancouver, BC, Canada

Jamie Horn, RMA, RPT, AHI
Medical Instructor
Medical Programs
Warren County Career Center
Warren, Pennsylvania

Konnie King Briggs, CCT, CCI; PBT(ASCP); CPCI, ACA
Healthcare Instructor
Healthcare Continuing Education
Houston Community College
Houston, Texas

Theresa Kittle, CPT
Adjunct Instructor
Healthcare
Rockford Career College
Rockford, Illinois

Judy Kline, NCMA, RMA
Medical Assistant Instructor
Health Science Medical Assisting
Miami Lakes Technical Education Center
Miami Lakes, Florida

Peggy Mayo, MEd
Associate Professor
Multi-Competency Health Technology
Columbus State Community College
Columbus, Ohio

Andrea Minaya, MA, CPT
MA/CPT Lab Assistant and CPT
  Administrator
Medical Assistant and Certified Phlebotomy
  Technician
Fortis Institute
Wayne, New Jersey

Linda Pace, CMA, CPC-A
Director, Medical Assisting/Phlebotomy
Medical Assisting and Phlebotomy
Red Rocks Community College
Lakewood, Colorado

Nicole Palmieri, BSN, RN; CCMA, CPT, CET, CPCT
Instructor
Medical Assistant, Phlebotomy, Cardiac/EKG
Patient Care Technician
Advantage Career Institute
Eatontown, New Jersey

Paula Phelps, RMA
Online Education Coordinator
Allied Health
Cowley County Community College
Arkansas City, Kansas

Deyal Riley, CPT, CHI(NHA)
Instructor
Healthcare
Washtenaw Community College
Ann Arbor, Michigan

Ann Robinson, BS, MA, RPBT, LPN
Laboratory Coordinator
Phlebotomy, CNA, RMA, Surg Tech, LPN
Sports Medication
Tulsa Technology Center
Tulsa, Oklahoma

Kristie Rose, MA, PBT(ASCP), CMP
Program Manager/Instructor
Phlebotomy-Health Sciences
Eastern Florida State College
Cocoa, Florida

Diana Ross, RPT(AMT)
Career Services Coordinator
Pima Medical Institute
Mesa, Arizona

Suzanne Rouleau, MSN, RN, HHS
Educator
Allied Health
Manchester Community College
Manchester, Connecticut

Michael Simpson, BA, MS, MT(ASCP)
Clinical Laboratory Instructor
Clinical Laboratory Science
College of Southern Nevada
Clark County, Nevada

Maria V. Suto, BA, CPT
Faculty
Medical Assisting/Certified Phlebotomy Technician
Fortis Institute
Wayne, New Jersey

Joseph Tharrington, CPT1, CPT2, CPT (AMT) RPT, MA
Northern & Central Coast Regional
Director/Instructor
Phlebotomy, Medical Assisting
Academy Education Services (DBA) Clinical
    Training Institute
Santa Maria, California

Tina Veith, MA
Phlebotomy Instructor
Phlebotomy
Allied Health Careers Institute
Murfreesboro, Tennessee

Amy Vogel, MHA
Program Director, Phlebotomy Technician
Allied Health
Harrisburg Area Community College
Harrisburg, Pennsylvania

Sharon F. Whetten, MEd, BS, MT(ASCP)
Education Coordinator
TriCore Reference Laboratories
Albuquerque, New Mexico

Kari Williams, BS, DC
Director, Medical Office Technology Program
Medical Office Technology
Front Range Community College
Westminster, Colorado

Rebecca C. Wilkins, MS, MT(ASCP), SM(ASCP)
Part-time Faculty Instructor
Health Science–MLT/Phlebotomy Program
San Juan College
Farmington, New Mexico

Preface

The demand for phlebotomists and other clinical healthcare professionals who perform phlebotomy to demonstrate competency through national certification continues to increase in light of ever-changing federal safety requirements and healthcare accrediting agency requirements for quality assurance. In addition, some states, such as California and Louisiana, require national certification by an approved certification agency as a condition of obtaining licensure.

Phlebotomy Exam Review, sixth edition, continues the tradition of the prior edition by providing a comprehensive review of current phlebotomy theory and offers an ideal way to study for phlebotomy licensing or national certification exams. It also makes an excellent study guide for students taking formal phlebotomy training programs.

By answering the questions in this review, you will be able to test your knowledge and application of current phlebotomy theory. Theory questions address recent federal safety standards, Clinical and Laboratory Standards Institute (CLSI) guidelines, and the National Accrediting Agency for Clinical Laboratory Sciences (NAACLS) phlebotomist competencies when applicable. Questions are standard multiple choice, like those used on national exams, with choices that often test your critical thinking abilities.

The question section of the book (Part 2) follows the same chapter sequence as that of the companion textbook, *Phlebotomy Essentials*, sixth edition, by the same authors. This format makes it an ideal chapter-by-chapter study reference when used in conjunction with the textbook and companion workbook in phlebotomy training programs.

Outstanding features include:

- A total of 1,640 multiple-choice questions including:
  - 1,385 chapter questions with detailed explanations of the correct answers
  - An additional 55 questions over Phlebotomy Essentials laboratory tests and laboratory math appendices
  - A pretest of 100 questions, with detailed answer explanations, and a pretest analysis to help you evaluate your knowledge and application of current phlebotomy theory
  - A comprehensive mock exam of 100 questions, with answers that provide the cognitive level of the question, the relevant exam topic covered, and the chapter of the textbook where the information can be found
- An online exam simulator of 150 additional questions that allows students to test themselves in review or test mode, with questions on three cognitive levels (application, recall, and analysis), available at http://thepoint.lww.com/McCallExamReview6e.
- An expanded table of contents for Part 2 that corresponds to the companion textbook, *Phlebotomy Essentials*, sixth edition
- Current information on the various exams, including names and contact information for seven organizations that offer phlebotomy certification exams
- A process for creating your very own study plan and way to track your study hours
- A section on study and test-taking skills to help ensure success on the exam
- An Overview and study tips for each chapter
- Preparation tips for test taking for ESL students
- Question choices that are concise, to lessen the chance of confusion, and similar in length, to enhance validity of results by minimizing guessing based on length

This book is designed to help you succeed by providing the information and tools you need to help you pass any national exam you choose to take. We have incorporated years of test-writing experience and major revisions to make this latest exam review book a stimulating learning experience. It is not intended to replace formal education in phlebotomy theory, nor is there any guarantee that using this exam review will ensure your success in passing any certification or licensing exam.

The authors wish to express their gratitude to all who assisted and supported this effort.

Ruth E. McCall
Cathee M. Tankersley

Acknowledgments

The authors would like to thank *Acquisitions Editor* **Jonathan Joyce** and the production and editorial staff at Wolters Kluwer, especially those with whom we worked most closely, with a special thank you to *Product Development Editor* **Paula Williams**, *Creative Services Art Director* **Jennifer Clements** and *Supervisor of Product Development* **Eve Malakoff-Klein** for their patience, support, and dedication to this endeavor, and an extra special thank you to Eve for stepping in and taking the lead when it was really needed. We also wish to give special recognition to our compositor **Indu Jawwad** and her team at Aptara for their patience and professionalism as they brought together the many components of all three texts.

Contents

The chapters in this part correspond to those of the companion textbook, *Phlebotomy Essentials* 6th edition by McCall, R.E., and Tankersley, C.M.

Part 1

Guide to Certification Success

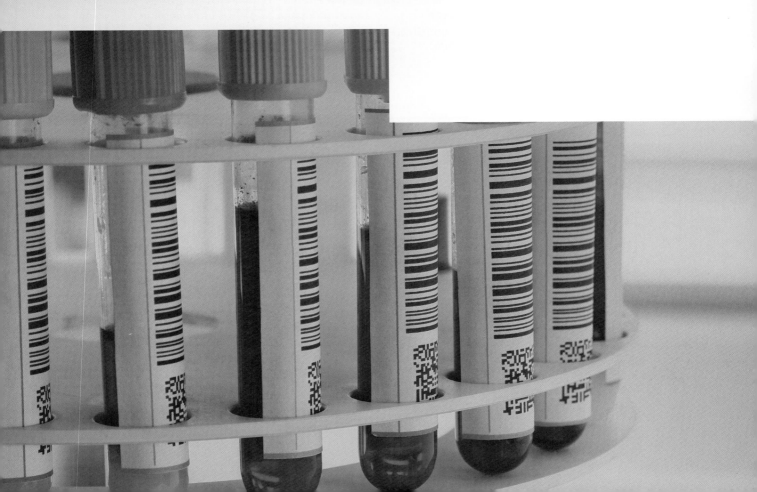

The Certification Process

CERTIFICATION

Certification is a process in which a national nongovernmental organization recognizes the competence of an individual in a particular profession or discipline. In today's healthcare climate, recognition through certification is becoming more popular because of the need for healthcare professionals to show evidence of proficiency in many different areas of practice. Most laboratory errors occur in the preanalytical phase, so it is essential that all healthcare workers who collect blood specimens prove their competence in an effort to ensure quality patient care. In addition, national certification in phlebotomy is required by many institutions to address federal safety and QA requirements and to meet licensing requirements in some states.

CREDENTIALS

Proof of certification is provided by credentials awarded to candidates who have met the educational or experiential requirements of a certifying organization and have successfully passed the organization's certification exam. Certification credentials provide evidence that the individual has mastered fundamental competencies in the profession. Certification credentials indicate competence at the time of the exam, and recertification is a mechanism used to demonstrate continued competence either through re-exam or continuing education.

ELIGIBILITY REQUIREMENTS

Eligibility requirements for obtaining certification vary according to the certifying organization; however, most certifying organizations recognize several eligibility routes. Eligibility routes typically include graduation from an approved educational program, other specific education requirements, or work experience. Requirements to maintain or renew certification also vary, from no requirements (meaning once certified, always certified) to submitting proof of a minimum number of hours of continuing education and payment of a renewal fee.

EXAM FORMAT

Although some certification exams are still traditional hard copy exams taken with pencil and paper, many exams are computer-based. Computer-based testing (CBT) is the equivalent of a paper test that is administered by computer and has the advantage of faster scoring. One example of a computer-based exam is the American Certification Agency (ACA) phlebotomy certification exam.

Some exams involve computer adaptive testing (CAT). When a question is answered correctly on a CAT exam, the very next question comes from a somewhat higher level of difficulty. The difficulty level of the questions presented to the examinee continues to increase until a question is answered incorrectly. At that time, a question that is a little easier is presented. Consequently, the test is tailored to the individual's ability level. CAT testing attempts to establish an appropriate level

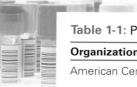

Table 1-1: Phlebotomy Certification Organizations

Organization	Address	Web site	Contact Person
American Certification Agency (ACA)	P.O. Box 58 Osceola, IN 46561	acacert.com	Shirley Evans Carole Mullins
American Medical Technologists (AMT)	10700 West Higgins Road, Suite 150 Rosemont, IL 60018	amt1.com	Geri Mulcahy Chris Damon Dr. James Fidler
American Society of Clinical Pathology (ASCP)*	33 West Monroe Street, Suite 1600 Chicago, IL 60603	ascp.org	Iris McLemore
American Society of Phlebotomy Technicians (ASPT)	P.O. Box 1831 Hickory, NC 28603	aspt.org	Helen Maxwell
National Center for Competency Testing (NCCT)	7007 College Blvd., Suite 385 Overland Park, KS 66211	ncctinc.com	Stan Adams Nancy Graham
National Healthcareer Association (NHA)	11161 Overbrook Road Leawood, KS 66211	nhanow.com	David Saben
National Phlebotomy Association (NPA)	1901 Brightseat Road Landover, MD 20785	nationalphlebotomy.org	Altonese Reese

*Note: Effective October 23, 2009, the National Credentialing Agency for Laboratory Personnel (NCA) was dissolved as a corporation. Certification for medical laboratory personnel is now offered through the ASCP Board of Certification. Current and active certifications will be transferred to the ASCP BOC; no examination is required for the transfer.

of performance and stops the test once the candidate's performance is determined to be at the highest sustainable level. Because CAT scoring takes into account which questions were correctly answered as well as how many, candidates who answer more difficult questions obtain higher scores than those who correctly answer easier questions. The American Society for Clinical Pathology (ASCP) phlebotomy certification exam is a CAT exam.

EXAM CONTENT

Regardless of the format, currently available exams are based on similar versions of accepted competencies for entry-level phlebotomists. Most often these competencies are determined through job/task analysis surveys. The National Accrediting Agency for Clinical Laboratory Sciences (NAACLS) outlines competencies for phlebotomy programs approved by their organization. Outlines reflecting exam content and references used in developing questions are available from most certifying organizations and are usually sent automatically to applicants. Exam questions typically are based on standards for venipuncture, skin puncture, and other phlebotomy procedures developed by the Clinical and Laboratory Standards Institute (CLSI). The number of questions varies from 80 to 250, depending on the offering agency. Some exams have a practical component. Examples are the American Certification Agency (ACA) and American Medical Technologists (AMT) phlebotomy certification exams.

CHOOSING AN EXAM

Once you have decided to become certified, your next job is to decide which organization's exam you would like to take. Currently, at least seven organizations offer certification in phlebotomy. All of these organizations have exam sites throughout the United States. Several of them also offer exams in United States territories, such as Puerto Rico, and in other countries such as Canada.

Generally speaking, employers do not favor any single certifying organization, but applicants may find that one exam better suits their needs than another. In addition, requirements vary by organization, so your choice may be limited depending on your ability to meet the eligibility requirements for the particular exam you choose. Table 1-1 (Phlebotomy Certification Organizations) has information that can help you decide which exam or exams you might be interested in taking. To find out if you are eligible for the exam of your choice, go to the agency's Web site listed in the table. Web sites have applications you can download, and in some cases, you can even apply online.

APPLICATION DEADLINES

Application deadlines for exams offered during a particular period vary according to organization policies. Applications can generally be submitted at any time throughout the year but will typically apply to the exam offering that corresponds with the deadline closest to

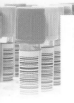

Telephone	E-mail	Fax	Testing Period	Testing Site
574-277-4538	info@acacert.com	574-277-4624	Contact office	Contact office
847-823-5169	RPT@amt1.com geri.mulcahy@amt1.com	847-823-0458	Self-scheduled; open all year	More than 200 test centers throughout the United States
312-541-4999	boc@ascp.org	312-541-4998	Self-scheduled; open all year	More than 200 test centers throughout the United States; current information regarding testing procedures can be found at: http://www.ascp.org/pdf/Procedures forExaminationCertification.aspx
828-294-0078	office@aspt.org	828-327-2969	Contact office for times; see http://96.36.117.186/ CeuExams.aspx for ASPT certification exam dates and times by state	Contact office for sites; see http://96.36.117.186/CeuExams. aspx for ASPT certification exam dates and times by state
800-875-4404;	stan@ncctinc.com; nancy@ncctinc.com	913-498-1243	Contact office	Contact office for nearest test site
800-499-9092 913-661-5592	info@nhanow.com	913-661-6291	Every day, as scheduled through specific sites	More than 1,000 national and international NHA-approved sites
301-386-4200	naltphle@aol.com	301-386-4203	As scheduled	Where requested

the date that the application is received. Applications can be submitted by mail or online, depending on the organization.

KNOWING WHAT TO STUDY

You have decided to become nationally certified. This is a worthy goal, but now where to start? Just what should be studied and how much time should it take? The pretest and pretest analysis that follow can help point out what subjects you need to study and how much time you will need to devote to each of those subjects.

The Pretest and Pretest Analysis

The pretest and pretest analysis help you determine your strengths and weaknesses in six major categories of phlebotomy: Anatomy and physiology, specimen collection, specimen handling, point-of-care testing (POCT), non-blood specimens, and laboratory operations. For study purposes, the categories have been divided into 36 subject areas. The pretest contains questions for each area.

THE PRETEST

This test is simply to indicate the subject areas in which you will need to study. Consequently, when you sit down to take it, do not rush and do not time yourself. Answer each question by writing the answer on a separate piece of paper. This allows you to retake the test as many times as you like. After taking the pretest found in Unit IV, perform the pretest analysis, which will show you how much review time to devote to each of the subject areas.

THE PRETEST ANALYSIS

The pretest analysis, which takes approximately 45 to 50 minutes, shows you which topics are in need of additional scrutiny and how much time should be allotted for each. You will find that time invested here saves you time in the long run. It is a three-step process, and when it is completed you will know minimum recommended study times for each subject and major category and a recommended total review time. The process involves filling out Tables 1-2 and 1-3. Copies of the tables have been provided in the back of the book so that you can perform the analysis more than once if you desire. You can also make additional copies of the tables.

Step 1

Each answer on the pretest has been assigned to a subject area that corresponds to 1 of the 36 subjects listed in Table 1-2. When you have finished the pretest, go back

and check each question. Put a check mark in the box provided by the question if the answer was incorrect or if you were unsure and it required a significant amount of time to decide on the answer.

Now review the pretest again and count the total boxes checked for each subject area. Write this number in the corresponding box in Table 1-2. For example, if you have three answers checked for Anatomy and Physiology, you would put a 3 in that box. Put a "happy face" in the subject box if there are no check marks for that subject.

Step 2

When you have reviewed all of the questions on the pretest and have filled in all of the boxes in Table 1-2, you can estimate your study time in the following way:

- 0–1 in a topic box implies reasonable knowledge of that particular topic and a recommended study time of a minimum of 1 hour. For every topic box that has a 0–1, place a "1" in the corresponding blank for recommended study time.
- 2 in a topic box implies partial knowledge of that particular topic and a recommended study time of a minimum of 2 hours. For every topic box that has a 2, place a "2" in the corresponding blank for recommended study time.
- 3 or more in a topic box implies limited knowledge of that particular topic and a recommended study time of a minimum of 3 hours. For every topic box that has a 3 or higher number, place a "3" in the corresponding blank for recommended study time.

Step 3

Add up all of the recommended study hours in Table 1-2 and write that total number in the appropriate blank in Table 1-3. Add up all hours in Table 1-3 and write that number in the "total suggested minimum study hours" blank.

Your pretest analysis is now complete. The results reveal your subject area strengths and weaknesses and provide a recommended minimum study time for each subject. In Table 1-3, Summary of Study Hours, you will see that the total review time includes suggested study hours for mock exams and final preparation hours. This summary has been tested and shows good results when followed.

Studying and Test-Taking Tips

Regardless of the type of test you are preparing for, you can use numerous techniques to study and review effectively and improve your test-taking ability. The following information is designed to help you develop a study plan, control the study and test-taking environment, and

Table 1-2: Exam Topics and Study Hours by Topics

Anatomy & Physiology (5–10%)	Specimen Collection (45–50%)	Specimen Handling & Processing (15–20%)	Point-of-Care Testing (3–8%)	Non-Blood Specimens (5–10%)	Lab Operations (15–20%)
Structure & Function ☐ Recommended study time ___ hr.	Review of Orders ☐ Recommended study time ___ hr.	Accessioning ☐ Recommended study time ___ hr.	Urinalysis ☐ Recommended study time ___ hr.	Physiology ☐ Recommended study time ___ hr.	Quality Control ☐ Recommended study time ___ hr.
Blood Composition & Function ☐ Recommended study time ___ hr.	Patient Communication, ID, & Assessment ☐ Recommended study time ___ hr.	Labeling ☐ Recommended study time ___ hr.	H & H ☐ Recommended study time ___ hr.	Patient Preparation ☐ Recommended study time ___ hr.	Quality Improvement ☐ Recommended study time ___ hr.
Blood Specimen Types ☐ Recommended study time ___ hr.	Patient Prep & Site Selection ☐ Recommended study time ___ hr.	Specimen Quality ☐ Recommended study time ___ hr.	Coagulation ☐ Recommended study time ___ hr.	Collection ☐ Recommended study time ___ hr.	Interpersonal Relations ☐ Recommended study time ___ hr
Body System Tests ☐ Recommended study time ___ hr.	Equipment & Techniques ☐ Recommended study time ___ hr.	Transport & Storage ☐ Recommended study time ___ hr.	Glucose ☐ Recommended study time ___ hr.	Handling & Processing ☐ Recommended study time ___ hr.	Professional Ethics ☐ Recommended study time ___ hr
Terminology ☐ Recommended study time ___ hr.	Additives & Order of Draw ☐ Recommended study time ___ hr.	Equipment ☐ Recommended study time ___ hr.	Test Performance ☐ Recommended study time ___ hr.	Terminology ☐ Recommended study time ___ hr.	Standards & Regs. ☐ Recommended study time ___ hr.
	Complications ☐ Recommended study time ___ hr.	Terminology ☐ Recommended study time ___ hr.	Test Operation ☐ Recommended study time ___ hr.		Terminology ☐ Recommended study time ___ hr.
	Terminology ☐ Recommended study time ___ hr.		Terminology ☐ Recommended study time ___ hr.		

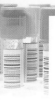

Table 1-3: Summary of Study Hours

Study Item	Hours
Pretest Suggested Study Hours	_____
Additional study hours added for Specimen Collection and Handling which is >60% of the test questions on all exams	4
Timed mock exam (computer or written) and final prep hours	4
Total suggested minimum study hours	_____

learn key ways to retain information while studying. The desired result is to be able to effectively express your knowledge of a subject while taking a test.

STRATEGIES FOR ESL STUDENTS

Studying for a national exam can be a challenge. It can be an even greater challenge if English is not your primary language. The following strategies are meant to help ESL (English as a Second Language) students meet that challenge.

- Fluency in English is obviously a plus when taking a national exam. If you have difficulty reading or speaking English, consider taking the Combined English Language Skills Assessment (CELSA) tests for non-English speakers. These tests, which are available at most community colleges, identify your level of English. Several Internet sites offer online English skills assessment tools and other resources for ESL students.

- Most exam agencies ask for proof of high school graduation or the equivalent as one of the requirements to sit for the exam. If your English skills are not at the level of a high school graduate, you may have a hard time passing a national exam and should consider taking an ESL course at a local community college or other school.

- Purchase or borrow an ESL dictionary (to help you with unfamiliar terms) and an ESL medical terminology book (to help you learn how to identify the meanings of basic elements of medical terms). Make flash cards for terms you need to work on.

- Most questions and choices in this exam review are short and concise to lessen confusion. However, you may still encounter problems understanding a question or choice. If so, focus on the words or parts of the question you do understand to lead you in the right direction when trying to figure it out. If it still doesn't make sense, work backwards by studying the explanation of the correct choice to see if that helps. Practicing this technique with the exam review questions will help prepare you to tackle difficult questions on the certification exam.

- The saying "two heads are better than one" is quite often true. Try to find a study partner whose native language is English or an ESL individual who is already fluent in English. Choose someone who is motivated and organized and who will encourage and inspire you to do your best.

- Wait to sign up for an exam until you are confident of your abilities. There is a big advantage to studying the material at your leisure without an exam deadline fast approaching. Use the studying and test-taking tips that follow, and you will be well on your way to a successful certification experience.

PREPARING TO STUDY

Cultivate a Positive Attitude

The adage, "You can do anything if you set your mind to it," makes a lot of sense. Those who think they can succeed at something and have a plan to achieve it are usually successful. Those who think they will fail often do. If your goal is to pass a national certification exam, tell yourself that you can pass it and visualize being successful. Your belief that you will be able to successfully pass the exam actually helps you achieve that goal. In addition, your attitude plays an important role in determining how you approach preparation for the exam and ultimately how well you do on the actual exam. A positive attitude during the study process will result in more effective studying and increase learning and retention. Bringing a positive attitude to the test will help relieve the stress associated with the testing process and leave your mind free to think logically, which will help you be a more successful test-taker.

Plan to Study

A key element of effective studying is the ability to manage your study or review time. Plan to study. Develop a routine by establishing a particular time and place to study. Committing yourself to a regular routine eliminates the continual need to decide when and where to study. This keeps you in control and helps eliminate procrastination.

Establish a Consistent Study Setting

The correct study environment is important to maximize learning. Choose a setting that is compatible with study activities, and study there on a regular basis. Make sure the site is comfortable and has adequate lighting to minimize eyestrain and fatigue. Be aware of other conditions such as temperature (i.e., warm or cool) and sound so you can manage them according to your preferences.

Identify your learning style. If you are a formal learner you tend to do your best when you study at a desk or table. Avoid beds or couches, where you may become too relaxed and fall asleep. If you are an informal learner, you may choose to study with a "mobile app" offered by ASCP. This will only work if you are disciplined and limit distractions.

Limit Distractions and Commitments

Select a place to study where you are less likely to be disturbed by family members, roommates, pets, TV, phones, and other distractions.

- Do not answer the phone. If you do not have an answering machine, consider unplugging the phone. Turn off your cell phone and put it where you cannot see it.
- Put a "Do Not Disturb" sign on the door.
- Do not disrupt your study schedule unless it is really important. Learn to say "no."

WHEN TO STUDY

Study When You Are Rested

You are more alert when you are rested. Do not study when you are already physically or emotionally tired, and never study to the point of exhaustion. Studies have shown that getting a good night's sleep soon after learning information helps retention, so avoid the temptation to stay up until the wee hours of the morning, especially on the day of the exam.

Follow Your Daily Biorhythm

If possible, study during a time of day when you are most alert and efficient. For example, if you are a morning person, try to arrange study time in the morning.

HOW TO STUDY

Have a Review Strategy

Decide in advance how you will review the material and allow adequate time to accomplish everything you want to do. Use whatever method works best for you. Effective study strategies include reviewing your notes, textbook, and study questions and taking practice tests or mock exams.

Consider Forming a Study Group

Set aside some time to study with other students or peers who are also preparing to take the same exam. Members of study groups tend to motivate each other. Members can also share study tips and techniques that work well for them. Socializing and conversations unrelated to the topic at hand are distracting and reduce actual study time. Agree ahead of time that you will limit socializing and other distractions to within the first few minutes of arriving and after the allotted study time is over.

Establish a Realistic Study Schedule

Avoid resorting to marathon study sessions. Short 1- to 3-hour study sessions on a regular basis are usually more beneficial than occasional long, drawn-out sessions.

Use Time Effectively

Copy information that needs to be memorized into a small notebook or on your smart phone and carry them with you. That way you can study small amounts while waiting in line, riding the bus, or waiting for appointments. Note cards can also be taped on mirrors or cupboards, for quick reviews in between work or other activities.

Take Breaks

Do not forget the old saying, "All work and no play makes Jack a dull boy." You by no means want to be "dull" on test day. Schedule breaks into your allotted study time. The ideal break should be short enough to relieve stress but not so extended that you lose focus, interest, or rhythm.

Watch the Time

Keep track of the time and do not waste it. If you get frustrated or your attention starts to wander, take a break.

Study What Is Appropriate

Try not to study more than necessary. Do not repeatedly go over material you already know. Review it every so often to make certain you still remember it, but do not spend a great deal of time on it. For example, it would be a waste of time to read the textbook or your class notes over and over. A more effective method would be to review your notes and refer to the textbook to clarify concepts or information you have forgotten or do not completely understand.

Study Difficult Topics First

Although the pretest will give you an idea of what subjects you need to study and a recommended amount of study time for each subject, you still have to decide the order in which to study them. It is usually advantageous to study difficult or boring concepts or topics first while your mind is clear. Trying to master a difficult topic at the end of your allotted study time can result in frustration because of a reduced ability to concentrate.

Don't Try to Study Everything At Once

Think about the answer to the joke, "How do you eat an elephant?" Answer: "One bite at a time!" Divide extensive topics into smaller portions.

Use the Exam Review Effectively

Once you feel that you are familiar with the material, try to answer the questions in the exam review. Refer to the textbook for information if you cannot answer a question or still need to clarify material after you read the explanation for the correct answer.

Take the Sample Exams

When you feel you have a good grasp of the material and have answered the review questions, take the sample exams. Again, refer to the text or class notes when you cannot answer a question. Never attempt to memorize questions and answers. The intent of the study questions and sample exams is to help you identify areas in which your knowledge is weak. In addition, because many exams are computer-based, taking the sample computer exam will help you feel more comfortable taking computer exams in the future.

HOW TO IMPROVE YOUR THINKING SKILLS

Multiple-choice questions usually cover six commonly recognized thinking levels. From lowest to highest they are memory, comprehension, application, analysis, synthesis, and evaluation. When studying for multiple-choice tests, many students mistakenly spend their study time learning at the lowest level, memorizing facts without understanding how to analyze and apply the information. Learning how to identify the various thinking levels and using the skills associated with them as you study should help to enhance your knowledge of the subject and help you be a successful test-taker.

Memory Skills

Memory questions require the lowest level of thinking and involve the ability to recall specific information such as terminology, structures, classifications, facts, or concepts. Information of this type is most commonly memorized using techniques involving constant repetition. Examples of memorization techniques include reciting information aloud, listing information, and using flash cards. Information learned this way is committed to short-term memory and may be forgotten unless reinforced using other study methods or practical application.

The following are ways to assist in the memorization of information and enhance recall.

ABCs

Associating information with letters of the alphabet is an effective means of recalling information. Each letter of the alphabet acts as a cue or hint to recall information. You can make up your own ABCs to remember information and use established ones such as the following: the ABCs of cardiopulmonary resuscitation are A = airway, open the airway; B = breathing, perform rescue breathing; and C = circulation, initiate chest compressions.

Acronyms

Another helpful technique used to recall information is the use of acronyms, or words formed by the first letter of a series of statements or facts. Each letter of the word jogs the memory to recall previously learned information. An example is the acronym RACE, used to remember action to take in the event of a fire: R = rescue, A = alarm, C = confine, E = extinguish.

Acrostics

Acrostics are catchy phrases or jingles in which the first letter of each word helps you to remember certain information. An example is the jingle used to help remember the order of draw for the evacuated tube method of venipuncture: Stop light red, stay put, green light, go. S = sterile collections such as blood culture bottles or tubes, L = light blue top tubes, R = red top tubes, S = serum separator tubes (SSTs), P = plasma separator tubes (PSTs), G = green top tubes, L = lavender top tubes, G = gray top tubes.

Imaging

Forming a mental picture associated with the information is another technique used to recall information. For example, one way to remember that a lipemic specimen is caused by fatty substances in the blood that make the serum appear cloudy or milky-looking is to visualize a fat, white cloud when thinking about or saying the term "lipemic."

Comprehension Skills

Comprehension questions test your ability to understand information. To answer comprehension questions, you not only must recall information but also be able to understand the significance of the information. Comprehension questions test your ability to interpret information to draw conclusions or determine consequences, effects, or implications. A good way to enhance comprehension of material is to ask yourself, "What is the significance of this information—how or why is this information useful?" Again, using the term "lipemic" as an example, once we know what the term lipemic means and what a lipemic specimen looks like, we can now ask ourselves, "What is the significance of a lipemic specimen? Why or how is this information useful?" One answer is that a lipemic specimen is a clue that the patient was not fasting. This is significant if the test was ordered fasting. Lipemia also interferes with the testing process for some chemistry tests. Now we not only can recall facts but are also learning to comprehend the significance of these facts.

Application Skills

Application questions test your ability to use information. Answering application questions requires that you not only remember and comprehend information but are also able to relate that information to a real-life situation. Again, using the example of the term "lipemic," an application question might be: "When processing a specimen for a fasting glucose test, you notice that the specimen is lipemic. What does this tell you about the specimen?" Thought process: Lipemia can occur after eating fatty foods. If the specimen is lipemic, the patient must have eaten recently, which means the specimen is probably not a fasting specimen.

Analysis Skills

Analysis questions test your ability to analyze or evaluate information. Analysis questions often require you to evaluate several options to reach an answer. You must be able to recognize differences and determine the significance of several choices before arriving at your answer.

Example: Which of the following specimens would most likely be rejected for testing? A:

a. lipemic specimen for glucose testing.

b. platelet count drawn in an EDTA tube.

c. routine UA in an unsterile container.

d. potassium specimen that is hemolyzed.

The following is a typical thought process used to analyze the choices for the question above and determine the correct answer:

a. A lipemic specimen is an indication that the patient was not fasting, but it does not say it was a fasting glucose. In addition, a few people have lipemic serum for other reasons, so the specimen would not necessarily be rejected.

b. A platelet count *should* be collected in EDTA, so it would not be rejected for that reason.

c. A urine C&S *must* be collected in a sterile container, but a routine UA *does not have to be,* so an unsterile container would not cause it to be rejected.

d. Hemolysis liberates potassium from the red blood cells. That means a hemolyzed potassium specimen would most likely be rejected. The correct answer is "d."

HOW TO ANSWER MULTIPLE-CHOICE QUESTIONS

- For written exams, jot down memory aids in the margins if you are allowed.
- Read the question carefully.
- Do not assume information that is not given.
- Eliminate choices that are clearly incorrect.
- Answer the easy questions first.
- Do not spend a great deal of time on questions you cannot answer.
- If you do not know the answer, skip the question and come back later. Information in other ques-

tions may remind you of the correct answer. If you still do not know the answer, try to make an educated guess.

- Do not change answers without a good reason. Your first guess is usually your best unless other questions remind you of the correct response.

Tips for Test Day

- Get a good night's sleep before the test. The more rested you are, the more you will be able to think clearly and do your best on the test.
- Collect the items that you must bring to the test, such as identification and test documents, ID, calculator, and pencils ahead of time so that you will not be scrambling to find them at the last minute.
- Wear comfortable clothes to the exam. Dress in layers so that you can adapt in case the room is too cold or too warm.
- Know your test site. If the test is in a location with which you are unfamiliar, drive by the testing site a day or two before the exam. If possible, travel during the same time of day as when you will be traveling to take the actual test. Allow yourself extra travel time the day of the test in case there are unexpected delays.
- Arrive early for the test. That way you can get yourself situated and mentally prepared. You also have the opportunity to situate yourself in a location that is comfortable for you and suits your needs, rather than having to choose quickly from the seats that are left.
- Listen carefully while test directions are given. Ask for clarification from the proctor if you do not understand something.
- Try to relax. Change positions, or pause to take a deep breath and stretch now and then.

Overcoming Test Anxiety

Keep in mind that some anxiety or tension before an exam is normal, although excessive anxiety is not. Being well prepared is an excellent way to keep anxiety levels low. Having familiarity with the material builds confidence. The more familiar you are with the material, the more confident you will be. The more confident you are, the better you will do on the exam. Confidence in your ability and a positive attitude about your chances of success go a long way toward relieving stress or anxiety about the testing process. So prepare yourself well, follow the tips for test day, approach the exam with confidence, banish negative thoughts, and visualize success.

Part 2

Exam Review

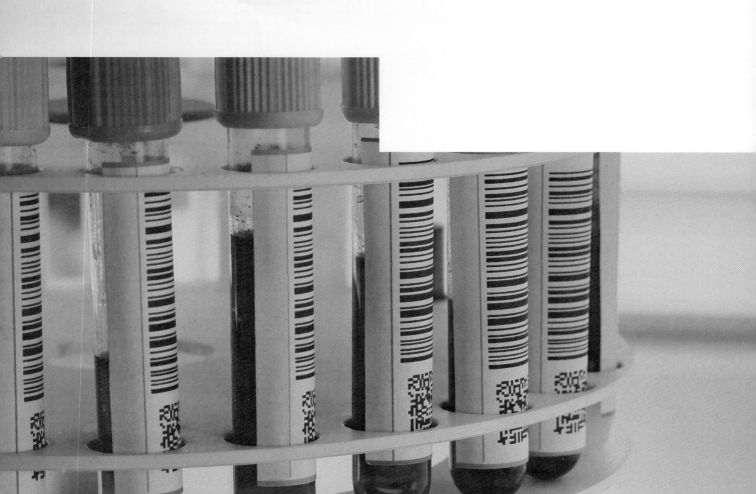

Chapter 1

Phlebotomy: Past and Present and the Healthcare Setting

Study Tips

- Study the key points in the corresponding chapter of the textbook.

- Make a list and describe or sketch the equipment used in early medical phlebotomy.

- Draw a stick-figure phlebotomist and surround him or her with a list of personal characteristics that make up the public's perception of the phlebotomist.

- Using Table 1-1, *Phlebotomist Title and Initials Awarded by Certification Agency,* in Chapter 1 of *Phlebotomy Essentials,* list the initials of the certification phlebotomy title from each national certifying organization.

- Draw a simple communication feedback loop and insert your name and the name of a friend as the sender and receiver. Using Figure 1-5 in the TEXTBOOK, the *Verbal Communication Feedback Loop,* write the most obvious communication barriers across the message and feedback lines between you and your friend when communicating.

- Draw a healthcare "delivery model" showing two general categories of healthcare facilities. See Box 1-3, Two Categories of Healthcare Facilities, in the TEXTBOOK and list the types of facilities that fall under each, e.g., urgent care, physician's office, hospice, etc.

- List 10 medical disorders and write the name of the physician who would specialize in each.

- Draw a flowchart showing all levels of laboratory personnel from the highest level of education to the least amount of education required.

- Complete the activities in Chapter 1 of the companion workbook.

Overview

Health care today has evolved into an integrated delivery system offering a full range of services intended to ensure that the patient gets what is needed at the right time and in the right way. In addition to physicians, nurses, and patient support personnel, allied health professionals such as clinical laboratory personnel play an important role in the delivery of patient care. The clinical laboratory provides physicians with some of medicine's most powerful diagnostic tests. The value of laboratory service has become even more important with the passage of new healthcare legislation. It is predicted the clinical laboratory providers' crucial diagnostic data will greatly influence physicians' decisions and positively affect those who manage patient outcomes and costs. Before patient test results can be reported to the physician, specimens must be collected and analyzed. The phlebotomist has been a key player in this process for some time and his or her role continues to expand. In addition to blood collection skills, successful specimen collection requires the phlebotomist to demonstrate competence, professionalism, good communication and public relations skills, thorough knowledge of the healthcare delivery system, and familiarity with clinical laboratory services.

Review Questions

Choose the BEST answer.

1. The Public Health Service's responsibilities are to
   a. administer programs for control of disease.
   b. implement national entitlement programs.
   c. provide emergency services and treatment.
   d. write laboratory regulations for CLIA '88.

2. This is an abbreviation for a healthcare provider that includes a number of associated medical facilities that furnish coordinated healthcare services from prebirth to death.
   a. CPT
   b. IDN
   c. PHS
   d. PPO

3. The abbreviation for the coding system used by physicians for patients seen in the ambulatory setting and for physician billing in hospitals is called
   a. CPT.
   b. DRGs.
   c. PPO.
   d. PPS.

4. It is the responsibility of the designated case manager or gatekeeper in managed care to
   a. know the patient's financial capabilities.
   b. manage the patient's extracurricular activities.
   c. provide early detection of a patient's disease.
   d. share this patient's information with the family.

5. A nationally endorsed principle ensuring that patients and their families understand their rights and responsibilities while in a healthcare facility can be found in
   a. federally mandated HIPAA regulations.
   b. prepaid healthcare insurance plans.
   c. Protected Health Information documents.
   d. the *Patient Care Partnership* brochure.

6. Managed care organizations control costs by
   a. discouraging patient visits.
   b. detecting risk factors early.
   c. eliminating case managers.
   d. limiting patient enrollment.

7. The term *third-party payer* is used to describe
   a. patient reimbursement.
   b. insurance portability.
   c. health insurance plans.
   d. public health services.

8. This is the abbreviation for a classification system that is only used to determine payment to hospitals for medicare services.
   a. APC
   b. DRGs
   c. ICD-10
   d. PPS

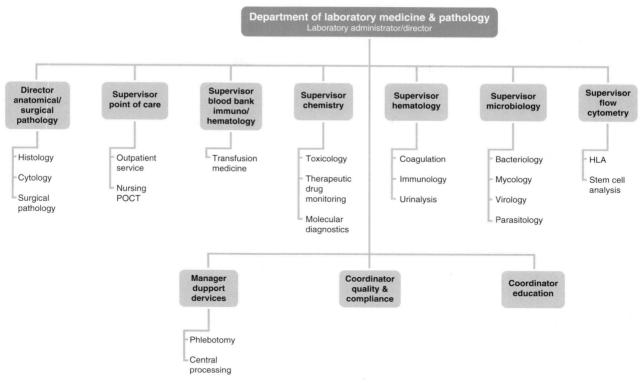

Figure 1-1 An example of a clinical laboratory organizational chart.

Use Figure 1-1 (An example of a clinical laboratory organizational chart) to answer the following five questions:

9. Which person would have the responsibility for seeing that nurses maintain quality bedside testing?
   a. Manager of Support Services
   b. Supervisor, Chemistry
   c. Supervisor, Hematology
   d. Supervisor, Point of Care

10. What person oversees the department that does the fungi and viral studies?
   a. Supervisor, Chemistry
   b. Supervisor, Hematology
   c. Supervisor, Microbiology
   d. Supervisor, Point of Care

11. Who is responsible for the personnel that prepare all specimens that are received for testing in the laboratory?
   a. Manager, Central Processing
   b. Supervisor, Immunohematology
   c. Supervisor, Immunology
   d. Supervisor, Outpatient Services

12. Which person alerts the personnel of the latest standards and regulations set by CAP?
   a. Coordinator, Quality and Compliance
   b. Manager, Central Processing

   c. Supervisor, Immunohematology
   d. Supervisor, Immunology

13. Which Supervisor oversees the typing and cross-matching of transfusion units in the laboratory?
   a. Supervisor, Cytology
   b. Supervisor, Flow Cytometry
   c. Supervisor, Immunohematology
   d. Supervisor, Immunology

14. Which phlebotomist's duty involves prioritizing specimens to achieve the desired TAT?
   a. Collecting routine venous specimens
   b. Performing point-of-care testing
   c. Preparing patient for specimen collection
   d. Preparing specimens for dispatching

15. Telephone etiquette involves
   a. keeping your statements simple and to the point.
   b. leaving a person on hold until you have the answer.
   c. referring an emotional caller to the administrator.
   d. remaining anonymous to avoid any problems.

16. Which of the following is an agency that certifies phlebotomists?
    a. ASCLS
    b. ASCP
    c. CLSI
    d. NAACLS

17. The *primary* duty of a phlebotomist is to
    a. answer all phone calls.
    b. collect blood specimens.
    c. document the workload.
    d. perform clerical duties.

18. Part of the phlebotomist's role is to promote good public relations because
    a. close personal relationships with the patients are essential.
    b. laboratorians are not recognized as part of the healthcare team.
    c. patients equate this interaction with the overall caliber of care.
    d. skilled public relations overcomes inexperience and insecurity.

19. *Primum non nocere* comes from the Hippocratic Oath and means
    a. do first things first.
    b. first do no harm.
    c. quality is foremost.
    d. ready to serve.

20. Which of the following is an example of good work ethic?
    a. Aggressiveness
    b. Indifference
    c. Dependability
    d. Self-interest

21. Phlebotomy is used as a therapeutic treatment for
    a. diabetes.
    b. leukemia.
    c. phlebitis.
    d. polycythemia.

22. A phlebotomist participates in continuing education programs to
    a. avoid state licensure or certification.
    b. eliminate the need for annual evaluation.
    c. explore other employment in health care.
    d. stay up to date on the latest procedures.

23. The term *phlebotomy* is derived from Greek words that, literally translated, mean to
    a. cut a vein.
    b. draw blood.
    c. stick a vein.
    d. withdraw blood.

24. One of a phlebotomist's duties is to
    a. assist with inserting IV cannulas.
    b. help nurses with direct patient care.
    c. inform patients of their test results.
    d. perform lab computer operations.

25. What are the credentials of an AMT-certified phlebotomist?
    a. CPT
    b. MLT
    c. PBT
    d. RPT

26. Which of the following ancient bloodletting instruments has a counterpart in a modern-day bleeding device?
    a. Bleeding bowl
    b. Cup
    c. Fleam
    d. Syringe

27. Proof of participation in a workshop to upgrade skills required by some agencies to renew certification is called
    a. accreditation verification.
    b. continuing education units.
    c. workload confirmation.
    d. reciprocity substantiation.

28. While staying in a healthcare facility, one of the patient's expectation as listed in *The Patient Care Partnership* brochure is the right to
    a. a 1:1 patient-to-nurse ratio.
    b. a secluded private room.
    c. help with billing claims.
    d. share confidential information.

29. The personal "zone of comfort" is a radius of
    a. 1 to 18 in.
    b. 1½ to 4 ft.
    c. 4 to 12 ft.
    d. over 12 ft.

30. The patient is very emotional and cannot understand what the phlebotomist is asking him to do. This is an example of
    a. a communication barrier.
    b. invasion of the intimate zone.
    c. lack of professionalism.
    d. all of the above.

31. Which of the following is an example of a confirming response to a patient?
    a. "I am on a tight schedule right now."
    b. "I do not know what you mean."
    c. "I have no idea how long it will take."
    d. "I understand how you must be feeling."

32. Which of the following is an example of negative kinesics?
    a. Eye contact
    b. Frowning
    c. Shouting
    d. Smiling

33. Which one of the following projects a professional image for a phlebotomist?
    a. A very strong-smelling scent
    b. Closed-toe, conservative shoes
    c. Long hair surrounding the face
    d. Natural-looking artificial nails

34. A patient loses trust in the phlebotomist when the phlebotomist
    a. brushes off patient concerns.
    b. conveys understanding.
    c. looks like a professional.
    d. makes good eye contact.

35. Which one of the following represents improper telephone protocol?
    a. Answering the phone promptly.
    b. Clarifying and recording information.
    c. Hanging up on hostile individuals.
    d. Restating information received.

36. Proxemics is the study of an individual's
    a. body language.
    b. concept of space.
    c. facial expressions.
    d. verbal communication.

37. One element of good communication in health care involves
    a. accepting patients as unique individuals with special needs.
    b. disguising the truth with statements like "this won't hurt."
    c. expressing disapproval when a patient refuses a blood draw.
    d. showing the patient that you are the one who is in control.

38. The best way to handle a "difficult" or "bad" patient is to
    a. help the patient to feel in control of the situation.
    b. leave the room without collecting the specimen.
    c. speak very firmly to maintain your dominance.
    d. threaten to report the patient to his or her doctor.

39. Which of the following is an example of proxemics?
    a. Eye contact
    b. Facial expression
    c. Personal contact
    d. Personal hygiene

40. Which of the following situations allows patients to feel in control?
    a. Agreeing with patients that it is their right to refuse a blood draw.
    b. Informing patients that you are going to collect a blood sample.
    c. Insisting that patients cooperate and let you draw needed samples.
    d. Telling patients they are not to eat or drink anything during a test.

41. What is the average speaking rate of a normal adult?
    a. 75 to 100 words per minute
    b. 125 to 150 words per minute
    c. 250 to 350 words per minute
    d. 500 to 600 words per minute

42. Another term for outpatient care is
    a. ambulatory care.
    b. nonambulatory care.
    c. nursing home care.
    d. rehabilitation care.

43. Which laboratory department performs tests to identify abnormalities of the blood and blood-forming tissues?
    a. Chemistry
    b. Hematology
    c. Microbiology
    d. Urinalysis

44. Which department is responsible for administering a patient's oxygen therapy?
    a. Cardiodiagnostics
    b. Electroencephalography
    c. Physical therapy
    d. Respiratory therapy

45. Which of the following tests would be performed in surgical pathology?
    a. Compatibility testing
    b. Differential cell count
    c. Frozen sections
    d. Viral studies

46. The phlebotomist is asked to collect a specimen from a patient in the nephrology department. A patient in this department is most likely being treated for a disorder of the
    a. joints.
    b. kidneys.
    c. lungs.
    d. nose.

47. The phlebotomy supervisor asked a phlebotomist to collect a specimen in the otorhinolaryngology department. The phlebotomist proceeded to go to the department that provides treatment for
    a. bone and joint disorders.
    b. ear, nose, and throat disorders.
    c. eye problems or diseases.
    d. skin problems and diseases.

48. Which of the following tests is performed in the coagulation department?
    a. BUN
    b. CBC
    c. D-dimer
    d. Glucose

49. Which medical specialty treats patients with tumors?
    a. Geriatrics
    b. Oncology
    c. Ophthalmology
    d. Orthopedics

50. The medical specialty that treats skeletal system disorders is
    a. gastroenterology.
    b. neurology.
    c. orthopedics.
    d. pediatrics.

51. The specialty of this physician is the treatment of newborns.
    a. Gerontologist
    b. Neonatologist
    c. Obstetrician
    d. Pediatrician

52. Another name for blood bank is
    a. immunohematology.
    b. immunology.
    c. microbiology.
    d. serology assays.

53. Which one of the following is a chemistry test?
    a. Hemoglobin A1c
    b. Hematocrit

    c. Hemoglobin
    d. Platelet count

54. These medical facilities were designed to bridge the gap between an injury that is too serious to wait for the primary care physician but not a life-threatening situation that calls for a trip to the ER.
    a. Hospice home care
    b. Public health clinics
    c. Surgical centers
    d. Urgent care centers

55. With which other hospital department would the laboratory coordinate therapeutic drug monitoring?
    a. Nuclear medicine
    b. Pharmacy
    c. Physical therapy
    d. Radiology

56. Which department processes and stains tissue samples for microscopic analysis?
    a. Chemistry
    b. Coagulation
    c. Histology
    d. Microbiology

57. Of the following personnel, only a high school diploma is required of which one?
    a. Laboratory scientist
    b. Medical technician
    c. Medical technologist
    d. Phlebotomist

58. An appendectomy performed in a freestanding ambulatory surgical center is an example of
    a. managed care.
    b. primary care.
    c. secondary care.
    d. tertiary care.

59. Which department performs blood cultures?
    a. Hematology
    b. Microbiology
    c. Serology
    d. Urinalysis

60. Electrolyte testing includes
    a. ALT and AST.
    b. BUN and creatinine.
    c. glucose and total protein.
    d. sodium and potassium.

61. Which hospital department performs diagnostic tests and monitors therapy of patients with heart problems?
    a. Cardiodiagnostics
    b. Electroneurodiagnostics
    c. Occupational therapy
    d. Respiratory therapy

62. Basic metabolic panels (BMPs) are performed in which department?
    a. Chemistry
    b. Hematology
    c. Histology
    d. Microbiology

63. Which laboratory department performs chromosome studies?
    a. Chemistry
    b. Coagulation
    c. Cytogenetics
    d. Hematology

64. A Pap smear is examined for the presence of cancer cells in this department.
    a. Cytology
    b. Hematology
    c. Histology
    d. Microbiology

65. The prepaid group healthcare organization in which members must have preauthorization for certain medical procedures is a
    a. DRG.
    b. HMO.
    c. IDN.
    d. SNF.

66. The term used to describe sophisticated and highly complex medical care is
    a. managed care.
    b. primary care.
    c. secondary care.
    d. tertiary care.

67. A patient in labor would normally be admitted to which of the following medical specialty departments?
    a. Cardiology
    b. Geriatrics
    c. Obstetrics
    d. Pediatrics

68. A primary care physician (PCP) is considered the patient's gatekeeper in this type of managed care plan.
    a. CMS
    b. HMO
    c. PHS
    d. PPO

69. Toxicology is often a part of which of the following laboratory departments?
    a. Chemistry
    b. Coagulation
    c. Hematology
    d. Urinalysis

70. This individual is a physician who is a specialist in diagnosing disease from laboratory findings.
    a. Administrative technologist
    b. Laboratory director
    c. Medical technologist
    d. Clinical pathologist

71. Which of the following is a hematology test?
    a. BMP
    b. C&S
    c. CBC
    d. HBsAg

72. The department that analyzes arterial blood gases and tests lung capacity is
    a. cardiodiagnostics.
    b. electroneurodiagnostics.
    c. diagnostic radiology.
    d. respiratory therapy.

73. Which department performs immunoglobulin testing?
    a. Chemistry
    b. Hematology
    c. Serology
    d. Urinalysis

74. Which department performs radiographic procedures and other imaging techniques to aid in detection of a problem?
    a. Occupational therapy
    b. Electroneurodiagnostics
    c. Diagnostic radiology
    d. Respiratory therapy

75. Which of the following is an example of an inpatient care facility?
    a. Day-surgery facility
    b. Dentist's office
    c. Children's hospital
    d. Physician's office

76. Which of the following would most likely be performed in the coagulation department?
    a. BUN
    b. CBC
    c. HCG
    d. PTT

77. Which of the following laboratory personnel has the same qualification as a medical technologist?
    a. MLS
    b. CLT
    c. MLT
    d. RPT

78. Which department would perform a hemogram?
    a. Chemistry
    b. Blood bank
    c. Hematology
    d. Immunology

79. This department examines specimens microscopically for the presence of crystals, casts, bacteria, and blood cells.
    a. Chemistry
    b. Hematology
    c. Microbiology
    d. Urinalysis

80. This hospital department provides treatment to restore patient mobility.
    a. Cardiodiagnostics
    b. Physical therapy
    c. Diagnostic radiology
    d. Respiratory therapy

81. Brain wave mapping and evoked potentials are performed by which department?
    a. Cardiodiagnostics
    b. Electroencephalography
    c. Physical therapy
    d. Respiratory therapy

82. All medical laboratories are regulated by
    a. AMT.
    b. CLIA.
    c. HIPAA.
    d. PHS.

83. This is the abbreviation for the recent healthcare legislation that deals primarily with insurance market reform.
    a. ACA
    b. ACO
    c. CLIA
    d. HIPAA

84. Which laboratory worker has a bachelor's degree or equivalent in medical technology?
    a. MLS
    b. CPT
    c. MLT
    d. PBT

85. Which of the following laboratory personnel has an associate's degree or equivalent?
    a. MLS
    b. MLT
    c. MT
    d. PBT

86. A specimen for ova and parasite testing would be sent to which department?
    a. Chemistry
    b. Coagulation
    c. Microbiology
    d. Urinalysis

87. The test to identify an organism and determine an appropriate antibiotic for treatment is called a
    a. compatibility screen.
    b. culture and sensitivity test.
    c. microscopic analysis.
    d. radioimmunoassay.

88. A glucose test would be performed in which department?
    a. Chemistry
    b. Hematology
    c. Microbiology
    d. Pathology

89. Which medical specialty treats patients with blood disorders?
    a. Dermatology
    b. Hematology
    c. Internal medicine
    d. Rheumatology

90. Which one of the following services is offered by local public health agencies?
    a. Licensure for healthcare workers.
    b. Immunization of the populace.
    c. Collection for donor blood.
    d. Therapy for patient mobility.

91. Which test suggests autoimmune hemolytic anemia, if positive?
    a. BMP
    b. DAT
    c. HCG
    d. PT

92. Blood typing and compatibility testing are performed in this department.
    a. Blood bank
    b. Chemistry
    c. Coagulation
    d. Hematology

93. A sample for fibrin degradation products (FSP) testing would be sent to which of the following departments?
    a. Blood bank
    b. Chemistry
    c. Coagulation
    d. Microbiology

94. Which immunology test detects rheumatoid arthritis?
    a. CMV
    b. EBV
    c. HCV
    d. RF

95. This is a federal program that provides medical care for the indigent.
    a. HIPAA
    b. Medicaid
    c. Medicare
    d. PHS

96. Which department performs chemical screening tests on urine specimens?
    a. Coagulation
    b. Hematology
    c. Microbiology
    d. Urinalysis

97. Which department monitors warfarin therapy?
    a. Chemistry
    b. Coagulation
    c. Immunology
    d. Microbiology

98. Diagnosis and treatment of diseases characterized by joint inflammation is part of which medical specialty?
    a. Dermatology
    b. Gastroenterology
    c. Internal medicine
    d. Rheumatology

99. Which phlebotomist's duty, if not complied with, has a penalty of possible fines or jail time?
    a. Maintain patient confidentiality
    b. Participate in continuing education
    c. Perform quality-control checks
    d. Promote good public relations

100. Which of the following factors is considered critical in understanding a diverse population's healthcare needs?
    a. Attitudes toward seeking help
    b. Knowledge of their customs
    c. Traditions related to healing
    d. All of the above

101. According to CLIA '88, the following is true.
    a. A CLIA certificate is required only for hospitals.
    b. All laboratories must follow the same standards.
    c. Personnel standards are not included in the law.
    d. Physicians' laboratories are exempt from CLIA.

102. Which of the following specimens would be analyzed in the anatomical pathology area?
    a. Biopsy tissue
    b. Stool sample
    c. Synovial fluid
    d. Urine sediment

103. Reference laboratories can offer tests that have
    a. an immediate TAT.
    b. more accurate results.
    c. reduced cost per test.
    d. all of the above.

104. A nurse practitioner may be considered the case manager in this category of care.
    a. Acute care
    b. Primary care
    c. Secondary care
    d. Tertiary care

105. The AMT, ASCP, and ACA are agencies that
    a. accredit phlebotomy programs.
    b. certify laboratory professionals.
    c. license allied health professionals.
    d. monitor communicable diseases.

106. A phlebotomist is told to take procedural shortcuts to save time in collecting specimens during morning sweeps. She disagrees and chooses to follow the rules. Which professional characteristic is she exhibiting?
    a. Compassion
    b. Diplomacy
    c. Integrity
    d. Motivation

107. Which of the following is the name or abbreviation of the federal law that established standards for the electronic exchange of patient information?
    a. CLIA
    b. HIPAA
    c. Medicare
    d. OSHA

108. Which of the following actions by a phlebotomist does not encourage good verbal communication?
    a. Active listening
    b. Giving feedback
    c. Watching nonverbals
    d. Using pat clichés

109. A phlebotomist who appears knowledgeable, honest, and sincere is creating in the patient a sense of
    a. control.
    b. dependency.
    c. empathy.
    d. trust.

110. After being discharged from the hospital, home-bound services offered to meet the needs of patients who require extended care typically include
    a. cancer screening.
    b. immunizations.
    c. physical therapy.
    d. tuberculosis screening.

Answers and Explanations

1. **Answer: a**

   WHY: Public Health Services (PHS), one of the principal units under the Department of Health and Human Services, have agencies at local and state levels. These agencies offer programs that are aimed at the prevention and control of infectious disease and drug abuse. PHS does not provide emergency services or treatment of infectious diseases. Responsibilities such as implementing national entitlement programs or writing laboratory regulation for CLIA '88 falls under the authority of the Centers for Medicare and Medicaid Services (CMS).

   REVIEW: Yes ☐ No ☐

2. **Answer: b**

   WHY: Integrated healthcare delivery systems (IDNs) have been developed to reduce health-care costs while maintaining patient satisfaction by directing the patient to the right provider for the right care. Preferred provider organizations (PPOs) are independent groups of physicians that negotiate contracts with employers for healthcare services at discounted rates in exchange for a guaranteed number of patients. The U.S. Public Health Service (PHS) deals with protection of the nation's mental and physical health, and CPT is a coding system for physician billing.

   REVIEW: Yes ☐ No ☐

3. **Answer: a**

   WHY: The current procedural terminology (CPT) codes were originally developed in the 1960s by the AMA to provide terminology and coding systems for physician billing. In 2014, CMS replaced ICD-9 with **ICD-10-PCS**, the *International Classification of Diseases–Tenth Revision, Procedural Coding System.* This new ICD must be used by all HIPAA-covered entities. ICD-9 diagnosis and procedure codes can no longer be used.

   REVIEW: Yes ☐ No ☐

4. **Answer: c**

   WHY: A case manager or gatekeeper in managed care is responsible for knowing and managing the patient well and recognizing early on changes in their health that could indicate a disease. It is not the responsibility or the right of the case manager to know the patient's financial status or extracurricular activities. Sharing information, even if it is with the family, is not allowed by HIPAA.

   REVIEW: Yes ☐ No ☐

5. **Answer: d**

   WHY: The Patient Care Partnership (Box 1-1) is an easy-to-read brochure and serves as an accepted statement of principle that encourages and guides healthcare institutions to put into writing what patients can expect during their hospital stay. It is designed to help patients understand their rights and responsibilities while being treated in that healthcare facility.

   REVIEW: Yes ☐ No ☐

6. **Answer: b**

   WHY: *Managed care* is a generic term for a payment system that manages costs and quality

Box 1-1

The Patient Care Partnership

Understanding Expectations, Rights, and Responsibilities

What to Expect during Your Hospital Stay

- High-quality hospital care
- A clean and safe environment
- Involvement in your care
- Protection of your privacy
- Help when leaving the hospital
- Help with your billing claims

Adapted from the American Hospital Association's brochure. *The Patient Care Partnership.* See complete document at http://www.aha.org.

by encouraging healthy lifestyles, detecting risk factors, and offering patient education. This payment system encourages patient enrollment rather than limiting it. The case manager or gatekeeper plays a vital role in managing care and the cost of services for the patient. Patient visits are not discouraged, but they are often less necessary if patients are encouraged to live in healthy ways.

REVIEW: Yes ☐   No ☐

7. **Answer: c**

WHY: The term *third-party payer* refers to any entity that insures healthcare costs. It involves multiple payers and numerous mechanisms of payment. It can be an insurance company, the federal government, a managed care program, or a self-insured company.

REVIEW: Yes ☐   No ☐

8. **Answer: a**

WHY: The Ambulatory Patient Classification (APC) method was implemented in 2000 for hospitals and outpatient services to use in determining payment for medicare and medicaid services only. Diagnosis-Related Groups (DRGs) and the *International Classification of Diseases,* 9th rev. (ICD-9), which were being used at that time, were designed for inpatient services only. Today, the new code ICD-10-PCS has replaced ICD-9. See Table 1-5, Methods of Payment and Diagnosis Coding, in the TEXTBOOK.

REVIEW: Yes ☐   No ☐

9. **Answer: d**

WHY: According to the lab organizational chart (Fig. 1-1), the supervisor of Point of Care Testing (POCT) has the responsibility to educate and supervise nursing personnel who do POCT at the bedside.

REVIEW: Yes ☐   No ☐

10. **Answer: c**

WHY: Mycology, the study of fungi, and virology, the study of viruses, are part of the microbiology department, and overseen by that supervisor (Fig. 1-1).

REVIEW: Yes ☐   No ☐

11. **Answer: a**

WHY: The manager of Central Processing is responsible for the personnel who receive, prepare, and dispatch lab specimens for testing (Fig. 1-1).

REVIEW: Yes ☐   No ☐

12. **Answer: a**

WHY: One of the responsibilities of the coordinator of the Quality and Compliance department is to make certain all lab personnel are aware at all times of the quality standards, regulations, and policies that pertain to their area of the laboratory (Fig. 1-1).

REVIEW: Yes ☐   No ☐

13. **Answer: c**

WHY: Figure 1-1 shows that the supervisor of Immunohematology or Blood Bank oversees all tests, such as typing and crossmatching that are performed to provide blood products to patients.

REVIEW: Yes ☐   No ☐

14. **Answer: d**

WHY: Phlebotomist's duties as seen in Box 1-2 involving collecting venous specimens, performing point-of-care testing, and preparing patients for specimen collection. It is when performing specimen processing or preparing specimens for dispatching that they must prioritize for desired turnaround time.

REVIEW: Yes ☐   No ☐

15. **Answer: a**

WHY: The phlebotomist should know laboratory procedures and policies and refer to them in answering callers' questions. In replying to the callers' inquiries, statements should be simple and to the point. A phlebotomist who uses proper telephone etiquette in the laboratory would

Box 1-2

Duties and Responsibilities of a Phlebotomist

Typical Duties

- Prepare patients and site for specimen collection following nationally recognized standards and institution's guidelines.
- Collect venipuncture and capillary specimens for testing following nationally recognized standards and institutional procedures.
- Prepare specimens for proper transport, ensuring the integrity and stability of the sample.
- Adhere to all HIPAA and confidentiality guidelines, including all Code of Conduct and Integrity programs instituted by the employer.
- Transport and dispatch samples efficiently by prioritizing specimens to ensure desired turnaround times.
- Comply with safety rules, policies, and guidelines for the area, department, and institution.
- Provide quality customer service for all internal and external customers.

Additional Duties as Required

- Assist in collecting and documenting monthly workload and record data.
- Perform quality-control protocols as specified in standard operating procedures, and perform and document instrument and equipment maintenance.
- Participate in continuing education programs such as Quality, Safety, Lean/Six Sigma, and Customer Service.
- Collect and perform point-of-care testing (POCT) following all standard operating procedures.
- Prepare drafts of procedures for laboratory tests according to standard format.
- Perform appropriate laboratory computer information operations.
- Provide proper instruction to patients/customers for container specimen collection.
- Perform front-office duties required by institution including scheduling, coding, itinerary updates, and obtaining Advance Beneficiary Notice (ABN).
- Train new technicians and students in duties and responsibilities.

identify himself or herself immediately and know how to handle an emotional caller and, unless absolutely necessary, avoid referring such a person to an administrator. Proper telephone etiquette involves not leaving a person on hold too long. If it will take some time to locate the requested information, the caller should be asked if he or she would like to be called back with the answer.

REVIEW: Yes ☐ No ☐

16. **Answer: b**

WHY: The American Society of Clinical Pathologists (ASCP) is one of several national organizations that certify phlebotomists. Certification is a process that indicates the completion of defined academic and training requirements and the attainment of a satisfactory score on a national exam. The Clinical and Laboratory Standards Institute (CLSI), the National Accrediting Agency for Clinical Laboratory Sciences (NAACLS), and the American Society for Clinical Laboratory Sciences (ASCLS) play a role in setting standards of care for healthcare professionals, including phlebotomists, but they do not certify individuals.

REVIEW: Yes ☐ No ☐

17. **Answer: b**

WHY: The phlebotomist has many duties, but the primary one is to collect high-quality blood specimens.

REVIEW: Yes ☐ No ☐

18. **Answer: c**

WHY: Positive public relations promote goodwill and harmonious relationships with employees and patients. Because the phlebotomist is an unofficial "public relations officer," everything the phlebotomist does reflects on the whole facility. The phlebotomist is often the only real contact patients have with the laboratory; therefore, it is important for the phlebotomist to know the difference between a professional relationship with a patient and a personal one. In many cases, patients equate their experience with phlebotomists with the quality of care they receive while in the hospital. However, being skilled at public relations does not compensate for inexperience and insecurity.

REVIEW: Yes ☐ No ☐

19. **Answer: b**

WHY: The primary objective in any healthcare professional's code of ethics must always be the patient's welfare: "first do no harm." This is the meaning of *primum non nocere*, from the

Hippocratic Oath, which is taken by physicians about to enter practice.

REVIEW: Yes ☐   No ☐

20. **Answer: c**

WHY: Having a good work ethic includes being dependable. A person with a good work ethic can be relied on to be there when scheduled or when needed. Dependability shows a determination to "hang in there" no matter what. This is not because of self-interest or indifference but because this conduct is desired and is the right choice for all involved. One's work ethic may include assertiveness, but that is not to be confused with aggressiveness, which is intended to be disruptive and cause harm.

REVIEW: Yes ☐   No ☐

21. **Answer: d**

WHY: Polycythemia is a condition caused by over-production of red blood cells; therapy includes occasionally removing some of the blood to bring blood cell levels back into the normal range.

REVIEW: Yes ☐   No ☐

22. **Answer: d**

WHY: Continuing education for a healthcare professional is important in order to maintain competency in all areas. It is necessary to remain current in the increasingly complex field of health care in order to maintain a high quality of care and avoid litigation. By staying current, the phlebotomist can maintain his or her certification through continuing education or by periodically retaking the certification exam, but continuing education does *not* eliminate the need for annual evaluations. Continuing education is not designed to prepare a person for different employment, since it is specifically designed for updating and reviewing the subject matter of the current job description.

REVIEW: Yes ☐   No ☐

23. **Answer: a**

WHY: The word *phlebotomy* comes from the Greek words *phlebos,* meaning "vein," and *tome,* meaning "incision." Literally translated, the word *phlebotomy* means to make an incision in (or cut) a vein.

REVIEW: Yes ☐   No ☐

24. **Answer: d**

WHY: With the advent of multiskilling in health care, phlebotomists' duties are expanding; however, tasks such as assisting with the insertion of

IV cannulas, helping nurses perform direct patient care, or informing patients of their test results are not considered within the phlebotomist's scope of practice. A routine and necessary part of the phlebotomist's duties is using the laboratory computer system to input patient data, access requests, and confirm collection. See Box 1-2.

REVIEW: Yes ☐   No ☐

25. **Answer: d**

WHY: Each certifying agency awards a designated title and initials to phlebotomists who successfully pass the national exam. The American Medical Technologists agency has chosen the initials RPT(AMT) to designate the title of Registered Phlebotomy Technician through AMT.

REVIEW: Yes ☐   No ☐

📖 **WORKBOOK Matching Exercise 1-2 will familiarize you with some national certification agencies.**

26. **Answer: c**

WHY: Today's lancet is the modern-day counterpart of the fleam. A typical fleam (Fig. 1-2) had a wide double-edged blade at a right angle to the handle and was used to slice a vein. During the 17th and 18th centuries, a suction device called a *cup* was placed on the skin to draw blood to the surface before making an incision. The specimen was collected in a "bleeding bowl." Today's *cupping* draws blood to the skin surface, but no incision is made to withdraw the blood.

REVIEW: Yes ☐   No ☐

27. **Answer: b**

WHY: Several organizations sponsor workshops and seminars to enable phlebotomists and other healthcare workers to earn credit required to renew their licenses or certification. Credits indicated on certificates that are awarded on

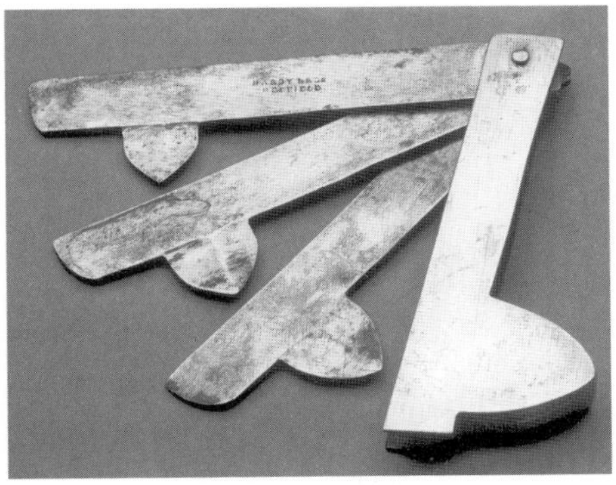

Figure 1-2 Typical fleams. (Courtesy of Robert Kravetz, MD, Chairman, Archives Committee, American College of Gastroenterology.)

completion of these events are called continuing education units (CEUs). The most widely accepted CEU standard, developed by the International Association for Continuing Education and Training, is that 10 contact hours equals 1 continuing education unit. Copies of the certificates can be sent to certifying agencies as "proof of continuing education."

REVIEW: Yes ☐ No ☐

28. **Answer: c**

WHY: *The Patient Care Partnership* brochure replaces the AHA Patient Bill of Rights and is designed to help patients understand their expectations during a hospital stay. One of the patient's expectations is the right to receive help concerning billing issues if required.

REVIEW: Yes ☐ No ☐

29. **Answer: b**

WHY: Every individual is surrounded by an invisible bubble of personal territory within which he or she feels most safe. This invisible bubble is known as the zone of comfort, which varies with each individual, depending largely on how well an intruder into the zone is known and other circumstances surrounding

the intrusion. One's personal zone of comfort is typically recognized as 1½ to 4 ft in diameter.

REVIEW: Yes ☐ No ☐

📖 *Check out Table 1-2 in the TEXTBOOK; it defines a person's territorial zones and the corresponding zone radius.*

30. **Answer: a**

WHY: Language, age, gender, and emotions can all be barriers to communication (Fig. 1-3) that require special communication techniques for an effective exchange of information to occur. The lack of professionalism displayed by invading a person's intimate zone inappropriately can come across as threatening, but if handled right, it is not considered a communication barrier.

REVIEW: Yes ☐ No ☐

31. **Answer: d**

WHY: Confirming responses help a patient feel recognized as an individual and not a number. "I understand how you must be feeling" is a response that communicates an effort on your part to view the patient as an individual and empathize with his or her situation.

REVIEW: Yes ☐ No ☐

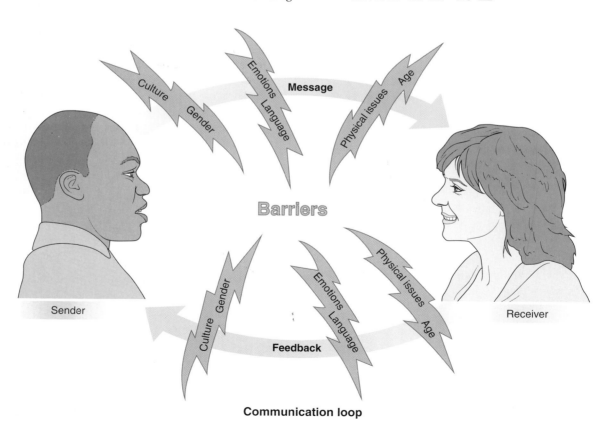

Figure 1-3 The verbal communication feedback loop.

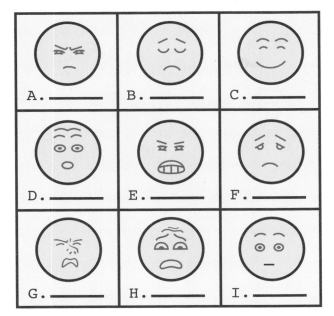

Figure 1-4 Nonverbal facial cues. Can you match the sketches with the correct affects? (1) Happy, (2) sad, (3) surprise, (4) fear, (5) anger, (6) disgust.

32. **Answer: b**

    WHY: Kinesics is the study of nonverbal communication or body language. Shouting is an example of a verbal response. Frowning is an example of negative kinesics or body language. Eye contact and smiling are all examples of positive body language. Examples of nonverbal facial cues are shown in Figure 1-4.

    REVIEW: Yes ☐ No ☐

33. **Answer: b**

    WHY: A neat, clean appearance plays a big part in presenting a professional image. A clean, pressed laboratory coat; closed-toe, conservative shoes; short, clean fingernails (artificial nails not allowed); and long hair pulled back contribute to a professional image. Giving off a strong scent is offensive to most people, especially those who are ill or allergic to perfume, and may interfere with their view of the individual who wears it as professional.

    REVIEW: Yes ☐ No ☐

34. **Answer: a**

    WHY: Making good eye contact, conveying sincere understanding, and presenting a professional appearance are all part of the professional image that will earn a patient's confidence or trust. Dismissing a patient's fears makes the phlebotomist seem insensitive to the situation and the patient's

needs and undermines the patient's confidence in the care received.

REVIEW: Yes ☐ No ☐

35. **Answer: c**

    WHY: Proper telephone protocol involves answering the phone promptly and restating what has been said to clarify information received before recording it. Callers who are upset and hostile should be handled carefully. Validating a hostile caller's feelings will often defuse the situation and allow the issue to be addressed. Never hang up on any caller.

    REVIEW: Yes ☐ No ☐

    📖 *See Table 1-3, Proper Telephone Etiquette, in the TEXTBOOK.*

36. **Answer: b**

    WHY: Proxemics is the study of an individual's concept and use of space. To better relate to the patient in a healthcare setting, it is important to understand this subtle part of nonverbal communication.

    REVIEW: Yes ☐ No ☐

37. **Answer: a**

    WHY: Elements of good communication in health care involve being truthful and accepting each patient as a unique individual with special needs. Showing facial expressions of disapproval is demeaning to the patient, your customer. The phlebotomist's words or actions that appear to be strict and controlling only serve to make the patient more uncomfortable. All communication by the phlebotomist reflects on the whole facility and therefore must be professional at all times.

    REVIEW: Yes ☐ No ☐

38. **Answer: a**

    WHY: A hospital is one of the few places where an individual gives up control over most of the personal tasks he or she normally performs. Because of this loss of control, the patient may respond by getting angry and is then characterized as a "difficult" or "bad" patient. The best way to deal with this is to help the patient feel in control of the situation.

    REVIEW: Yes ☐ No ☐

39. **Answer: c**

    WHY: Proxemics is the study of an individual's concept and use of space. It involves four categories of naturally occurring territorial zones (Table 1-2 in TEXTBOOK), referred to as zones of comfort, that are very obvious in human interaction. Personal contact involves one of these zones. Entering a patient's personal zone is often necessary in a healthcare setting, and if this is not carefully handled, the patient may feel threatened, insecure, or out of control.

REVIEW: Yes ☐ No ☐

40. **Answer: a**

WHY: Feeling in control is essential to a patient's well-being. Informing, insisting, and telling patients what to do are actions that may cause the patient to feel as if he or she had no control over the situation. Allowing the patient the right to either agree to a procedure or to refuse it allows the patient to exercise control over the situation and generally makes him or her more agreeable.

REVIEW: Yes ☐ No ☐

41. **Answer: b**

WHY: The average speaking rate of an adult is 125 to 150 words per minute. Because the average person absorbs verbal messages at 500 to 600 words per minute (which is approximately four times the speaking rate), the listener must make an effort to stay actively involved in what the speaker is saying to communicate effectively.

REVIEW: Yes ☐ No ☐

42. **Answer: a**

WHY: The term "outpatient care" is synonymous with "ambulatory care." Ambulatory, or outpatient, care is offered to those who are able to come to the facility for care and go home the same day. Nonambulatory or inpatient care is found in tertiary facilities, where patients must stay over one or more nights. Nursing home or rehabilitation care is considered inpatient care for the reasons stated above.

REVIEW: Yes ☐ No ☐

43. **Answer: b**

WHY: The hematology department identifies abnormalities of the blood by analyzing whole blood specimens in automated analyzers (Fig. 1-5).

REVIEW: Yes ☐ No ☐

📖 *WORKBOOK Matching Exercise 1-4 will help you learn laboratory tests and the laboratory departments associated with them.*

44. **Answer: d**

WHY: Respiratory means relating to respiration or the act of breathing, which provides lungs with oxygen. The respiratory therapy department is responsible for administering oxygen therapy to patients with respiratory disorders.

REVIEW: Yes ☐ No ☐

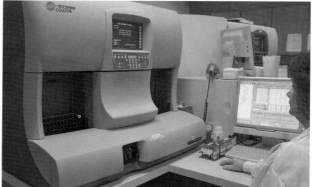

Figure 1-5 A medical technologist checks CBC results from the Beckman Coulter LH780 Hematology Analyzer.

45. **Answer: c**

WHY: A frozen section is a test performed by a pathologist in the surgical pathology department. Tissue removed during surgery is quickly frozen, and a thin slice of the specimen is microscopically examined for abnormalities while the patient is still under anesthesia. Results of the frozen section analysis determine what further action is to be taken by the surgeon.

REVIEW: Yes ☐ No ☐

46. **Answer: b**

WHY: Nephrology is the study of the kidneys. A patient being treated in the nephrology department is most likely being treated for a disorder associated with the kidneys.

REVIEW: Yes ☐ No ☐

47. **Answer: b**

WHY: "Oto" means ear, "rhino" means nose, and the "larynx" is a structure in the throat. The otorhinolaryngology department treats disorders of the ear, nose, and throat. Skin disorders are treated in the dermatology department. Eye problems are treated in the ophthalmology department, and bone and joint disorders are treated in the orthopedics department.

REVIEW: Yes ☐ No ☐

48. **Answer: c**

WHY: D-dimer is a test used in the diagnosis of disseminated intravascular coagulation (DIC) and will be performed in the coagulation department. The D-dimer test verifies the breakdown of fibrinogen in the body and is more specific for DIC than other tests for fibrin split products (FSP). Blood urea nitrogen (BUN) and glucose tests are performed in the chemistry

department. A complete blood count (CBC) is performed in the hematology department.
REVIEW: Yes ☐ No ☐

49. **Answer: b**

WHY: The word "onco" means tumor, and the suffix "ology" denotes the study of. The term "oncology" is used to describe the medical specialty that treats patients who have tumors. Geriatrics is the branch of medicine that deals with problems of aging. Ophthalmology deals with eye disorders, and orthopedics deals with musculoskeletal system disorders.
REVIEW: Yes ☐ No ☐

50. **Answer: c**

WHY: The term "orthopedics" is used to describe the medical specialty that treats disorders of the musculoskeletal system. Gastroenterology is the specialty that treats disorders of the digestive tract and related structures; neurology is the specialty that treats disorders of the brain, spinal cord, and nerves; and pediatrics is the specialty that treats children from birth to adolescence.
REVIEW: Yes ☐ No ☐

51. **Answer: b**

WHY: A neonate is a newborn up to the age of 1 month. A neonatologist is a physician who specializes in the study, treatment, and care of newborns. A gerontologist specializes in disorders related to aging; an obstetrician/gynecologist specializes in pregnancy, childbirth, and treatment of disorders of the reproductive system; and a pediatrician treats children from birth to adolescence.
REVIEW: Yes ☐ No ☐

52. **Answer: a**

WHY: The blood bank department is sometimes called immunohematology. Immunology is another name for the serology department. An earlier name for the microbiology department was bacteriology.
REVIEW: Yes ☐ No ☐

53. **Answer: a**

WHY: Hemoglobin A1c is another way to say glycosylated hemoglobin, which is a chemistry test. Glycosylated hemoglobin is formed when glucose and hemoglobin combine, and it is tested to provide the physician with a time-averaged picture of the patient's blood glucose over the past 3 months. The most common glycosylated hemoglobin is hemoglobin A1.
REVIEW: Yes ☐ No ☐

54. **Answer: d**

WHY: Urgent care centers are the medical facilities that were specifically designed to bridge the gap between an injury that is too urgent to wait for the primary care physician but not a life-threatening situation that calls for a trip to the ER. They are seen as a way to decrease the overcrowded emergency rooms and assist the primary care physician. Even though they are for ambulatory patients, they do not offer the same services as public health clinics or surgical centers. Hospice is a program that provides palliative or special care to relieve pain and stress for terminally ill patients.
REVIEW: Yes ☐ No ☐

55. **Answer: b**

WHY: Therapeutic drug monitoring is a team effort and requires cooperation between nursing, pharmacy, and the laboratory for quality results.
REVIEW: Yes ☐ No ☐

56. **Answer: c**

WHY: The histology department prepares tissue samples for microscopic exam by a pathologist.
REVIEW: Yes ☐ No ☐

57. **Answer: d**

WHY: A phlebotomist is not required to have a college degree and may not even be required to show any type of certification or proof of training to practice. A few states require licensing of phlebotomists, and many employers require their phlebotomists to be nationally certified. To become nationally certified, a phlebotomist must have a high school diploma or GED and have completed a formal, structured phlebotomy program or have a minimum of 1 year of full-time experience as a phlebotomist. A medical technologist (MT) or medical laboratory scientist (MLS) is normally required to have a minimum of a bachelor's degree in medical technology or chemical or biological science. A medical laboratory technician (MLT) is normally required to have a minimum of an associate's degree or equivalent.
REVIEW: Yes ☐ No ☐

58. **Answer: c**

WHY: Secondary care involves care by specialists in a particular area of health care. An appendectomy performed in an ambulatory surgical center is an example of secondary care. Managed care is a system of healthcare delivery and financing that involves primary, secondary, and tertiary care. Primary care entails initial consultation and

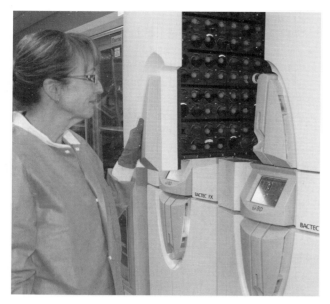

Figure 1-6 A microbiologist reviews blood cultures processed by the BACTEC™ FX blood culture instrument.

treatment by a family physician or other caregiver. Tertiary care implies highly complex or specialized services delivered primarily in inpatient facilities to patients who stay overnight.

REVIEW: Yes ☐   No ☐

59. **Answer: b**

WHY: Blood cultures are performed in the microbiology department and are blood specimens collected in special nutrient substance or media designed to encourage the growth of microorganisms that might be present in a patient's bloodstream. The process is often automated using a special system such as the BACTEC™ FX (Fig. 1-6).

REVIEW: Yes ☐   No ☐

60. **Answer: d**

WHY: Sodium and potassium are both electrolytes. They can be ordered as individual tests or as part of an electrolyte panel that includes sodium, potassium, chloride, and bicarbonate (commonly measured as carbon dioxide [CO_2]). Alanine aminotransferase (ALT), aspartate aminotransferase (AST), blood urea nitrogen (BUN), creatinine, glucose, and total protein are tests that are performed in the chemistry department and are ordered to check the status of various organs or body systems.

REVIEW: Yes ☐   No ☐

61. **Answer: a**

WHY: The cardiodiagnostic department diagnoses and monitors patients with heart problems. The

most common test performed by this department is the electrocardiogram (ECG). The electroneurodiagnostic technology department—also called the electroencephalography department assists neurologists in detection, diagnosis, and treatment of neurological disorders. The occupational therapy department assists mentally, physically, or emotionally disabled patients to maintain daily living skills and the respiratory therapy department diagnoses and treats lung deficiencies and administers oxygen therapy.

REVIEW: Yes ☐   No ☐

📖 *See Matching 1-5 in the WORKBOOK, Patient Conditions and Medical Specialties, for more review.*

62. **Answer: a**

WHY: Basic metabolic panel (BMP) is a term used for one of the CMS-approved disease and organ-specific panels that evaluate the functioning of various body systems. It includes glucose, blood urea nitrogen (BUN), creatinine, sodium, potassium, chloride, carbon dioxide (CO_2), and calcium. These tests can all be performed on a highly automated computerized analyzer (Fig. 1-7) in the chemistry department.

REVIEW: Yes ☐   No ☐

63. **Answer: c**

WHY: The cytogenetics department performs chromosome studies; however, not all laboratories have a cytogenetics department, in which case these studies are sent to a reference laboratory.

REVIEW: Yes ☐   No ☐

64. **Answer: a**

WHY: Cytology is the study of the formation, structure, and function of cells. The cells in body fluids and tissues are analyzed in the cytology department to detect signs of cancer. The Pap smear test is named after a cytology staining technique

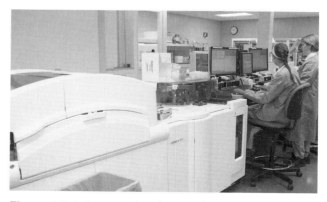

Figure 1-7 Laboratory chemists monitor and review chemistry results from the cobas® 6000 chemistry analyzer.

used to detect cancerous cells in specimens obtained from the cervix in the vagina.

REVIEW: Yes ☐ No ☐

65. **Answer: b**

WHY: A type of managed care organization is the prepaid healthcare plans such as HMOs. Enrollees must comply with managed care policies such as preauthorization for certain medical procedures and approved referral to specialists for claims to be paid.

REVIEW: Yes ☐ No ☐

📖 *Find out more about managed care organizations and integrated healthcare delivery in the section called "The Changing Healthcare System" in the TEXTBOOK.*

66. **Answer: d**

WHY: There are three basic levels of care offered in the United States: primary (basic) care through the physician, secondary (specialist) care offered on an outpatient basis, and tertiary (highly sophisticated and complex) care requiring a stay in an inpatient facility.

REVIEW: Yes ☐ No ☐

67. **Answer: c**

WHY: Obstetrics is the medical specialty that includes treating women throughout pregnancy and childbirth. This specialty also treats disorders of the female reproductive system and menopause.

REVIEW: Yes ☐ No ☐

68. **Answer: b**

WHY: A primary care physician (PCP) is one of the most important concepts in the managed care organizations called HMOs. In HMOs, the physician (or in his or her place, a nurse practitioner) serves as a gatekeeper because directives to other physicians and services must be accompanied by his request or referral. This type of coordination reduces the time and cost of care. In PPOs, a patient does not need to select a PCP and referrals to see other providers in the network are not needed. CMS and PHS are healthcare organizations not involved directly to manage care.

REVIEW: Yes ☐ No ☐

69. **Answer: a**

WHY: Toxicology is a subsection of the chemistry department. Toxicology tests determine the presence of poisons or toxic substances in blood or urine specimens.

REVIEW: Yes ☐ No ☐

70. **Answer: d**

WHY: A clinical pathologist is a physician who specializes in diagnosing disease from abnormal changes detected in blood, body fluid, and tissue specimens.

REVIEW: Yes ☐ No ☐

71. **Answer: c**

WHY: A complete blood count (CBC) is the most common test performed in the hematology department. Culture & sensitivity (C&S) testing is performed in the microbiology department. HBsAg is analyzed in the serology department and demonstrates the presence of hepatitis B antigen if positive. A BMP is a disease and organ-specific diagnostic panel that is performed in the automated chemistry area of the laboratory.

REVIEW: Yes ☐ No ☐

72. **Answer: d**

WHY: The respiratory therapy department diagnoses, treats, and manages patient lung deficiencies, tests capacity of the lungs, and administers oxygen therapy. This department may also analyze arterial blood gas (ABG) specimens, although in some instances, ABGs are performed in the clinical laboratory.

REVIEW: Yes ☐ No ☐

73. **Answer: c**

WHY: Immunoglobulin testing is performed in the serology/immunology department and is used to help diagnose immunodeficiencies. Testing is done for five subclasses of antibodies (IgA, IgG, IgM, IgE, IgD) made by immune system to neutralize foreign antigens, such as bacteria or toxins.

REVIEW: Yes ☐ No ☐

74. **Answer: c**

WHY: X-ray procedures and other imaging techniques are functions of the radiology department. The occupational therapy department assists mentally, physically, or emotionally disabled patients in maintaining daily living skills. The pharmacy prepares and dispenses drugs, provides advice on selection and side effects of drugs, and helps coordinate therapeutic drug monitoring. The respiratory therapy department aids in the diagnosis, treatment, and management of lung deficiencies.

REVIEW: Yes ☐ No ☐

75. **Answer: c**

WHY: There are two main types of healthcare facilities: inpatient and outpatient. An inpatient facility is designed for patients who stay overnight. A hospital is primarily an inpatient facility. Outpatient facilities are places where patients receive treatment and go home the same day. Physician and dentist offices and day-surgery centers are examples of outpatient facilities.

REVIEW: Yes ☐ No ☐

76. **Answer: d**

WHY: HCG is a common serology test performed on serum or urine and is used to determine pregnancy. BUN is a chemistry test; CBC, a hematology test; and the partial thromboplastin time (PTT), a coagulation test used to screen bleeding abnormalities.

REVIEW: Yes ☐ No ☐

77. **Answer: a**

WHY: Both the medical technologist (MT) and the medical laboratory scientist (MLS) have the same qualifications, including a bachelor's degree in medical technology or a chemical or biological science. The title depends on which national certification exam was chosen and passed. A medical laboratory technician (MLT) is required to have a minimum of a 2-year associate's degree or equivalent. A pathologist is a physician with a specialty in laboratory diagnosis.

REVIEW: Yes ☐ No ☐

78. **Answer: c**

WHY: A hemogram is a hematology test. It is the name given to the graph or printed results of complete blood cell count (CBC) on an automated blood cell counter. It generally includes the major components of a CBC except a manual differential.

REVIEW: Yes ☐ No ☐

📖 *Learn more about laboratory tests as you write out the associated test names and lab departments using WORKBOOK Skills Drill 1-1.*

79. **Answer: d**

WHY: The urinalysis department performs urinalysis testing, a routine exam of urine that includes a microscopic exam of urine sediment for the presence of blood cells, bacteria, crystals, and other substances.

REVIEW: Yes ☐ No ☐

📖 *See Table 1-12, Common Urinalysis Tests, in the TEXTBOOK, for more information about this department.*

80. **Answer: b**

WHY: The physical therapy department provides many types of assistance to patients who have

physical handicaps, including therapy to restore mobility. The cardiodiagnostics department provides diagnosis, monitoring, and therapy for patients with cardiovascular problems. The radiology department diagnoses medical conditions using x-rays and other imaging techniques. The respiratory therapy department provides testing, therapy, and monitoring of patients with respiratory disorders.

REVIEW: Yes ☐ No ☐

81. **Answer: b**

WHY: The electroencephalography (EEG) or electroneurodiagnostic technology (ENT) department performs evoked potential testing to determine muscle function and brain wave mapping to diagnose and monitor neurologic disorders. The cardiodiagnostic department is where electrocardiograms (ECGs) are performed for diagnosis and therapy. The physical therapy (PT) department diagnoses physical impairment to determine appropriate therapy. The respiratory therapy (RT) department provides testing, therapy, and monitoring of patients with respiratory disease.

REVIEW: Yes ☐ No ☐

82. **Answer: b**

WHY: Clinical Laboratory Improvement Amendments of 1988 (CLIA '88) mandate that all laboratories must be regulated using the same standards regardless of the location, type, or size. American Medical Technologists (AMT) is a certification agency for allied health professionals. Public Health Services (PHS) agencies function at local and state level to provide services for the entire population of the region. The Health Insurance Portability and Accountability Act (HIPAA) is a bill that established standards for electronic data exchange, including coding systems.

REVIEW: Yes ☐ No ☐

83. **Answer: a**

WHY: The Patient Protection and Affordable Care Act was passed in March 2013. This recent healthcare legislation, better known as the Affordable Care Act (ACA) is primarily about insurance market reform. This new law is to provide the consumer with insurance options and an increased accessibility to *affordable* health care. One of the goals of the ACA is to streamline the delivery of health care by reducing duplication through a new kind of integrated care offered by an Accountable Care Organization (ACO), a group of hospitals, physicians, and other healthcare providers who *voluntarily* offer to coordinate care for their Medicare patients and others. HIPAA is a national law that sets national standards for the security of electronic protected health information and CLIA regulates all laboratory medicine except research.

REVIEW: Yes ☐ No ☐

84. **Answer: a**

WHY: A medical laboratory scientist (MLS) and a medical technologist (MT) are equivalent and are required to have a bachelor's degree in medical technology or a chemical or biological science. A medical laboratory technician (MLT) normally has an associate's degree from a 2-year college or equivalent, or certification from a military or proprietary (private) college. A certified phlebotomy technician (CPT)ACA or phlebotomy technician (PBT)ASCP are required to have a high school diploma or GED to sit for the exam.

REVIEW: Yes ☐ No ☐

Information about the title change for Medical Technologist can be found in the section called "Clinical Laboratory Personnel" in the TEXTBOOK.

85. **Answer: b**

WHY: A medical laboratory technician (MLT) normally has an associate's degree from a 2-year college or equivalent, or certification from a military or proprietary (private) college. A medical laboratory scientist (MLS) and a medical technologist (MT) are required to have a bachelor's degree in medical technology or a chemical or biological science. Phlebotomy technician (PBT) is the title awarded to those who successfully pass the ASCP phlebotomy certification exam. To apply for certification, a phlebotomist is typically required to have a high school diploma or GED at a minimum.

REVIEW: Yes ☐ No ☐

86. **Answer: c**

WHY: A subsection of the microbiology department is parasitology, where stool specimens are carefully examined for the presence of parasites or their eggs (ova).

REVIEW: Yes ☐ No ☐

87. **Answer: b**

WHY: The process used to identify microorganisms and determine the appropriate antibiotic for treatment is called culture and sensitivity (C&S) testing.

REVIEW: Yes ☐ No ☐

88. **Answer: a**

WHY: The chemistry department performs tests to evaluate analytes such as glucose that are dissolved in the plasma. Glucose levels are evaluated to diagnose or monitor diabetes.

REVIEW: Yes ☐ No ☐

89. **Answer: b**

WHY: The word root "hemato" means blood, and the suffix "logy" means the study of; therefore, hematology is the medical specialty that treats patients with blood disorders. Dermatology is the medical specialty that treats skin disorders. Internal medicine treats disorders of the internal organs and general medical conditions. Urology treats disorders of the urinary tract and male reproductive organs.

REVIEW: Yes ☐ No ☐

WORKBOOK Matching Exercise 1-5 will familiarize you with medical specialties and patient conditions.

90. **Answer: b**

WHY: Public health agencies take care of large-scale healthcare problems at the federal, state, and local levels. Their designated services are to be used by the entire populace of an area and include immunization programs. Licensure of personnel, blood donor collections, and therapy for patient mobility are not part of public health service responsibilities.

REVIEW: Yes ☐ No ☐

91. **Answer: b**

WHY: Autoimmune hemolytic anemia is caused by a person producing antibodies against their own RBC antigens. The direct antiglobulin test (DAT), also called the Coombs test, performed in immunohematology may be used to help diagnose hemolytic disease of the newborn (HDN) due to an incompatibility between the blood types of a mother and baby and transfusion incompatibility.

REVIEW: Yes ☐ No ☐

92. **Answer: a**

WHY: Blood typing and compatibility testing are performed in the blood bank department, which is sometimes called immunohematology.

REVIEW: Yes ☐ No ☐

93. **Answer: c**

WHY: Fibrin degradation products (FDP), also called fibrin split products (FSP), are the end products of the breakdown of fibrin formed during the coagulation process. The test is performed in the coagulation department and is most commonly ordered to diagnose disseminated intravascular coagulation (DIC).

REVIEW: Yes ☐ No ☐

94. **Answer: d**

WHY: Rheumatoid factor (RF) is an autoantibody that is found in rheumatoid arthritis and is an immunoglobulin. EBV, CMV, and HCV are tests that are performed in the serology/immunology department and each is specific for a type of viral condition.

REVIEW: Yes ☐ No ☐

95. **Answer: b**

WHY: Medicaid is a state-based, federal program that provides medical care for the poor (indigent). Medicare, a federal program, provides medical care to patients of age 65 and older. HIPAA, a law that sets national standards for the security of electronic protected health information, and PHS is a federal government service that promotes public health and safety of our nation.

REVIEW: Yes ☐ No ☐

96. **Answer: d**

WHY: The urinalysis department performs chemical screening tests on urine specimens as part of a urinalysis test. Chemical screening involves dipping a special strip (dipstick) impregnated with chemical reagents into the urine and interpreting color reactions that take place on the strip.

REVIEW: Yes ☐ No ☐

97. **Answer: b**

WHY: Warfarin is an anticoagulant that is used to prevent heart attacks, strokes, and blood clots. It is monitored closely by the prothrombin time test which is performed in the coagulation department.

REVIEW: Yes ☐ No ☐

98. **Answer: d**

WHY: The medical specialty of rheumatology is involved in the diagnosis and treatment of diseases characterized by joint inflammation. Dermatology involves the treatment of skin disorders. Gastroenterology involves the treatment of disorders of the digestive tract and related structures. Internal medicine involves the treatment of disorders of the internal organs and general medical conditions.

REVIEW: Yes ☐ No ☐

99. **Answer: a**

WHY: The Health Insurance Portability and Accountability Act (HIPAA) established national standards for protecting patient health information. Maintaining patient confidentiality is a major concern, and all healthcare workers must sign a confidentiality and nondisclosure agreement affirming that they understand HIPAA and will keep all patient information confidential. Penalties for HIPAA violations include disciplinary action, fines, and possible jail time.

REVIEW: Yes ☐ No ☐

100. **Answer: d**

WHY: Critical factors in the provision of healthcare services that meet the needs of diverse populations include understanding the beliefs that shape their approach to illness and traditions that relate to their healing. The family living environment is another factor that needs to be considered whether the patient is from a diverse population or not.

REVIEW: Yes ☐ No ☐

101. **Answer: b**

WHY: CLIA '88 mandates that all laboratories that test human specimens must be regulated using the same standard measurement regardless of the location, type, or size. Qualifications for laboratory personnel performing moderate- and high-complexity tests are stated in the regulations.

REVIEW: Yes ☐ No ☐

102. **Answer: a**

WHY: Biopsy tissue is analyzed by a physician in the anatomical pathology area (Box 1-3). All other specimens listed above will be processed and analyzed in the clinical area of the laboratory.

REVIEW: Yes ☐ No ☐

Box 1-3

Two Major Divisions in the Clinical Laboratory

Clinical Analysis Areas	Anatomical and Surgical Pathology
Specimen processing, hematology, microbiology, blood bank/immunohematology, immunology/serology, and urinalysis	Tissue analysis, cytologic exam, surgical biopsy, frozen sections, and performance of autopsies

103. **Answer: c**

    WHY: Reference laboratories are large, independent facilities that receive specimens from many different areas. They provide specialized testing that is not cost-effective in smaller labs and they offer faster turnaround time (TAT) on those specialized tests, but does not mean they do STAT or immediate testing. The high volume of tests they perform allows them to reduce costs but does not necessarily mean they have more accurate results than in any other laboratory facility.

    REVIEW: Yes ☐ No ☐

104. **Answer: b**

    WHY: The primary care nurse practitioner can fill the role of gatekeeper/case manager and serves as the patient's advocate to advise and coordinate services for each individual, including advising the patient on care offered through secondary and tertiary sources.

    REVIEW: Yes ☐ No ☐

105. **Answer: b**

    WHY: American Medical Technologists (AMT), American Society of Clinical Pathologists (ASCP), and the American Certification Agency (ACA) are among the agencies that offer certification for all levels of laboratory professionals. Licensure of health care and allied health professionals is the responsibility of the states that have passed licensure laws. Phlebotomy programs are approved by the National Accrediting Agency for Clinical Laboratory Sciences (NAACLS). State and local Public Health Services (PHS) monitor communicable diseases.

    REVIEW: Yes ☐ No ☐

106. **Answer: c**

    WHY: Professional standards of integrity and honesty require a person to do what is right regardless of the circumstances.

    REVIEW: Yes ☐ No ☐

    📖 *WORKBOOK Knowledge Drill 1-7 will be helpful in defining your perception of a professional attitude.*

107. **Answer: b**

    WHY: The Health Information Portability and Accountability Act (HIPAA) is a federal law that was enacted to more closely secure protected health information (PHI) and regulate patient privacy. The law established national standards for the electronic exchange of PHI.

    REVIEW: Yes ☐ No ☐

108. **Answer: d**

    WHY: Using clichés or overused expressions is not a form of good communication because they could be misunderstood, especially by those who have language limitations. Using clichés often indicates that the speaker is not using active listening.

    REVIEW: Yes ☐ No ☐

109. **Answer: d**

    WHY: A very important professional characteristic that a phlebotomist should exhibit is that of being trustworthy. Patients appear comfortable and relaxed when interacting with a sincere, honest, and knowledgeable phlebotomist they feel they can trust.

    REVIEW: Yes ☐ No ☐

110. **Answer: c**

    WHY: Many homebound older adults require respiratory therapy, nursing care, phlebotomy, and physical therapy. Immunizations and screening services are not considered extended care after discharge.

    REVIEW: Yes ☐ No ☐

Chapter 2

Quality Assurance and Legal Issues in Healthcare

Study Tips

- Study the key points in the corresponding chapter of the textbook.

- Write the abbreviations of the four national agencies that deal with quality assurance for the clinical laboratory.

- List The Joint Commission's three NPSGs for the laboratory as of 2014.

- Divide a sheet of paper into two columns and, in the first column, list all the forms, reports, and manuals used in the laboratory, such as test catalogs. In the second column, write why it is used for quality assurance.

- Describe the difference between GLPs and NPSGs.

- List tort actions. Give an example of each.

- List six types of consent and why each is necessary.

- Differentiate between "breach of confidentiality" and "invasion of privacy."

- Complete the activities in Chapter 2 of the companion workbook.

Overview

This chapter focuses on quality assurance (QA) and legal issues in health care, including the relationship of both to the practice of phlebotomy. Consumer awareness has increased lawsuits in all areas of society. This is especially true in the healthcare industry. Consequently, it is essential for phlebotomists to recognize the importance of following QA guidelines and understand the legal implications of not doing so.

Review Questions

Choose the BEST answer.

1. Legal actions in which the alleged injured party sues for monetary damages are
   a. civil actions.
   b. criminal actions.
   c. malpractice.
   d. vicarious liability.

2. Significant gaps in the quality of testing practices in physicians' offices resulted in the recent development of
   a. behavioral competencies.
   b. good laboratory practices.
   c. quality indicators.
   d. test threshold values.

3. The level of care that a person of ordinary intelligence and good sense would exercise under the given circumstances is the definition of
   a. due care.
   b. quality care.
   c. critical care.
   d. standard of care.

4. Deceitful practice or false portrayal of facts either by words or conduct is the definition of
   a. battery.
   b. discovery.
   c. fraud.
   d. negligence.

5. Continuous quality improvement means
   a. accepting unionization by the hourly employees.
   b. being committed to ongoing process monitoring.
   c. overseeing employees' investments and retirement.
   d. providing annual salary increases and bonuses.

6. The Joint Commission
   a. accredits or approves schools of phlebotomy.
   b. created a toll-free line for customer complaints.
   c. offers proficiency testing for the laboratory.
   d. writes guidelines for purchasing equipment.

7. One of the responsibilities of the Center for Medicare and Medicaid Services (CMS) is to
   a. accredit all educational facilities.
   b. operate risk management programs.
   c. oversee administration of CLIA '88.
   d. provide healthcare worker insurance.

8. A process in which one party questions another under oath while a court reporter records every word is a
   a. civil action.
   b. deposition.
   c. discovery.
   d. tort.

9. Which one of the following is found in a procedure manual?
   a. Description of QC checks for equipment used.
   b. Instruction for reporting errors in specimen handling.
   c. Listing of all revision dates for the procedure.
   d. References to the applicable CLIA regulations.

10. An internal process focused on identifying and minimizing situations throughout the organization that pose danger to patients and employees is
    a. a performance improvement plan.
    b. decision criteria for accreditation.
    c. facility-wide risk management.
    d. the delta check procedure.

11. CLIA categorizes certificates for laboratories according to
    a. the complexity of testing.
    b. personnel qualifications.
    c. quality-control standards.
    d. the size of the laboratory.

12. CLIA laboratories that perform high-complexity testing
    a. are funded by the federal government.
    b. are subjected to routine inspections.
    c. must hire PhDs as supervisors.
    d. must renew their certificates annually.

13. The Joint Commission's Sentinel Event program's purpose is to
    a. demonstrate flexibility in setting QC measures.
    b. prevent unfavorable events from happening again.
    c. research healthcare organizations' collection of data.
    d. standardize measurements of quality performance.

14. If a sentinel event occurs, the healthcare organization is required to
    a. develop new personnel guidelines and standards.
    b. incorporate a complaint procedure into the process.
    c. monitor improvements to see if they are effective.
    d. send a complete report to the Joint Commission.

15. In the central processing area of a large clinical laboratory
    a. computers monitor refrigerator and freezer temperatures.
    b. periodic reports on equipment are required by CDC and OSHA.
    c. QC checks on the centrifuges are done by phlebotomists.
    d. refrigerator temperature are monitored by the Lab Manager.

16. Guides used to monitor all aspects of patient care are called
    a. IQCP tools.
    b. PI standards.
    c. QA indicators.
    d. QC deficiencies.

17. What is the abbreviation for an agency that has an approval process for phlebotomy programs?
    a. CLIAC
    b. CLSI
    c. NAACLS
    d. NCCT

18. A very busy phlebotomist misidentifies the patient when collecting a specimen for transfusion preparation. The possible misdiagnosis of blood type could cause the patient's death. If the phlebotomist's action results in injury, this wrongful act is called
    a. assault.
    b. battery.
    c. fraud.
    d. negligence.

19. The abbreviation for the federal regulations that established quality standards for all laboratories that test human specimens is
    a. BBP standard.
    b. CLIA '88.
    c. HazCom.
    d. OSHA.

20. The abbreviation for a national agency that sets standards for phlebotomy procedures is the
    a. ASCP.
    b. CLSI.
    c. NAACLS.
    d. NCCT.

21. Which of the following is *not* subject to quality-control (QC) procedures by a phlebotomist?
    a. Patient identification
    b. Patient IV adjustment
    c. Phlebotomy technique
    d. Specimen labeling

22. A laboratory technician asked a phlebotomist to recollect a specimen on a patient. When the phlebotomist asked what was wrong with the specimen, the technician replied, "The specimen was OK, but the results were inconsistent." How would the laboratory technician have decided that the results were questionable? The results did not
    a. compare with previous results after delta check.
    b. match results of patients with the same diagnosis.
    c. measure up to the results on the control specimens.
    d. relate well to other patients tested at the same time.

23. Which organization provides voluntary laboratory inspections and proficiency testing?
    a. ASCP
    b. CAP
    c. CLSI
    d. OSHA

24. QC protocols prohibit use of outdated evacuated tubes because
    a. additives that speed up clotting become crystallized in the tube.
    b. bacteria begin to grow in these tubes, yielding erroneous results.
    c. stoppers may shrink, allowing specimen leakage if the tube is inverted.
    d. tubes may not fill completely, changing additive-to-sample ratios.

25. The Joint Commission
    a. accredits healthcare organizations.
    b. approves phlebotomy programs.
    c. certifies laboratory personnel.
    d. develops phlebotomy standards.

26. An example of a QC measure in phlebotomy is
    a. checking the expiration dates of evacuated tubes.
    b. documenting every missed venipuncture.
    c. logging hours worked on your time sheet daily.
    d. recording patient census daily in the computer.

27. When the threshold value of a QA clinical indicator is exceeded and a problem is identified
    a. a corrective action plan is implemented.
    b. an incident report must be filed immediately.
    c. patient specimens must always be redrawn.
    d. the patient's physician must be notified.

28. Which of the following is a phlebotomy QA procedure?
    a. Checking needles for blunt tips and small barbs
    b. Keeping a record of employee paid sick leave
    c. Recording chemistry instrument maintenance
    d. Tracking all of the laboratory OSHA violations

29. Which preanalytical factor that can affect validity of test results is not always under the phlebotomist's control?
    a. Patient identification
    b. Patient preparation
    c. Specimen collection
    d. Specimen handling

30. Which of the following contains a chronological record of a patient's care?
    a. Delta check
    b. Internal report
    c. Medical record
    d. Test catalog

31. After a failed venipuncture attempt and before deciding to switch to the other arm, the phlebotomist moves the needle around several times in search of the vein without knowing exactly where the needle is in relationship to the desired vein. No blood was obtained. At the new site, blood easily flows and the venipuncture is completed. The patient later complains of pain in the antecubital area where the phlebotomist was unsuccessful. What claim can be made against the phlebotomist?
    a. Assault
    b. Fraud
    c. Negligence
    d. *Res ipsa loquitur*

32. A specimen was mislabeled on the floor by the same phlebotomist for the second time. You, as the phlebotomist's supervisor, are required to fill out a *performance improvement plan.* Which of the following is the only information that would *not* be included?
    a. Explanation of the deficiency
    b. Description of the consequence
    c. Detailed corrective action plan
    d. Suggestion for new guidelines

33. Which of the following is an example of a QA indicator?
    a. All phlebotomists' absences will be reviewed and recorded.
    b. Laboratory personnel will not wear lab coats when on break.
    c. No eating, drinking, or smoking is allowed in lab work areas.
    d. The contamination rate for BCs will not exceed the national rate.

34. What laboratory document describes in detail the steps to follow for specimen collection?
    a. OSHA safety manual
    b. Policy guidelines
    c. Procedure manual
    d. Safety manual

35. Drawing a patient's blood without his or her permission can result in a charge of
    a. assault and battery.
    b. breach of confidentiality.
    c. malpractice.
    d. negligence.

36. The term *tort* means a
    a. criminal action.
    b. felony charge.
    c. personal injury.
    d. wrongful act.

37. One of the steps in the risk management process is
    a. approving rule variations.
    b. educating employees.
    c. sharing issues with patients.
    d. validating new treatments.

38. Which of the following would violate a patient's right to confidentiality?
    a. Discussing the nature of a patient's test results with the family.
    b. Giving the patient a physician's name that you know and trust.
    c. Sharing information on a "difficult draw" with a coworker.
    d. Showing a patient his or her lab results when requested.

39. Unauthorized release of confidential patient information is called
    a. a type of negligence.
    b. failure to use due care.
    c. invasion of privacy.
    d. violation of discovery.

40. Civil actions involve
    a. legal proceedings between private parties.
    b. offenses that can lead to imprisonment.
    c. regulations established by governments.
    d. violent crimes against the state or nation.

41. Malpractice is a claim of
    a. breach of confidentiality.
    b. improper treatment.
    c. invasion of privacy.
    d. *res ipsa loquitur.*

42. An example of negligence is when the phlebotomist
    a. fails to report significant changes in a patient's condition.
    b. forgets to sign out at the nurses' station when draws are complete.
    c. is unable to obtain a specimen from a very combative patient.
    d. misses the vein and has to redirect twice to complete the draw.

43. A patient is told that she must remain still during blood collection or she will be restrained. Which tort is involved in this example?
    a. Assault
    b. Battery
    c. Fraud
    d. Malpractice

44. A patient agrees to undergo treatment after the method, risks, and consequences are explained to him. This is an example of
    a. implied consent.
    b. informed consent.
    c. respondent superior.
    d. standard of care.

45. The period within which an injured party may file a lawsuit is known as
    a. binding arbitration.
    b. discovery period.
    c. litigation process.
    d. statute of limitations.

46. The definition of a minor is anyone
    a. who is not self-supporting.
    b. who is not the age of majority.
    c. younger than 18 years of age.
    d. younger than 21 years of age.

47. Performing one's duties in the same manner as any other reasonable and prudent person with the same experience and training is referred to as
    a. required care.
    b. res ipsa loquitur.
    c. standard of care.
    d. vicarious liability.

48. Doing something that a reasonable and prudent person *would not* do or failing to do something that a reasonable and prudent person *would* do is
    a. battery.
    b. discovery.
    c. fraud.
    d. negligence.

49. A phlebotomist explains to an inpatient that he has come to collect a blood specimen. The patient extends his arm and pushes up his sleeve. This is an example of
    a. expressed consent.
    b. implied consent.
    c. informed consent.
    d. refusal of consent.

50. A 12-year-old inpatient who refused to have his blood collected was restrained by a healthcare worker while the phlebotomist collected the specimen. This could be considered an example of
    a. assault and battery.
    b. implied consent.
    c. malpractice.
    d. negligence.

51. The standard of care used in phlebotomy malpractice cases is often based on guidelines from this organization.
    a. CAP
    b. CLSI
    c. OSHA
    d. NAACLS

52. Which one of the following actions points to negligence?
    a. Causing harm as a result of a violation of duty.
    b. Documenting an unusual happening during a draw.
    c. Informing the patient of a scheduled lab procedure.
    d. Watching for implied consent from the patient.

53. The process of gathering information by taking statements and interrogating parties involved in a lawsuit is called
    a. collaboration.
    b. deposition.
    c. discovery.
    d. litigation.

54. The "standard of care" in the practice of phlebotomy is influenced by which of the following organizations?
    a. The Environmental Protection Agency
    b. The Health Insurance Privacy Agency
    c. The Joint Commission & CAP
    d. The U.S. Food and Drug Administration

55. A lawsuit is filed against the phlebotomist after a patient claimed an injury occurred during a venipuncture. In litigation proceedings, the phlebotomist is the
    a. client.
    b. defendant.
    c. plaintiff.
    d. prosecutor.

Use Figure 2-1 (QA form for microbiology) to answer questions 56 to 59.

56. This quality assessment and tracking tool shows the number of contaminated blood cultures to be highest in what month?
    a. April
    b. May
    c. June
    d. September

57. Which hospital department's blood culture collections exceeded the threshold for each month of the quarter?
    a. Emergency room
    b. Laboratory
    c. Outpatient services
    d. Radiology

HOSPITAL & HEALTH CENTER
QUALITY ASSESSMENT AND IMPROVEMENT TRACKING
CONFIDENTIAL A.R.S. 36-445 et. seq.

STANDARD OF CARE/SERVICE:

IMPORTANT ASPECT OF CARE/SERVICE:
LABORATORY SERVICES
COLLECTION/TRANSPORT

SIGNATURES:

_____
DIRECTOR

_____
MEDICAL DIRECTOR

_____
VICE PRESIDENT/ADMINISTRATOR

DEPARTMENTS:
DATA SOURCE(S):
METHODOLOGY: [X] RETROSPECTIVE [   ] CONCURRENT
TYPE: [   ] STRUCTURE [   ] PROCESS [X] OUTCOME
PERSON RESPONSIBLE FOR:
• DATA COLLECTION: J. HERRIG
• DATA ORGANIZATION: J. HERRIG
• ACTION PLAN: J. HERRIG
• FOLLOW-UP: J. HERRIG
DATE MONITORING BEGAN: 1990
TIME PERIOD THIS MONITOR: 2ND QUARTER 2009
MONITOR DISCONTINUED BECAUSE:
FOLLOW-UP:

INDICATORS	THLD	ACT	PREV	CRITICAL ANALYSIS/EVALUATION	ACTION PLAN
Blood Culture contamination rate will not exceed 3%				**Population: All patients** All monthly indicators were under threshold, 3%	Share results and analysis with Lab staff and ER staff.
APR - # of Draws: 713 # Contaminated: 13	3.00%	1.8%	1.2%	% Contamination from draws other than Line draws, by unit:	
MAY - # of Draws: 710 # Contaminated: 23	3.00%	2.8%	2.3%	APR: ER = 4.7% Lab = 0.7% MAY: ER = 11.5% Lab = 1.0%	
JUN - # of Draws: 702 # Contaminated: 17	3.00%	2.4%	1.9%	JUN: ER = 8.6% Lab = 1.1% ER was over threshold for each month of quarter.	
Total for 1st Quarter - # of Draws: 2125 # Contaminated: 50	3.00%	2.4%	1.9%		

Figure 2-1 A microbiology quality assessment form.

58. The use of the microbiology quality assessment form for tracking and evaluating blood cultures began in what year?
    a. 1985
    b. 1990
    c. 2000
    d. 2004

59. In which month did the laboratory blood culture collections actually exceed 3% contamination?
    a. April
    b. May
    c. June
    d. None of the above

Use Figure 2-2 (A reference manual page) to answer questions 60 to 62.

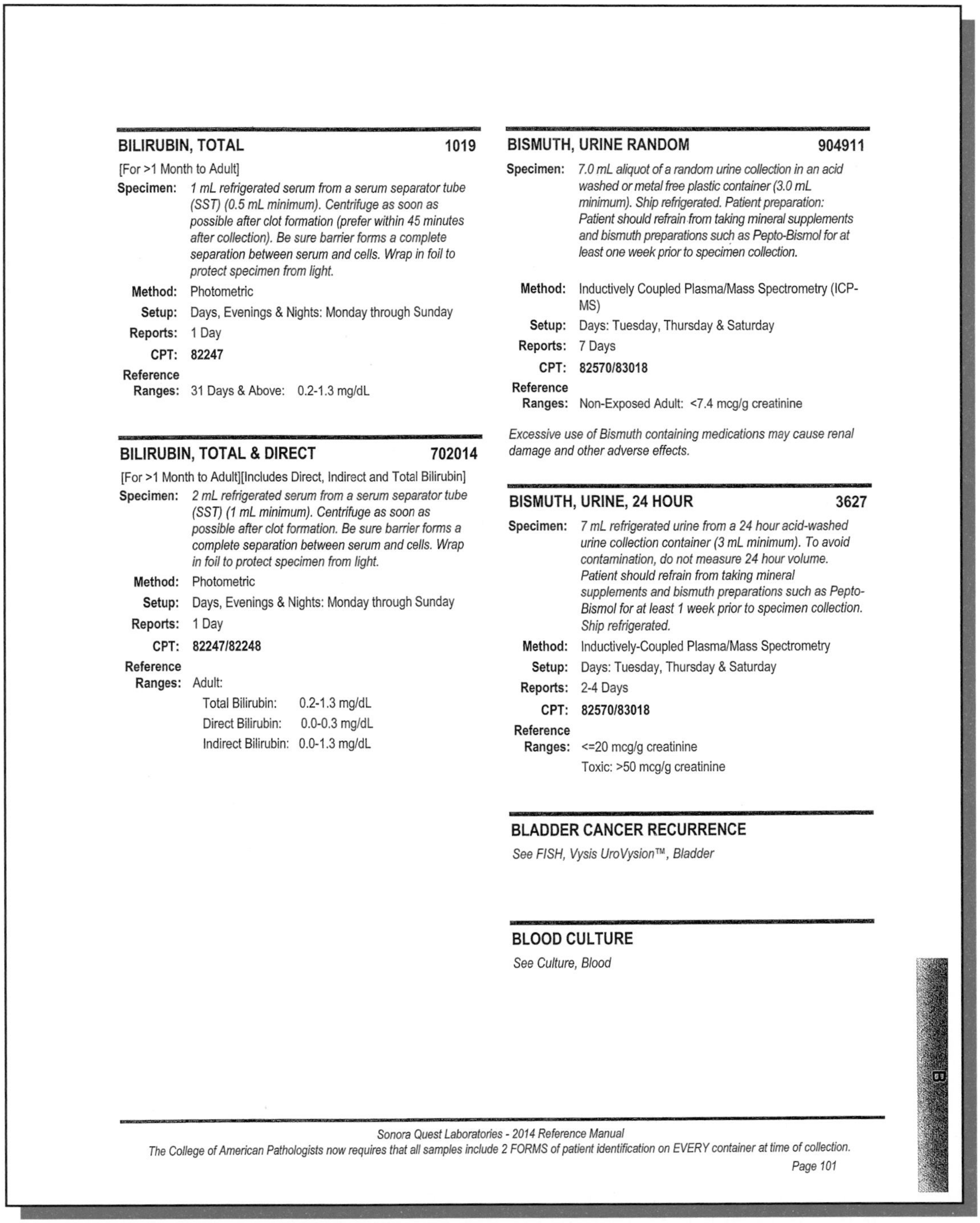

BILIRUBIN, TOTAL   1019

[For >1 Month to Adult]

Specimen: *1 mL refrigerated serum from a serum separator tube (SST) (0.5 mL minimum). Centrifuge as soon as possible after clot formation (prefer within 45 minutes after collection). Be sure barrier forms a complete separation between serum and cells. Wrap in foil to protect specimen from light.*

Method: Photometric

Setup: Days, Evenings & Nights: Monday through Sunday

Reports: 1 Day

CPT: **82247**

Reference Ranges: 31 Days & Above: 0.2-1.3 mg/dL

BILIRUBIN, TOTAL & DIRECT   702014

[For >1 Month to Adult][Includes Direct, Indirect and Total Bilirubin]

Specimen: *2 mL refrigerated serum from a serum separator tube (SST) (1 mL minimum). Centrifuge as soon as possible after clot formation. Be sure barrier forms a complete separation between serum and cells. Wrap in foil to protect specimen from light.*

Method: Photometric

Setup: Days, Evenings & Nights: Monday through Sunday

Reports: 1 Day

CPT: **82247/82248**

Reference Ranges: Adult:

Total Bilirubin:	0.2-1.3 mg/dL
Direct Bilirubin:	0.0-0.3 mg/dL
Indirect Bilirubin:	0.0-1.3 mg/dL

BISMUTH, URINE RANDOM   904911

Specimen: *7.0 mL aliquot of a random urine collection in an acid washed or metal free plastic container (3.0 mL minimum). Ship refrigerated. Patient preparation: Patient should refrain from taking mineral supplements and bismuth preparations such as Pepto-Bismol for at least one week prior to specimen collection.*

Method: Inductively Coupled Plasma/Mass Spectrometry (ICP-MS)

Setup: Days: Tuesday, Thursday & Saturday

Reports: 7 Days

CPT: **82570/83018**

Reference Ranges: Non-Exposed Adult: <7.4 mcg/g creatinine

Excessive use of Bismuth containing medications may cause renal damage and other adverse effects.

BISMUTH, URINE, 24 HOUR   3627

Specimen: *7 mL refrigerated urine from a 24 hour acid-washed urine collection container (3 mL minimum). To avoid contamination, do not measure 24 hour volume. Patient should refrain from taking mineral supplements and bismuth preparations such as Pepto-Bismol for at least 1 week prior to specimen collection. Ship refrigerated.*

Method: Inductively-Coupled Plasma/Mass Spectrometry

Setup: Days: Tuesday, Thursday & Saturday

Reports: 2-4 Days

CPT: **82570/83018**

Reference Ranges: <=20 mcg/g creatinine

Toxic: >50 mcg/g creatinine

BLADDER CANCER RECURRENCE

See FISH, Vysis UroVysion™, Bladder

BLOOD CULTURE

See Culture, Blood

Sonora Quest Laboratories - 2014 Reference Manual
The College of American Pathologists now requires that all samples include 2 FORMS of patient identification on EVERY container at time of collection.
Page 101

Figure 2-2 A page from a reference manual.

60. Which test specimen has to be collected in metal-free plastic container?
    a. Direct bilirubin
    b. Indirect bilirubin
    c. Total bilirubin
    d. Urine bismuth

61. Special handling of specimens for bilirubin testing means to
    a. collect in a metal-free container.
    b. refrigerate sample 1 hour after collection.
    c. ship specimen in refrigerated container.
    d. wrap in foil to protect from the light.

62. Why would a physician order a test for bismuth in the urine?
    a. An abnormal quantity of this substance may cause renal failure.
    b. Mineral supplements and bismuth preparations cause diarrhea.
    c. Pepto-Bismol can become addictive and cause stomach ulcers.
    d. Too much bismuth causes inflammation of the digestive track.

63. One of the Joint Commission's screening criteria used to determine accreditation of the clinical laboratory is the category *Immediate Threat to Health and Safety.* An example of not meeting this criteria would be
    a. absence of a QC program for each area of laboratory.
    b. lack of documentation of ongoing education for staff.
    c. recurrent problems with proper patient identification.
    d. use of unlicensed personnel in state that requires it.

64. One of NPSG's specified 2014 goals for the laboratory is to
    a. decrease sick days.
    b. identify safety issues.
    c. improve communication.
    d. increase proficiency testing.

65. CLIAC's role in assisting CMS to administer CLIA is to
    a. advise.
    b. educate.
    c. inspect.
    d. manage.

66. The purpose of the Office of Quality Monitoring is to
    a. evaluate and track complaints related to care.
    b. implement immediate response to safety issues.
    c. inspect healthcare facilities for accreditation.
    d. set specific patient safety goals to improve care.

67. National Patient Safety Goals address
    a. healthcare-associated infections.
    b. proficiency testing in the laboratory.
    c. tracking methods for complaints.
    d. waived testing practices and protocol.

68. The guidelines from this organization are the basis for national certification exam questions and the standards of care for the laboratory.
    a. ACO
    b. CLSI
    c. HIPAA
    d. PHS

Use Figure 2-3 (Near Miss/Occurrence Report Form) to answer questions 69 to 70.

69. If a glucose specimen is collected above an IV, under what category would this error be listed on the occurrence form?
    a. Disposition
    b. Patient order information
    c. Specimen identification
    d. Specimen integrity

70. If a specimen label was not completely filled out, which category does that fall under on the occurrence form?
    a. Disposition
    b. Patient order information
    c. Specimen identification
    d. Specimen integrity

Clinical Laboratory
Near Miss/Occurrence Report Form

Patient Name: _____ Patient Location: _____
Medical Rec. #: _____ Occurrence Date: _____ Occurrence Time: _____
Accession #: _____
Test (s): _____
Type of Spec.: _____
Problem Description: _____
_____
_____

Initial steps performed. Mark all that apply:

SPECIMEN INTEGRITY	RESULT (Process/Equipment/Environment)
____ Hemolysis ____ Clotted ____ QNS ____ Incorrect container ____ Leaking/contaminated ____ Transport time exceeded ____ Collected above IV ____ Fluid contaminated from line draw ____ Lipemia ____ Other	____ Repeat – same specimen, new specimen, previous specimen ____ Check patient history ____ Verify QC/instrument ____ Dilution error ____ Wrong cup/specimen/accession ____ Check ABO Acc# _____ ABO/RH_____ Acc# _____ ABO/RH_____ ____ Other:

SPECIMEN IDENTIFICATION	DISPOSITION
____ Unlabeled ____ Mislabeled (wrong) ____ Improperly labeled (alignment) ____ Transposed letters/numbers ____ Incomplete label ____ Incorrect collection time ____ Other:	____ Incorrect result ____ Procedure cancelled ____ Erroneous results corrected ____ Procedure credited ____ Notification to _____ date/time_____ _____ date/time_____ ____ Specimen recollected ____ Unlabeled/leaking specimen discarded ____ Mislabeled specimen in ERROR rack

PATIENT ORDER/INFORMATION	LABORATORY USE ONLY
____ Ordered on wrong patient ____ Wrong procedure ordered ____ Wrong encounter ____ Wrong date/time ____ Missing or incorrect requisition ____ Wrong therapy Other Departments affected by Near Miss Occurrence: ☐No ☐Yes	Date:_____ Employee Name: _____ Counseled By: _____ Repeat Error: Yes No Other Corrective Action Needed: Yes No ____ Written PIP ____ Final Written

	OFFICE USE ONLY
Occurrence by (username): _____ Report completed by: _____ Date: _____ Report Reviewed by: _____Date: _____	Midas NMOR: _____ Date: _____ Midas Follow up: _____ Date: _____ Spec Mislabel: _____ Date: _____ FDA Report: _____ Date: _____

Figure 2-3 Near Miss/Occurrence Report Form.

Answers and Explanations

1. **Answer: a**

   WHY: Civil lawsuits are concerned with actions between private parties, such as individuals or organizations, and constitute the bulk of the legal actions dealt within health care. Almost all legal actions against healthcare workers are civil actions in which the alleged injured party sues for monetary damages. Criminal action deals with felonies and misdemeanors. Malpractice, a type of negligence, would constitute a civil action. Vicarious liability is a liability imposed by law on one person for acts committed by another.

   REVIEW: Yes ☐ No ☐

2. **Answer: b**

   WHY: Good Laboratory Practices (GLPs), as seen in Box 2-1, are 10 QA recommendations developed by the Clinical Laboratory Improvement Advisory Committee (CLIAC) for Certificate of Waiver (CoW) labs because of problems with the quality of their testing practices. These GLPs emphasize QA when collecting and performing blood work using waived testing kits.

   REVIEW: Yes ☐ No ☐

   📖 *See the WORKBOOK Case Study 2-1: Quality Assurance in the CoW, for better understanding of CLIA and CLIAC.*

3. **Answer: a**

   WHY: Due care is a level of care that is expected to be exercised by a person of ordinary intelligence and good sense under the given circumstances. The standard of care is the level of skill and care that is expected to be performed to provide due care. Quality care and critical care are phrases that might be used in health care to describe types of assistance or supervision given to a patient.

   REVIEW: Yes ☐ No ☐

4. **Answer: c**

   WHY: Fraud is a deliberate deception carried out for unlawful gain and is in the form of a deceitful practice or false portrayal of facts, either by words or by conduct. Battery is defined as intentional harmful or offensive touching of or use of force on a person without consent or legal justification. Negligence is failure to exercise due care. If any of these torts make it to court, a formal discovery will occur, which involves taking depositions and interrogating parties involved.

   REVIEW: Yes ☐ No ☐

Box 2-1

Good Laboratory Practices

1. Keep the manufacturer's current product insert for the laboratory test in use and be sure it is available to the testing personnel. Use the manufacturer's product insert for the kit currently in use; do not use old product inserts.
2. Follow the manufacturer's instructions for specimen collection and handling.
3. Be sure to properly identify the patient.
4. Be sure to label the patient's specimen for testing with an identifier unique to each patient.
5. Inform the patient of any test preparation such as fasting, clean-catch urines, etc.
6. Read the product insert before performing a test and achieve the optimal result.
7. Follow the storage requirements for the test kit. If the kit can be stored at room temperature but this changes the expiration date, write the new expiration date on the kit.
8. Do not mix components of different kits.
9. Record the patient's test results in the proper place, such as the laboratory test log or the patient's chart, but not on unidentified Post-it notes or pieces of scrap paper that can be misplaced.
10. Perform any instrument maintenance as directed by the manufacturer.

Adapted from U.S. Department of Health and Human Services, Centers for Medicare and Medicaid Services, Clinical Laboratory Improvement Amendments, Good Laboratory Practices. Retrieved April 14, 2010 from http://www.cms.hhs.gov/clia/downloads/wgoodlab.pdf. See that document for more information.

5. **Answer: b**

   WHY: Continuous quality improvement means the institution is committed to an ongoing effort to improve all necessary processes so as to provide better service to their customers, the patients.

   Normally, unionization, employee investments, and financial issues do not fall under the institution's CQI plans.

   REVIEW: Yes ☐ No ☐

6. **Answer: b**

   WHY: The Joint Commission created an Office of Quality Monitoring to track and evaluate complaints about healthcare organizations and their quality of care. The office has a toll-free line that can help people register their complaints.

   REVIEW: Yes ☐   No ☐

7. **Answer: c**

   WHY: The Center for Medicare and Medicaid Services (CMS) is an agency of the U.S. government that administers or manages federal healthcare programs for Medicare and Medicaid. The supervision of federal regulations passed by Congress such as the Clinical Laboratory Improvement Amendments of 1988 (CLIA '88) also falls under its scope of authority. Although the CMS manages federal healthcare programs, it is not in the business of insuring medical personnel, operating risk management programs, or accrediting educational programs.

   REVIEW: Yes ☐   No ☐

8. **Answer: b**

   WHY: Giving a deposition is a process in which one party questions another under oath with both defense and prosecuting attorneys present. A court reporter records every word. Discovery is the process during which the attorneys for the defendant and plaintiff interrogate all parties involved in the legal dispute to determine the facts, which will be used in the trial phase. Civil actions are procedures in which the alleged injured party sues for monetary damages, and the tort is the most common civil action in health care.

   REVIEW: Yes ☐   No ☐

9. **Answer: c**

   WHY: The *Procedure Manual* states the policies and procedures that apply to each test or practice performed in the laboratory. It is a QA document that must be made available to all employees of the laboratory for standardization purposes. It contains, among other things, equipment used, purpose of the procedure, and all revision dates (Fig. 2-4).

   REVIEW: Yes ☐   No ☐

10. **Answer: c**

    WHY: Risk is managed in two ways: controlling risk to avoid incidents and paying for occurrences after they have happened. Risk management focuses on minimizing the situations that could lead to occurrences for patients and employees. Sentinel event policies signal the need for immediate investigation and response to an occurrence that had unexpected results. Performance improvement plans and delta checks in an institution deal with QA rather than risk management.

    REVIEW: Yes ☐   No ☐

11. **Answer: a**

    WHY: Not all laboratories perform the same level of testing. All laboratories subject to CLIA '88 regulations are required to obtain a CLIA certificate according to the complexity of testing performed there. Complexity of testing is based on the level of difficulty involved in performing a test and the degree of risk of harm to the patient if the test is performed incorrectly. The higher the complexity of testing performed, the more stringent the CLIA requirements are. Personnel qualifications are spelled out in the regulations but do not determine the type of certificate the laboratory will be awarded. In addition, QC standards and the size of the laboratory do not play a part in determining CLIA certification.

    REVIEW: Yes ☐   No ☐

12. **Answer: b**

    WHY: CLIA requirements are stringent for laboratories that perform moderate- and high-complexity testing. These laboratories are subject to routine inspections and must have written protocols for all procedures used. The laboratories are not federally funded. Personnel standards do not dictate that PhDs be hired as supervisors. The certificates do not need to be renewed annually.

    REVIEW: Yes ☐   No ☐

13. **Answer: b**

    WHY: The Joint Commission is committed to improving the safety of patients. The Joint Commission's quality improvement sentinel event policy is intended to identify unfavorable occurrences, initiate an immediate response, and take steps to prevent it from happening again. It stresses early identification of serious physical or psychological injury or any deviation from practice that increases the chance that an undesirable outcome might recur. Because the intent of this policy is to protect the patients and residents, it can never be considered flexible. Researching healthcare organizations' (HCOs') data collection and working to standardize QA is not the goal of the Sentinel Event QI program.

    REVIEW: Yes ☐   No ☐

    📖 *Learn more about Sentinel Event Policies and other Joint Commission CQI programs in Chapter 2 of the TEXTBOOK.*

Patient Identification

Content Applies To:
The Best Clinic: Support Services, Division of Laboratory Medicine
Scope
This procedure applies to all Support Services areas involved with patient identification.
Purpose
Patient Identification is paramount in the laboratory setting. Not properly identifying a patient seriously compromises patient safety. The purpose of this procedure is to provide instructions on how to properly identify patients prior to specimen collection to ensure an accurate match will be made to the laboratory order received.
Revision date: 1/22/2015
Synopsis of Change: Revised to include latest patient ID policies.

Procedure

Step	Action		Detail

01	Ask patient to state his/her first and last name and date of birth.		Identification of patient is required by using two patient identifiers before specimens are collected. Preferred patient identifiers are:
			 o Full name (first, last and middle initial as needed)
			 o Date of birth
			 o MRN
			 o Other acceptable identifiers:
			   o Address
			   o Legal photo ID
			   o Verification by a family member or caregiver

02	Compare and confirm information provided by the patient match the patient order received: o Inpatient – patient's armband and the LIS Soft PC/PDA o Outpatient – Cerner notification sheet and LIS Soft PC/PDA		
03	If no discrepancies found	Proceed with patient sample draw	Inpatient Venipuncture Collection Procedure **Or** Outpatient Venipuncture Collection Procedure
	If patient information requires correction	**Inpatient:** go to nurse to have information corrected **Outpatient:** Use *Correction of Patient Demographics* Procedure	

Figure 2-4 A procedure manual page.

14. Answer: c

WHY: The intent of this policy is to help healthcare organizations identify sentinel events and take steps to prevent them from happening again. The steps involve conducting a thorough analysis of the cause, initiating improvements to reduce the risk, and monitoring improvements for effectiveness. HCOs are not expected to develop new personnel standards or create a complain procedure. After an event, the HCO is not required to report these incidents to the Joint Commission.

REVIEW: Yes ☐   No ☐

15. Answer: a

WHY: In a large laboratory, items such as refrigerators, freezers, and centrifuges are monitored by computers and reports are sent to the Facilities Department. Inspections on the reliability and consistency of these items are done by TJC or CAP.

REVIEW: Yes ☐   No ☐

16. Answer: c

WHY: QA indicators are specific markers that can measure quality, adequacy, accuracy, timeliness, and customer satisfaction. They are designed to

look at all areas of care and are used in conjunction with process improvement tools, such as LEAN or Six Sigma, to monitor workflow and outcomes. Individual Quality Control Plans (IQCP) are the latest addition to the CLIA quality system and allow laboratories to customize their QA programs.
REVIEW: Yes ☐ No ☐

17. **Answer: c**
WHY: The National Accrediting Agency for Clinical Laboratory Sciences (NAACLS) is an agency that approves phlebotomy programs. The Clinical Laboratory Improvement Advisory Committee (CLIAC) was formed to advise CMS in regards to CLIA '88. The Clinical and Laboratory Standards Institute (CLSI) develops standards for laboratory procedures, including phlebotomy. The National Center for Competency Testing (NCCT) is one of the several organizations that certify laboratory personnel, including phlebotomists.
REVIEW: Yes ☐ No ☐

18. **Answer: d**
WHY: Failure to exercise the level of care that a person of ordinary intelligence and good sense would exercise under the given circumstances is called negligence. If a medical procedure results in injury, the injured person has the right to sue for damages. Because the phlebotomist did not threaten or intend to harm the patient, there are no assault and battery charges, nor did the phlebotomist commit fraud because there was not a willful plan to deceive the patient.
REVIEW: Yes ☐ No ☐

19. **Answer: b**
WHY: The Clinical Laboratory Improvement Amendments of 1988 (CLIA '88) are federal regulations aimed at ensuring the accuracy, reliability, and timeliness of patient test results regardless of the size, type, or location of the laboratory. CLIA regulations pertain to all laboratories in the United States that perform laboratory testing used for the assessment of human health or the diagnosis, treatment, or prevention of disease. The Occupational Safety and Health Act (OSHA) mandates safe working conditions for employees and is enforced by the Occupational Safety and Health Administration (OSHA). The Bloodborne Pathogen (BBP) Standard was instituted by OSHA to protect employees from exposure to blood-borne pathogens. The Hazard Communication Standard (HazCom) was developed by OSHA to protect employees from exposure to hazardous chemicals.
REVIEW: Yes ☐ No ☐

20. **Answer: b**
WHY: The Clinical and Laboratory Standards Institute (CLSI), formerly known as the National Committee for Clinical Laboratory Standards (NCCLS), is a global, nonprofit, standards-developing organization with representatives from the profession, industry, and government who use a consensus process to develop guidelines and standards for all areas of the laboratory. The American Society for Clinical Pathology (ASCP), NCCT, and NAACLS are organizations that contribute to the standards of phlebotomy practices by offering continuing education, certification exams, and phlebotomy program approval, respectively.
REVIEW: Yes ☐ No ☐
📖 *Learn more about all of these organization in Chapter 2 of the TEXTBOOK.*

21. **Answer: b**
WHY: Patient identification, phlebotomy technique, and specimen handling are all areas of phlebotomy that are subject to QC procedures. Adjusting a patient's IV is not in the scope of practice for a phlebotomist. Even though it is necessary at times to have blood specimens withdrawn from intravenous devices, such as heparin or saline locks, it is not in the phlebotomist's scope of practice to handle such procedures unless specifically trained by the facility to do so. It is never appropriate to adjust an IV in a patient's arm or to put a tourniquet near that area.
REVIEW: Yes ☐ No ☐

22. **Answer: a**
WHY: Delta checks compare current results of a test with previous results for the same test on the same patient. Although some variation is to be expected, a major difference in results could indicate error and require investigation.
REVIEW: Yes ☐ No ☐

23. **Answer: b**
WHY: The College of American Pathologists (CAP) is a national organization of board-certified pathologists that offers laboratory inspection and proficiency testing. OSHA inspections involve safety violations. The American Society for Clinical Pathology is an organization that certifies laboratory personnel. The Clinical and Laboratory Standards Institute (CLSI) develops standards and guidelines for laboratory procedures, including phlebotomy. OSHA mandates and enforces safe working conditions for employees.
REVIEW: Yes ☐ No ☐

24. **Answer: d**

WHY: Outdated tubes should never be used. The tube vacuum and the integrity of any additive that might be in the tube are guaranteed by the manufacturer but only if the tube is used before the expiration date. After that date, the additive may break down and no longer function as intended. In addition, outdated tubes may lose some of the vacuum and no longer fill completely changing the additive-to-sample ratio. In either situation, the results may be incorrect or erroneous. It has not been shown that the tube stoppers actually shrink when held past the expiration date or that bacteria start to grow in outdated tubes. It is important to note that some additives can be seen on the sides of tubes before blood is added because they are made this way at the factory.

REVIEW: Yes ☐   No ☐

📖 *Learn more about QA in the phlebotomy area of the laboratory in Chapter 2 of the TEXTBOOK.*

25. **Answer: b**

WHY: The Joint Commission is a nongovernmental agency that establishes standards and provides accreditation for healthcare organizations. Their standards focus on improving the quality and safety of care provided and stress performance improvement by requiring healthcare facilities to be directly accountable to their customers. The Clinical and Laboratory Standards Institute (CLSI) develops standards for laboratory procedures, including phlebotomy. NAACLS develops phlebotomy competencies and has an approval process for phlebotomy programs. Laboratory personnel are certified by organizations such as ASCP, AMT, and NCA.

REVIEW: Yes ☐   No ☐

26. **Answer: a**

WHY: QC procedures involve checking all operational procedures to make certain they are performed correctly. This includes checking expiration dates of evacuated tubes. Phlebotomy QC does not mean documenting every missed venipuncture or recording patient census daily. Filling out your time sheet is important but is not considered a QC procedure.

REVIEW: Yes ☐   No ☐

27. **Answer: a**

WHY: If the threshold of an indicator is exceeded, data are collected and organized to see if there is a problem. If a problem is identified, a corrective action plan is established and implemented (Fig. 2-1).

REVIEW: Yes ☐   No ☐

28. **Answer: a**

WHY: QA procedures include checking for needle defects before use. It is not part of the phlebotomy QA to track all of the laboratory OSHA violations or to record any of the chemistry instrument maintenance. Keeping a record of employee paid sick leave is an important personnel issue but is not a part of laboratory QA.

REVIEW: Yes ☐   No ☐

29. **Answer: b**

WHY: Preparing a patient for testing is not generally under the control of the phlebotomist. However, it is up to the phlebotomist to determine that preparation procedures have been followed. For example, if a test is ordered fasting, the phlebotomist must check to see that the patient is indeed fasting. The phlebotomist is responsible for obtaining proper patient identification, collecting the specimen, and handling the specimen properly after collection until turning it over to the laboratory for testing.

REVIEW: Yes ☐   No ☐

30. **Answer: c**

WHY: The medical record is a chronological record of a patient's care and serves as a valuable tool in evaluating medical treatment and communicating with all of the patient's caregivers. A delta check compares current results of a lab test with previous results for the same test on the same patient. A major difference in results could indicate error and requires investigation. An internal report is used for specific incidents and the test catalog gives specimen requirements and collection information.

REVIEW: Yes ☐   No ☐

31. **Answer: c**

WHY: Negligence is failure to exercise due care or perform duties according to the standards of the profession. If a medical procedure such as phlebotomy results in injury, a claim of negligence can be made by the injured party. Redirecting the needle multiple times in an attempt to locate a vein without knowing where the vein and needle are currently located in the arm is called probing and is not considered due care because it can result in damage to nerves, arteries, and other tissues. Pain in the area where the venipuncture attempt was unsuccessful is an indication that the patient may have been physically harmed by the probing.

REVIEW: Yes ☐   No ☐

HOSPITAL & HEALTH CENTER
PERFORMANCE IMPROVEMENT PLAN

Employee Name:	Facility	Department	Job Title
Previous Action:	Type	Reason	Date

Current Action: ☐ Verbal Counseling   ☐ Written Warning   ☐ Final Written Warning
(please check one)   ☐ Suspension – Date   ☐ Termination (check reason below)

Termination   ☐ Unexcused   ☐ Job Performance   ☐ Conduct   ☐ Other
Reason: Absence/Tardiness

  I.   Describe the performance deficiency giving rise to the counseling (include specific dates, times and policies violated, etc.):

  II.   Describe specific job performance expectations and areas for improvement:

  III.   Describe the agreed upon action plan for improvement including date of follow-up to review progress, if applicable:

  IV.   State the next step if job performance does not improve (warning, discharge, etc.):

  V.   Department director/supervisor Comments:

Department Director/Supervisor Signature:	Date

  VI.   **Employee Comments:**

I understand that all corrective action notices other than a verbal counseling will be placed in my personnel file. My signature below does not indicate agreement regarding the contents of the document; only that I have received a copy for my records.

Employee	Date	Witness	Date
Human Resources	Date	Reason	

Figure 2-5 A performance improvement form.

---

32. Answer: d

WHY: A document called a Performance Improvement Plan (Fig. 2-5) is used in counseling a person or when suspension is necessary. The document states the deficiency, describes a specific action plan for improvement, or indicates consequences such as termination or suspension. New guidelines are sometimes implemented as a result of an incident but are not included on the incident report form. REVIEW: Yes ☐   No ☐

33. Answer: d

WHY: Following standard precaution guidelines, not wearing lab coats outside of work areas, and

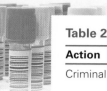

Table 2-1: Criminal and Civil Actions

Action	Definition	Punishment
Criminal	Concerned with laws designed to protect all members of society from unlawful acts by others, e.g., felonies and misdemeanors.	• A felony is a crime (e.g., murder, assault, and rape) punishable by death or imprisonment. • Misdemeanors are considered lesser offenses and usually carry a penalty of a fine or less than 1 year in jail.
Civil	Concerned with actions between two private parties, such as individuals or organizations; constitute the bulk of the legal actions dealt within the medical office or other healthcare facilities.	• Damages may be awarded in a court of law and result in monetary penalties.

not eating, drinking, or smoking in lab work areas are all safety rules. QA indicators are not considered rules but are statements that serve as monitors of patient care. By setting a limit or threshold value, they serve as initiators of action plans, as shown in Figure 2-1.

REVIEW: Yes ☐ No ☐

34. **Answer: c**

WHY: The laboratory procedure manual is a reference book that describes in detail the step-by-step processes for specimen collection and other procedures performed in the laboratory. An example of a page from a procedure manual is shown in Figure 2-4. Other manuals may contain information on safety, details on administrative duties, or data for the QC program.

REVIEW: Yes ☐ No ☐

35. **Answer: a**

WHY: Attempting to collect a person's blood without permission can be perceived as assault, which is the act or threat of intentionally causing a person to be in fear of harm to his or her person. If the act or threat is actually carried out, then it can also be perceived as battery. Battery is defined as the intentional harmful or offensive touching of a person without consent or legal justification. Breach of confidentiality involves failure to keep medical information private or confidential. Negligence requires doing something that a reasonable person would not do or not doing something a reasonable person would do. Malpractice is negligence by a professional.

REVIEW: Yes ☐ No ☐

36. **Answer: d**

WHY: A "tort" is a wrongful act resulting in injury for which a civil, rather than criminal, action can be brought. A tort is committed against one's

property, reputation, or other legally protected right, for which an individual is entitled to damages awarded by the court. Damages are generally in the form of monetary awards. See Table 2-1 for more information about tort law.

REVIEW: Yes ☐ No ☐

37. **Answer: b**

WHY: Risk management is a *process* that focuses on identifying and minimizing situations that pose a risk to patients and employees by using education and following procedures that are already in place. Sharing issues and information with patients is unauthorized and can lead to the issues with personnel but it is not one of the designated steps in the process. Approving rule variations and validating new treatments is not part of the risk management process.

REVIEW: Yes ☐ No ☐

38. **Answer: a**

WHY: As a professional, the phlebotomist should recognize that patient information, including disease status is private or confidential. A recent ruling by Health and Human Services states that patients may request to see their laboratory test results, but it is not a phlebotomist's duty to give them out unless that is the institution's policy. However, letting other phlebotomists know where the best site is to obtain a blood sample on a patient who is a "difficult draw" is part of proper patient care and not considered a violation of patient confidentiality.

REVIEW: Yes ☐ No ☐

39. **Answer: c**

WHY: Unauthorized release of confidential patient information is called invasion of privacy and can result in a civil lawsuit. It may also be considered breach of confidentiality if medical information is involved. It is not considered a type of negligence or failure to use due care, nor is it called a violation of discovery.

REVIEW: Yes ☐   No ☐

40. **Answer: a**

WHY: Civil actions involve legal proceedings between private parties. The most common civil actions involve tort. For example, a claim of malpractice because of harm or injury to a patient by a phlebotomist is a civil wrong or tort. Crimes against the state or that violate laws established by governments are criminal actions for which a guilty individual may be imprisoned.

REVIEW: Yes ☐   No ☐

41. **Answer: b**

WHY: Malpractice can be described as improper or negligent treatment resulting in injury, loss, or damage. Breach of confidentiality involves failure to keep medical information private or confidential, as opposed to invasion of privacy, which involves physical intrusion or the unauthorized publishing or releasing of private information. *Res ipsa loquitur* is a Latin phrase meaning "the thing speaks for itself" and applies to the rule of evidence in cases of negligence in which a breach of duty is obvious.

REVIEW: Yes ☐   No ☐

42. **Answer: a**

WHY: Not reporting an obvious problem with a patient's condition (such as severe breathing difficulties or inability to awaken) could lead to serious consequences and are examples of negligence or failure to exercise reasonable care. Inability to obtain a specimen from a patient is not negligence, especially if the patient is very combative and not willing to cooperate. It is not a major issue if the patient is not signed out as the phlebotomist leaves the nursing area. A quick call can inform the nursing staff of the patient's phlebotomy status.

REVIEW: Yes ☐   No ☐

43. **Answer: a**

WHY: Assault involves the act or threat of causing an individual to be in fear of harm. Threatening to restrain the patient can be considered assault. Restraining the patient and collecting a blood specimen can be considered assault and battery.

REVIEW: Yes ☐   No ☐

44. **Answer: b**

WHY: Informed consent implies voluntary and competent permission for a medical procedure, test, or medication and requires that the patient be given adequate information as to the method, risks, and consequences involved before consent is given. In implied consent, the patient's actions or condition (as in an emergency situation in which the patient is unconscious) indicate consent rather than a verbal or written statement.

REVIEW: Yes ☐   No ☐

📖 *For more practice in learning the different types of consent, see Matching Exercise 2-2 in the WORKBOOK.*

45. **Answer: d**

WHY: Statute of limitations is the particular number of years within which one party can sue another. Binding arbitration is a way that equitable settlements over a controversy are made outside the courts. It is one of the pathways used in the litigation process, which is defined as a course of action used to settle legal disputes. One of the steps in the litigation process is the discovery period.

REVIEW: Yes ☐   No ☐

46. **Answer: b**

WHY: The definition of a minor is anyone who has not reached the age of majority. The age of majority is determined by state law and normally ranges from 18 to 21 years of age regardless of whether the individual is self-supporting.

REVIEW: Yes ☐   No ☐

47. **Answer: c**

WHY: The standard of care is defined as a level of care that protects clients from harm because it follows established standards of the profession and expectations of society. It requires that duties be performed the same way any other reasonable and prudent person with the same experience and training would perform those duties.

REVIEW: Yes ☐   No ☐

48. **Answer: d**

WHY: Negligence involves doing something that a reasonable and prudent person would not do or not doing something that a reasonable and prudent person would do. Battery is the intentional harmful or offensive touching of another person without consent or legal justification. Discovery is the process of taking depositions or interrogating parties involved in a lawsuit. Fraud is deceitful practice or false portrayal of facts by word or conduct.

REVIEW: Yes ☐   No ☐

49. **Answer: b**

    WHY: With implied consent, the patient's actions or condition (as in an emergency situation in which the patient is unconscious) indicate consent, rather than a verbal or written statement. A patient who extends his arm and rolls up his sleeve after being told that the phlebotomist is there to collect a blood specimen is implying consent with his actions. The patient is obviously not refusing consent, or he might have pulled his arm away and kept his sleeve down. To give expressed consent, the patient would have to provide a written or verbal statement of consent. Implied consent can be informed consent; however, implied consent is the best choice because it is a more specific answer to the situation.

    REVIEW: Yes ☐ No ☐

50. **Answer: a**

    WHY: A 12-year-old is not old enough to give consent for a medical procedure such as phlebotomy. A phlebotomist who collects a blood specimen from a minor without permission from a parent risks being charged with assault and battery. As long as no harm to the patient was involved, this would not be considered negligence or malpractice. The patient refused blood collection, so this is not considered implied consent.

    REVIEW: Yes ☐ No ☐

51. **Answer: b**

    WHY: The Clinical and Laboratory Standards Institute (CLSI) is a global, nonprofit organization that publishes standards for phlebotomy procedures. These standards are recognized as the legal standard of care for phlebotomy procedures. CAP sets standards for laboratories, but not specifically for phlebotomy procedures. OSHA sets and enforces standards regarding the safety of employees. NAACLS approves phlebotomy programs.

    REVIEW: Yes ☐ No ☐

52. **Answer: a**

    WHY: To claim negligence, the following elements must be present: a legal obligation or duty owed by one person to another, a breaking of that duty or obligation, and harm done as a result of that breach of duty. Informing the patient of a scheduled lab procedure is the responsibility of the person who ordered the test. Watching for implied consent from a patient is necessary in some cases. Documenting an unusual happening

during venipuncture is a good habit to get into in case there are future complaints.

REVIEW: Yes ☐ No ☐

53. **Answer: c**

    WHY: The process of gathering information by taking statements and interrogating parties involved in a lawsuit is called discovery. It involves taking depositions (questioning parties under oath). Some collaboration may be involved but it is not the term used to describe this process. Litigation is the process used to settle disputes, and discovery is part of this process.

    REVIEW: Yes ☐ No ☐

54. **Answer: c**

    WHY: The Joint Commission and CAP are presently standards-setting bodies throughout the world. All departments of a healthcare facility, including the laboratory, must comply with its standards to receive accreditation. The Environmental Protection Agency (EPA) and the U.S. Food and Drug Administration (FDA) are agencies of the federal government that are designed to protect the public in their respective areas.

    REVIEW: Yes ☐ No ☐

55. **Answer: b**

    WHY: The person against whom a complaint has been filed is the defendant. The person who complains of injury is the plaintiff and will become the prosecuting attorney's client.

    REVIEW: Yes ☐ No ☐

56. **Answer: b**

    WHY: The number of contaminated blood culture draws was highest in May (Fig. 2-1).

    REVIEW: Yes ☐ No ☐

57. **Answer: a**

    WHY: The report on the form in Figure 2-1 clearly states that the emergency room (ER) is over threshold for each month of the quarter. The percentage of contaminated draws for the ER went as high as 11.5% in May. The report shows the comparison between laboratory draws and those in the ER. This QA indicator tool is an objective measurement of phlebotomist technique.

    REVIEW: Yes ☐ No ☐

    📖 *For more understanding of the Quality Assessment and Improvement Tracking form, do the Labeling Exercise 2-1 in the WORKBOOK.*

58. Answer: b

WHY: The date this QA monitoring began was in 1990 (Fig. 2-1). This long-term tracking serves to point out valuable patterns in collection and gives insight into corrective actions that can be taken.

REVIEW: Yes ☐ No ☐

59. Answer: d

WHY: As shown in the report (Fig. 2-1), during the 3 months being monitored, the laboratory staff did not exceed the allowable contamination rate of 3% during blood culture collection.

REVIEW: Yes ☐ No ☐

60. Answer: d

WHY: A urine sample for bismuth must be collected in a metal-free plastic container to avoid interfering substances from the container when tested.

REVIEW: Yes ☐ No ☐

61. Answer: d

WHY: The bilirubin sample is most often ordered by the physician to check liver function. For the most accurate results, the tube of blood should be protected from sunlight and manufactured light so as to stop the breakdown of bilirubin in the sample. If not protected, the test results could be flawed. By carefully placing a foil around the specimen after collection, light cannot get to the specimen.

REVIEW: Yes ☐ No ☐

62. Answer: a

WHY: Elevated levels of bismuth in the body can cause renal damage and neurological problems, such as dementia. Any medications and mineral supplements containing bismuth should be stopped 1 week prior to the test so as to not affect the results.

REVIEW: Yes ☐ No ☐

63. Answer: c

WHY: One of the four scoring categories used to screen pre- and postanalytical processes in the laboratory is "immediate threat to health and safety." Because of the severity of this category, Preliminary Denial of Accreditation (PDA) would be issued until corrective action was validated. If patient identification is not carefully and methodically performed, it is a critical threat to the health and safety of patients.

REVIEW: Yes ☐ No ☐

64. Answer: c

WHY: The annually updated goals address several critical areas of concern that contribute to patient safety and describe expert-based solutions. For 2014, the National Safety Patient Goals for the clinical laboratory are (a) identifying patients correctly, (b) improving staff communication, and (c) preventing infection through the use of hand hygiene guidelines specified by CDC or WHO.

REVIEW: Yes ☐ No ☐

65. Answer: a

WHY: To assist in administering Clinical Laboratory Improvement Amendments (CLIA) regulations, the Clinical Laboratory Improvement Advisory Committee (CLIAC) was formed. Its purpose is to provide technical and scientific guidance or advice to the appropriate people in the Center of Medicare and Medicare Services (CMS) who are administering the regulations. CLIAC's advice centers on the need for revisions to the standards.

REVIEW: Yes ☐ No ☐

66. Answer: a

WHY: To evaluate and track complaints about healthcare organizations relating to quality of care, the Commission's Office of Quality Monitoring was created. The office has a toll-free line that can help people register their complaints. Information and concerns often come from patients, their families, and healthcare employees.

REVIEW: Yes ☐ No ☐

67. Answer: a

WHY: The National Patient Safety Goals address several areas of health care. A safety expert panel as well as physician, nurse, and risk managers review and update the CQI-required safety goals. Examples of the goals addressed are patient identification, communication, medication, safety, and health-associated infections (HAI).

REVIEW: Yes ☐ No ☐

68. Answer: b

WHY: The Clinical and Laboratory Standards Institute is a global, nonprofit standards-developing organization with representatives from the profession, industry, and government. CLSI uses a widespread agreement process to develop voluntary guidelines and standards for all areas of the laboratory.

REVIEW: Yes ☐ No ☐

69. **Answer: d**

    WHY: On the Near Miss/Occurrence Report Form, the error in the collection process is listed under "Specimen Integrity." The test results for glucose drawn above an IV containing glucose will be completely out of normal range. The result is out of integrity or untrue because the process used to obtain the specimen did not follow the collection standard regarding IVs.

    REVIEW: Yes ☐   No ☐

70. **Answer: c**

    WHY: On the Near Miss/Occurrence Report Form, the error in the collection process is listed under "Specimen Identification" because anything to do with the patient name and other identifying information must be correct. A mislabeled specimen cannot be tested and must be redrawn. The phlebotomist and the error are well documented and corrective action is noted.

    REVIEW: Yes ☐   No ☐

Chapter 3

Infection Control, Safety, First Aid, and Personal Wellness

Study Tips

- Complete the activities in Chapter 3 of the companion workbook.

- Draw a representation of the chain of infection, identifying the components in order starting with the infectious agent and including examples of each component.

- Find a partner and drill yourself on the principles of biohazard, chemical, electrical, fire, and radiation safety.

- Go over the cautions and key points in the textbook.

- Learn proper hand washing procedure by practicing or simulating each step.

- Make flash cards with biohazard exposure routes on one side and examples and how to protect yourself on the other. Do the same with the components of the chain of infection.

- Quiz yourself on the meanings of abbreviations found in the key terms throughout the textbook.

- Study the factors that contribute to personal wellness and list and describe the importance of those listed in the textbook.

Overview

This chapter covers infection control, safety, first aid, and personal wellness. A thorough knowledge in these areas is necessary for phlebotomists to protect themselves, patients, coworkers, and others from infection or injury, react quickly and skillfully in emergency situations, and stay healthy both physically and emotionally, all without compromising the quality of patient care. This chapter explains the process of infection, identifies the components of the chain of infection, lists required safety equipment, and describes infection control procedures. Also covered are biological, electrical, fire, radiation, and chemical hazards and the safety precautions, rules, and procedures necessary to eliminate or minimize them. First aid issues covered include control of external hemorrhage and how to recognize and treat shock victims. Wellness issues addressed include the prevention of back injury, benefits of exercise, and dealing with stress.

Review Questions

Choose the BEST answer.

1. These are the initials of the United States government agency that mandates and enforces safe working conditions for employees.
   a. CDC
   b. HICPAC
   c. NIOSH
   d. OSHA

2. The series of components that lead to infection are referred to as the
   a. chain of infection.
   b. immune response.
   c. infection cycle.
   d. pathogenic series.

3. The pathogen responsible for causing an infection is called the infectious
   a. agent.
   b. host.
   c. vector.
   d. vehicle.

4. The term pathogenic means
   a. highly communicable.
   b. possessing virulence.
   c. productive of disease.
   d. systemic in nature.

5. A specimen processor removes the stopper from a tube without barrier protection and feels a mist of specimen touch the eyes. What type of exposure occurs through eye contact?
   a. Airborne
   b. Nonintact skin
   c. Percutaneous
   d. Permucosal

6. Isolation procedures are used to separate patients from contact with others if they
   a. are a carrier of a blood-borne pathogen.
   b. have highly transmissible infections.
   c. require blood or body fluid precautions.
   d. were exposed to a contagious disease.

7. Which of the following is something other than a microbe?
   a. Bacteria
   b. Fungi
   c. Ova
   d. Viruses

8. Which of the following makes a patient less susceptible to a particular infection?
   a. Antibiotic treatment
   b. Chemotherapy drugs
   c. Previous vaccination
   d. Surgical procedures

9. An individual who has little resistance to an infectious microbe is referred to as a susceptible
   a. agent.
   b. host.
   c. pathway.
   d. reservoir.

10. SDS information includes
    a. general and emergency information.
    b. highly technical chemical formulas.
    c. information on competitor products.
    d. product manufacturing conditions.

11. Transmission-based precautions must be followed for patients with
    a. compromised immune systems.
    b. highly transmissible diseases.
    c. severe gastrointestinal distress.
    d. symptoms of acute appendicitis.

12. Which of the following patients would require contact precautions pending a diagnosis?
    a. Child with a maculopapular rash highly suggestive of rubeola (measles)
    b. Diapered patient with symptoms of infection with an enteric pathogen
    c. HIV-positive patient who has a cough, fever, and pulmonary infiltrate
    d. Man with a severe persistent cough indicative of *Bordetella pertussis*

13. An individual is infected with *E. Coli* after eating contaminated spinach. What type of infection transmission is involved?
    a. Contact
    b. Droplet
    c. Vector
    d. Vehicle

14. An avulsion is a
    a. hematoma in an extremity.
    b. situation that is repulsive.
    c. tearing away of a body part.
    d. type of operation on a bone.

15. This type of precautions is required for a patient with *mycoplasma pneumonia.*
    a. Airborne
    b. Contact
    c. Droplet
    d. Standard

16. Which type of precautions would be used for a patient who has pulmonary tuberculosis?
    a. Airborne
    b. Droplet
    c. Contact
    d. Reverse

17. What does the NFPA codeword *RACE* mean?
    a. React, activate, cover, extinguish
    b. Rescue, alarm, confine, extinguish
    c. Respond, activate, confine, escape
    d. Run, alarm, counter, extinguish

18. Which of the following statements concerning an employee blood-borne pathogen exposure incident is true?
    a. Exposures need not be documented if no transmission occurs.
    b. Incidents must be promptly reported to the CDC and OSHA.
    c. Source patients, if known, must be tested for HIV and HBV.
    d. The employee is entitled to a confidential medical evaluation.

19. When the chain of infection is broken an
    a. individual is immune to that microbe.
    b. individual is susceptible to infection.
    c. infection is prevented from happening.
    d. infection will most likely be the result.

20. The focus of infection control turned from preventing patient-to-patient transmission to preventing patient-to-personnel transmission with the introduction of this concept.
    a. Body substance isolation (BSI)
    b. Category-specific isolation
    c. Disease-specific isolation
    d. Universal precautions (UP)

21. The term used to describe an infection that infects the entire body is
    a. communicable.
    b. local.
    c. nosocomial.
    d. systemic.

22. Which of the following is proper neonatal ICU blood-drawing procedure?
    a. Clean hands and put on new gloves for each patient.
    b. Do not awaken an infant to collect a blood specimen.
    c. Place the phlebotomy tray right next to the isolette.
    d. Use povidone-iodine to cleanse skin puncture sites.

23. Exercise reduces stress by
    a. decreasing buildup of lactic acid.
    b. increasing utilization of glucose.
    c. promoting glycogen production.
    d. triggering release of endorphins.

24. The abbreviation for the virus that causes acquired immune deficiency syndrome (AIDS) is
    a. HAV.
    b. HBV.
    c. HCV.
    d. HIV.

25. A person who has recovered from a particular virus and has developed antibodies against that virus is said to be
    a. a carrier.
    b. immune.
    c. infectious.
    d. susceptible.

26. According to standard first aid procedures, severe external hemorrhage is *best* controlled by
    a. applying direct firm pressure to the wound.
    b. keeping the injured extremity well below heart level.
    c. placing a tourniquet directly above the affected area.
    d. raising the victim's head above the level of the injury.

27. The main purpose of an infection control program is to
    a. identify the source of communicable infections.
    b. separate infectious patients from other patients.
    c. prevent the spread of infection in the hospital.
    d. protect patients from outside contamination.

28. All pathogens are
    a. communicable microorganisms.
    b. microbes that can cause disease.
    c. microorganisms that live in soil.
    d. normal flora found on the skin.

29. Which one of the following diseases involves a blood-borne pathogen?
    a. Diphtheria
    b. Hepatitis B
    c. Meningitis
    d. Pneumonia

30. Which of the following is part of proper hand washing procedure?
    a. Apply a generous amount of soap to dry hands.
    b. Stand as close to the water source as possible.
    c. Use one towel to dry hands and turn off faucets.
    d. Wash hands thoroughly for at least 20 seconds.

31. An example of a disease requiring droplet isolation is
    a. pertussis.
    b. rubeola.
    c. scabies.
    d. varicella.

32. Class C fires involve
    a. combustible metals.
    b. electrical equipment.
    c. flammable liquids.
    d. ordinary materials.

33. Standard precautions should be followed
    a. for anyone with hepatitis B.
    b. if a patient is HIV-positive.
    c. while a patient is in isolation.
    d. with all patients, at all times.

34. Hepatitis B vaccination for adults normally involves
    a. a first shot of vaccine, one a month later, and one 6 months after the first.
    b. a single shot of vaccine that confers immunity for the individual's lifetime.
    c. three shots of vaccine, each 3 months apart, then yearly booster shots.
    d. two shots of vaccine 6 months apart, then a booster shot every 5 years.

35. Objects that can harbor and transmit infectious material are called
    a. fomites.
    b. hosts.
    c. pathogens.
    d. vectors.

36. The HazCom Standard is also commonly called the
    a. Full Disclosure Law.
    b. Material Safety Law.
    c. Right to Know Law.
    d. Universal Safety Law.

37. The body organ targeted by HBV is the
    a. brain.
    b. heart.
    c. liver.
    d. lungs.

38. These are the initials of the two organizations responsible for the *Guideline for Isolation Precautions in Hospitals.*
    a. CDC and HICPAC
    b. CLSI and OSHA
    c. HICPAC and NIOSH
    d. NIOSH and OSHA

39. The primary purpose of wearing gloves during phlebotomy procedures is to protect the
    a. patient from contamination by the phlebotomist.
    b. phlebotomist from exposure to the patient's blood.
    c. specimen from contamination by the phlebotomist.
    d. venipuncture site from contamination by the hands.

40. The first three components of fire that were traditionally referred to as the fire triangle are
    a. carbon, air, and static.
    b. fuel, oxygen, and heat.
    c. oxygen, energy, and fuel.
    d. vapor, heat, and static.

41. This would contribute to the chain of infection rather than help break it.
    a. Implementing isolation procedures.
    b. Opening exit pathways for pathogens.
    c. Practicing stress reduction techniques.
    d. Washing hands and wearing gloves.

42. Which of the following statements complies with electrical safety guidelines?
    a. Electrical equipment should be unplugged while being serviced.
    b. Extension cords should be used to conveniently place equipment.
    c. It is safe to use a frayed electrical cord if that area has been taped.
    d. Use electrical equipment carefully if it is starting to malfunction.

43. Which body fluid is exempt from standard precautions?
    a. Joint fluid
    b. Saliva
    c. Sweat
    d. Urine

44. The ability of a microorganism to survive on contaminated articles and equipment has to do with its
    a. susceptibility.
    b. transmission.
    c. viability.
    d. virulence.

45. The fourth component that turns the fire triangle into a fire tetrahedron is a
    a. chain of ignition.
    b. chemical reaction.
    c. combustible item.
    d. temperature boost.

46. This equipment is required when collecting a specimen from a patient in airborne isolation.
    a. Eye protection
    b. Full face shield
    c. Mask and goggles
    d. N95 respirator

47. The majority of exposures to HIV in healthcare settings are the result of
    a. accidental needlesticks.
    b. splashes during surgery.
    c. tainted blood transfusions.
    d. touching AIDS patients.

48. The most common type of HAI in the United States is
    a. bedsore infection.
    b. hepatitis B infection.
    c. respiratory infection.
    d. urinary tract infection.

49. These are the initials of the organization that instituted and enforces the Bloodborne Pathogens Standard.
    a. CAP
    b. CDC
    c. NIOSH
    d. OSHA

50. The only unsafe laboratory practice in the following list would be to
    a. keep your lab coat on at all times.
    b. never eat or apply makeup in the lab.
    c. secure long hair away from the face.
    d. wear closed-toe shoes when in the lab.

51. You accidentally splash a bleach solution in your eyes while preparing it for cleaning purposes. What is the first thing to do?
    a. Dry your eyes quickly with a clean paper towel or tissue.

    b. Flush your eyes with water for a minimum of 15 minutes.
    c. Proceed to the emergency room as quickly as possible.
    d. Put 10 to 20 drops of saline in your eyes immediately.

52. What is the best way to clean up blood that has dripped on the arm of a phlebotomy chair?
    a. Absorb it with a gauze pad and clean the area with disinfectant.
    b. Rub it with a damp cloth and wash the area with soap and water.
    c. Wait for it to dry and then scrape it into a biohazard container.
    d. Wipe it with an alcohol pad using an outward circular motion.

53. An example of employee screening for infection control is requiring employees to have
    a. hepatitis B vaccinations.
    b. measles vaccinations.
    c. PPD (or TB) testing.
    d. tetanus booster shots.

54. Which mode of infection transmission occurs from touching contaminated bed linens?
    a. Direct contact
    b. Droplet contact
    c. Indirect contact
    d. Vehicle contact

55. Which of the following diseases or microbes can be transmitted through blood transfusion?
    a. Bubonic plague
    b. Diabetes mellitus
    c. *Clostridium difficile*
    d. *Treponema pallidum*

56. Which of the following is required by the Bloodborne Pathogens (BBP) Standard?
    a. Isolation of patients known to be HIV-positive.
    b. Gowning before entering rooms of AIDS patients.
    c. Warning labels on specimens from AIDS patients.
    d. Wearing gloves when performing phlebotomy.

57. A laboratory or patient care activity that requires goggles to prevent exposure from sprays or splashes also requires this protective attire.
    a. Earplugs
    b. Gown
    c. Mask
    d. Respirator

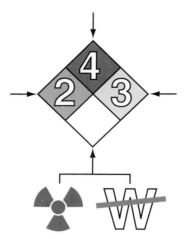

Figure 3-1 National Fire Protection Association 704 marking system.

58. Neutropenic isolation is a type of reverse isolation used for patients with
    a. a low WBC count.
    b. tuberculosis (TB).
    c. very severe burns.
    d. viral meningitis.

59. What should the phlebotomist do if the outside of a patient specimen tube has blood on it?
    a. Discard it and draw a new tube.
    b. Label it with a biohazard sticker.
    c. Put the specimen in a new tube.
    d. Wipe the tube with disinfectant.

60. What is the meaning of the symbol W in Figure 3-1?
    a. Water based
    b. Water neutral
    c. Water reactive
    d. Water soluble

61. Which of the following conditions seldom leads to work restrictions for a hospital employee?
    a. A positive PPD test
    b. Acute conjunctivitis
    c. German measles
    d. Mononucleosis

62. How many classes of fire are identified by the National Fire Protection Association (NFPA)?
    a. Two
    b. Three
    c. Four
    d. Five

63. Which of the following is considered one of the most important means of preventing healthcare-associated infections?
    a. Current immunization
    b. Glove use if indicated
    c. Isolation procedures
    d. Proper hand hygiene

64. The purpose of "reverse" isolation is to
    a. prevent airborne transmission of infectious microbes.
    b. protect susceptible patients from outside contamination.
    c. provide the safest environment for psychiatric patients.
    d. separate contagious patients from contact with others.

65. Which of the following could result in exposure to a blood-borne pathogen by a "percutaneous" exposure route?
    a. Drawing blood without using a needle safety device.
    b. Handling specimens with ungloved, chapped hands.
    c. Licking your fingers while turning lab manual pages.
    d. Rubbing your eyes while processing blood specimens.

66. In which instance could an electrical shock to a patient most likely occur?
    a. Collecting a blood specimen during a bad electrical storm.
    b. Performing phlebotomy while the patient is on the phone.
    c. Standing on a wet floor while drawing a blood specimen.
    d. Touching some electrical equipment during a blood draw.

67. The "Right to Know" law primarily deals with
    a. electrical safety issues.
    b. exposure to pathogens.
    c. hazard communication.
    d. labeling of specimens.

68. The *best* course of action to take before entering an isolation room is
    a. ask the patient's nurse what to do.
    b. do whatever you did the last time.
    c. follow the posted precautions.
    d. put on gloves and a respirator.

69. Which one of the following diseases involves a blood-borne pathogen?
    a. Diphtheria
    b. Influenza
    c. Malaria
    d. Rubella

70. The degree to which a microorganism is capable of causing disease is the definition of
    a. resistance.
    b. susceptibility.
    c. viability.
    d. virulence.

71. A material or substance harmful to health is the definition of a
    a. biohazard.
    b. contaminant.
    c. pathogen.
    d. toxic agent.

72. What is the proper order for putting on protective clothing?
    a. Gloves first, then gown, mask last
    b. Gown first, then gloves, mask last
    c. Gown first, then mask, gloves last
    d. Mask first, then gown, gloves last

73. The blue quadrant of the NFPA diamond-shaped symbol for hazardous materials (Fig. 3-1) indicates a
    a. fire hazard.
    b. health hazard.
    c. reactivity hazard.
    d. specific hazard.

74. These are the initials of the agency that developed a hazard labeling system that is a diamond-shaped sign containing a United Nations hazard class number and a symbol representing the hazard.
    a. CDC
    b. DOT
    c. NFPA
    d. OSHA

75. Which of the following actions violates a chemical safety rule?
    a. Adding the acid to the water when diluting an acid.
    b. Adding bleach to a cleaner to make it more effective.
    c. Making a 1:10 dilution of bleach to clean a counter.
    d. All of the above.

76. Federal law requires that hepatitis B vaccination be made available to employees assigned to duties with occupational exposure risk
    a. after any probationary period is over.
    b. immediately or as soon as possible.
    c. within 1 month of their employment.
    d. within 10 working days of assignment.

77. What is the *first* thing a phlebotomist should do if he or she is accidentally stuck by a needle used to draw blood from a patient?
    a. Check the patient's medical records for HIV test results.
    b. Clean the site with soap and water for at least 30 seconds.
    c. Go to employee health service and get a tetanus booster.
    d. Leave the area so the patient does not notice the injury.

78. One of the following symptoms of shock is wrong. Which one is it?
    a. An expressionless face
    b. Increased shallow breathing
    c. Pale, cold, clammy skin
    d. Slow, strong, pulse rate

79. The main principles involved in radiation exposure are
    a. exposure rate, dose, and shelter.
    b. distance, shielding, and time.
    c. source, amount, and duration.
    d. strength, location, and protection.

80. Which of the following is a role of the Joint Commission?
    a. Accreditation of healthcare facilities
    b. Development of BBP exposure plans
    c. Enforcement of safety requirements
    d. Prevention of work-related injuries

81. Which of the following would be considered a healthcare-associated infection?
    a. Catheter site of an ICU patient becomes infected
    b. Child breaks out with measles on admission day
    c. Healthcare worker comes down with hepatitis B
    d. Patient is admitted with *Hantavirus* infection

82. According to the CDC prevalence survey, how many hospital patients have at least one HAI on any given day?
    a. 1 out of 5
    b. 1 out of 10
    c. 1 out of 25
    d. 1 out of 50

83. The free availability of personal protective equipment (PPE) for employee use in the medical laboratory is mandated by the
    a. Clinical Laboratory Improvement Amendments.
    b. Guideline for Isolation Precautions in Hospitals.
    c. OSHA Bloodborne Pathogens (BBP) Standard.
    d. OSHA Hazard Communication (HazCom) Standard.

84. Current AHA recommendations for CPR by laypersons emphasize performing
    a. compressions only.
    b. eight pulse checks.
    c. fewer compressions.
    d. more rescue breaths.

85. The most frequently occurring laboratory-acquired infection is caused by
    a. HAV.
    b. HBV.
    c. HCV.
    d. HIV.

86. All of the following are required parts of an exposure control plan EXCEPT
    a. an exposure determination.
    b. communication of hazards.
    c. isolation procedure policies.
    d. methods of implementation.

87. Which class of fire occurs with combustible metals?
    a. Class A
    b. Class B
    c. Class C
    d. Class D

88. What precautions are to be used for a patient who has an enteric pathogen?
    a. Airborne
    b. Contact
    c. Droplet
    d. Standard

89. Which of the following is an example of possible "parenteral" means of transmission?
    a. Drinking water from a glass that is contaminated.
    b. Licking your fingers as you turn pages of a book.
    c. Not washing your hands before eating your lunch.
    d. Rubbing your eyes without washing hands first.

90. A person's general susceptibility to infection is unaffected by
    a. age.
    b. gender.
    c. health.
    d. immunity.

91. An example of vector infection transmission is contracting
    a. HBV from a contaminated countertop.
    b. HIV from a tainted blood transfusion.
    c. the plague from the bite of a rodent flea.
    d. tuberculosis after inhaling droplet nuclei.

92. A patient might be placed in protective isolation if he or she has
    a. chickenpox.
    b. hepatitis C.
    c. severe burns.
    d. tuberculosis.

93. What is the correct order for removing protective clothing?
    a. Gloves, mask, gown
    b. Gown, gloves, mask
    c. Gown, mask, gloves
    d. Mask, gown, gloves

94. The substance abbreviated as HBsAg when detected in a patient's serum confirms
    a. active hepatitis B infection.
    b. some hepatitis B immunity.
    c. susceptibility to hepatitis B.
    d. vaccination for hepatitis B.

95. A radiation hazard symbol (Fig. 3-2) on a patient's door signifies a patient who
    a. has been sent to the radiology department.
    b. has had x-rays taken in the past few days.
    c. is being treated with radioactive isotopes.
    d. is scheduled for a radiology procedure.

96. Which of the following is an example of a work practice control that reduces risk of exposure to blood-borne pathogens?
    a. Ordering self-sheathing needles
    b. Reading the exposure control plan
    c. Receiving an HBV vaccination
    d. Mandated use of PPE in the lab

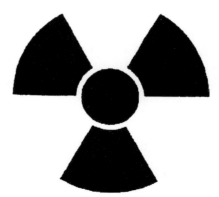

Figure 3-2 Radiation hazard symbol.

97. These are the initials of the organization that instituted Universal Precautions, the precursor to standard precautions.
    a. CAP
    b. CDC
    c. NIOSH
    d. OSHA

98. Healthcare workers are considered immune to a disease if they
    a. eat right, and get enough rest and exercise.
    b. have a normal number of white blood cells.
    c. have contracted the disease and recovered.
    d. received gamma globulin in the past year.

99. What is the best way to extinguish a flammable liquid fire?
    a. Douse it with large amounts of water.
    b. Smother it with a special fire blanket.
    c. Spray it with a Class A extinguisher.
    d. Spray it with a Class B extinguisher.

100. These are the initials of the federal agency that instituted and enforces regulations requiring the labeling of hazardous materials.
    a. CDC
    b. EPA
    c. NFPA
    d. OSHA

101. Which mode of infection transmission involves transfer of an infective microbe to the mucous membranes of a susceptible individual by means of a cough or sneeze?
    a. Contact
    b. Droplet
    c. Fomite
    d. Vehicle

102. All of the following are links (component) in the chain of infection EXCEPT
    a. exit pathway.
    b. reservoir.
    c. surveillance.
    d. susceptible host.

103. This is the abbreviation for the organization that is specifically charged with the investigation and control of disease.
    a. CDC
    b. HICPAC
    c. NIOSH
    d. OSHA

104. What is the first action to take to help a victim in shock?
    a. Call for assistance.
    b. Control any bleeding.
    c. Keep victim lying down.
    d. Maintain an open airway.

105. Which of the following would be an unhealthy way to deal with stress?
    a. Exercise regularly.
    b. Learn how to relax.
    c. Make a major life change.
    d. Take time to plan your day.

106. A nosocomial infection is one that is
    a. acquired while in a hospital.
    b. caught by a healthcare worker.
    c. highly contagious in nature.
    d. present without any symptoms.

107. This mode of transmission involves contaminated food, water, drugs, or blood transfusions.
    a. Airborne
    b. Contact
    c. Vector
    d. Vehicle

108. A phlebotomist who has been diagnosed with strep throat should be
    a. allowed to work if no symptoms are currently being exhibited.
    b. evaluated by an employee health nurse before resuming duties.
    c. off work until on an antibiotic for 24 hours and symptom-free.
    d. required to wear a mask when having any contact with patients.

109. The manufacturer must supply a safety data sheet for
    a. distilled water.
    b. laboratory coats.
    c. isopropyl alcohol.
    d. isotonic saline.

110. OSHA-required devices that remove BBP hazards from the workplace are called
    a. biohazard controls.
    b. engineering controls.
    c. pathogen controls.
    d. work practice controls.

111. Chemical manufacturers are required to supply safety data sheets for hazardous products by the
    a. Chemical Manufacturers Association Guideline.
    b. National Fire Protection Association Act.
    c. OSHA Hazard Communication Standard.
    d. United Nations Placard Recognition System.

112. What term is used to describe a type of infection that can be spread from person to person?
    a. Communicable
    b. Nonpathogenic
    c. Nosocomial
    d. Systemic

113. Which class of fire occurs with flammable liquids?
    a. Class B
    b. Class C
    c. Class D
    d. Class K

114. The first thing to do in the event of electrical shock to a coworker or patient is
    a. call for medical assistance.
    b. keep the victim warm.
    c. shut off electricity source.
    d. start CPR, if indicated.

115. The main purpose of PPE is to
    a. help project a professional appearance.
    b. prevent infection transmission to patients.
    c. protect street clothes from getting soiled.
    d. provide the user a barrier against infection.

116. The acronym used to remember the actions to take when using a fire extinguisher is
    a. ACT.
    b. HELP.
    c. PASS.
    d. RACE.

117. Which of the following is the *best* action to take if a coworker's clothing is on fire?
    a. Have the individual roll on the floor.
    b. Smother the fire with a fire blanket.
    c. Spray it with a Class A extinguisher.
    d. Tear off everything that is burning.

118. What type of hazard is identified by the symbol in Figure 3-3?
    a. Biohazard
    b. Electrical
    c. Explosive
    d. Radiation

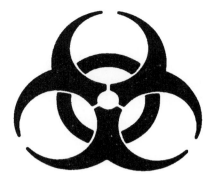

Figure 3-3

119. Which of the following bleach dilutions is recommended for cleaning specimen collection area surfaces?
    a. 1:1
    b. 1:2
    c. 1:10
    d. 1:25

120. Alcohol-based antiseptic hand cleaners can be used in place of hand washing if
    a. gloves were worn during the prior activity.
    b. hands are first cleaned with detergent wipes.
    c. hands were washed after the prior activity.
    d. no dirt or organic matter is seen on the hands.

121. Which of the following actions violate laboratory safety rules?
    a. Chewing on a pencil while processing specimens.
    b. Stashing your lunch in a lab specimen refrigerator.
    c. Wearing open-toed shoes while working in the lab.
    d. All of the above.

122. Approximately how many workplace injuries and illness are related to back injuries?
    a. 10%
    b. 20%
    c. 30%
    d. 40%

123. HBV in dried blood on work surfaces, equipment, telephones, and other objects can survive up to
    a. 24 hours.
    b. 3 days.
    c. 7 days.
    d. 2 months.

124. The most common chronic blood-borne illness in the United States is
   a. HAV.
   b. HBV.
   c. HCV.
   d. HDV.

125. Respirators used to enter rooms of patients with airborne diseases must be approved by this agency.
   a. CDC
   b. HICPAC
   c. NIOSH
   d. OSHA

126. Personal wellness means
   a. accepting chronic illnesses.
   b. being covered by insurance.
   c. eating like a vegan would.
   d. making exercise a priority.

127. Which of the following microbes is a gram-negative pathogen?
   a. *Acinetobacter baumannii*
   b. *Clostridium difficile*
   c. *Staphyloccus aureas*
   d. *all of the above*

128. CLSI guidelines say pants worn in the laboratory should be this much off of the floor.
   a. ½ to ¾ in.
   b. 1 to 1½ in.
   c. 1 to 2½ in.
   d. 2 to 2¼ in.

129. This microbe is unaffected by alcohol-based hand cleaners.
   a. *Bordetella pertussis*
   b. *Clostridium difficile*
   c. *Klebsiella pneumoniae*
   d. *Staphyloccus aureas*

130. The most accurate measurements of fitness consist of evaluating these three components.
   a. Body mass, agility, and willpower
   b. Diet, immune status, and resilience
   c. Limberness, fortitude, and intensity
   d. Strength, flexibility, and endurance

131. The Needlestick Safety and Prevention Act directed OSHA to revise the BBP Standard to include
   a. asking for community input on safety devices.
   b. changing the definition of work practice control.

   c. having exposure control plans updated monthly.
   d. the requirement to maintain a sharps injury log.

132. OSHA developed this standard to protect employees from exposure to hazardous chemicals.
   a. SDS
   b. HCS
   c. GHS
   d. EPA

133. Tests used to screen employees for TB include a
   a. blood TB test (QFT-G).
   b. chest x-ray if positive TST.
   c. tuberculin skin test (TST).
   d. all of the above.

134. A change needed to the HazCom Standard to align it with the Globally Harmonized System of Classification and Labeling of Chemicals (GHS) was
   a. decreasing known chemical hazards.
   b. eliminating paper safety data sheets.
   c. enacting new labeling requirements.
   d. renaming every hazardous chemical.

135. Which of the following helps healthcare facilities eliminate HAIs by tracking and identifying problem areas across the United States?
   a. HCS
   b. NHSN
   c. OSHA
   d. WHO

136. Good infection control practices include
   a. Scrubs pants that do not touch the HC facility's floor.
   b. Artificial nails if they are less than 0.5 cm long.
   c. Using only alcohol-based antiseptic hand cleaners.
   d. Taking precautions if infectious microbes are visible.

137. Which of the following situations would be considered an HAI?
   a. A bedridden nursing home resident catches a very bad cold.
   b. An employee periodically gets a cold sore on his upper lip.
   c. A patient acquires diarrhea from taking too much laxative.
   d. A visitor begins vomiting right after visiting her sick aunt.

138. Which of the following would be considered aseptic technique?
    a. Hanging a mask around the neck between uses.
    b. Keeping phlebotomy supplies within easy reach.
    c. Removing a respirator before exiting isolation.
    d. Letting blood spills dry before cleaning them up.

139. Back injuries can happen when
    a. heavy items are lifted improperly.
    b. patients are moved incorrectly.
    c. undue stress causes back spasms.
    d. all of the above.

140. One of the features of the new healthcare law is its focus on
    a. a holistic integrative food pyramid.
    b. increasing wellness businesses.
    c. providing free preventative services.
    d. eliminating all processed foods.

Answers and Explanations

1. **Answer: d**

    WHY: OSHA stands for the Occupational Safety and Health Administration. This agency enforces the Occupational Safety and Health ACT (also OSHA), a federal law that requires employers to ensure safe working conditions. The Centers for Disease Control and Prevention (CDC) is charged with the investigation and control of certain communicable diseases with epidemic potential. The Healthcare Infection Control Practices Advisory Committee (HICPAC) is a federal committee of experts who provide advice and guidance to the CDC and the Department of Health and Human Services (HHS) regarding infection control. The National Institute for Occupational Safety and Health (NIOSH), a federal agency that is part of the CDC, is responsible for conducting research and making recommendations for the prevention of work-related injury and illness.
    REVIEW: Yes ☐ No ☐

2. **Answer: a**

    WHY: Infection transmission requires the presence of six key components which form the links in what is commonly referred to as the chain of infection (Fig. 3-4). The components are an infectious agent, reservoir, exit pathway, means of transmission, entry pathway, and susceptible host.
    REVIEW: Yes ☐ No ☐

3. **Answer: a**

    WHY: A pathogen is a microbe that is capable of causing disease. The microbe that is responsible for an infection is referred to as the infectious or causative agent. In human infection transmission, a host is a susceptible individual or one that harbors an infectious agent. A vector is an insect, arthropod, or animal that harbors an infectious agent. A vehicle is food, water, or drugs that are contaminated with the infectious agent.
    REVIEW: Yes ☐ No ☐

4. **Answer: c**

    WHY: The term pathogenic means "causing or productive of disease." A microorganism that is capable of causing disease is said to be pathogenic. Communicable is an adjective used to describe infections that can spread from person to person. Virulence is the degree to which an organism is capable of causing disease. Systemic means pertaining to the entire body.
    REVIEW: Yes ☐ No ☐

5. **Answer: d**

    WHY: Permucosal means through or across mucous membranes, moist tissue layers that line areas of the body open to the environment such as eyes, nose, and mouth. Mucous membranes can be an entry pathway for infectious agents if aerosols or splashes land on them. Airborne exposure occurs if an infectious agent is inhaled. Nonintact skin exposure occurs through visible or invisible pre-existing breaks in the skin. Percutaneous exposure occurs when a sharp object penetrates previously intact skin.
    REVIEW: Yes ☐ No ☐

6. **Answer: b**

    WHY: Isolation procedures minimize the spread of infection by separating patients with highly transmissible infections from contact with other patients, and limiting their contact with hospital personnel and visitors. Simply being a carrier of a blood-borne pathogen or having been exposed to a contagious disease does not warrant isolation

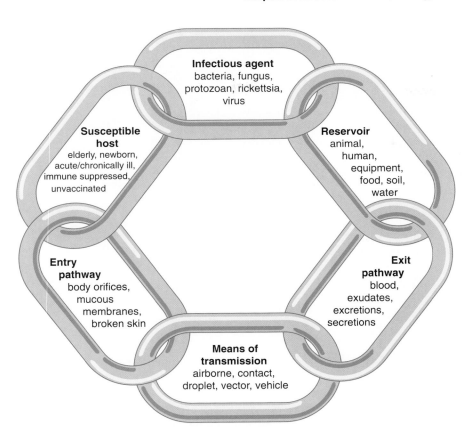

Figure 3-4 The chain of infection.

procedures. Standard precautions, which encompass blood and body fluid precautions, are used in the care of all patients.

REVIEW: Yes ☐　No ☐

7. **Answer: c**

WHY: Microbes (a short term for microorganisms) are tiny life forms that cannot be seen with the naked eye. They include bacteria, fungi, protozoa, and viruses. Ova (gametes or eggs) are reproductive cells, and although they may be microscopic they are not microorganisms.

REVIEW: Yes ☐　No ☐

8. **Answer: c**

WHY: Antibiotic treatment, chemotherapy drugs, and surgical procedures can all increase a patient's susceptibility to infection. Vaccination against a particular microbe decreases the likelihood of infection (i.e., makes them less susceptible to infection) with that microbe. Previous vaccination does not increase an individual's present susceptibility to other types of infection.

REVIEW: Yes ☐　No ☐

9. **Answer: b**

WHY: In health care, a susceptible host is someone with decreased ability to resist infection. A microbe responsible for an infection is called the causative or infectious agent. An exit or entry pathway is the way an infectious microbe is able respectively, to leave or to enter a host. A reservoir is a place where an infectious microbe can survive and multiply, and includes humans, animals, food, water, soil, contaminated articles, and equipment.

REVIEW: Yes ☐　No ☐

10. **Answer: a**

WHY: SDS stands for safety data sheet, a document that contains general, precautionary, and emergency information for a product with a hazardous warning on the label. The OSHA Hazard Communication (HazCom) Standard requires manufacturers to supply safety data sheets for their products. Employers are required to obtain the SDS for every hazardous chemical present in the workplace and have them readily accessible to employees.

REVIEW: Yes ☐　No ☐

11. **Answer: b**

WHY: Transmission-based precautions are used in addition to standard precautions only for patients who are known or suspected to be infected or colonized with highly transmissible or epidemiologically significant pathogens.

REVIEW: Yes ☐　No ☐

12. **Answer: b**

    WHY: According to transmission-based precautions, symptoms of infection with an enteric pathogen in an incontinent or diapered patient warrant contact precautions pending diagnosis. A child with a rash suggestive of rubeola requires airborne precautions. A cough, fever, and pulmonary infiltrate in an HIV patient are suggestive of TB infection and require airborne precautions. A cough indicative of *Bordetella pertussis* requires droplet precautions.

    REVIEW: Yes ☐ No ☐

13. **Answer: d**

    WHY: Transmission of an infective agent through contaminated food, water, or drugs is called vehicle transmission. Contact transmission involves direct transmission of an infectious microbe to a susceptible host through close or intimate contact such as kissing, or indirect transmission of the microbe by personal contact with a contaminated inanimate object. Droplet transmission involves the transfer of the microbe to the mucous membranes of a susceptible host by activities such as sneezing, coughing, or talking by an infected person. Vector transmission typically involves the transfer of the microbe by an insect, arthropod, or animal.

    REVIEW: Yes ☐ No ☐

14. **Answer: c**

    WHY: An avulsion is the forceful tearing away or amputation of a body part.

    REVIEW: Yes ☐ No ☐

15. **Answer: c**

    WHY: A patient with mycoplasma pneumonia requires droplet precautions, one of three types of transmission-based precautions used for patients known or suspected to be colonized or infected with certain highly transmissible pathogens. Droplet precautions protect against microbes transmitted in droplets generated when a person talks, coughs, or sneezes, and during certain procedures such as suctioning. The other two transmission-based precautions are airborne and contact. Airborne precautions protect against microbes transmitted in droplet nuclei, which are the residue of evaporated droplets. Contact precautions protect against microbes transmitted by contact with a patient, or contaminated items and surfaces. Transmission-based precautions are used in addition to the standard precautions, which are used in the care of all patients.

    REVIEW: Yes ☐ No ☐

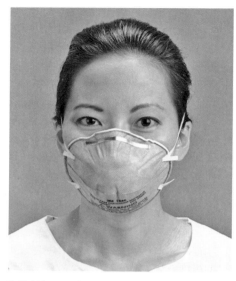

Figure 3-5 N95 respirator.

16. **Answer: a**

    WHY: Under transmission-based precautions, airborne isolation is required in addition to standard precautions for a patient who has pulmonary tuberculosis (TB). With airborne precautions, anyone entering the patient's room is required to wear an N95 respirator (Fig. 3-5).

    REVIEW: Yes ☐ No ☐

17. **Answer: b**

    WHY: The code word or acronym *RACE* was established by the National Fire Protection Association (NFPA) as a way to remember the order of action steps in the event of a fire. The "R" stands for *rescue* individuals in danger (Step 1). The "A" stands for sound the *alarm* (Step 2). The "C" stands for *confine* the fire by closing doors and windows (Step 3). The "E" stands for *extinguish* the fire with the nearest fire extinguisher (Step 4).

    REVIEW: Yes ☐ No ☐

18. **Answer: d**

    WHY: According to the BBP standard employees are entitled to a confidential medical evaluation. Exposures must be documented whether or not transmission of an infectious agent occurs. OSHA requires the facility to keep a log of exposure incidents, but they do not have to be reported independently to the CDC or OSHA. It is not mandatory for the source patient to submit to HIV or HBV testing. The source patient will be asked to submit to testing, and it is hoped that he or she will do so.

    REVIEW: Yes ☐ No ☐

19. **Answer: c**

    WHY: The process of infection requires the chain of infection (Fig. 3-4) to be complete. Stopping or interrupting the process by such things as wearing gloves, immunization of susceptible individuals, or instituting isolation procedures, breaks the chain and prevents infection.

    REVIEW: Yes ☐ No ☐

20. **Answer: d**

    WHY: The concept that the blood and certain body fluids of all patients potentially contain blood-borne pathogens originated with the introduction of universal precautions (UP) by the CDC. This concept changed the focus of infection control from prevention of patient-to-patient transmission to prevention of patient-to-personnel transmission. Category-specific and disease-specific precautions focused on patient-to-patient transmission. BSI focused on patient-to-personnel transmission, but came after UP.

    REVIEW: Yes ☐ No ☐

21. **Answer: d**

    WHY: Systemic means "pertaining to a whole body rather than one of its parts." A systemic infection infects the entire body. A communicable infection is one that is spread from person to person. A local infection is restricted to a small area of the body. A nosocomial infection is a hospital-acquired infection.

    REVIEW: Yes ☐ No ☐

22. **Answer: a**

    WHY: Because newborns are more susceptible to infection than older children or adults, strict infection control techniques are required for those working with them. Typical nursery and neonatal ICU infection control techniques include decontaminating hands and putting on new gloves for each patient. Infants sometimes have to be awakened to collect specimens. Only the equipment needed is brought into the room, not the phlebotomy tray. Povidone-iodine (e.g., Betadine) should not be used to clean a skin puncture site as it interferes with some tests.

    REVIEW: Yes ☐ No ☐

23. **Answer: d**

    WHY: Exercise reduces stress by triggering the release of substances called endorphins, which create an exhilarating, yet peaceful state.

    REVIEW: Yes ☐ No ☐

24. **Answer: d**

    WHY: Human immunodeficiency virus (HIV) is the leading cause of AIDS. Hepatitis A virus (HAV), hepatitis B virus (HBV), and hepatitis C virus (HCV) cause hepatitis A, hepatitis B, and hepatitis C, respectively.

    REVIEW: Yes ☐ No ☐

25. **Answer: b**

    WHY: Immunity to a particular virus normally exists when a person's blood has antibodies directed against that virus. A person who has recovered from infection with a virus has antibodies directed against it and is considered immune. Such a person would no longer be infectious, or able to transmit the virus to others. A person who does not display symptoms of a virus such as hepatitis B, but whose blood contains the virus, is capable of transmitting it to others and is called a carrier. A person who is susceptible to a virus has no antibodies against it.

    REVIEW: Yes ☐ No ☐

26. **Answer: a**

    WHY: Control of external profuse bleeding (hemorrhage) is most effectively accomplished by applying direct firm pressure to the wound.

    REVIEW: Yes ☐ No ☐

27. **Answer: c**

    WHY: An infection control program is responsible for implementing procedures designed to break the chain of infection and prevent the spread of infection in the hospital.

    REVIEW: Yes ☐ No ☐

28. **Answer: b**

    WHY: Microorganisms (microbes) that are capable of causing disease are called pathogens. Communicable microorganisms are pathogens that can be spread from person to person. Only some pathogenic microbes live in the soil. Normal flora (microorganisms that live on the skin) do not cause disease under normal conditions.

    REVIEW: Yes ☐ No ☐

29. **Answer: b**

    WHY: The microbe that causes hepatitis B is a blood-borne pathogen. Diphtheria meningitis and pneumonia are not transmitted through the blood.

    REVIEW: Yes ☐ No ☐

30. **Answer: d**

    WHY: According to the CDC, proper hand washing procedure requires hands to be washed thoroughly for at least 20 seconds. Hands should be wet before applying soap to minimize drying, chapping, and cracking. One should stand back from the sink to prevent touching it, since it may be contaminated. A clean paper towel should be used to turn off the faucet after hand washing. Using the same paper towel to dry the hands and turn off the faucets can contaminate the faucet handles and the hands.

    REVIEW: Yes ☐   No ☐

31. **Answer: a**

    WHY: Pertussis (whooping cough) is a respiratory disease transmitted by droplets. Varicella (chickenpox) and rubeola are highly contagious and require airborne precautions. Varicella requires contact precautions in addition to airborne precautions. Scabies requires contact precautions.

    REVIEW: Yes ☐   No ☐

32. **Answer: b**

    WHY: Fires are classified by fuel source. Class C fires occur with electrical equipment. Class A fires involve ordinary combustible materials, Class B fires involve flammable liquids, and Class D fires involve combustible metals. Class K fires involve cooking oils, fat, or grease.

    REVIEW: Yes ☐   No ☐

33. **Answer: d**

    WHY: Standard precautions should be followed for all patients at all times with no exceptions. When standard precautions are followed it is not necessary to know if the patient has hepatitis B or is HIV-positive. Patients in normal isolation require transmission-based precautions in addition to standard precautions. Reverse isolation requires precautions to protect the patient in addition to standard precautions.

    REVIEW: Yes ☐   No ☐

34. **Answer: a**

    WHY: Hepatitis B vaccination for adults normally involves three separate injections: an initial dose, another dose 1 month later, and a final dose 6 months from the original dose.

    REVIEW: Yes ☐   No ☐

35. **Answer: a**

    WHY: Fomites are objects capable of adhering to infectious material and transmitting disease. Fomites can include telephones, computer terminals, and counter tops. Hosts, as related to healthcare infection control, are individuals who harbor infectious agents. A pathogen is a microbe that is capable of causing disease. A vector is an insect arthropod or animal involved in the transmission of an infective microbe.

    REVIEW: Yes ☐   No ☐

36. **Answer: c**

    WHY: The OSHA Hazardous Communication Standard (HCS), which is also called the HazCom Standard, is known as the "Right to Know" Law because it requires all chemicals to be evaluated for health hazards, all chemicals found to be hazardous to be labeled as such, and the information communicated to employees. Recent changes to the standard now also give employees the ability to understand the chemical hazards they may face.

    REVIEW: Yes ☐   No ☐

37. **Answer: c**

    WHY: Hepatitis means inflammation of the liver. (The word root "hepat" means *liver,* and the suffix "itis" means *inflammation.*) Hepatitis B virus (HBV) and the other hepatitis viruses target the liver, causing liver inflammation.

    REVIEW: Yes ☐   No ☐

38. **Answer: a**

    WHY: The CDC and HICPAC together developed and jointly issued the *Guideline for Isolation Precautions in Hospitals.* An update to the guideline identifies two tiers of precautions; standard precautions to be used in the care of all patients, and transmission-based precautions to be used in addition to standard precautions for patients with certain highly transmissible diseases.

    REVIEW: Yes ☐   No ☐

39. **Answer: b**

    WHY: The OSHA Bloodborne Pathogens (BBP) Standard requires glove use during phlebotomy procedures to protect the phlebotomist from blood-borne pathogen contamination. Gloves do not necessarily protect the patient; in fact they can be a source of contamination to the patient if the phlebotomist touches contaminated articles before touching the patient's arm. Gloves can also be a source of contamination to capillary puncture specimens. Rather than protecting the venipuncture site, gloves can contaminate it if the phlebotomist touches the site after it is cleaned.

    REVIEW: Yes ☐   No ☐

Fire tetrahedron

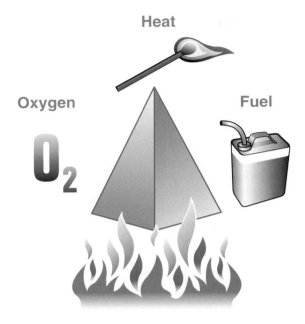

Figure 3-6 Fire tetrahedron.

40. **Answer: b**

    WHY: Four components must be present for fire to occur. Three of them are the traditional fire triangle components of fuel (material that will burn), heat (to raise the temperature of the material to a point where it will ignite), and oxygen (to maintain combustion). The fourth component is the chemical reaction that produces the fire. Addition of the fourth component to the original fire triangle created the fire tetrahedron (Fig. 3-6).
    REVIEW: Yes ☐   No ☐

41. **Answer: b**

    WHY: An exit pathway is the way an infectious agent is able to leave a reservoir host and be transmitted to a new susceptible individual, and should be blocked, not opened. Infectious agents can exit a reservoir host in secretions from the eyes, nose, or mouth; exudates from wounds; tissue specimens; blood from venipuncture and skin puncture sites; and excretions of feces, and urine. Blocking a pathogen exit pathway by protecting yourself from secretions, excretions, exudates, and other potentially infectious body substances can break the chain of infection. Implementing isolation procedures, practicing stress reduction, and washing hands and wearing gloves all help break the chain of infection.
    REVIEW: Yes ☐   No ☐

42. **Answer: a**

    WHY: Electrical equipment should be unplugged before servicing to avoid electrical shock. The use of extension cords should be avoided because they lead to circuit overload, incomplete connections, and potential clutter in the path of workers. Frayed electrical cords are dangerous and should be replaced rather than used, even if the frayed area has been taped. Malfunctioning equipment should be unplugged and not used until fixed.
    REVIEW: Yes ☐   No ☐

43. **Answer: c**

    WHY: Standard precautions apply to all body fluids, excretions, and secretions except sweat, whether or not they contain visible blood.
    REVIEW: Yes ☐   No ☐

44. **Answer: c**

    WHY: The ability of a microorganism to survive on contaminated articles and equipment has to do with its viability, which is the ability to survive, or live, grow, and develop.
    REVIEW: Yes ☐   No ☐

45. **Answer: b**

    WHY: Fuel, oxygen, and heat make up the fire triangle. The fourth component, the chemical reaction that produces fire, creates a fire tetrahedron (Fig. 3-6), the latest way of looking at the chemistry of fire.
    REVIEW: Yes ☐   No ☐

46. **Answer: d**

    WHY: Anyone entering the room of a patient with airborne precautions must wear an N95 respirator (Fig. 3-5), unless the precautions are for rubeola or varicella and the individual entering the room is immune.
    REVIEW: Yes ☐   No ☐

47. **Answer: a**

    WHY: Statistics compiled by the CDC have shown that accidental needlesticks are the leading cause of HIV exposures that have occurred so far among healthcare workers.
    REVIEW: Yes ☐   No ☐

48. **Answer: d**

    WHY: The most widely used HAI tracking system is provided by the CDC National Healthcare Safety Network (NHSN). Data provided by NHSN helps United States healthcare facilities eliminate HAIs by identifying problem areas and measuring progress of prevention efforts. The most common type

of HAI reported to the HSN is urinary tract infection (UTI), accounting for over 30% of all HAIs.
REVIEW: Yes ☐   No ☐

49. Answer: d

WHY: The BBP Standard was instituted by OSHA when it was determined that healthcare employees face a serious health risk as a result of occupational exposure to blood-borne pathogens. The standard is part of Federal law, and OSHA is responsible for its enforcement.
REVIEW: Yes ☐   No ☐

50. Answer: a

WHY: Laboratory safety procedures include securing long hair away from the face; never eating, drinking, or applying makeup in the laboratory; and wearing closed-toe shoes. A laboratory coat is considered personal protective equipment and as such may become contaminated. It should be worn during procedures that require it, but it should not be worn on break, to lunch, or when leaving the lab to go home.
REVIEW: Yes ☐   No ☐

51. Answer: b

WHY: The immediate thing to do in the event of a chemical splash to the eyes is to flush them with water for a minimum of 15 minutes at the nearest eyewash station (Fig. 3-7).
REVIEW: Yes ☐   No ☐

52. Answer: a

WHY: The best way to clean up small amounts of blood is to absorb them with a paper towel or gauze pad and then clean the area with a disinfectant, being careful not to spread the blood over a wider area than the original spill. Dried spills should be moistened with disinfectant to avoid scraping, which could disperse infectious organisms into the air. Do not wipe in an outward circular motion as it can spread the contamination. Alcohol is not a disinfectant, nor is soap and water.
REVIEW: Yes ☐   No ☐

53. Answer: c

WHY: Purified protein derivative (PPD) is the antigen used in a tuberculosis (TB) test. Both PPD and TB are abbreviations used for the test, which screens for exposure to tuberculosis. Hepatitis B vaccination, measles vaccinations, and tetanus booster shots are examples of employee immunizations that prevent the spread of infection.
REVIEW: Yes ☐   No ☐

54. Answer: c

WHY: The indirect contact mode of infection transmission occurs when a susceptible individual touches contaminated inanimate objects such as bed linens. Direct contact transmission involves direct, physical transfer of an infective microbe through close or intimate contact such as touching or kissing. Droplet transmission involves the transfer of an infective microbe to the mucous membranes of a susceptible individual through sneezing, coughing, or talking. Vehicle transmission involves contaminated food, water, drugs, or blood for transfusion.
REVIEW: Yes ☐   No ☐

55. Answer: d

WHY: *Treponema pallidum,* the organism that causes syphilis, is a blood-borne pathogen that can be transmitted through blood transfusion if present in the transfused blood. Bubonic plague is a vector-borne disease caused by *Yersinia pestis.* Diabetes mellitus is an endocrine disorder involving improper carbohydrate metabolism. *Clostridium difficile* is an enteric pathogen.
REVIEW: Yes ☐   No ☐

56. Answer: d

WHY: According to the OSHA Bloodborne Pathogens Standard, gloves are to be worn when performing vascular access procedures. This means that gloves are required for phlebotomy procedures. HIV-positive patients are not normally isolated unless they have AIDS and their immune systems are severely weakened, in which case

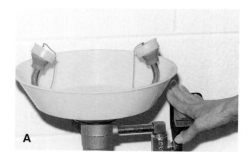 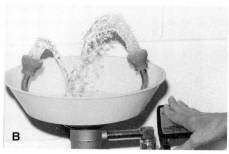

Figure 3-7 Eyewash station. **A:** Press the lever at the right side of the basin. **B:** The stream of water forces the caps from the nozzles. Lower your face and eyes into the stream and continue to wash the eye area until your eyes are clear. (Reprinted from Kronenberger J. *Comprehensive Medical Assisting.* 3rd ed. Baltimore, MD: Lippincott Williams & Wilkins; 2008.)

they may be placed in protective isolation. A gown may be required in certain situations but is not normally required when working with AIDS patients. It is against the law to label specimens from patients with blood-borne pathogens any differently than other specimens.

REVIEW: Yes ☐ No ☐

57. **Answer: c**

WHY: If a laboratory or patient care activity requires a healthcare worker to wear goggles to prevent exposure from sprays or splashes, a mask must also be worn to prevent mucous membrane exposure of the nose and mouth.

REVIEW: Yes ☐ No ☐

58. **Answer: a**

WHY: Reverse isolation is designed to protect patients who have compromised immune systems. Neutropenic is a term used to describe a condition in which there is an abnormally low number of white blood cells (neutrophils). A patient with a low white blood cell count has increased susceptibility to infection and may be placed in a type of protective or reverse isolation called neutropenic isolation. A person with severe burns may be put in reverse isolation because the burns make them susceptible to infection, but it is not called neutropenic isolation.

REVIEW: Yes ☐ No ☐

59. **Answer: d**

WHY: To prevent contamination of other workers who may handle it, a tube that has blood on it should be wiped with disinfectant.

REVIEW: Yes ☐ No ☐

60. **Answer: c**

WHY: Figure 3-1 represents the National Fire Protection Association (NFPA) 704 marking system used to identify areas where hazardous chemicals are present. The symbol ₩ means "water reactive" and identifies material that should not come in contact with water (Fig. 3-8).

REVIEW: Yes ☐ No ☐

61. **Answer: a**

WHY: A positive PPD test means that an individual has been exposed to TB and developed antibodies against it. It does not necessarily mean that the individual has TB. An employee with a positive PPD test would not have restrictions on working if the results of chest x-rays to detect signs of TB were negative. An employee with pink eye (acute conjunctivitis), German measles,

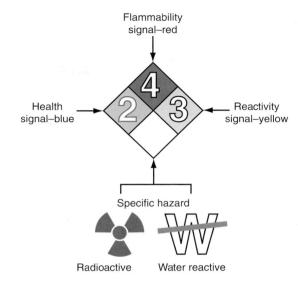

Figure 3-8 National Fire Protection Association 704 marking system.

or mononucleosis could spread the infection to others and would have work restrictions.

REVIEW: Yes ☐ No ☐

62. **Answer: d**

WHY: There are five classes of fire recognized by the NFPA. Fires are classified by fuel source. Class C fires occur with electrical equipment. Class A fires involve ordinary combustible materials. Class B fires involve flammable liquids. Class D fires involve combustible metals. Class K fires (the newest class) occur with cooking oils, grease, or fat.

REVIEW: Yes ☐ No ☐

63. **Answer: d**

WHY: Healthcare-associated infections can result from contact with infected personnel, other patients, visitors, or equipment. Studies have shown that the best way to prevent transmission of pathogenic microorganisms is proper hand hygiene, which includes the frequent use of antiseptic hand cleaners or hand washing, depending upon the degree of contamination. Following isolation procedures and being up-to-date on immunizations are important in preventing specific infections. Wearing gloves when required plays a role in infection control, but proper hand hygiene measures are still required after glove removal.

REVIEW: Yes ☐ No ☐

64. **Answer: b**

WHY: Also called "protective" isolation, reverse isolation is a special kind of isolation that is used for patients who are highly susceptible to infections. Examples of patients requiring protective isolation are patients with compromised immune systems such as neutropenic patients (those with abnormally low white blood cell counts), severely burned patients, and patients with compromised immune systems such as AIDS patients.

REVIEW: Yes ☐ No ☐

65. **Answer: a**

WHY: Percutaneous means "through the skin." Percutaneous exposure routes involve direct inoculation of infectious material through previously intact skin, such as occurs with accidental needlesticks and injuries from other sharp objects. Drawing blood without using a needle safety device increases the risk of an accidental needlestick. The exposure route involved when handling blood specimens with ungloved, badly chapped hands is nonintact skin contact. Licking your fingers before turning pages of a lab manual could lead to ingestion of infectious material. Rubbing your eyes during specimen processing activities could lead to mucous membrane contact with infectious material, or permucosal route of exposure.

REVIEW: Yes ☐ No ☐

66. **Answer: d**

WHY: Touching electrical equipment while drawing a patient's blood could conceivably cause a short to travel through the needle and shock the patient. Drawing a patient's blood when he or she is talking on the phone, during an electrical storm, or while you are standing on a wet floor will not cause electrical shock to the patient.

REVIEW: Yes ☐ No ☐

67. **Answer: c**

WHY: The OSHA HazCom Standard, which is called the "Right to Know Law," requires manufacturers of hazardous materials to provide an SDS for every hazardous product they make. An SDS contains general, precautionary, and emergency information about the product.

REVIEW: Yes ☐ No ☐

68. **Answer: c**

WHY: Because different types of isolation require the use of different types of personal protective equipment, the *best* thing to do before entering an isolation room is to follow the directions on the precaution sign on the door. Precautions needed are usually indicated on the sign, or you may be directed to check with the patient's nurse before entering the room. You must check the sign even if you have entered that room before, as precautions may have changed.

REVIEW: Yes ☐ No ☐

69. **Answer: c**

WHY: Blood-borne pathogen is a term applied to any infectious microorganism present in blood and other body fluids and tissues. It most commonly refers to HBV and HIV but also includes the organisms that cause syphilis, malaria, relapsing fever, and Creutzfeldt–Jakob disease. The microorganisms that cause diphtheria, influenza, and rubella are not found in the blood.

REVIEW: Yes ☐ No ☐

70. **Answer: d**

WHY: The virulence of a microorganism is the degree to which it is capable of causing disease. Resistance and susceptibility have to do with the immune system of the host and are affected by such things as age and health. Viability is the ability of the microorganism to survive on a source.

REVIEW: Yes ☐ No ☐

71. **Answer: a**

WHY: Biohazard is defined as any material or substance that is harmful to health. Federal regulations require any material that is a biohazard to be marked with a special biohazard symbol (Fig. 3-9).

REVIEW: Yes ☐ No ☐

72. **Answer: c**

WHY: When putting on protective clothing, the healthcare worker puts on the gown first, being careful to touch only the inside surface. The mask is put on next. Gloves are applied last and pulled over the cuffs of the gown.

REVIEW: Yes ☐ No ☐

73. **Answer: b**

WHY: In the NFPA hazardous materials rating system (Fig. 3-8), health hazards are indicated in the blue quadrant on the left. The upper red quadrant indicates fire hazards. Stability or reactivity

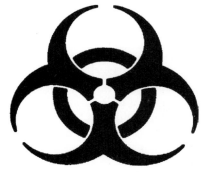

Figure 3-9 Biohazard symbol.

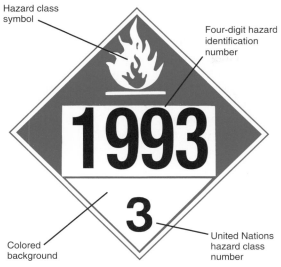

Hazard class symbol

Four-digit hazard identification number

Colored background

United Nations hazard class number

Figure 3-10 Example of DOT hazardous material label.

hazards are indicated in the yellow quadrant on the right, and other specific hazards are indicated in the white quadrant on the bottom.

REVIEW: Yes ☐ No ☐

74. **Answer: b**

WHY: The Department of Transportation (DOT) labeling system (Fig. 3-10) uses a diamond-shaped warning sign incorporating a United Nations hazard class number and symbol as well as a four-digit identification number. This symbol should not be confused with the NFPA diamond-shaped sign divided into four quadrants used to signify specific hazards.

REVIEW: Yes ☐ No ☐

75. **Answer: b**

WHY: Bleach or bleach solutions should never be mixed with other cleaners because doing so can release dangerous gases.

REVIEW: Yes ☐ No ☐

76. **Answer: d**

WHY: OSHA regulations require employers to offer HBV vaccination free of charge to employees within 10 days of their assignment to duties with risk of exposure.

REVIEW: Yes ☐ No ☐

77. **Answer: b**

WHY: If an accidental needlestick occurs, it is very important to decontaminate the site immediately. The exposure should then be reported to the supervisor and an incident report filled out. The phlebotomist should also report to the employee

health department for medical evaluation and possible treatment. Checking the patient's medical record cannot be done as it would violate HIPAA confidentiality regulations.

REVIEW: Yes ☐ No ☐

78. **Answer: d**

WHY: The symptoms of shock are an expressionless face and staring eyes; increased shallow breathing; pale, cold, clammy skin; and a rapid, weak pulse, not a slow, strong pulse.

REVIEW: Yes ☐ No ☐

79. **Answer: b**

WHY: Distance, shielding, and time are the principles involved in radiation exposure. This means that the amount of radiation you are exposed to depends on how far you are from the source of radioactivity, what protection you have from it, and how long you are exposed to it.

REVIEW: Yes ☐ No ☐

80. **Answer: a**

WHY: The Joint Commission (formerly JCAHO, the Joint commission on the accreditation of Healthcare Organizations) accredits healthcare facilities. Development of BBP exposure plans is a healthcare facility obligation. OSHA enforces safety requirements. NIOSH conducts research and makes recommendations for the prevention of work-related disease and injury.

REVIEW: Yes ☐ No ☐

81. **Answer: a**

WHY: A healthcare-associated infection (HAI) is an infection that is acquired by a patient after admission to a healthcare facility. Consequently, a catheter site that becomes infected while a patient is in the intensive care unit (ICU) is an HAI. Because the incubation period for measles is longer than 1 day, the patient with measles acquired the infection before being admitted to the hospital. Infection of a healthcare worker is an occupationally acquired infection, not an HAI. The patient admitted with *Hantavirus* obviously acquired the virus before admission.

REVIEW: Yes ☐ No ☐

82. **Answer: c**

WHY: An HAI prevalence survey of United States acute care hospitals conducted by the CDC in 2011, found that on any given day, about 1 in 25 patients has at least one HAI.

REVIEW: Yes ☐ No ☐

83. **Answer: c**

    WHY: Availability of PPE for use in the laboratory is mandated by the BBP Standard to minimize occupational exposure to HBV, HIV, and other blood-borne pathogens. The Clinical Laboratory Improvement Amendments of 1988 (CLIA '88) are concerned with laboratory testing. The CDC and HICPAC Guideline for Isolation Precautions in Hospitals describes what PPE to use for the different categories of precautions but has no authority to regulate availability of PPE. The OSHA HazCom Standard deals with communicating chemical hazards to employees.

    REVIEW: Yes ☐ No ☐

84. **Answer: a**

    WHY: Current American Heart Association (AHA) recommendations simplify CPR for lay rescuers by advocating Hands-Only™ (compressions only) CPR, and stressing the need for early chest compressions for victims of cardiac arrest.

    REVIEW: Yes ☐ No ☐

85. **Answer: b**

    WHY: According to OSHA, thousands of healthcare workers contract hepatitis B (HBV) every year and approximately 200 die as a result. This makes HBV the most frequently occurring laboratory-associated infection and a major infectious health hazard. Hepatitis A virus (HAV), hepatitis C Virus (HCV), and human immunodeficiency virus (HIV) are also hazards to healthcare workers but they do not occur as frequently as HBV.

    REVIEW: Yes ☐ No ☐

86. **Answer: c**

    WHY: To comply with OSHA standards, an exposure control plan must contain an exposure determination, communication of hazards, and methods of implementation. Isolation guidelines are not a required part of an exposure control plan.

    REVIEW: Yes ☐ No ☐

87. **Answer: d**

    WHY: Class D fires occur with combustible or reactive metals such as sodium, potassium, magnesium, and lithium. Class A fires occur with ordinary combustible materials. Class B fires occur with flammable liquids, and Class C fires occur with electrical equipment.

    REVIEW: Yes ☐ No ☐

88. **Answer: b**

    WHY: The word "enteric" is defined as pertaining to the small intestine. The route of exposure for enteric pathogens is ingestion. According to guidelines for transmission-based precautions, contact precautions should be followed in addition to standard precautions for patients with enteric pathogens.

    REVIEW: Yes ☐ No ☐

89. **Answer: d**

    WHY: The word "parenteral" means *other than the digestive tract*. Drinking water, ingesting contaminates by licking fingers, or failing to wash hands before eating food all involve the digestive tract and therefore are *not* parenteral. Rubbing your eyes without washing hands first does not involve the digestive tract and is therefore a possible parenteral means of transmission.

    REVIEW: Yes ☐ No ☐

90. **Answer: b**

    WHY: Gender does not play a role in a person's general susceptibility to infection. Age, health, and immune status do. Gender may, however, play a role in the site of infection because of differences in male and female anatomy.

    REVIEW: Yes ☐ No ☐

91. **Answer: c**

    WHY: Vector transmission involves transfer of the microbe by an insect, arthropod, or animal, for example, the bite of a rodent flea. HIV acquired from a blood transfusion is vehicle transmission. Contracting hepatitis B infection from a contaminated countertop is indirect contact transmission involving a fomite. Contracting tuberculosis from droplet nuclei is airborne transmission.

    REVIEW: Yes ☐ No ☐

92. **Answer: c**

    WHY: Protective or reverse isolation is used for patients who are highly susceptible to infections as in the case with a severely burned patient. Hepatitis C requires standard precautions. Chickenpox and tuberculosis require airborne precautions in addition to standard precautions.

    REVIEW: Yes ☐ No ☐

93. **Answer: a**

    WHY: Protective clothing is removed in the opposite order that it is put on. For phlebotomy procedures, the gloves are considered the most contaminated article and are removed first. They are removed by grasping one glove below the wrist and pulling it inside-out off the hand and holding it in the gloved hand. The second glove is removed by slipping several fingers under it at the wrist and pulling it inside-out over the first glove, which ends up inside of it. The mask is removed next, by touching only the strings. The gown is removed last by sliding one's arms out of the sleeves, holding the gown away from the body, and folding it with the outside (contaminated side) in.

REVIEW: Yes ☐ No ☐

94. **Answer: a**

WHY: Active HBV infection is indicated by the presence of hepatitis B surface antigen (HBsAg) in the patient's serum. HBV immunity and proof of successful vaccination are both indicated by a certain titer (level) of hepatitis B antibody (HBsAb) in the patient's serum. HBV susceptibility is indicated by the absence of hepatitis antibody or an insufficient level of antibody to confer immunity.

REVIEW: Yes ☐ No ☐

95. **Answer: c**

WHY: A radiation hazard sign on a patient's door means the patient has been injected with radioactive dyes or has radioactive implants. Although they are inside the patient, these radioactive isotopes can be hazardous to the fetus of a pregnant healthcare worker. In addition, a blood specimen collected at this time may be radioactive.

REVIEW: Yes ☐ No ☐

96. **Answer: d**

WHY: Work practice controls are routines that alter the manner in which a task is performed to reduce likelihood of exposure to blood-borne pathogens (BBPs). Wearing gloves to draw blood reduces the chance of exposure to BBPs. Ordering self-sheathing needles, reading the exposure control plan, and receiving an HBV vaccination are all important in reducing the risk of exposure to BBPs, but do not in themselves alter the actual performance of a task and are not considered work practice controls.

REVIEW: Yes ☐ No ☐

97. **Answer: b**

WHY: The CDC introduced the concept of Universal Precautions (UP) because it is not always possible to know if a patient is infected with a blood-borne pathogen. Under UP the blood and certain body fluids of all patients are considered potentially infectious.

REVIEW: Yes ☐ No ☐

98. **Answer: c**

WHY: Immunity to a particular disease is conferred by having had the disease and therefore developing antibodies against the disease-causing organism, or by vaccination against the particular organism. Eating right, getting enough rest, and exercising are all important to staying healthy and reducing susceptibility to disease, but will not make an individual immune to a disease. A normal white blood cell count is necessary to fight infection but it is not an indication of immunity. A shot of gamma globulin or immune globulin confers temporary immunity.

REVIEW: Yes ☐ No ☐

99. **Answer: d**

WHY: The Class B fire extinguisher was designed to put out flammable liquid fires. A flammable liquid or vapor fire requires blocking the source of oxygen or smothering the fuel to extinguish the fire. Class B extinguishers use dry chemicals to smother the fire.

REVIEW: Yes ☐ No ☐

100. **Answer: d**

WHY: OSHA instituted and enforces the Hazard Communication (HazCom) Standard (HCN). This federal law requires the labeling of hazardous materials. The HCS was recently revised to align it with the Globally Harmonized System of Classification and Labeling of Chemicals (GHS) that is being promoted for use worldwide.

REVIEW: Yes ☐ No ☐

101. **Answer: b**

WHY: Droplet contact transmission involves the transfer of infective microbes to the mucous membranes of the mouth, nose, or eyes of a susceptible individual by the sneezing, coughing, or talking by an infected person. The common cold is an example of infection that can be transmitted by droplets through coughing or sneezing.

REVIEW: Yes ☐ No ☐

102. **Answer: c**

WHY: An exit pathway, a reservoir where the organism can survive, and a susceptible host are all "links" in the chain of infection (Fig. 3-4). Surveillance is a means of monitoring and preventing infection or breaking the chain of infection.

REVIEW: Yes ☐ No ☐

103. **Answer: a**

WHY: The CDC is a division of the U.S. Public Health Service that is charged with the investigation and control of various diseases, especially those that are communicable and have epidemic potential.

REVIEW: Yes ☐ No ☐

104. **Answer: d**

WHY: An immediate and proper first aid response to shock is important and includes the following in order: maintain an open airway, call for assistance, keep the victim lying down with the head lower than the rest of the body, attempt to control bleeding or other cause of shock if known, and keep the victim warm until help arrives.

REVIEW: Yes ☐ No ☐

105. **Answer: c**

WHY: Healthy ways to deal with stress include exercising regularly, learning how to relax, and planning your day. Making a major life change can be a source of stress.

REVIEW: Yes ☐ No ☐

106. **Answer: a**

WHY: Nosocomial is a term applied to infections acquired after admission to a hospital. (A newer term that applies to infections acquired in any healthcare setting is healthcare-associated infection). An infection caught by a healthcare worker would be an occupationally acquired infection, but it could become a source of nosocomial infection in patients. A nosocomial infection can be, but is not normally, a communicable infection. Nosocomial infections are not normally without symptoms.

REVIEW: Yes ☐ No ☐

107. **Answer: d**

WHY: Vehicle transmission involves the transmission of an infective microbe through contaminated food, water, drugs, or blood products. Shigella infection from contaminated water and hepatitis infection from blood products are examples of vehicle transmission. Airborne infection involves droplet nuclei. Contact transmission involves close or intimate contact with an infectious patient or articles contaminated by the patient. Vector transmission involves the transfer of an infectious microbe by an insect, arthropod, or animal.

REVIEW: Yes ☐ No ☐

108. **Answer: c**

WHY: A phlebotomist diagnosed with strep throat is not allowed to work until he or she has taken antibiotics for a minimum of 24 hours and is not exhibiting symptoms. Once allowed to return to work, a mask is not necessary and neither is an evaluation by infection control personnel.

REVIEW: Yes ☐ No ☐

109. **Answer: c**

WHY: Any product that has a hazardous warning on the label must have an SDS supplied by the manufacturer. Isopropyl alcohol has a hazardous warning on the label and requires an SDS. Laboratory coats, saline, and most medications do not have hazard warnings and do not require an SDS.

REVIEW: Yes ☐ No ☐

110. **Answer: b**

WHY: The Bloodborne Pathogens Standard requires the use of engineering controls to reduce the risk of blood-borne pathogen (BBP) exposure. OSHA defines engineering controls as items or devices that isolate or remove a BBP hazard from the workplace. Examples of engineering controls include sharps containers and self-sheathing needles.

REVIEW: Yes ☐ No ☐

111. **Answer: c**

WHY: The OSHA HazCom Standard (HCS) requires chemical manufacturers to supply an SDS for any product with a hazardous warning on the label. In addition to the identity of a chemical, the label of a hazardous chemical must include a precautionary statement and a GHS hazard statement, signal word, and pictogram for each hazard class and category. A signal word specifies the severity of the hazard faced. A pictogram is an easily recognized and universally accepted symbol that alerts users to the type of chemical hazard they may face.

REVIEW: Yes ☐ No ☐

112. **Answer: a**

WHY: An infection or disease that can spread from person to person is called a communicable infection. A nonpathogenic microorganism is not capable of causing disease or infection. A nosocomial infection is a hospital-acquired infection. Systemic is a term used to describe an infection that infects the entire body.

REVIEW: Yes ☐ No ☐

113. **Answer: a**

WHY: Class B fires occur with flammable liquids and vapors such as paint, oil, grease, or gasoline. Class C fires occur with electrical equipment, Class D fires occur with combustible or reactive metals, and Class K fires occur with cooking oils, grease, or fat.

REVIEW: Yes ☐ No ☐

114. **Answer: c**

     WHY: The first thing to do when someone is the victim of electrical shock is shut off the source of electricity. (A typical first reaction is to try to remove the person from the source of the electricity, but that can result in shock to the rescuer if the source of electricity is still there). Other actions to take after the source of electricity is shut off are to call for medical assistance, start CPR if indicated, and keep the victim warm.

     REVIEW: Yes ☐   No ☐

115. **Answer: d**

     WHY: Personal protective equipment (PPE) includes all items worn to provide a barrier against infection and other hazards in situations where exposure to hazardous agents is likely. PPE includes gloves, gowns, lab coats, aprons, face shields, masks, and resuscitation mouthpieces that minimize the risk of BBP infection. OSHA requires PPE in situations where there is potential exposure to blood-borne pathogens.

     REVIEW: Yes ☐   No ☐

116. **Answer: c**

     WHY: The acronym PASS provides an easy way to remember the actions to take when using a fire extinguisher. The "P" stands for "Pull the Pin"; the "A" stands for "Aim Nozzle"; the first "S" stands for "Squeeze the Trigger"; and the second "S" stands for "Sweep Nozzle."

     REVIEW: Yes ☐   No ☐

117. **Answer: b**

     WHY: The best way to extinguish a fire in a coworker's clothing is to smother the fire by wrapping him or her in a fire blanket (Fig. 3-11). Although it could be an option if no fire blanket

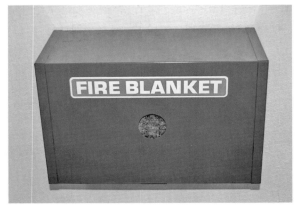

Figure 3-11 Fire blanket storage box.

were available, rolling on the floor is not the best option because it could spread the fire. Spraying the person with a fire extinguisher could injure him or her. Trying to take off a coworker's burning clothes could spread the fire to you or surrounding areas, and could even result in your actions being misinterpreted as assault or harassment.

     REVIEW: Yes ☐   No ☐

118. **Answer: a**

     WHY: The symbol in Figure 3-3 is a biohazard symbol (Fig. 3-9), which identifies something that is hazardous to health.

     REVIEW: Yes ☐   No ☐

119. **Answer: c**

     WHY: OSHA requires surfaces in specimen collection and processing areas to be decontaminated at the end of each shift and whenever surfaces are visibly contaminated by cleaning them with a 1:10 bleach solution or other EPA-approved disinfectant. Bleach solutions should be prepared daily.

     REVIEW: Yes ☐   No ☐

120. **Answer: d**

     WHY: CDC and HICPAC infection control recommendations allow the use of alcohol-based antiseptic hand cleaners such as foams, gels, and lotions in place of hand washing if there is no visible dirt or organic material such as blood or other body substances on the hands. Hands must be cleaned even if gloves are worn because gloves can have defects that allow contaminants to leak through them. Cleaning with detergent-containing wipes followed by the use of an alcohol-based cleaner is recommended if hands are heavily contaminated and hand washing facilities are not available. Hand washing after a prior activity has no bearing on how hands should be decontaminated for a current activity.

     REVIEW: Yes ☐   No ☐

121. **Answer: d**

     WHY: Chewing on pencils or pens, and putting your lunch in a reagent or specimen refrigerator risk exposure to toxic or infectious substances. Open-toed shoes leave the wearer vulnerable to spills of hazardous or infectious substances, or sharps injury from broken glass and other sharp objects.

     REVIEW: Yes ☐   No ☐

122. **Answer: b**

     WHY: It has been estimated that approximately 20% of all workplace injuries and illnesses involve back injuries. Healthcare workers are at risk of back injuries from work they are required to do (such as lift and move patients) and the stressful environment often associated with health care.

REVIEW: Yes ☐ No ☐

123. **Answer: c**

WHY: Studies have shown that hepatitis B virus (HBV) can survive up to a week in dried blood on work surfaces, equipment, telephones, and other objects.

REVIEW: Yes ☐ No ☐

124. **Answer: c**

WHY: According to the CDC, hepatitis C (HCV infection), has become the most widespread chronic blood-borne illness in the United States. Infection primarily occurs after large or multiple exposures. HCV symptoms are similar to HBV infection, although only 25% to 30% of infections even display symptoms. No vaccine is currently available, although research and development of a vaccine is underway.

REVIEW: Yes ☐ No ☐

125. **Answer: c**

WHY: NIOSH conducts research and makes recommendations for the prevention of work-related injury and illness. CDC and HICPAC transmission-based precautions recommend the wearing of properly fitting, NIOSH-approved N95 respirators when entering rooms of patients with airborne infections. Manufacturers apply to NIOSH for certificates of approval for their respirators. NIOSH-approved respirators are marked with the manufacturer's name, the part number (PN), the protection provided by the filter (e.g., N95), and "NIOSH."

REVIEW: Yes ☐ No ☐

126. **Answer: d**

WHY: Personal wellness is not just about what you eat, it requires a holistic approach, one that meets the physical, emotional, social, spiritual, and economic needs. Studies show that being physically fit increases the chance of staying healthy and living longer. Today our most serious health threats are chronic illnesses such as heart disease or cancer—diseases that we have the power to prevent. By taking aim on prevention and creating a well-balanced life through knowledge, self-awareness, and self-care, personal wellness is something that is achievable.

REVIEW: Yes ☐ No ☐

127. **Answer: a**

WHY: *Acinetobacter baumannii* is a gram-negative bacterium. Gram-negative bacteria are so named because of the way they stain with a type of stain called the Gram stain. Both *Clostridium difficile* and *Staphyloccus aureas* are gram-positive bacteria.

REVIEW: Yes ☐ No ☐

128. **Answer: b**

WHY: Scrubs or other pants that touch the floor can easily pick up infectious material. According to CLSI laboratory safety guidelines, pants worn by laboratory personnel should be 1 to 1½ in off of the floor to prevent contamination.

REVIEW: Yes ☐ No ☐

129. **Answer: b**

WHY: *Clostridium difficile* is a bacterium that forms spores. The spores of some microbes such as *C. difficile* are not killed by alcohol-based hand cleaners.

REVIEW: Yes ☐ No ☐

130. **Answer: d**

WHY: Studies show that being physically fit increases the chance of staying healthy and living longer. The most accurate measurements of fitness consist of evaluating three components—strength (the ability to carry, lift, push, or pull a heavy load), flexibility (the ability to bend, stretch, and twist), and endurance (the ability to maintain effort for an extended period of time).

REVIEW: Yes ☐ No ☐

131. **Answer: d**

WHY: The Needlestick Safety and Prevention Act directed OSHA to revise the BBP Standard to include the requirement to keep a sharps injury log. It required updating of the exposure control plan, but not monthly. It modified the definition of engineering controls, not work practice controls. It also required solicitation of employee input in selecting safety devices, but not community input.

REVIEW: Yes ☐ No ☐

132. **Answer: b**

WHY: The OSHA Hazard Communication Standard (HCS) was developed and put into force to protect employees from hazardous chemicals in the workplace. Safety Data Sheets (SDSs) are a requirement of the HCS. Elements of The Globally Harmonized System of Classification and Labeling of Chemicals (GHS) used worldwide have been incorporated in the updated HCS. EPA stands for the Environmental Protection Agency, a government agency that implements and enforces environmental laws.

REVIEW: Yes ☐ No ☐

133. **Answer: d**

    WHY: Tests used to screen for tuberculosis (TB) include a relatively new blood test called the QuantiFERON®-TB Gold (QFT-G), the traditional tuberculin skin test (TST), and a chest x-ray when a TST is positive.

    REVIEW: Yes ☐ No ☐

134. **Answer: c**

    WHY: One of the changes made to the HCS to align it with GHS was to enact new labeling requirements. In addition to the identity of a chemical, the label of a hazardous chemical must now include a precautionary statement and a GHS hazard statement, signal word to identify the severity of the hazard, and a universally recognized symbol called a pictogram for each hazard class and category. It did not decrease the number of known hazards, or rename chemicals. Safety data sheets can be in paper, or electronic form, or both.

    REVIEW: Yes ☐ No ☐

135. **Answer: b**

    WHY: The most widely used HAI tracking system is provided by the CDC National Healthcare Safety Network (NHSN). Data provided by NHSN helps United States healthcare facilities eliminate HAIs by identifying problem areas and measuring progress of prevention efforts.

    REVIEW: Yes ☐ No ☐

136. **Answer: a**

    WHY: Scrubs or other pants that touch the floor can easily pick up infectious material. According to CLSI laboratory safety guidelines, pants worn by laboratory personnel should be 1 to 1½ in off of the floor to prevent contamination. Studies have shown that artificial nails harbor more pathogenic microbes than natural nails. The World Health Organization (WHO) consensus recommendations in the 2009 Guidelines on Hand Hygiene in Health Care are that HCWS do not wear artificial fingernails or extenders when having direct contact with patients and *natural* nails should be kept short (0.5 cm long or approximately ¼ in long). If hands become visibly soiled or feel as if something is on them they should be washed with soap and water. Hand washing is also required when a patient is known to have a *C. difficile* infection because the spores of this bacterium are not killed by alcohol-based hand cleaners. Microbes are not visible to the naked eye.

    REVIEW: Yes ☐ No ☐

137. **Answer: a**

    WHY: A healthcare-associated infection (HAI) is an infection that is acquired after admission to a healthcare facility. The bedridden nursing home resident undoubtedly caught the cold while in the facility. A healthcare employee infection is not considered an HAI. Diarrhea from too much laxative is not an infection and thus not an HAI. A visitor infection is not considered an HAI but if the vomiting is due to an infection it could become a source of an HAI to patients in the facility.

    REVIEW: Yes ☐ No ☐

138. **Answer: b**

    WHY: Keeping supplies within reach is aseptic technique because it keeps them from dropping on the floor and becoming contaminated. Masks should be for one use only, if hung around the neck for reuse they can become reservoirs for bacteria and viruses. A respirator should be removed after exiting an isolation room and closing the door. Blood spills should be cleaned up right away.

    REVIEW: Yes ☐ No ☐

139. **Answer: d**

    WHY: A healthy back is necessary to lead an active and healthy life. The spine is designed to withstand everyday movement, including the demands of exercise. Improper lifting (Fig. 3-12) and poor posture habits, however, can reveal weaknesses. Healthcare workers are at risk for back injury because of activities they are required to do (i.e., lift and move patients) and because of the stressful environment often associated with health care today. Stress can make a person vulnerable to back problems because of muscle spasms.

    REVIEW: Yes ☐ No ☐

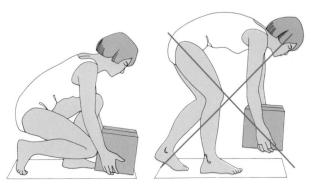

Figure 3-12 Lifting techniques. Left, correct technique; Right, incorrect technique.

140. **Answer: c**

     WHY: Today our most serious health threats are chronic illnesses such as heart disease or cancer—diseases that we have the power to prevent. The good news is that prevention has become a greater focus now than ever before. As the country moves into reforming health care by controlling costs, streamlining services, and pursuing consolidation, the uniting of primary prevention and primary/ambulatory care is inevitable. Insurance plans must now provide free preventive services to all members as part of Health Care Reform.

     REVIEW: Yes ☐   No ☐

Chapter 4

Medical Terminology

Study Tips

- Review the tables of word parts, abbreviations, and symbols in Chapter 4 of the textbook.

- Match the word elements with their meanings in Chapter 4 of the accompanying workbook.

- Make flashcards with their meanings and examples so you can drill yourself or have others drill you.

- Practice deciphering the meaning of medical terms from the text or a medical dictionary, and pronouncing terms in their singular and plural forms. (Remember: It is generally best to start with the suffix, go to the prefix next, and identify the meaning of the word root last).

- Hurriedly write the abbreviations and symbols on the "Do Not Use List" to see why they can be misinterpreted.

Overview

Medical terminology is a special vocabulary of scientific and technical terms used in the healthcare professions to speak and write effectively and precisely. It is based on an understanding of three basic word elements (word roots, prefixes, and suffixes) that are often derived from Greek and Latin words. Most medical terms are formed from two or more of these elements. If the meanings of the word elements are known, the general meaning of most medical terms can be established (although the actual definition may differ slightly). This chapter covers the three basic word elements, related elements called combining vowels and combining forms, unique plural endings, and pronunciation guidelines for medical terms. Common abbreviations and symbols used in health care, including those found on the Joint Commission's Do Not Use Lists are also covered.

Review Questions

Choose the BEST answer.

1. A suffix is an element of a word that
   a. establishes its basic meaning.
   b. follows the root of the word.
   c. makes pronunciation easier.
   d. precedes the root of the word.

2. The meaning of a medical term is usually determined by identifying the
   a. combining form first, suffix next, and prefix last.
   b. prefix first, word root next, and suffix last.
   c. suffix first, prefix next, and word root last.
   d. word root first, suffix next, and prefix last.

3. What word is used to describe the breakdown of red blood cells?
   a. Erythema
   b. Erythrocytosis
   c. Hemostasis
   d. Hemolysis

4. The balanced or "steady state" of the body is called
   a. hematology.
   b. homeostasis.
   c. hemopoiesis.
   d. hemostasis.

5. The combining form *erythro* means
   a. cell.
   b. earthlike.
   c. oxygen.
   d. red.

6. The singular form of atria is
   a. atris.
   b. atrium.
   c. atrion.
   d. atrius.

7. The plural form of lumen is
   a. lumena.
   b. lumeni.
   c. lumina.
   d. lumini.

8. What word means "large cell"?
   a. Acromegaly
   b. Cystocele
   c. Macrocyte
   d. Myelocyte

9. What word means "controlling blood flow"?
   a. Hemolysis
   b. Hemostasis
   c. Homeostasis
   d. Venostasis

10. In which of the following pairs of letters is each letter pronounced separately?
    a. "ae" as in venae cavae
    b. "ch" as in chloride
    c. "pn" as in dyspnea
    d. "ps" in psychology

11. The "e" at the end is pronounced separately in
    a. centriole.
    b. clavicle.
    c. supine.
    d. syncope.

12. Which of the following is a suffix?
    a. an
    b. neo
    c. osis
    d. ren

13. In the term *bicuspid,* "bi-" is a
    a. combining form.
    b. prefix.
    c. suffix.
    d. word root.

14. The "c" has the sound of "s" in the term
    a. brachial.
    b. cirrhosis.
    c. glycolysis.
    d. pancreas.

15. Which of the following is the abbreviation for a type of cell?
    a. CMV
    b. ESR
    c. RBC
    d. TSH

16. *Myalgia* means
    a. bone condition.
    b. muscle pain.
    c. nerve sheath.
    d. small algae.

17. Which of the following word roots means "vessel"?
    a. Arteri
    b. Bronch
    c. Vas
    d. Ven

18. This prefix means "outside."
    a. anti
    b. exo
    c. dys
    d. mal

19. Which of the following word parts means "recording" or "writing"?
    a. gram
    b. meter
    c. rrhage
    d. tomy

20. A hematologist is a specialist in the branch of medicine that deals with
    a. blood disorders.
    b. eye problems.
    c. lung diseases.
    d. benign tumors.

21. According to the meanings of its word parts, *phlebotomy* means
    a. cutting a vein.
    b. drawing blood.
    c. piercing a vessel.
    d. suctioning of fluid.

22. What is the meaning of the word root in the term *hyperglycemia*?
    a. Condition
    b. Sugar
    c. Low
    d. Under

23. Which of the following terms means "pertaining to the skin"?
    a. Dermal
    b. Dermatitis
    c. Epidermis
    d. Scleroderma

24. Which of the following abbreviations is on the Joint Commission's Do Not Use List?
    a. diff
    b. IU
    c. mL
    d. QNS

25. Which of the following can be both a word root and a prefix?
    a. arthr
    b. chondr
    c. erythr
    d. gastr

26. The Greek word root *nephr* means kidney. What is the Latin word root for kidney?
    a. cyst
    b. kid
    c. nep
    d. ren

27. The prefix *inter* means
    a. between.
    b. entrance.
    c. inside.
    d. within.

28. Which of the following word parts are prefixes?
    a. al, lysis, pnea
    b. gastr, lip, onc
    c. ices, ina, nges
    d. iso, neo, tachy

29. Identify the combining form among the following word parts.
    a. iso
    b. hypo
    c. lipo
    d. neo

30. Which of the following abbreviations identifies a type of blood cell?
    a. diff
    b. Hct
    c. seg
    d. trig

31. The meanings of the suffix, prefix, and word root (in that order) of the medical term *anisocytosis* are
    a. condition, unequal, cell.
    b. deficiency, blue, skin.
    c. disorder, without, cold.
    d. pertaining to, many, bladder.

32. Which of the following word parts means "blood condition"?
    a. emia
    b. ism
    c. oma
    d. osis

33. Which of the following is the word part of *cardiomyopathy* that means "disease"?

    a. cardio
    b. diom
    c. myo
    d. pathy

34. Which of the following are abbreviations for lab tests?

    a. ABGs, ASO, LDL, TIBC
    b. CAD, CML, COPD, SLE
    c. CCU, OR, PEDs, RR
    d. PP, PRN, Sx, TPR

35. Which body organ is primarily affected in a person with pulmonary disease?

    a. Brain
    b. Kidney
    c. Lungs
    d. Stomach

36. *Hepatitis* means

    a. blood cell disorder.
    b. kidney infection.
    c. liver inflammation.
    d. muscle weakness.

37. The lab abbreviation PT stands for

    a. partial thromboplastin.
    b. patient temperature.
    c. prothrombin time.
    d. prenatal therapy.

38. The word root of the term *oncologist* means

    a. cancer.
    b. tumor.
    c. study of.
    d. without.

39. The word root of the medical term *thoracic* is

    a. acic.
    b. oraci.
    c. racic.
    d. thorac.

40. Which of the following word parts means "cold"?

    a. cry
    b. cyan
    c. hypo
    d. sub

41. A trailing zero is

    a. a zero that is to the right of a decimal point.
    b. indicated by digits before a decimal point.
    c. must not be used in reporting test results.
    d. used when precision is not necessary.

42. The word part *later-* means

    a. late.
    b. last.
    c. side.
    d. wide.

43. The word root *sphygm* means

    a. muscle.
    b. pulse.
    c. spit.
    d. tight.

44. *Squamous* is a medical term used to describe skin cells that are

    a. flat.
    b. oval.
    c. round.
    d. smooth.

45. *Cubit* is a word element that means

    a. cube.
    b. elbow.
    c. patch.
    d. size.

Answers and Explanations

1. **Answer: b**
   WHY: A suffix is a word ending. It follows a word root and either changes or adds to the meaning of the word root.
   REVIEW: Yes ☐　No ☐
   📖 *Can you match other word elements with their descriptions in WORKBOOK activity Matching 4-1?*

2. **Answer: c**
   WHY: Generally the best way to determine the meaning of a medical term is to start with the meaning of the suffix, then the prefix, and identify the meaning of the word root or roots last.
   REVIEW: Yes ☐　No ☐

3. **Answer: d**
   WHY: Hemolysis is the breakdown of red blood cells. The combining form *hemo* means blood. The suffix *-lysis* means "breakdown."
   REVIEW: Yes ☐　No ☐
   📖 *Practice word building skills with WORKBOOK activity Skills Drill 4-2.*

4. **Answer: b**
   WHY: *Homeostasis* is the term used to describe the state of equilibrium or "steady state" that the body strives to maintain. The word part *homeo* means "the same," and *stasis* means controlling, standing, or stopping.
   REVIEW: Yes ☐　No ☐

5. **Answer: d**
   WHY: The combining form *erythro* means "red," as in the word "erythrocyte," which means "red blood cell."
   REVIEW: Yes ☐　No ☐

6. **Answer: b**
   WHY: Atrium is the singular form for atria, the name for the upper chambers of the heart.
   REVIEW: Yes ☐　No ☐

7. **Answer: c**
   WHY: *Lumina* is the plural form of *lumen*, which means the internal space of a tubular structure such as a vein or a blood collection needle.
   REVIEW: Yes ☐　No ☐
   📖 *Unique plural endings and examples can be found in Table 4-4 in Chapter 4 of the TEXTBOOK.*

8. **Answer: c**
   WHY: The term *macrocyte* means "large cell," from *macro*, meaning "large," and *cyte*, which means "cell."
   REVIEW: Yes ☐　No ☐

9. **Answer: b**
   WHY: *Hemostasis* means the stoppage or control of bleeding and is another name for the coagulation process. The combining form *hemo* means "blood." The suffix *-stasis* means controlling, standing, or stopping.
   REVIEW: Yes ☐　No ☐

10. **Answer: c**
    WHY: When "pn" is in the middle of a word, it is pronounced as a "p" and an "n," as in dyspnea and apnea. Only the "e" of the "ae" at the end of vena cavae is pronounced. The "ch" in chloride is pronounced as a "k." The "p" in psychology is silent, only the "s" is pronounced.
    REVIEW: Yes ☐　No ☐
    📖 *Pronunciation guidelines can be found in Table 4-5 in Chapter 4 of the TEXTBOOK.*

11. **Answer: d**
    WHY: The "e" at the end of some words such as syncope and systole is pronounced separately. The "e" at the end of centriole, clavicle, and supine is silent.
    REVIEW: Yes ☐　No ☐

12. **Answer: c**
    WHY: The word part *-osis* is a suffix, as in the word *necrosis*, which means "the death of cells, tissues, or organs." The word part *an* is a prefix meaning "without" that is used before a word beginning with a vowel, as in anaerobic. The word part *neo* is also a prefix meaning new, as in neonatal. The word part *ren* is a word root meaning kidney, as in *renal*.
    REVIEW: Yes ☐　No ☐

13. **Answer: b**
    WHY: In the term *bicuspid, bi-* is a prefix that means "two." *Bicuspid* means having two cusps.
    REVIEW: Yes ☐　No ☐

14. **Answer: b**
    WHY: The letter "c" before an "e," "i," or "y" is pronounced like an "s," as in the term "cirrhosis." The

letter "c" before other vowels has the sound of a "k," as in brachial, glycolysis, and pancreas.

REVIEW: Yes ☐ No ☐

15. **Answer: c**

WHY: RBC is the abbreviation for "red blood cell." CMV is the abbreviation for cytomegalovirus. ESR is the abbreviation for erythrocyte sedimentation rate. TSH is the abbreviation for thyroid-stimulating hormone.

REVIEW: Yes ☐ No ☐

16. **Answer: b**

WHY: "Myalgia" means muscle pain. The word root *my* means "muscle." The suffix *algia* means pain.

REVIEW: Yes ☐ No ☐

17. **Answer: c**

WHY: The word root *vas* means vessel, as in *vascular,* which means "pertaining to or composed of blood vessels." The word root *arteri* means "artery," *bronch* means "bronchus," and *ven* means "vein."

REVIEW: Yes ☐ No ☐

📖 *See if you know the meanings of the word roots in WORKBOOK activity Matching 4-2.*

18. **Answer: b**

WHY: The prefix *exo-* means "outside," as in *exocrine,* a term used to describe a gland that secretes to the outside of the body through ducts. The prefix *anti-* means "against," *dys-* means "difficult," and *mal* means "poor."

REVIEW: Yes ☐ No ☐

19. **Answer: a**

WHY: The word part *gram* means recording or writing, as in the term *electrocardiogram,* which is a recording of the electrical activity of the heart. The word part *meter* means "an instrument that measures," *rrhage* means "bursting forth," and *tomy* means "cutting or incision."

REVIEW: Yes ☐ No ☐

20. **Answer: a**

WHY: The word *hematologist* means a specialist in the study of blood disorders. The word root *hemat* means "blood." The suffix *ologist* means "specialist in the study of."

REVIEW: Yes ☐ No ☐

21. **Answer: a**

WHY: The word *phleb* means "vein." The term *tomy* means "cutting" or "incision."

REVIEW: Yes ☐ No ☐

22. **Answer: b**

WHY: The word root of the term *hyperglycemia* is *glyc,* which means "sugar or glucose." *Hyperglycemia* means a condition of too much glucose (sugar) in the blood.

REVIEW: Yes ☐ No ☐

23. **Answer: a**

WHY: *Dermal* means "pertaining to the skin." The word root *derm* means "skin." The suffix *-al* means "pertaining to." Dermatitis is inflammation of the skin. Epidermis is the outer layer of the skin. Scleroderma is a skin disorder that causes abnormal thickening of the skin.

REVIEW: Yes ☐ No ☐

24. **Answer: b**

WHY: The abbreviation for international units (IU) is on the Joint Commission's Do Not Use List because it can be mistaken for IV, the abbreviation for "intravenous," or it can be mistaken for the number 10. The Joint Commission wants it to be written out as "international units" instead.

REVIEW: Yes ☐ No ☐

📖 *The Do Not Use List is shown in Figure 4-1 in the TEXTBOOK.*

25. **Answer: c**

WHY: Some word elements may be classified one way in one term and a different way in another. The word element *erythr,* which means "red," is classified as a word root in the term *erythema.* It functions as a prefix, however, in the word *erythrocyte,* which means "red blood cell." Either way, the meaning of the word part is basically the same.

REVIEW: Yes ☐ No ☐

26. **Answer: d**

WHY: The Latin word root for kidney is *ren,* as in *renal,* which means "pertaining to the kidney."

REVIEW: Yes ☐ No ☐

27. **Answer: a**

WHY: The prefix *inter-* means between, as in "interstitial fluid," which is fluid between the cells.

REVIEW: Yes ☐ No ☐

28. **Answer: d**

WHY: The word parts *iso-, neo-,* and *tachy-* are prefixes. The word parts *-al, -lysis,* and *-pnea* are suffixes; *gastr, lip,* and *onc* are word roots; and *ices, ina,* and *nges* are plural endings.

REVIEW: Yes ☐ No ☐

29. **Answer: c**

    WHY: A combining form is a word root combined with a vowel. The word part *lipo* is the word root *lip*, which means "fat," combined with the vowel "o." The word parts *iso-*, *hypo-*, and *neo-* are prefixes that end in "o."

    REVIEW: Yes ☐ No ☐

30. **Answer: c**

    WHY: The abbreviation "seg" stands for segmented neutrophil, a type of white blood cell. The abbreviation "diff" stands for differential, a test that determines the number and type of blood cells in a specimen. Hct is the abbreviation for hematocrit, a test that determines the percentage by volume of red blood cells in whole blood. Trig is the abbreviation for triglycerides, a type of fat, or lipid, in the blood.

    REVIEW: Yes ☐ No ☐

    📖 *Check out the list of abbreviations in Chapter 4 of the TEXTBOOK.*

31. **Answer: a**

    WHY: Anisocytosis is a condition in which the red blood cells are unequal in size. The suffix is *-osis*, which means "condition." The prefix is *aniso-*, which means "unequal." The word root is *cyte*, which means "cell."

    REVIEW: Yes ☐ No ☐

32. **Answer: a**

    WHY: The suffix *-emia* means "blood condition." It is more specific than the suffix *-ism*, which simply means "condition." The suffix *-osis* means "state of." The suffix *-oma* means tumor.

    REVIEW: Yes ☐ No ☐

33. **Answer: d**

    WHY: *Cardiomyopathy* means "disease of the myocardium (heart muscle)." *Cardio* is a combining form that means "heart," *myo* is a combining form that means "muscle," and *-pathy* is a suffix that means "disease." *Diom* is not a recognized word part.

    REVIEW: Yes ☐ No ☐

34. **Answer: a**

    WHY: Arterial blood gases (ABGs), antistreptolysin O (ASO), low-density lipoprotein (LDL), and total iron binding capacity (TIBC) are laboratory tests. CAD, CML, COPD, and SLE are abbreviations for diseases. CCU, OR, PEDs, and RT are abbreviations for hospital departments. PP, PRN, Sx, and TPR are abbreviations seen in physician's orders and notes.

    REVIEW: Yes ☐ No ☐

35. **Answer: c**

    WHY: Pulmonary disease affects the lungs. The word root *pulmon* means "lungs." The suffix *-ary* means "pertaining to."

    REVIEW: Yes ☐ No ☐

36. **Answer: c**

    WHY: *Hepatitis* means "liver inflammation." The word root *hepat* means "liver." The suffix *-itis* means "inflammation."

    REVIEW: Yes ☐ No ☐

37. **Answer: c**

    WHY: PT is a laboratory abbreviation for prothrombin time (or protime for short).

    REVIEW: Yes ☐ No ☐

38. **Answer: b**

    WHY: The word root of the medical term *oncologist* is *onc*, which means "tumor." An oncologist is a physician who is a specialist in the study of tumors, both malignant and benign.

    REVIEW: Yes ☐ No ☐

39. **Answer: d**

    WHY: *Thoracic* means "pertaining to the chest." The word root is *thorac*, which means "chest." The suffix *-ic* means "pertaining to."

    REVIEW: Yes ☐ No ☐

40. **Answer: a**

    WHY: The word part *cry* means cold. An example is *cryoglobulin*, an abnormal protein (globulin) that precipitates when cooled. The word part *cyan* means "blue." The word part *hypo* means "low" or "under." The word part *sub* means "below" or "under."

    REVIEW: Yes ☐ No ☐

41. **Answer: a**

    WHY: A trailing zero is a zero to the right of a decimal point. It is on the Joint Commission's "Do Not Use" list. However, it is allowed in reporting laboratory test results because the precision of a numeric value is often indicated by the digits after the decimal point, even if the trailing digit is a zero. For example, it would be acceptable to report a serum potassium level as 4.0 mEq/L, rather than 4 mEq/L.

    REVIEW: Yes ☐ No ☐

42. **Answer: c**

    WHY: *Later* is a word element that means "side" as in the directional term lateral which means toward the side of the body.

    REVIEW: Yes ☐ No ☐

43. **Answer: b**

    WHY: The word root *sphygm* originated from the Greek word *sphygmos* which means "pulse." An example of a term with *sphygm* as a word root is sphygmomanometer, a blood pressure cuff.

    REVIEW: Yes ☐ No ☐

44. **Answer: a**

    WHY: *Squamous* is derived from the Latin term *squama* which means "scale." It is a medical term used to describe skin cells that are thin and flat like a scale.

    REVIEW: Yes ☐ No ☐

45. **Answer: b**

    WHY: *Cubit* is a word element that is derived from the Latin word *cubitum* which means elbow. It is the word root of the medical term antecubital which means "in front of the elbow" and is used to describe the primary area where venipuncture is performed.

    REVIEW: Yes ☐ No ☐

Chapter 5

Human Anatomy and Physiology Review

Study Tips

- Make an outline or table that lists the functions, structures, disorders, and diagnostic tests associated with each body system described in Chapter 5 of the TEXTBOOK. Allow sufficient time to study each system.

- Complete and study the matching and labeling exercises in Chapter 5 of the WORKBOOK.

- Review the memory joggers and key points in the TEXTBOOK.

- Point out the various planes and directional terms on a friend or fellow student.

- Identify the word elements of medical terms in the chapter to help remember what they mean and how to spell them.

Overview

The human body consists of over 30 trillion cells, 206 bones, 700 muscles, approximately 5 L of blood, and around 25 miles of blood vessels. To fully appreciate the workings of this wonder, it is necessary to have a basic understanding of human anatomy (structural composition) and physiology (function). A fundamental knowledge of anatomy and physiology (A&P) is an asset to anyone working in a healthcare setting, and especially helps the phlebotomist understand the nature of the various disorders of the body, the rationale for the laboratory tests associated with them, and the importance of the role that laboratory tests play in monitoring body system functions and diagnosing disorders. This chapter covers general body organization and function, anatomic terminology, and the functions, structures, disorders, and diagnostic tests associated with nine body systems. Because of its special importance to phlebotomy, a tenth system (circulatory) is covered separately in Chapter 6.

Review Questions

Choose the BEST answer.

1. Human anatomy deals with
   a. chemical reactions within the body.
   b. functioning of all the body systems.
   c. homeostatic equilibrium processes.
   d. structural composition of the body.

2. A person who is standing erect with arms at the side and eyes and palms facing forward is said to be in the
   a. anatomic position.
   b. prone position.
   c. supine position.
   d. syncope position.

3. Pronation of the hand is the act of
   a. extending the hand out to the side.
   b. flexing the hand at the wrist.
   c. rotating the hand so that it is vertical.
   d. turning the hand palm down.

4. Which body plane divides the body into equal portions?
   a. Frontal
   b. Midsagittal
   c. Sagittal
   d. Transverse

5. When you are facing someone in normal anatomical position, at which body plane are you looking?
   a. Frontal
   b. Midsagittal
   c. Sagittal
   d. Transverse

6. Which body plane divides the body into upper and lower portions?
   a. Frontal
   b. Midsagittal
   c. Sagittal
   d. Transverse

7. Which of the following is a true statement?
   a. A man who is supine is lying on his stomach.
   b. The big toe is on the medial side of the foot.
   c. The hand is at the proximal end of the arm.
   d. The posterior curvature is a heelstick site.

8. Which of these statements is true?
   a. The abdominal cavity is inferior to the diaphragm.
   b. The elbow is on the ventral surface of the forearm.
   c. The head is described as being inferior to the neck.
   d. The little finger is on the medial surface of the hand.

9. The term "distal" means
   a. farthest from the point of attachment.
   b. higher or above, or toward the head.
   c. nearest the central portion of the body.
   d. to the back of the body or body part.

10. The plantar surface of the foot is the
    a. area of the arch.
    b. heel portion.
    c. sole or bottom.
    d. top of the foot.

11. An example of a dorsal body cavity is the
    a. abdominal cavity.
    b. pelvic cavity.
    c. spinal cavity.
    d. thoracic cavity.

12. The heart and lungs are located in this body cavity.
    a. Abdominal
    b. Cranial
    c. Spinal
    d. Thoracic

13. Which body cavities are separated by the diaphragm?
    a. Abdominal and thoracic
    b. Cranial and spinal
    c. Pelvic and abdominal
    d. Thoracic and cranial

14. Simple compounds are transformed by the body into complex substances in the process called
    a. anabolism.
    b. catabolism.
    c. digestion.
    d. homeostasis.

15. This term describes the balanced or "steady state" condition normally maintained by the body.
    a. Anabolism
    b. Catabolism
    c. Hemostasis
    d. Homeostasis

16. The result of all chemical and physical reactions in the body that are necessary to sustain life is called
    a. anabolism.
    b. cannibalism.
    c. catabolism.
    d. metabolism.

17. Human chromosomes are
    a. networks of tubules in the cytosol.
    b. rod-shaped bodies near the nucleus.
    c. strands of deoxyribonucleic acid.
    d. structures within the cytoplasm.

18. Which one of the following cellular structures plays a role in assembling proteins from amino acids?
    a. Lysosome
    b. Mitochondria
    c. Nucleus
    d. Ribosome

19. This cellular structure contains the chromosomes and is called the command center of the cell.
    a. Centriole
    b. Cytoplasm
    c. Nucleus
    d. Nucleolus

20. These are oval or rod-shaped organelles that play a role in energy production.
    a. Golgi apparatus
    b. Lysosomes
    c. Mitochondria
    d. Ribosomes

21. Which of the following is adipose tissue?
    a. Bone
    b. Cells
    c. Fat
    d. Skin

22. The skeletal system produces
    a. blood cells.
    b. calcium.
    c. lactic acid.
    d. vitamin D.

23. Which of the following is a disorder associated with the skeletal system?
    a. Atrophy
    b. Cholecystitis
    c. Multiple sclerosis
    d. Osteochondritis

24. Which of the following laboratory tests is associated with the skeletal system?
    a. Alkaline phosphatase
    b. Creatine kinase (CK)
    c. Cholinesterase
    d. Lactic dehydrogenase

25. Skeletal system structures include
    a. dendrites.
    b. papillae.
    c. phalanges.
    d. ureters.

26. Which of the following bones are categorized as short bones?
    a. Carpals
    b. Femurs
    c. Ribs
    d. Vertebrae

27. Which of the following is one way muscle type is determined?
    a. Enzymes released
    b. Heat production
    c. Layer thickness
    d. Nervous control

28. Which of the following is an abbreviation for a test that is associated with the muscular system?
    a. BUN
    b. CK
    c. CSF
    d. TSH

29. Wasting or decrease in size of a muscle because of inactivity is called
    a. atrophy.
    b. myalgia.
    c. rickets.
    d. uremia.

30. Which type of muscle is under voluntary nervous control?
    a. Cardiac
    b. Skeletal
    c. Smooth
    d. Visceral

31. Which of the following is a function of the muscular system?
    a. Absorption of nutrients
    b. Creation of blood cells
    c. Maintenance of posture
    d. Production of vitamin D

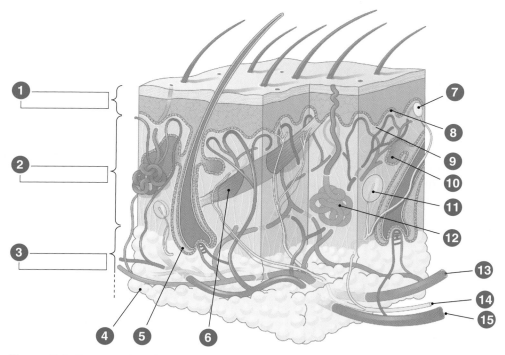

Figure 5-1 Cross-section of the skin. (Adapted with permission from Cohen BJ, Hull KL. *Study Guide for Memmler's the Human Body in Health and Disease*. 12th ed. Philadelphia, PA: Lippincott Williams & Wilkins; 2013:89.)

32. In numerical order, the skin layers or structures identified by numbers 1, 2, and 3 in Figure 5-1 are the
    a. corium, stratum basale, and epidermis.
    b. dermis, epidermis, and adipose tissue.
    c. epidermis, dermis, and subcutaneous.
    d. papillary dermis, dermis, and corneum.

33. The skin structures identified by numbers 6, 5, 12, and 10 in Figure 5-1 are the
    a. arrector pili muscle, hair follicle, sweat gland, and oil gland.
    b. nerve ending, sweat gland, hair follicle, and pressure receptor.
    c. papilla, sebaceous gland, sudoriferous gland, and pore opening.
    d. touch receptor, nerve ending, sweat gland, and dermal papilla.

34. Which of the following is a function of the skin?
    a. Hormone production
    b. Maintenance of posture
    c. Temperature regulation
    d. Vitamin C production

35. Which skin structures give rise to fingerprints?
    a. Arrector pili
    b. Hair follicles
    c. Oil glands
    d. Papillae

36. Blood vessels of the skin are found only in the
    a. corium and subcutaneous tissue.
    b. dermis and germinativum.
    c. epidermis and adipose layer.
    d. germinativum and corneum.

37. Which of the following tests is often associated with the integumentary system?
    a. Aldosterone
    b. Occult blood
    c. Fungal culture
    d. Serum gastrin

38. Mitosis takes place in this skin structure.
    a. Adipose tissue layer
    b. Papillary dermis
    c. Stratum germinativum
    d. Subcutaneous tissue

39. Which of the following is an integumentary system disorder?
    a. Diabetes
    b. Impetigo
    c. Meningitis
    d. Rhinitis

40. This skin layer is avascular.
    a. Corneum
    b. Dermis
    c. Epidermis
    d. Subcutaneous

41. The integumentary system produces
    a. melanin.
    b. melatonin.
    c. surfactant.
    d. trypsin.

42. Cells in this skin structure can be described as stratified and keratinized epithelial cells.
    a. Adipose tissue
    b. Dermis
    c. Epidermis
    d. Subcutaneous

43. The brain and spinal cord comprise the
    a. autonomic nervous system.
    b. central nervous system.
    c. peripheral nervous system.
    d. somatic nervous system.

44. Which of the following is a nervous system test?
    a. AFB culture
    b. CK isoenzymes
    c. C-reactive protein
    d. CSF analysis

45. In numerical order, the structures identified by numbers 1, 2, 3, and 4 in Figure 5-2 are
    a. axons, dendrites, cell body, and myelin sheath.
    b. dendrites, cell body, cell nucleus, and axon.
    c. myelin sheath, cell body, axon branch, and node.
    d. neurilemma, nodes, nucleus, and axon branches.

46. Which of the following is a nervous system disorder?
    a. Encephalitis
    b. Gigantism
    c. Myxedema
    d. Pediculosis

47. The spinal cavity is enclosed and protected by three layers of connective tissue called
    a. bursae.
    b. calcaneous.
    c. glomeruli.
    d. meninges.

48. Which of the following structures belong in the peripheral nervous system?
    a. Afferent nerves
    b. Brain
    c. Meninges
    d. Spinal cord

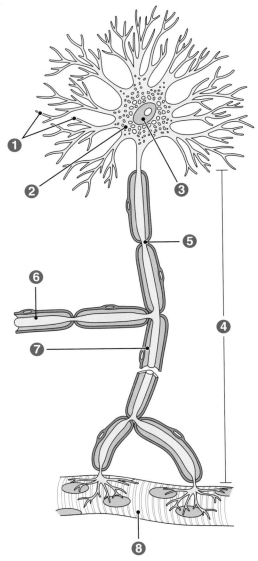

Figure 5-2 Diagram of a motor neuron. (Adapted with permission from Cohen BJ, Hull KL. *Study Guide for Memmler's the Human Body in Health and Disease.* 12th ed. Philadelphia, PA: Lippincott Williams & Wilkins; 2013:150.)

49. The fundamental units of the nervous system are the
    a. axons.
    b. meninges.
    c. nephrons.
    d. neurons.

50. This disorder involves destruction of the myelin sheath of nerves.
    a. Cushing syndrome
    b. Hydrocephalus
    c. Multiple sclerosis
    d. Parkinson disease

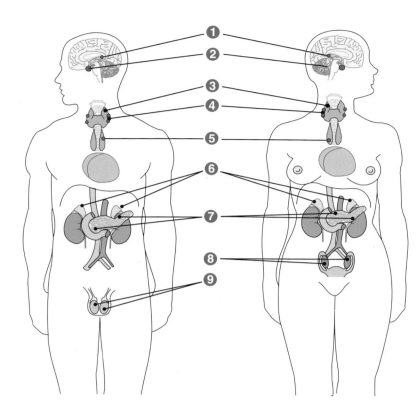

Figure 5-3 Endocrine system. (Adapted with permission from Cohen BJ, Hull KL. *Study Guide for Memmler's the Human Body in Health and Disease*. 12th ed. Philadelphia, PA: Lippincott Williams & Wilkins; 2013:203.)

51. Which of the following glands is an integumentary system structure?

    a. Adrenal
    b. Pituitary
    c. Sebaceous
    d. Thyroid

52. Erythropoietin is a hormone secreted by the

    a. adrenals.
    b. kidneys.
    c. ovaries.
    d. thyroid.

53. Excessive growth hormone in adulthood can cause

    a. acromegaly.
    b. emphysema.
    c. encephalitis.
    d. myxedema.

54. A disorder in which the pancreas is unable to produce insulin is

    a. diabetes insipidus.
    b. diabetes mellitus type I.
    c. diabetes mellitus type II.
    d. gestational diabetes.

55. Although they are not glands, these body structures secrete a hormone called B-type natriuretic peptide (BNP).

    a. Glomeruli
    b. Intestines

    c. Meninges
    d. Ventricles

56. In numerical order, the glands identified by numbers 2, 3, 5, and 6 in Figure 5-3 are the

    a. adrenals, pineal, thymus, and parathyroids.
    b. hypophysis, thyroid, thymus, and adrenals.
    c. pineal, adrenals, parathyroids, and thymus.
    d. pituitary, parathyroid, thymus, and pineal.

57. T_4 and TSH are abbreviations for tests that measure the function of the

    a. adrenals.
    b. ovaries.
    c. pancreas.
    d. thyroid.

58. This gland is called the "master gland" of the endocrine system.

    a. Pineal
    b. Pituitary
    c. Thymus
    d. Thyroid

59. Growth hormone (GH) levels test the function of the

    a. adrenals.
    b. ovaries.
    c. pancreas.
    d. pituitary.

60. Which of the following substances is secreted by the islets of Langerhans?
    a. Adrenaline
    b. Cortisol
    c. Estrogen
    d. Glucagon

61. Antidiuretic hormone (ADH) is also called
    a. aldosterone.
    b. epinephrine.
    c. noradrenaline.
    d. vasopressin.

62. This gland produces "fight-or-flight" hormones.
    a. Adrenal
    b. Pancreas
    c. Pituitary
    d. Thyroid

63. Calcitonin levels test the function of the
    a. adrenals.
    b. pituitary.
    c. thymus.
    d. thyroid.

64. Which gland is most active before birth and during childhood?
    a. Pineal
    b. Pituitary
    c. Thymus
    d. Thyroid

65. This gland is affected by light and helps create the diurnal rhythm of the sleep–wake cycle.
    a. Adrenal
    b. Pineal
    c. Thymus
    d. Thyroid

66. This hormone increases metabolism.
    a. Cortisol
    b. Glucagon
    c. Melatonin
    d. Thyroxine

67. Which of the following structures is part of the digestive system?
    a. Arrector pili
    b. Bronchiole
    c. Gallbladder
    d. Glomerulus

68. Which of the following is a test of a digestive system organ?
    a. Bilirubin
    b. Cortisol

c. Myoglobin
d. Uric acid

69. Hepatitis is a disorder that primarily affects the
    a. colon.
    b. kidneys.
    c. liver.
    d. spleen.

70. Bile is stored in the
    a. duodenum.
    b. epididymis.
    c. gallbladder.
    d. glomerulus.

71. Diagnostic tests of the digestive system include
    a. amylase and lipase.
    b. calcium and uric acid.
    c. cortisol and glucagon.
    d. Dilantin and serotonin.

72. Digestive system structures include the
    a. esophagus and salivary glands.
    b. neurilemma and axon branches.
    c. seminal ducts and vas deferens.
    d. stratum corneum and papillae.

73. Reproductive system functions include production of
    a. gametes.
    b. gastrin.
    c. melanin.
    d. sputum.

74. Which of the following is a structure of the male reproductive system?
    a. Alveolar sac
    b. Epididymis
    c. Fallopian tube
    d. Renal artery

75. Which of the following is an abbreviation for a test of the male but not the female reproductive system?
    a. ALP
    b. BMP
    c. PSA
    d. RPR

76. Which of the following are male gametes?
    a. Gonads
    b. Ovum
    c. Sperm
    d. Testes

77. Female gametes are produced in the
    a. cervix.
    b. fallopian tubes.
    c. ovaries.
    d. uterus.

78. Which of the following is an abbreviation for a female reproductive system test?
    a. CEA
    b. FSH
    c. GTT
    d. PSA

79. Which of the following is a structure of the female reproductive system?
    a. Oviduct
    b. Pharynx
    c. Sacrum
    d. Ureter

80. This disease is associated with the reproductive system.
    a. Cholecystitis
    b. Gonorrhea
    c. Myxedema
    d. Shingles

81. Which of the following is a urinary system test?
    a. Alkaline phosphatase
    b. Creatinine clearance
    c. Lactic dehydrogenase
    d. Rapid plasma reagin

82. Which of the following are urinary system structures?
    a. Axons, myelin sheath, prostate
    b. Centriole, nuclei, Golgi apparatus
    c. Glomeruli, nephrons, ureters
    d. Neurons, renal arteries, urethra

83. Which of the following is a function of the urinary system?
    a. Electrolyte balance
    b. Heat production
    c. Stimuli reception
    d. Removal of gases

84. Which of the following is normally a urinary system disorder?
    a. Cystitis
    b. Gastritis
    c. Neuritis
    d. Pruritus

85. This substance, secreted by the kidneys, plays a role in increasing blood pressure.
    a. Melanin
    b. Renin
    c. Sebum
    d. Uric acid

86. These tufts of capillaries are the filtering components of the urinary system.
    a. Fallopian tubes
    b. Glomeruli
    c. Nephrons
    d. Ureters

87. Which of the following is an abbreviation for a respiratory system test?
    a. ABG
    b. KOH
    c. TSH
    d. UA

88. During internal respiration
    a. carbon dioxide enters the tissue cells.
    b. carbon dioxide exits the bloodstream.
    c. oxygen enters the blood in the lungs.
    d. oxygen enters the cells in the tissues.

89. During normal respiratory function, bicarbonate ion acts as a buffer to keep blood pH within a steady range of
    a. 7.25 to 7.75.
    b. 7.35 to 7.45.
    c. 7.50 to 8.00.
    d. 8.00 to 8.10.

90. Acidosis can result from
    a. high carbon dioxide levels.
    b. increased blood pH levels.
    c. an increased rate of respiration.
    d. prolonged hyperventilation.

91. The ability of oxygen to combine with this substance in the red blood cells increases by up to 70 times the amount of oxygen that can be carried in the blood.
    a. Carbon dioxide
    b. Glucose
    c. Hemoglobin
    d. Potassium

92. A major cause of respiratory distress in infants and young children is
    a. airway blockage associated with emphysema.
    b. dyspnea as a consequence of cystic fibrosis.
    c. infection with *Mycobacterium tuberculosis*.
    d. infection with respiratory syncytial virus (RSV).

93. Which of the following are respiratory system structures?
    a. Bronchioles, epiglottis, pleura
    b. Calcaneus, mandible, phalanges
    c. Corium, corneum, adipose cells
    d. Neurons, meninges, myelin sheath

94. The exchange of O_2 and CO_2 in the lungs takes place in the
    a. alveoli.
    b. bronchi.
    c. larynx.
    d. trachea.

95. Decreased partial pressure of oxygen (PO_2) in the capillaries of the tissues causes
    a. carbon dioxide to diffuse into the tissues.
    b. carbon dioxide to be released from hemoglobin.
    c. oxygen to associate with hemoglobin.
    d. oxygen to disassociate from hemoglobin.

96. Infant respiratory distress syndrome (IRDS) in premature infants is most often caused by a lack of
    a. alveolar sacs.
    b. carbon dioxide.
    c. hemoglobin.
    d. surfactant.

97. This is the abbreviation for a respiratory system disorder caused by an acid-fast bacillus.
    a. COPD
    b. IRDS
    c. RSV
    d. TB

98. A person is having difficulty breathing. The term used to describe this condition is
    a. asthma.
    b. dyspnea.
    c. emphysema.
    d. pneumonia.

99. Which body system controls and coordinates the activities of all the other body systems?
    a. Muscular
    b. Nervous
    c. Respiratory
    d. Skeletal

100. Elimination of waste products is a function of this body system.
    a. Digestive
    b. Endocrine
    c. Nervous
    d. Skeletal

101. The medical term for elevated blood sugar is
    a. diabetes mellitus.
    b. diabetes insipidus.
    c. hyperglycemia.
    d. hyperinsulinism.

102. This body system is responsible for releasing hormones directly into the bloodstream.
    a. Circulatory
    b. Endocrine
    c. Integumentary
    d. Respiratory

103. Pancreatitis is a disorder of this system.
    a. Digestive
    b. Reproductive
    c. Respiratory
    d. Skeletal

104. Powerful chemical substances secreted directly into the bloodstream by certain glands are called
    a. electrolytes.
    b. hormones.
    c. lysosomes.
    d. surfactants.

105. Hematopoiesis is a function of this body system.
    a. Endocrine
    b. Muscular
    c. Skeletal
    d. Urinary

Answers and Explanations

1. **Answer: d**

   WHY: Human anatomy is defined as the branch of science that deals with the structural composition of the body. Human physiology deals with body function, including chemical reactions and homeostatic processes.

   REVIEW: Yes ☐   No ☐

   📖 *A quick review of human anatomy can be found in Chapter 5 in the TEXTBOOK.*

2. **Answer: a**

   WHY: Anatomic position is defined as standing erect, arms at the side, with eyes and palms facing forward. In describing the direction or the location of a given point on the body, medical personnel normally refer to the body as if the patient were in the anatomical position, regardless of actual body position. Prone is lying face down. Supine is lying face up. *Syncope* is a medical term for fainting.

   REVIEW: Yes ☐   No ☐

3. **Answer: d**

   WHY: *Pronation* is defined as the condition of being prone or the act of assuming a prone position. A hand that is prone is palm down. Consequently, pronation of the hand can be defined as the act of turning the hand palm down. Extending the hand out to the side of the body is called abduction. The act of flexing the hand at the wrist is called flexion of the wrist. The act of rotating the hand is called rotation.

   REVIEW: Yes ☐   No ☐

4. **Answer: b**

   WHY: A sagittal plane (Fig. 5-4) divides the body into right and left portions, but they are not necessarily equal. A midsagittal plane is a type of sagittal plane that divides the body into equal right and left portions. A frontal plane divides the body vertically into front and back portions. A transverse plane divides the body into upper and lower portions.

   REVIEW: Yes ☐   No ☐

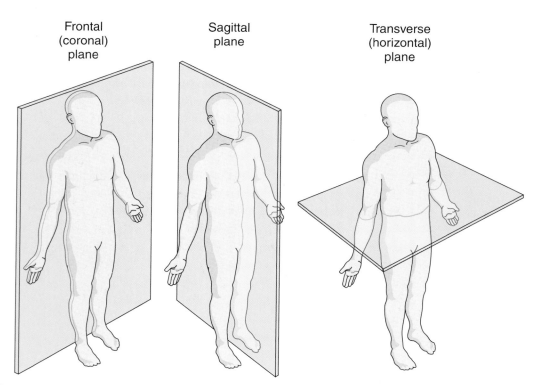

Frontal (coronal) plane   Sagittal plane   Transverse (horizontal) plane

Figure 5-4 Body planes. (Adapted with permission from Cohen BJ. *Memmler's the Human Body in Health and Disease.* 12th ed. Philadelphia, PA: Lippincott Williams & Wilkins; 2009:9.)

5. **Answer: a**

   WHY: The frontal plane (Fig. 5-4) divides the body vertically into front and back portions. When you are facing someone in normal anatomical position, he or she is also facing you, which means that you are seeing a frontal plane. A midsagittal plane divides a body into equal right and left portions. A sagittal plane divides the body into right and left portions that are not necessarily equal. A transverse plane divides the body into upper and lower portions.

   REVIEW: Yes ☐ No ☐

   📖 *Check out Labeling Exercise 5-1 in the WORKBOOK to remind yourself how the planes divide the body.*

6. **Answer: d**

   WHY: A transverse plane (Fig. 5-4) is defined as a plane that divides the body into upper and lower portions. A frontal plane divides the body vertically into front and back portions. A sagittal plane divides the body into right and left portions. A midsagittal plane divides the body into equal right and left portions.

   REVIEW: Yes ☐ No ☐

7. **Answer: b**

   WHY: Medial means "toward the midline of the body" (Fig. 5-5). The big toe is on the inner side of the foot, which is the side closest to the midline of the body. A man who is in a supine position is lying on his back. The hand is at the distal end of the arm. The posterior curvature of the heel is *not* a recommended site for heel puncture.

   REVIEW: Yes ☐ No ☐

8. **Answer: a**

   WHY: The diaphragm separates the thoracic cavity from the abdominal cavity. The meaning of *inferior* is "beneath or lower." The abdominal cavity is beneath the thoracic cavity and therefore beneath the diaphragm also. The elbow is on the back, or dorsal, surface of the arm. The head is above or superior to the neck. The little finger is on the lateral side of the hand.

   REVIEW: Yes ☐ No ☐

9. **Answer: a**

   WHY: *Distal* is defined as farthest from the center of the body, origin, or point of attachment. *Superior* means "higher or above." *Proximal* means "nearest to the center of the body." *Dorsal* refers to the back (Fig. 5-5).

   REVIEW: Yes ☐ No ☐

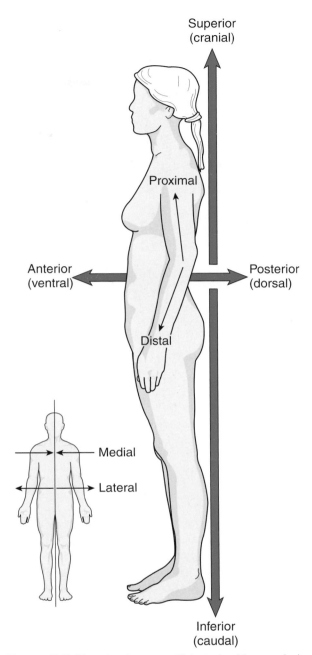

Figure 5-5 Directional terms. (Adapted with permission from Cohen BJ. *Memmler's the Human Body in Health and Disease.* 12th ed. Philadelphia, PA: Lippincott Williams & Wilkins; 2013:8.)

10. **Answer: c**

    WHY: *Plantar* means "concerning the sole or bottom of the foot."

    REVIEW: Yes ☐ No ☐

11. **Answer: c**

    WHY: *Dorsal* refers to the back (Fig. 5-5). Dorsal cavities (Fig. 5-6) are at the back of the body. The spinal and cranial cavities are dorsal cavities.

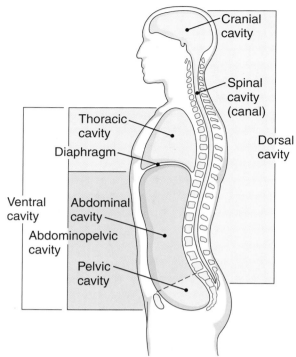

Figure 5-6 Body cavities, lateral view. (Adapted with permission from Cohen BJ. *Memmler's the Human Body in Health and Disease.* 12th ed. Philadelphia, PA: Lippincott Williams & Wilkins; 2013:12.)

The abdominal, pelvic, and thoracic cavities are ventral cavities.

REVIEW: Yes ☐   No ☐

12.   **Answer: d**

WHY: The heart and lungs are located in a cavity in the chest called the *thoracic* cavity (Fig. 5-6). The word *thoracic* comes from thorac, which means "chest," and -*ic*, which means "pertaining to."

REVIEW: Yes ☐   No ☐

13.   **Answer: a**

WHY: The diaphragm (Fig. 5-6) is the name of the muscular partition between the thoracic cavity and the abdominal cavity.

REVIEW: Yes ☐   No ☐

14.   **Answer: a**

WHY: Anabolism is the name for the constructive process in which simple compounds are transformed into complex substances. Catabolism is a destructive process by which complex substances are broken into simple ones. Digestion is the process by which food is broken into simple usable components. *Homeostasis* means "staying the same" and is the term used to describe the state of equilibrium or balance that the body strives to maintain.

REVIEW: Yes ☐   No ☐

15.   **Answer: d**

WHY: *Homeostasis* means "staying the same." The term is used to describe the state of equilibrium or balance, referred to as "steady state," that the body strives to maintain. Anabolism is the part of the metabolic process whereby the body converts simple compounds into complex substances. Catabolism is the process by which the body breaks complex substances into simple ones. *Hemostasis* refers to the stagnation or stopping of the flow of blood within the circulatory system.

REVIEW: Yes ☐   No ☐

16.   **Answer: d**

WHY: *Metabolism* is defined as the sum of all the chemical and physical reactions necessary to sustain life. Anabolism is the part of the metabolism process in which the body converts simple compounds into complex substances. Cannibalism is the eating of human flesh. Catabolism is the process by which the body breaks complex substances into simple ones.

REVIEW: Yes ☐   No ☐

17.   **Answer: c**

WHY: Chromosomes are the genetic material of the cell found in the nucleus. They are long strands of deoxyribonucleic acid (DNA) that are organized into units called genes. Humans normally have 23 identical pairs of chromosomes (46 individual ones). The endoplasmic reticulum is a network of tubules in the cytosol (fluid of the cytoplasm). The rod-shaped bodies near the nucleus are the centrioles. Structures within the cytoplasm are called organelles.

REVIEW: Yes ☐   No ☐

18.   **Answer: d**

WHY: Ribosomes (Fig. 5-7) are tiny organelles in the fluid portion of cells where amino acid assembly takes place. Lysosomes digest substances within the cell. The mitochondria play a role in energy production. The nucleus is the command center of the cell and contains the chromosomes.

REVIEW: Yes ☐   No ☐

19.   **Answer: c**

WHY: The chromosomes are found in the large, dark-staining organelle called the nucleus that is found near the center of the cell (Fig. 5-7). Because the nucleus contains the chromosomes, which govern all cellular activities, it is referred to as the command center of the cell.

REVIEW: Yes ☐   No ☐

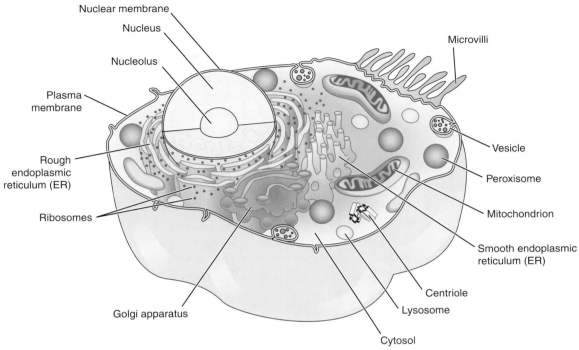

Nuclear membrane
Nucleus
Nucleolus
Plasma membrane
Rough endoplasmic reticulum (ER)
Ribosomes
Golgi apparatus
Cytosol
Lysosome
Centriole
Smooth endoplasmic reticulum (ER)
Mitochondrion
Peroxisome
Vesicle
Microvilli

Figure 5-7 Cell diagram. (Adapted with permission from Cohen BJ. *Memmler's the Human Body in Health and Disease*. 12th ed. Philadelphia, PA: Lippincott Williams & Wilkins; 2013:37.)

20. **Answer: c**

WHY: Organelles are specialized structures in the fluid portion of the cell (Fig. 5-7). Although mitochondria, Golgi apparatus, lysosomes, and ribosomes are all organelles, the mitochondria are oval or rod-shaped and are the site of energy production. The Golgi apparatus comprises layers of membranes that make, sort, and prepare protein compounds for transport. Lysosomes are small sacs of enzymes that digest substances within the cell. Ribosomes are tiny bodies that play a role in assembling proteins from amino acids.

REVIEW: Yes ☐ No ☐

21. **Answer: c**

WHY: *Adipose* means "fat or pertaining to fat." Adipose tissue consists mainly of fat cells. Adipose tissue, bone, and blood are types of connective tissue. Cells are the basic structural unit of all life. Skin is epithelial tissue.

REVIEW: Yes ☐ No ☐

22. **Answer: a**

WHY: Blood cells are produced in the bone marrow, which is part of the skeletal system (Fig. 5-8). The skeletal system does not produce calcium; it stores calcium. Lactic acid is produced in muscle and other tissues in the process of carbohydrate metabolism. Vitamin D is produced in the skin.

REVIEW: Yes ☐ No ☐

23. **Answer: d**

WHY: *Osteochondritis* means "inflammation of the bone and cartilage," structures that are part of the skeletal system (Fig. 5-8). Atrophy, a disorder of the muscular system, is muscle wasting. Cholecystitis is gallbladder inflammation. The gallbladder is an accessory organ of the digestive system. Multiple sclerosis is an inflammatory disease of the nervous system that causes degeneration of the myelin sheaths of the nerves.

REVIEW: Yes ☐ No ☐

📖 *Check out Matching Exercise 5-2 in the WORKBOOK to see if you can match other disorders with the appropriate body systems.*

24. **Answer: a**

WHY: Alkaline phosphatase is an enzyme that functions in the mineralization of bone. Creatine kinase and lactic dehydrogenase are muscular system tests. Cholinesterase is a nervous system test.

REVIEW: Yes ☐ No ☐

25. **Answer: c**

WHY: Phalanges are finger bones and part of the skeletal system (Fig. 5-8). Dendrites are nervous system structures. Papillae are integumentary system structures. Ureters are urinary system structures.

REVIEW: Yes ☐ No ☐

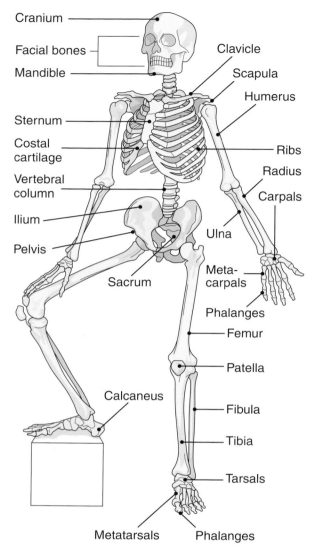

Cranium

Facial bones

Mandible

Clavicle

Scapula

Humerus

Sternum

Costal cartilage

Vertebral column

Ilium

Pelvis

Ribs

Radius

Carpals

Ulna

Sacrum

Meta-carpals

Phalanges

Femur

Patella

Calcaneus

Fibula

Tibia

Tarsals

Metatarsals   Phalanges

Figure 5-8 Human skeleton. (Adapted with permission from Cohen BJ. *Memmler's the Human Body in Health and Disease.* 12th ed. Philadelphia, PA: Lippincott Williams & Wilkins; 2013:128.)

26. **Answer: a**

WHY: Bones are categorized by shape. Carpals (wrist bones) are categorized as short bones. Femurs are categorized as long bones. Ribs are categorized as flat bones. Vertebrae are categorized as irregular bones (see Fig. 5-8).

REVIEW: Yes ☐ No ☐

27. **Answer: d**

WHY: Muscle type (Table 5-1) is determined according to where the muscle is located, its histological (microscopic) cellular characteristics, and whether nervous control of the muscle is voluntary or involuntary.

REVIEW: Yes ☐ No ☐

28. **Answer: b**

WHY: Creatine kinase (CK) is an enzyme present in skeletal and heart muscle. Blood urea nitrogen (BUN) is a urinary system test. CSF stands for cerebrospinal fluid. CSF analysis is a nervous system test. Thyroid-stimulating hormone (TSH) is an endocrine system test.

REVIEW: Yes ☐ No ☐

29. **Answer: a**

WHY: *Atrophy* means "muscle wasting." *Myalgia* means "muscle pain." Rickets is abnormal bone formation from lack of vitamin D. Uremia is impaired kidney function with a buildup of waste products in the blood.

REVIEW: Yes ☐ No ☐

30. **Answer: b**

WHY: Skeletal muscles are made to contract by conscious thought, which means that their nervous control is voluntary. Cardiac and visceral (smooth) muscles function automatically, which means that their nervous control is involuntary (see Table 5-1).

REVIEW: Yes ☐ No ☐

31. **Answer: c**

WHY: Muscular system functions include maintaining posture, producing heat, and enabling movement. Nutrient absorption is a function of the digestive system. Blood cells are produced in the skeletal system. Vitamin D is manufactured in the skin of the integumentary system.

REVIEW: Yes ☐ No ☐

32. **Answer: c**

WHY: There are two main layers of the skin (Fig. 5-9) and a subcutaneous (under the skin) layer. The epidermis is the outer layer of the skin. The dermis is the inner layer of the skin. The subcutaneous layer connects the skin to the surface of muscles.

REVIEW: Yes ☐ No ☐

📖 *Practice labeling skin and other body system structures in the WORKBOOK Labeling Exercises.*

33. **Answer: a**

WHY: The skin structures identified in Figure 5-1 are an arrector pili muscle (6), a hair follicle (5), a sudoriferous (sweat) gland (12), and a sebaceous (oil) gland (10) (see Fig. 5-9).

REVIEW: Yes ☐ No ☐

Table 5-1: Comparison of the Different Types of Muscle

	Smooth	**Cardiac**	**Skeletal**
Location	Wall of hollow organs, vessels, respiratory passageways	Wall of heart	Attached to bones
Cell characteristics	Tapered at each end, branching networks, nonstriated	Branching networks; special membranes (intercalated disks) between cells; single nucleus; lightly striated	Long and cylindrical; multinucleated heavily striated
	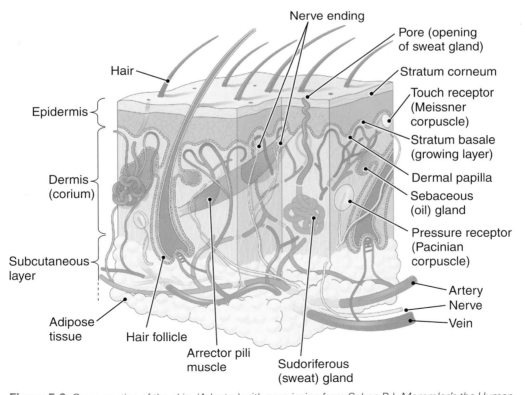		
Control	Involuntary	Involuntary	Voluntary
Action	Produces peristalsis; contracts and relaxes slowly; may sustain contraction	Pumps blood out of heart; self-excitatory but influenced by nervous system and hormones	Produces movement at joints; stimulated by nervous system; contracts and relaxes rapidly

Figure 5-9 Cross-section of the skin. (Adapted with permission from Cohen BJ. *Memmler's the Human Body in Health and Disease*. 12th ed. Philadelphia, PA: Lippincott Williams & Wilkins; 2013:108.)

34. **Answer: c**

    WHY: The skin plays a role in temperature regulation by helping give off excess heat and protecting the body against the cold. Hormones are produced by endocrine system glands and tissues with endocrine function. The muscular system gives the body the ability to maintain posture. The skin manufactures vitamin D, not vitamin C.

    REVIEW: Yes ☐ No ☐

35. **Answer: d**

    WHY: Elevations called papillae (Fig. 5-9), and resulting depressions in the dermis where it meets the epidermis, form the ridges, and grooves of fingerprints.

    REVIEW: Yes ☐ No ☐

36. **Answer: a**

    WHY: Blood vessels are found in the corium (dermis) and subcutaneous layers of the skin (Fig. 5-9). The epidermis is avascular, which means that it does not contain blood vessels. The stratum germinativum (syn., stratum basale) and stratum corneum are layers of the epidermis. Adipose (fat) cells are found in the subcutaneous layer.

    REVIEW: Yes ☐ No ☐

37. **Answer: c**

    WHY: Fungal cultures are often performed on skin scrapings. The skin is part of the integumentary system. Aldosterone is an endocrine system test. Occult blood (a test for hidden blood in feces) and serum gastrin are digestive system tests.

    REVIEW: Yes ☐ No ☐

38. **Answer: c**

    WHY: Mitosis occurs in the stratum germinativum (syn., stratum basale), the deepest layer of cells in the epidermis and its only layer of living cells.

    REVIEW: Yes ☐ No ☐

39. **Answer: b**

    WHY: Impetigo is an inflammatory condition of the skin most often caused by staphylococcal or streptococcal infection. It is characterized by isolated blisters that rupture and crust over. The skin is part of the integumentary system. Diabetes is an endocrine system disorder. Meningitis is a nervous system disorder. Rhinitis is a respiratory system disorder.

    REVIEW: Yes ☐ No ☐

40. **Answer: c**

    WHY: *Avascular* means "without blood vessels." The epidermis of the skin (Fig. 5-9) does not contain blood vessels. The blood vessels are in the dermis (corium) and subcutaneous layers of the skin.

    REVIEW: Yes ☐ No ☐

41. **Answer: a**

    WHY: Melanin is a skin pigment produced in the stratum germinativum (syn., stratum basale) of the epidermis (Fig. 5-9). Melatonin plays a role in promoting sleep and is secreted by the pineal gland of the endocrine system. Surfactant is a substance that coats the walls of the alveoli of the respiratory system. Trypsin is a digestive system enzyme.

    REVIEW: Yes ☐ No ☐

42. **Answer: c**

    WHY: The epidermis consists mainly of stratified (layered) epithelial cells. New cells form in the stratum germinativum (syn., stratum basale), its deepest layer. As the cells push to the surface of the skin, they become keratinized (hardened), which helps to thicken and protect the skin.

    REVIEW: Yes ☐ No ☐

43. **Answer: b**

    WHY: The central nervous system (Fig. 5-10) is composed of the brain and spinal cord. The

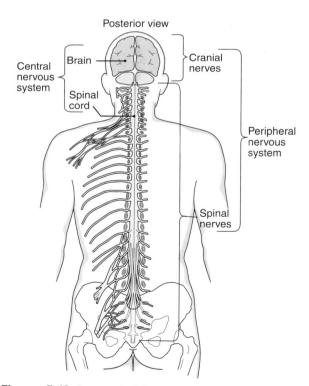

Figure 5-10 Structural divisions of the nervous system. (Adapted with permission from Cohen BJ. *Memmler's the Human Body in Health and Disease.* 11th ed. Philadelphia, PA: Lippincott Williams & Wilkins; 2013:188.)

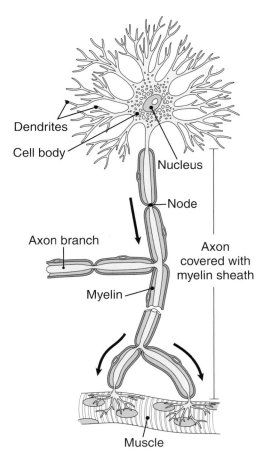

Dendrites

Cell body

Nucleus

Node

Axon branch

Axon covered with myelin sheath

Myelin

Muscle

Figure 5-11 Diagram of a motor neuron. (Adapted with permission from Cohen BJ. *Memmler's the Human Body in Health and Disease.* 12th ed. Philadelphia, PA: Lippincott Williams & Wilkins; 2013:189.)

autonomic and somatic nervous systems are part of the peripheral nervous system.

REVIEW: Yes ☐ No ☐

44. **Answer: d**

WHY: Cerebrospinal fluid (CSF) is the fluid that surrounds and cushions the brain and spinal cord. Acid-fast bacillus (AFB) culture is a respiratory system test. The CK isoenzymes test is a muscular system test. C-reactive protein (CRP) is a substance that is often elevated in the serum of individuals with certain inflammatory and infectious diseases.

REVIEW: Yes ☐ No ☐

45. **Answer: b**

WHY: Figure 5-2 is a motor neuron. Dendrites (1) carry messages to the nerve cell body (2). The cell nucleus (3) is the nerve cell command center. The axon (4), which has a myelin sheath, carries messages away from the nerve cell body (see Fig. 5-11).

REVIEW: Yes ☐ No ☐

46. **Answer: a**

WHY: *Encephalitis* means "inflammation of the brain," a nervous system structure. Gigantism is a pituitary disorder. Myxedema is a thyroid disorder. The pituitary and thyroid are endocrine system glands. Pediculosis (louse infestation) is an integumentary system disorder.

REVIEW: Yes ☐ No ☐

47. **Answer: d**

WHY: The meninges are layers of connective tissue that completely surround and protect the brain and spinal cavities. Bursae are synovial fluid–filled sacs near joints. *Calcaneus* is the medical term for the heel bone. Glomeruli are filtering structures in the nephrons of the kidneys.

REVIEW: Yes ☐ No ☐

📖 *See if you can unscramble the answer in Knowledge Drill 5-2 in the WORKBOOK.*

48. **Answer: a**

WHY: The peripheral nervous system (PNS) consists of all the nerves outside of the central nervous system (CNS). Afferent (sensory) nerves, which conduct impulses toward the brain, are part of the peripheral nervous system. The brain, spinal cord, and meninges are structures of the central nervous system.

REVIEW: Yes ☐ No ☐

49. **Answer: d**

WHY: Neurons (Fig. 5-11) are highly complex cells that are the primary functioning components of the nervous system. Axons are structural parts of neurons. The meninges are the covering of the brain and spinal cord. Nephrons are the functional units of the kidneys.

REVIEW: Yes ☐ No ☐

50. **Answer: c**

WHY: Multiple sclerosis is a disorder of the nervous system in which there is destruction of portions of the myelin sheath and disruption of the conduction of nerve impulses within several regions of the brain and spinal cord. Cushing syndrome is an endocrine system disorder involving excess production of cortisone. Hydrocephalus is the accumulation of cerebrospinal fluid in the brain. Parkinson disease is a chronic nervous system disease characterized by muscle weakness and tremors.

REVIEW: Yes ☐ No ☐

51. **Answer: c**

WHY: Sebaceous glands are located in the skin (Fig. 5-9), which is a major part of the integumentary system. They secrete an oily substance called sebum that helps lubricate the skin. The adrenal, pituitary, and thyroid glands secrete hormones and are part of the endocrine system.

REVIEW: Yes ☐ No ☐

52. **Answer: b**

WHY: The kidneys secrete erythropoietin, a hormone that stimulates red blood cell production.

REVIEW: Yes ☐ No ☐

53. **Answer: a**

WHY: Acromegaly is a condition characterized by the overgrowth of bones in the hands, feet, and face caused by excessive growth hormone in adulthood. Emphysema is chronic obstructive pulmonary disease. *Encephalitis* means "inflammation of the brain." Myxedema is a hypothyroid syndrome, a disorder caused by decreased functioning of the thyroid gland.

REVIEW: Yes ☐ No ☐

54. **Answer: b**

WHY: Diabetes mellitus type I, also called insulin-dependent diabetes, is a disorder in which the body is unable to produce insulin. In diabetes mellitus type II, or non–insulin-dependent diabetes, the body is able to produce insulin, but either the amount produced is not sufficient or the insulin is

not properly used by the body. Diabetes insipidus, a condition characterized by increased thirst and increased urine production, is caused by inadequate secretion of antidiuretic hormone. Gestational diabetes is impaired glucose tolerance that develops during pregnancy.

REVIEW: Yes ☐ No ☐

55. **Answer: d**

WHY: Although the heart is not an endocrine gland, the ventricles have endocrine function in that they secrete the hormone B-type natriuretic peptide (BNP) in response to ventricular volume expansion and pressure overload. Measurement of BNP levels helps the physician differentiate congestive heart failure (CHF) from chronic obstructive pulmonary disease (COPD). The kidneys produce the hormone erythropoietin (EPO), but it is produced in the tubular cells, not the glomeruli. The small intestine secretes hormones that play a role in the digestive process, but not BNP. The meninges do not have endocrine function.

REVIEW: Yes ☐ No ☐

56. **Answer: b**

WHY: The hypophysis (2) is another name for the pituitary gland, which is located in the brain. The thyroid (3) is located in the neck. The thymus (5) is located in the chest behind the sternum

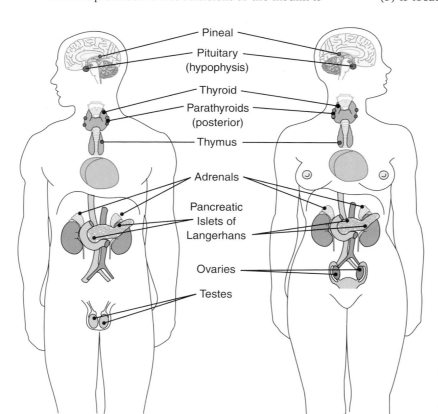

Figure 5-12 Endocrine system. (Adapted with permission from Cohen BJ. *Memmler's the Human Body in Health and Disease*. 12th ed. Philadelphia, PA: Lippincott Williams & Wilkins; 2013:261.)

(breastbone). There are two adrenals (6), one on top of each kidney. All of the choices in this question are adrenal system glands (Fig. 5-12).
REVIEW: Yes ☐ No ☐

57. **Answer: d**
WHY: Thyroxine (T_4) is a hormone released by the thyroid gland (Fig. 5-12) that increases metabolic rate. TSH is released by the pituitary to stimulate the thyroid. Both T_4 and TSH are common tests of thyroid function.
REVIEW: Yes ☐ No ☐

58. **Answer: b**
WHY: The pituitary gland (Fig. 5-12) is referred to as the "master gland" of the endocrine system because it releases hormones that stimulate other glands.
REVIEW: Yes ☐ No ☐

59. **Answer: d**
WHY: Growth hormone (GH) is secreted by the pituitary gland. The adrenals secrete several hormones, including epinephrine, norepinephrine, cortisol, and aldosterone. The ovaries secrete several hormones, including estrogen and progesterone. The islets of Langerhans in the pancreas secrete insulin and glucagon (see Fig. 5-12).
REVIEW: Yes ☐ No ☐

60. **Answer: d**
WHY: The islets of Langerhans are located in the pancreas and are part of the endocrine system (Fig. 5-12). They secrete insulin and glucagon. Insulin reduces blood glucose levels by helping move glucose into the cells. Glucagon increases blood glucose levels by stimulating the liver to release glucose into the bloodstream. Adrenaline and cortisol are secreted by the adrenal glands. Estrogen is secreted by the reproductive system.
REVIEW: Yes ☐ No ☐

61. **Answer: d**
WHY: Vasopressin is another name for antidiuretic hormone (ADH), which is secreted by the pituitary (Fig. 5-12) and decreases urine production.
REVIEW: Yes ☐ No ☐

62. **Answer: a**
WHY: The adrenals secrete the hormones epinephrine (adrenaline) and norepinephrine (noradrenaline), also referred to as the "fight-or-flight" hormones because of their effects on the body when it is under stress. There are two adrenal glands, one atop each kidney (Fig. 5-12).
REVIEW: Yes ☐ No ☐

63. **Answer: d**
WHY: Calcitonin is a hormone secreted by the thyroid (Fig. 5-12) that regulates the amount of calcium in the blood.
REVIEW: Yes ☐ No ☐

64. **Answer: c**
WHY: The thymus gland (Fig. 5-12), located in the chest behind the sternum, functions in the development of immunity and is most active before birth and during childhood until puberty, when it begins to shrink.
REVIEW: Yes ☐ No ☐

65. **Answer: b**
WHY: The pineal gland (Fig. 5-12) secretes the hormone melatonin. Melatonin secretion is inhibited by light and enhanced by darkness. Blood levels of melatonin create the diurnal (daily) rhythm of the sleep–wake cycle, with levels lowest around noon and highest at night.
REVIEW: Yes ☐ No ☐

66. **Answer: d**
WHY: Thyroxine is a hormone released by the thyroid (Fig. 5-12) that increases the metabolic rate. Cortisol is an adrenal hormone that suppresses inflammation. Glucagon is produced by the islets of Langerhans of the pancreas and stimulates the liver to release glucose (from glycogen stores) into the bloodstream. Melatonin, a hormone released by the pineal gland, plays a role in diurnal (daily) rhythms.
REVIEW: Yes ☐ No ☐

67. **Answer: c**
WHY: The gallbladder stores and concentrates bile, which is needed for the digestion of fat. Consequently, it is considered an accessory organ of the digestive system (Fig. 5-13). Arrector pili are structures in the skin. A bronchiole is a structure of the respiratory system. The glomerulus (plural, glomeruli) is a structure of the urinary system.
REVIEW: Yes ☐ No ☐

68. **Answer: a**
WHY: Bilirubin is a liver function test. The liver is an accessory organ of the digestive system (Fig. 5-13). Cortisol is an adrenal function test. The adrenals are endocrine system glands. Myoglobin is a muscular system test. Uric acid is a skeletal system test.
REVIEW: Yes ☐ No ☐

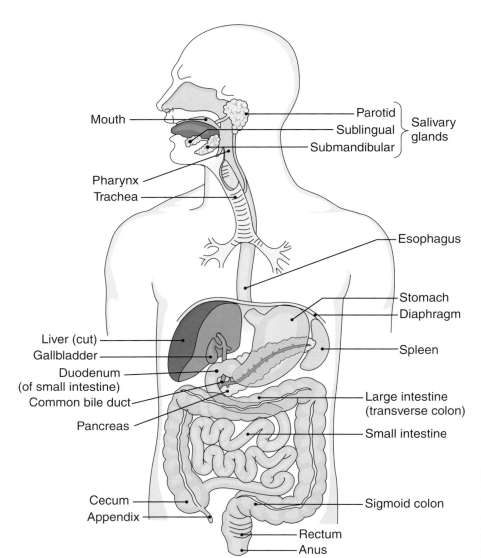

Mouth

Parotid ⎫
Sublingual ⎬ Salivary glands
Submandibular ⎭

Pharynx
Trachea

Esophagus

Stomach
Diaphragm

Liver (cut)
Gallbladder
Duodenum
(of small intestine)
Common bile duct
Pancreas

Spleen

Large intestine
(transverse colon)

Small intestine

Cecum
Appendix

Sigmoid colon

Rectum
Anus

Figure 5-13 The digestive system. (Adapted with permission from Cohen BJ. *Memmler's the Human Body in Health and Disease.* 12th ed. Philadelphia, PA: Lippincott Williams & Wilkins; 2013:413.)

69. **Answer: c**

WHY: *Hepatitis* means "liver inflammation." The term comes from the Greek word *hepatos*, meaning "liver." The suffix *-itis* means "inflammation." The term for inflammation of the colon is *colitis*. Kidney inflammation is called nephritis. Splenitis is inflammation of the spleen.

REVIEW: Yes ☐ No ☐

70. **Answer: c**

WHY: Bile is secreted by the liver and stored in the gallbladder, an accessory organ of the digestive system (Fig. 5-13). Bile emulsifies fats and facilitates their digestion.

REVIEW: Yes ☐ No ☐

71. **Answer: a**

WHY: Amylase and lipase are tests for digestive enzymes produced by the pancreas. Calcium and

uric acid are skeletal system tests. Cortisol and glucagon are endocrine system tests. Dilantin (phenytoin) and serotonin are nervous system tests.

REVIEW: Yes ☐ No ☐

72. **Answer: a**

WHY: The esophagus is part of the gastrointestinal (GI) tract (Fig. 5-13). Salivary glands are accessory structures of the digestive system. Neurilemma and axon branches are nervous system structures. Seminal ducts and the vas deferens are male reproductive system structures. The stratum corneum and papillae are integumentary system structures.

REVIEW: Yes ☐ No ☐

73. **Answer: a**

WHY: Gametes are the sex cells needed to create a new human being. They are produced by the reproductive system (Fig. 5-14). The male reproductive

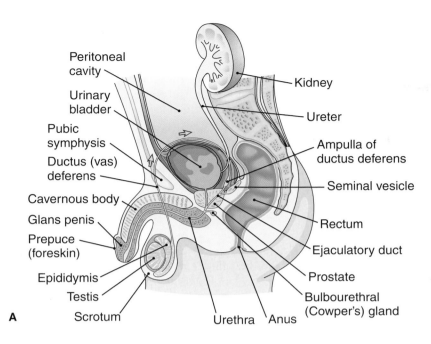

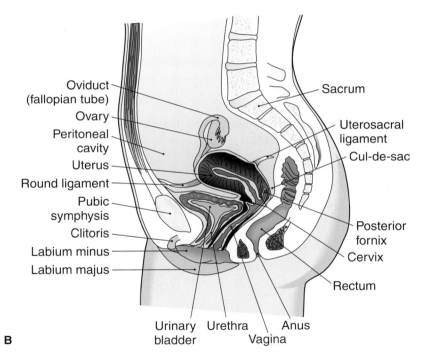

Figure 5-14 Reproductive system. **A:** Male. **B:** Female. (Adapted with permission from Cohen BJ. *Memmler's the Human Body in Health and Disease.* 12th ed. Philadelphia, PA: Lippincott Williams & Wilkins; 2013:486, 495.)

system produces gametes called sperm. The female reproductive system produces gametes called ova (eggs). Gastrin is produced by endocrine tissue in the stomach. Melanin is produced in the skin. Sputum is produced by the respiratory system.

REVIEW: Yes ☐ No ☐

74. **Answer: b**

WHY: The epididymis is a tightly coiled duct in the male reproductive system (Fig. 5-14A) that carries sperm from the testes to the vas deferens. An

alveolar sac is a cluster of alveoli in the lungs of the respiratory system. A fallopian tube is a structure of the female reproductive system (Fig. 5-14B). The renal artery carries blood to the kidneys and is part of the urinary system.

REVIEW: Yes ☐ No ☐

75. **Answer: c**

WHY: The prostate-specific antigen (PSA) test identifies the level of a protein produced by the prostate, a male reproductive system structure.

ALP is an abbreviation for alkaline phosphatase, a test associated with the skeletal system. A basic metabolic panel or profile (BMP) is a group of tests that cover several body systems. The rapid plasma reagin (RPR) test is a syphilis test and is a test of both the male and female reproductive systems.

REVIEW: Yes ☐ No ☐

76. **Answer: c**

WHY: Male gametes (sex cells) are called spermatozoa (sperm). An ovum is a female gamete. Gonads are the glands that produce gametes. The male gonads are the testes.

REVIEW: Yes ☐ No ☐

77. **Answer: c**

WHY: Female gametes (ova) are produced in the ovaries. The cervix is the neck of the uterus. The fallopian tubes are the pathway through which the ova reach the uterus. *Uterus* is another name for the womb (see Fig. 5-14B).

REVIEW: Yes ☐ No ☐

78. **Answer: b**

WHY: Follicle-stimulating hormone (FSH) is a female reproductive system test. Carcinoembryonic antigen (CEA) is a digestive system test associated with the diagnosis of colon cancer. A glucose tolerance test (GTT) is a digestive and an endocrine system test. Prostate-specific antigen (PSA) is a male reproductive system test.

REVIEW: Yes ☐ No ☐

79. **Answer: a**

WHY: *Oviduct* is another name for fallopian tube, a structure of the female reproductive system (Fig. 5-14B). Each ovary has an oviduct that extends from the ovary to the uterus. The pharynx is a digestive system structure. The sacrum is a skeletal system structure. A ureter is a urinary system structure.

REVIEW: Yes ☐ No ☐

80. **Answer: b**

WHY: Gonorrhea is a sexually transmitted disease (STD). Cholecystitis is inflammation of the gallbladder, which is an accessory organ of the digestive system. Myxedema is an endocrine system disorder that results from decreased thyroid function. Shingles, a nervous system disorder, is an acute eruption of herpes blisters along the length of a peripheral nerve.

REVIEW: Yes ☐ No ☐

81. **Answer: b**

WHY: Creatinine, a by-product of muscle metabolism, is produced at a constant rate and is cleared from the blood by the kidneys. The creatinine clearance test measures the rate that creatinine is cleared from the blood by the kidneys as a test of kidney function. Alkaline phosphatase is a skeletal system test. Lactic dehydrogenase is a muscular system test. Rapid plasma reagin is a reproductive system test.

REVIEW: Yes ☐ No ☐

82. **Answer: c**

WHY: Glomeruli are the filtering structures in the nephrons. Ureters are the tubes that carry urine from the kidneys to the bladder (see Fig. 5-15). The prostate is a structure of the male reproductive system, but the axons and myelin sheath are nervous system structures. Centrioles, nuclei, and the Golgi apparatus are all structures within cells. Renal arteries and the urethra are structures of the urinary system, but neurons are nervous system structures.

REVIEW: Yes ☐ No ☐

📖 *Practice naming structures in the urinary system in WORKBOOK Labeling Exercise 5-14.*

83. **Answer: a**

WHY: The primary function of the kidneys, which are part of the urinary system (Fig. 5-15), is to maintain water and electrolyte balance. (Electrolytes include sodium, potassium, chloride, and bicarbonate.) Heat production is a function of the muscular system. The nervous system and structures in the skin receive environmental stimuli. The circulatory system removes carbon dioxide gas.

REVIEW: Yes ☐ No ☐

84. **Answer: a**

WHY: Cystitis is inflammation of the urinary bladder. Gastritis is inflammation of the stomach lining, a digestive system disorder. Neuritis is nerve inflammation, a nervous system disorder. Pruritus (itching) is typically an integumentary system disorder.

REVIEW: Yes ☐ No ☐

85. **Answer: b**

WHY: Renin is an enzyme secreted by the kidneys that plays a role in the formation of angiotensin, a family of substances that cause vasoconstriction, and an increase in blood pressure. Melanin is a pigment produced in the skin. Sebum is an oily substance produced by the sebaceous glands in the skin. Uric acid is an end product of purine

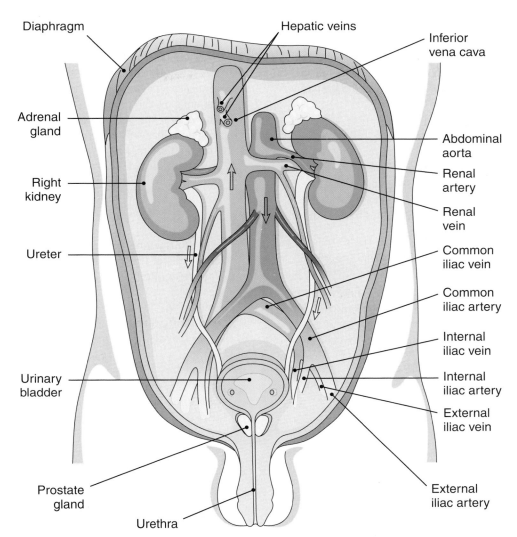

Diaphragm

Hepatic veins

Inferior vena cava

Adrenal gland

Abdominal aorta

Renal artery

Right kidney

Renal vein

Common iliac vein

Ureter

Common iliac artery

Internal iliac vein

Internal iliac artery

Urinary bladder

External iliac vein

Prostate gland

External iliac artery

Urethra

Figure 5-15 Urinary system (male). (Adapted with permission from Cohen BJ. *Memmler's the Human Body in Health and Disease.* 12th ed. Philadelphia, PA: Lippincott Williams & Wilkins; 2013:465.)

metabolism that increases in certain disorders such as gout, a skeletal system disorder.
REVIEW: Yes ☐ No ☐

86. **Answer: b**
WHY: Glomeruli are tufts of capillaries within the nephrons of the kidneys that filter water and dissolved substances, including wastes, from the blood. Fallopian tubes are structures of the female reproductive system. Ureters are the two tubes (one per kidney) that carry urine from the kidneys to the bladder.
REVIEW: Yes ☐ No ☐

87. **Answer: a**
WHY: An arterial blood gas (ABG) test assesses a patient's oxygenation and ventilation, which are respiratory system functions. A potassium

hydroxide (KOH) prep is typically an integumentary system test. Thyroid-stimulating hormone (TSH) is a thyroid function test. Urinalysis (UA) is a urinary system test.
REVIEW: Yes ☐ No ☐

88. **Answer: d**
WHY: Internal respiration takes place in the tissues. During internal respiration, oxygen from the bloodstream enters the cells in the tissues, and carbon dioxide from the tissues enters the bloodstream to be carried back to the lungs. During external respiration, oxygen enters the blood in the lungs and carbon dioxide exits the bloodstream in the lungs.
REVIEW: Yes ☐ No ☐

📖 *For a visual of this process, see Figure 5-15 in the TEXTBOOK.*

89. **Answer: b**

WHY: Normal blood pH is maintained within a narrow range of 7.35 to 7.45. A decrease below normal levels results in acidosis. An increase above normal levels is alkalosis. Both are dangerous conditions.

REVIEW: Yes ☐ No ☐

90. **Answer: a**

WHY: Carbon dioxide (CO_2) levels play a major role in acid–base balance. As CO_2 levels increase, blood pH decreases (becomes more acidic), which can lead to a condition called acidosis.

REVIEW: Yes ☐ No ☐

91. **Answer: c**

WHY: The ability of oxygen to combine with a protein in red blood cells called hemoglobin increases the oxygen-carrying capacity of the blood. Hemoglobin combined with oxygen is called oxyhemoglobin.

REVIEW: Yes ☐ No ☐

92. **Answer: d**

WHY: Infection with respiratory syncytial virus causes acute respiratory problems in children. Cystic fibrosis, emphysema, and *Mycobacterium tuberculosis* can cause respiratory distress in children, but they are not nearly as common.

REVIEW: Yes ☐ No ☐

93. **Answer: a**

WHY: Bronchioles are small branches of the bronchi. The epiglottis is the structure that covers the entrance of the larynx during swallowing. The pleura are thin layers of membrane that encase the lungs. All of these structures are part of the respiratory system (Fig. 5-16). The calcaneus, mandible, and phalanges are skeletal system bones. The corium, corneum, and adipose cells are structures of the skin. The neurons, meninges, and myelin sheath are nervous system structures.

REVIEW: Yes ☐ No ☐

94. **Answer: a**

WHY: The alveoli, bronchi, larynx, and trachea are all structures of the respiratory system (Fig. 5-16), but the exchange of oxygen and carbon dioxide occurs through the walls of the alveoli in the lungs.

REVIEW: Yes ☐ No ☐

95. **Answer: d**

WHY: Partial pressure (P) is the pressure exerted by one gas in a mixture of gases. Whether oxygen or carbon dioxide associates (combines) with or disassociates (releases) from hemoglobin depends on the partial pressure of each gas. In the tissues, the PaO_2 of oxygen is decreased, so oxygen releases from hemoglobin and defuses into the tissues. Pco_2 is increased in the tissues, so carbon dioxide from the tissues associates with hemoglobin.

REVIEW: Yes ☐ No ☐

96. **Answer: d**

WHY: Surfactant is a fluid substance that coats the thin walls of the alveoli to help keep them from collapsing. Premature infants often lack or do not have sufficient surfactant to keep their lungs from collapsing. The resulting condition is called infant respiratory distress syndrome (IRDS).

REVIEW: Yes ☐ No ☐

97. **Answer: d**

WHY: Tuberculosis (TB) is caused by *Mycobacterium tuberculosis*. This microorganism is called an acid-fast bacillus (AFB) because it is not decolorized by acid alcohol after being stained with a dark dye. Chronic obstructive pulmonary disease (COPD) is a condition associated with breathing difficulties resulting from lung damage. Infant respiratory distress syndrome (IRDS) is a condition caused by a lack of surfactant. RSV stands for respiratory syncytial virus, a virus that affects the lungs.

REVIEW: Yes ☐ No ☐

98. **Answer: b**

WHY: *Dyspnea* is the medical term for difficult breathing. (The prefix *dys-* means "difficult." *Pnea* means "breathing.") Asthma is a condition characterized by dyspnea accompanied by wheezing. Emphysema is a chronic obstructive pulmonary disease. Pneumonia is inflammation of the lungs most commonly caused by bacteria, viruses, or chemical irritation.

REVIEW: Yes ☐ No ☐

99. **Answer: b**

WHY: The nervous system controls and coordinates the activities of all body systems by means of electrical impulses and chemical substances sent to and received from all parts of the body.

REVIEW: Yes ☐ No ☐

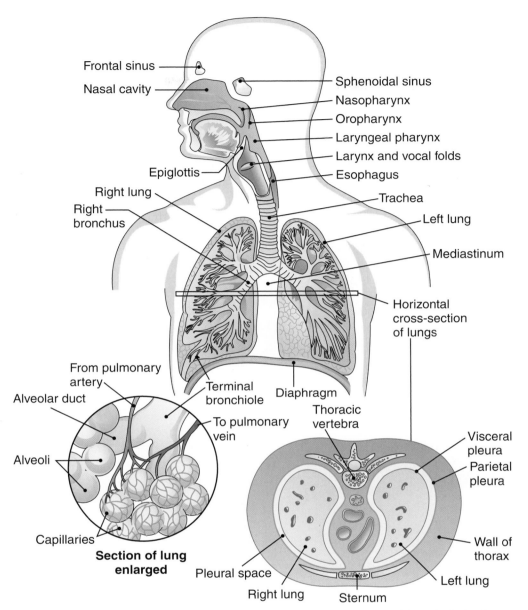

Frontal sinus

Nasal cavity

Sphenoidal sinus

Nasopharynx

Oropharynx

Laryngeal pharynx

Larynx and vocal folds

Epiglottis

Esophagus

Right lung

Trachea

Right bronchus

Left lung

Mediastinum

Horizontal cross-section of lungs

From pulmonary artery

Alveolar duct

Terminal bronchiole

Diaphragm

Thoracic vertebra

To pulmonary vein

Alveoli

Visceral pleura

Parietal pleura

Capillaries

Wall of thorax

Section of lung enlarged

Pleural space

Left lung

Right lung

Sternum

Figure 5-16 Respiratory system. (Adapted with permission from Cohen BJ. *Memmler's the Human Body in Health and Disease.* 12th ed. Philadelphia, PA: Lippincott Williams & Wilkins; 2013:387.)

100. **Answer: a**

WHY: Functions of the digestive system (Fig. 5-13) include taking in food, breaking it down into usable components, and eliminating waste products from this process.

REVIEW: Yes ☐ No ☐

101. **Answer: c**

WHY: Hyperglycemia is the medical term for abnormally increased blood sugar. The prefix *hyper*- means "too much" or "too high." *Glyc* is the word root for glucose (sugar). The suffix *-emia* means "blood condition." Diabetes mellitus is a disorder characterized by abnormal glucose metabolism.

Diabetes insipidus is a disorder characterized by abnormally increased urination. Hyperinsulinism is an excess of insulin in the blood.

REVIEW: Yes ☐ No ☐

102. **Answer: b**

WHY: The endocrine system is a series of glands that produce hormones and release them directly into the bloodstream. The circulatory system is primarily composed of the heart, blood, and lymph vessels. The glands of the integumentary system release their substances through ducts leading to the surface of the skin. The respiratory system is responsible for delivering oxygen to the cells and removing carbon dioxide from the cells.

REVIEW: Yes ☐   No ☐

103. **Answer: a**

WHY: *Pancreatitis* means inflammation of the pancreas, which is an accessory organ of the digestive system (Fig. 5-13).

REVIEW: Yes ☐   No ☐

104. **Answer: b**

WHY: Hormones are powerful chemical substances secreted directly into the bloodstream by endocrine system glands. Individual endocrine glands secrete unique hormones that control specific body functions.

REVIEW: Yes ☐   No ☐

105. **Answer: c**

WHY: Hematopoiesis (also called hemopoiesis) is the production and development of the formed elements (blood cells and platelets). Hematopoiesis occurs in the bone marrow of the skeletal system. The urinary system produces the hormone erythropoietin, which stimulates erythrocyte (red blood cell) production.

REVIEW: Yes ☐   No ☐

Chapter 6

The Circulatory System

Study Tips

- Make flash cards of the circulatory system components and the associated structures, functions, disorders, and diagnostic tests described in Chapter 6 of the TEXTBOOK.

- Study the diagrams of the arm, hand, and leg in the TEXTBOOK and memorize the names of the major veins, visualizing their locations.

- Locate the major antecubital veins on a friend or fellow student.

- Complete and study the labeling exercises in the workbook.

- Review the chapter memory joggers, key points, and cautions.

- Create a diagram that illustrates the flow of blood throughout the body, labeling the chambers of the heart and identifying the various blood vessels it passes through.

Overview

The circulatory system carries oxygen and food to the cells of the body, and it carries carbon dioxide and other wastes away from the cells to the excretory organs, the kidneys, lungs, and skin. It also aids in the coagulation process, assists in defending the body against disease, and plays an important role in the regulation of body temperature. A thorough knowledge of this system is especially important to the phlebotomist, who must access it to collect blood specimens for analysis. It also helps the phlebotomist appreciate the importance of the many tests associated with it. This chapter covers the two main components of the circulatory system, the cardiovascular system (heart, blood, and blood vessels) and the lymphatic system (lymph, lymph vessels, and nodes) and describes the structures, functions, disorders, and diagnostic tests associated with them, including the coagulation process, which helps protect the system from blood loss.

Review Questions

Choose the BEST answer.

1. In numerical order, the structures indicated by numbers 1 and 8 in Figure 6-1 are the
   a. aortic arch and the left pulmonary arteries.
   b. aortic arch and the right pulmonary arteries.
   c. left pulmonary artery and left pulmonary veins.
   d. superior vena cava and right pulmonary arteries.

2. In numerical order, the structures indicated by numbers 11 and 17 in Figure 6-1 are the
   a. left pulmonary arteries and right pulmonary veins.

   b. left pulmonary veins and the arch of the aorta.
   c. right pulmonary arteries and superior vena cava.
   d. right pulmonary veins and inferior vena cava.

3. In numerical order, the structures indicated by numbers 4 and 15 in Figure 6-1 are the
   a. aortic valve and the bicuspid valve.
   b. mitral valve and the pulmonic valve.
   c. right and left atrioventricular valves.
   d. tricuspid valve and the aortic valve.

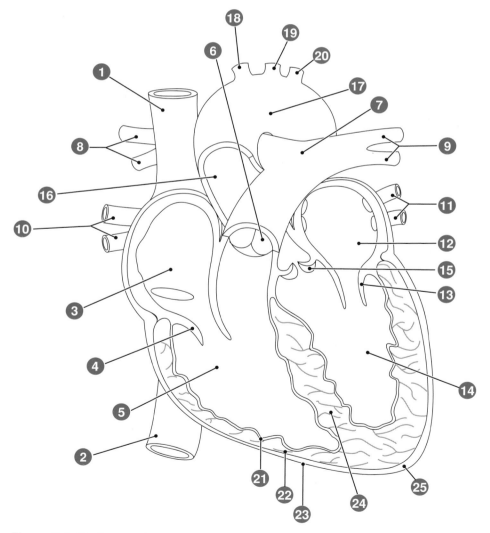

Figure 6-1 The heart and great vessels. (Adapted with permission from Cohen BJ, Hull KL. Study Guide for *Memmler's the Human Body in Health and Disease.* 12th ed. Philadelphia, PA: Lippincott Williams & Wilkins; 2013:268.)

4. In numerical order, the structures indicated by numbers 5 and 12 in Figure 6-1 are the
   a. left atrium and right ventricle.
   b. left ventricle and right atrium.
   c. right atrium and left ventricle.
   d. right ventricle and left atrium.

5. Which of the following is a function of the circulatory system?
   a. Carrying oxygen to the tissue cells
   b. Conveying afferent nerve impulses
   c. Excreting wastes from the body
   d. Producing the formed elements

6. The heart is surrounded by a thin fluid-filled sac called the
   a. endocardium.
   b. epicardium.
   c. myocardium.
   d. pericardium.

7. The middle layer of the heart is called the
   a. endocardium.
   b. epicardium.
   c. myocardium.
   d. pericardium.

8. How many chambers are there in the human heart?
   a. 1
   b. 2
   c. 4
   d. 6

9. This heart chamber delivers oxygen-rich blood to the ascending aorta.
   a. Left atrium
   b. Left ventricle
   c. Right atrium
   d. Right ventricle

10. This heart chamber receives blood from the systemic system.
    a. Left atrium
    b. Left ventricle
    c. Right atrium
    d. Right ventricle

11. The semilunar valves are located
    a. at the exits of both of the ventricles.
    b. between the atria and the ventricles.
    c. where the aortic arch becomes the aorta.
    d. within the veins of the systemic system.

12. The right atrioventricular valve is also called the
    a. bicuspid valve.
    b. pulmonic valve.
    c. semilunar valve.
    d. tricuspid valve.

13. This valve gets its name from its resemblance to a bishop's hat.
    a. Aortic valve
    b. Mitral valve
    c. Pulmonic valve
    d. Tricuspid valve

14. The structure that separates the right and left ventricles of the heart is called the
    a. atrioventricular septum.
    b. interatrial septum.
    c. interventricular septum.
    d. myocardial septum.

15. The heart muscle gets its blood supply from the
    a. carotid arteries.
    b. coronary arteries.
    c. pulmonary arteries.
    d. pulmonary veins.

16. These structures keep the atrioventricular valves from flipping back into the atria.
    a. Chordae tendineae
    b. Myocardial septa
    c. Purkinje fibers
    d. Semilunar cusps

17. Myocardial ischemia is a condition that results from
    a. complete blockage of a coronary artery.
    b. death of a portion of myocardial tissue.
    c. malfunction of an atrioventricular valve.
    d. partial obstruction of a coronary artery.

18. The medical term for a heart attack is myocardial
    a. arrhythmia.
    b. infarction.
    c. ischemia.
    d. tachycardia.

19. The heart's "pacemaker" is the
    a. bundle of His.
    b. chorda tendinea.
    c. papillary muscle.
    d. sinoatrial node.

20. This is an abbreviation for a test that traces the electrical impulses of the heart.
    a. ALT
    b. ECG
    c. EEG
    d. TnT

21. One complete contraction and subsequent relaxation of the heart is called one cardiac
    a. cycle.
    b. diastole.
    c. output.
    d. systole.

22. Systole is the
    a. closing of the semilunar valves.
    b. completion of one cardiac cycle.
    c. contracting phase of the heart.
    d. relaxation stage of the heart.

23. A cardiac cycle lasts approximately
    a. 0.5 seconds.
    b. 0.8 seconds.
    c. 1.5 seconds.
    d. 8.0 seconds.

24. On an electrocardiogram, atrial activity is represented by the
    a. P wave.
    b. QRS complex.
    c. T wave.
    d. T and P waves.

25. On an electrocardiogram, which wave represents the activity of the ventricles?
    a. P
    b. P and T
    c. QRS and P
    d. QRS and T

26. The first sound of the heartbeat is created by the
    a. closing of the atrioventricular valves.
    b. opening of the semilunar valves.
    c. resonation of the chordae tendineae.
    d. ventricular muscle contraction echo.

27. Abnormal heart sounds are called
    a. arrhythmias.
    b. extrasystoles.
    c. fibrillations.
    d. murmurs.

28. The average normal heart rate is
    a. 63 beats per minute.
    b. 72 beats per minute.
    c. 81 beats per minute.
    d. 96 beats per minute.

29. An abnormally fast heart rate is called
    a. bradycardia.
    b. extrasystole.
    c. fibrillation.
    d. tachycardia.

30. A person's pulse is created by a wave of pressure caused by
    a. atrial contraction.
    b. atrial relaxation.
    c. ventricular contraction.
    d. ventricular relaxation.

31. The force exerted by the blood on the walls of the blood vessels is called
    a. blood pressure.
    b. cardiac output.
    c. heart rhythm.
    d. pulse rate.

32. The technical term for this device is sphygmomanometer.
    a. Artificial pacemaker
    b. Brain wave detector
    c. Blood pressure cuff
    d. Heart wave monitor

33. Which of the following is a normal blood pressure reading?
    a. 60/90 mm Hg
    b. 80/120 mm Hg
    c. 100/120 mm Hg
    d. 118/79 mm Hg

34. Systolic pressure measures pressure in the arteries during
    a. atrial contraction.
    b. atrial relaxation.
    c. ventricular contraction.
    d. ventricular relaxation.

35. An infection of the lining of the heart is called
    a. angina pectoris.
    b. aortic stenosis.
    c. endocarditis.
    d. pericarditis.

36. Which of the following are abbreviations for cardiac enzyme tests?
    a. ALP, ALT
    b. BUN, PT
    c. CK, LDH
    d. GTT, ESR

37. The pulmonary circulation takes blood to the
    a. arteries in the heart muscle.
    b. heart from the body tissues.
    c. internal organs to the body.
    d. lungs and back to the heart.

38. Which of the following veins is found in the leg?
    a. Brachial
    b. Cephalic
    c. Femoral
    d. Median

39. Blood vessels that carry blood away from the heart are called
    a. arteries.
    b. capillaries.
    c. veins.
    d. venules.

40. Which of the following veins carry oxygen-rich blood?
    a. Pulmonary
    b. Saphenous
    c. Subclavian
    d. Vena cava

41. Normal systemic arterial blood is
    a. dark blue.
    b. bright red.
    c. bluish red.
    d. dark red.

42. The largest artery in the body is the
    a. aorta.
    b. carotid.
    c. femoral.
    d. vena cava.

43. The longest vein in the body is the
    a. great saphenous.
    b. median cubital.
    c. inferior vena cava.
    d. right pulmonary.

44. What keeps the blood moving through the venous system?
    a. Expansion and contraction of the systemic arteries
    b. Movement of fluid throughout the lymphatic system
    c. Pressure caused by contraction of the ventricles
    d. Skeletal muscle movement and valves in the veins

45. The smallest branches of veins are called
    a. arterioles.
    b. capillaries.
    c. lumina.
    d. venules.

46. These are tiny blood vessels that are only one cell thick.
    a. Arteries
    b. Arterioles
    c. Capillaries
    d. Venules

47. The tunica adventitia is the
    a. external layer of a blood vessel.
    b. inside lining of a blood vessel.
    c. internal layer of a blood vessel.
    d. middle layer of a blood vessel.

48. The internal space of a blood vessel is called the
    a. interna.
    b. intima.
    c. lumen.
    d. media.

49. The layers of arteries differ from the layers of veins in that the
    a. inner lining is much thicker in veins.
    b. middle layer of veins is more elastic.
    c. muscle layer is thicker in arteries.
    d. outer layer of arteries is thinner.

50. Oxygen and nutrients diffuse through the walls of the
    a. alveoli.
    b. arterioles.
    c. capillaries.
    d. venules.

51. Identify the structure on the right in Figure 6-2 from the following choices.
    a. Artery
    b. Capillary
    c. Lymph vessel
    d. Vein

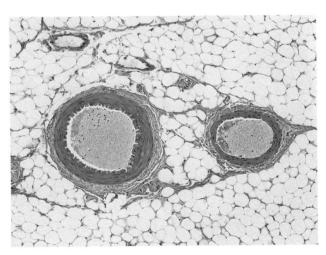

Figure 6-2 Cross-section of two circulatory system vessels as seen through a microscope. (Reprinted with permission from Cormack DH. *Essential Histology.* Philadelphia, PA: JB Lippincott; 1993: Plate 11–1.)

52. The right ventricle delivers blood to the
    a. aortic arch.
    b. left atrium.
    c. pulmonary artery.
    d. pulmonary vein.

53. Which of the following blood vessels carries oxygenated blood?
    a. Brachial vein
    b. Pulmonary vein
    c. Pulmonary artery
    d. Inferior vena cava

54. Which of the following blood vessels are listed in the proper direction of blood flow?
    a. Arteries, arterioles, capillaries
    b. Arterioles, venules, capillaries
    c. Capillaries, arterioles, arteries
    d. Veins, venules, capillaries

55. The antecubital (AC) fossa is located
    a. anterior and distal to the elbow.
    b. anterior and distal to the wrist.
    c. posterior and proximal to the elbow.
    d. posterior and proximal to the wrist.

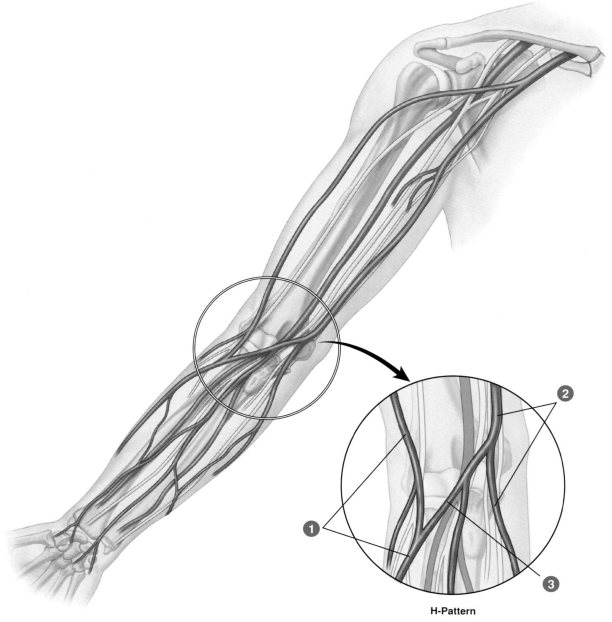

H-Pattern

Figure 6-3 The principal veins of the right arm in anatomical position displaying the H-shaped pattern of antecubital veins.

56. Which one of the following veins is found only in or below the AC fossa?
    a. Basilic
    b. Cephalic
    c. Median
    d. Subclavian

57. In numerical order, the veins identified by numbers 1, 2, and 3 in Figure 6-3 are the
    a. basilic, median cubital, and cephalic.
    b. cephalic, basilic, and median cubital.
    c. median cubital, cephalic, and basilic.
    d. subclavian, median cubital, and basilic.

58. In numerical order, the veins identified by numbers 1, 2, and 3 in Figure 6-4 are the
    a. accessory cephalic, median, and median basilic.
    b. cephalic, median basilic, and accessory basilic.
    c. median basilic, accessory cephalic, and median.
    d. median cephalic, median basilic, and median.

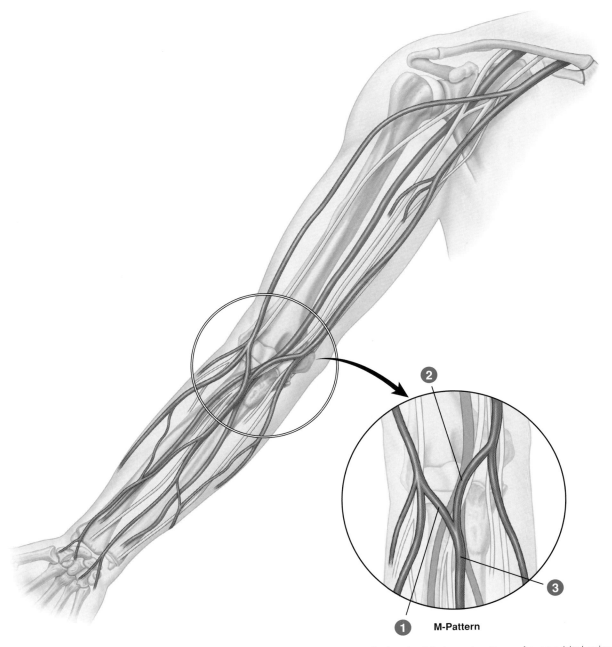

Figure 6-4 The principal veins of the right arm in anatomical position displaying the M-shaped pattern of antecubital veins.

Dorsal Forearm, Wrist, and Hand Veins

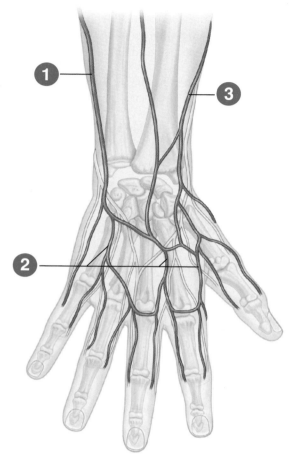

Figure 6-5 Veins of the right forearm, wrist, and hand in prone position.

59. In numerical order, the veins identified by numbers 1, 2, and 3 in Figure 6-5 are the
    a. basilic, dorsal metacarpal, and cephalic.
    b. brachial, dorsal metacarpal, and basilic.
    c. cephalic, dorsal metacarpal, and basilic.
    d. median, dorsal metacarpal, and cephalic.

60. The basilic vein is the last choice for venipuncture because it is
    a. deeply buried in the AC fossa.
    b. fixed in the surrounding tissue.
    c. located close to a major nerve.
    d. the hardest AC vein to palpate.

61. This major vein merges with the brachiocephalic vein in the chest.
    a. Cephalic
    b. Popliteal
    c. Saphenous
    d. Subclavian

62. Two median cutaneous nerves lie close to this vein.
    a. Basilic
    b. Cephalic
    c. Median
    d. Radial

63. Which of the following veins are listed in the proper order of selection for venipuncture?
    a. Basilic, cephalic, median cubital
    b. Cephalic, median cubital, basilic
    c. Median, median basilic, cephalic
    d. Median cubital, cephalic, basilic

64. When the hand is prone, the antecubital portion of the cephalic vein is normally located in line with the
    a. index finger.
    b. little finger.
    c. radial artery.
    d. thumb.

65. According to the Clinical and Laboratory Standards Institute (CLSI), venipuncture should not be performed on leg, ankle, or foot veins unless
    a. both arms have IVs or other intravascular devices.
    b. permission of the patient's physician has been obtained.
    c. there are no acceptable antecubital or hand veins.
    d. the patient does not have any coagulation problems.

66. The popliteal vein is found in the
    a. arm.
    b. hand.
    c. heart.
    d. leg.

67. This is the medical term for a blood clot circulating in the bloodstream.
    a. Aneurysm
    b. Embolism
    c. Embolus
    d. Thrombus

68. The medical term for vein inflammation is
    a. embolism.
    b. hemostasis.
    c. phlebitis.
    d. thrombosis.

69. Which of the following is an abbreviation used for a vascular system test?
    a. ADH
    b. CSF
    c. DIC
    d. RPR

70. Lipid accumulation on the intima of an artery is called
    a. atherosclerosis.
    b. cholesterol.
    c. endocarditis.
    d. lipemia.

71. Which of the following is a localized dilation or bulging of an artery?
    a. Aneurysm
    b. Embolism
    c. Phlebitis
    d. Thrombus

72. Inflammation of a vein in conjunction with formation of a blood clot is called
    a. atherosclerosis.
    b. phlebosclerosis.
    c. thrombophlebitis.
    d. vasculitis.

73. Normal adult blood volume is approximately
    a. 2 L.
    b. 4 L.
    c. 5 L.
    d. 8 L.

74. The normal composition of blood is approximately
    a. 10% plasma, 90% formed elements.
    b. 30% plasma, 70% formed elements.
    c. 55% plasma, 45% formed elements.
    d. 91% plasma, 09% formed elements.

75. Normal plasma is a
    a. clear, colorless, watery fluid containing about 10% solutes.
    b. clear or slightly hazy, pale-yellow fluid that is 90% water.
    c. cloudy, completely colorless fluid containing 45% solutes.
    d. slightly hazy, pale-yellow fluid that is close to 55% water.

76. Which of the following is an abnormal finding in the blood?
    a. Antibodies
    b. Bacteria
    c. Blood cells
    d. Platelets

77. Which blood cell contains a nucleus?
    a. Erythrocyte
    b. Leukocyte
    c. Thrombocyte
    d. Reticulocyte

78. A reticulocyte count identifies immature
    a. lymphocytes.
    b. neutrophils.
    c. red blood cells.
    d. white blood cells.

79. Which blood cell increases in allergic reactions and pinworm infestations?
    a. Basophil
    b. Eosinophil
    c. Lymphocyte
    d. Neutrophil

80. How large is a normal erythrocyte?
    a. 4 to 5 microns
    b. 7 to 8 microns
    c. 8 to 10 microns
    d. 10 to 12 microns

81. Which of the following would be considered a normal erythrocyte count?
    a. 4.5 million/mm^3
    b. 6.0 million/mm^3
    c. 10.5 million/mm^3
    d. 20.0 million/mm^3

82. Red blood cells are produced in the
    a. bloodstream.
    b. bone marrow.
    c. lymph nodes.
    d. thymus gland.

83. The primary function of red blood cells is to
    a. deliver nutrients to the body tissues.
    b. produce antibodies to combat infection.
    c. transport carbon dioxide to the lungs.
    d. transport oxygen to cells in the body.

84. A leukocyte is a
    a. lymphatic cell.
    b. platelet stem cell.
    c. red blood cell.
    d. white blood cell.

85. Which blood cell has the ability to pass through blood vessel walls?
    a. Erythrocyte
    b. Leukocyte
    c. Reticulocyte
    d. Thrombocyte

86. Which type of cell destroys pathogens by phagocytosis?
    a. Erythrocyte
    b. Neutrophil
    c. Red blood cell
    d. Thrombocyte

87. Which of the following is a short term for neutrophils?
    a. Eos
    b. Basos
    c. Monos
    d. Polys

88. Which formed element is the first to play a role in sealing an injury to a blood vessel?
    a. Erythrocyte
    b. Leukocyte
    c. Platelet
    d. Reticulocyte

89. Which of the following is an anuclear biconcave disc?
    a. Erythrocyte
    b. Granulocyte
    c. Leukocyte
    d. Thrombocyte

90. Which type of cell is sometimes called a macrophage?
    a. Eosinophil
    b. Basophil
    c. Lymphocyte
    d. Monocyte

91. Some of these cells give rise to plasma cells.
    a. Eosinophils
    b. Lymphocytes
    c. Monocytes
    d. Neutrophils

92. Which of the following would be considered a normal platelet count?
    a. 20,000/mm^3
    b. 70,000/mm^3
    c. 300,000/mm^3
    d. 600,000/mm^3

93. Platelets are also called
    a. erythrocytes.
    b. leukocytes.
    c. neutrophils.
    d. thrombocytes.

94. A platelet is actually a part of a bone marrow cell called a
    a. granulocyte.
    b. macrophage.
    c. megakaryocyte.
    d. T lymphocyte.

95. Which of the following are normally the most numerous of the formed elements?
    a. Platelets
    b. Red blood cells

    c. Reticulocytes
    d. White blood cells

96. A person's blood type is determined by the presence or absence of certain types of
    a. antibodies on the surfaces of the red blood cells.
    b. antibodies on the surfaces of the white blood cells.
    c. antigens on the surfaces of the red blood cells.
    d. antigens on the surfaces of the white blood cells.

97. To prevent sensitization, Rh immunoglobulin is given to
    a. pregnant women who bleed throughout the pregnancy.
    b. Rh-negative mothers who deliver Rh-positive babies.
    c. Rh-positive babies immediately after they are born.
    d. Rh-positive mothers who deliver Rh-negative babies.

98. A woman who becomes "sensitized" to the Rh factor
    a. can produce antibodies against the Rh antigen.
    b. has Rh antigen circulating in her bloodstream.
    c. should not try to have more than one child.
    d. will test Rh-positive for months afterward.

99. A person who has A-negative blood has red blood cells that
    a. have the A antigen and lack the Rh antigen.
    b. have both the A antigen and the Rh antigen.
    c. lack the A antigen and have the Rh antigen.
    d. lack both the A antigen and the Rh antigen.

100. Hemolytic disease of the newborn is most often caused by
    a. ABO incompatibility between mother and infant.
    b. incompatible blood given to the infant in utero.
    c. previous sensitization of an Rh-negative mother.
    d. Rh incompatibility between the infant and the father.

101. A whole-blood specimen consists of
    a. aggregated blood cells and water.
    b. blood cells suspended in serum.
    c. plasma and the formed elements.
    d. serum and clotted red blood cells.

102. The liquid portion of a clotted blood specimen is called
    a. fibrinogen.
    b. plasma.
    c. saline.
    d. serum.

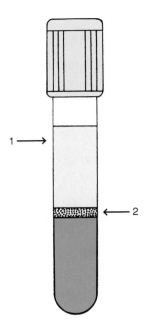

Figure 6-6 A centrifuged whole-blood specimen.

103. A whole-blood specimen has an abnormally large buffy coat. This is an indication that the patient has:
    a. an elevated leukocyte or platelet count.
    b. an increased amount of red blood cells.
    c. large numbers of bacteria in the blood.
    d. recently eaten a meal with a lot of fat.

104. Figure 6-6 shows a centrifuged whole-blood specimen. Identify the portion of the specimen indicated by arrow 1.
    a. Buffy coat
    b. Plasma
    c. Serum
    d. Red blood cells

105. Identify the portion of the specimen indicated by arrow 2 in Figure 6-6.
    a. Buffy coat
    b. Plasma
    c. Serum
    d. Red blood cells

106. How can you visually tell serum from plasma?
    a. Plasma is yellow, serum is colorless.
    b. Serum is clear, plasma is cloudy.
    c. Serum is fluid, plasma is gel-like.
    d. You cannot visually tell them apart.

107. On a blood smear made using Wright stain, the granules of eosinophils stain this color.
    a. Dark blue
    b. Lavender

    c. Orange-pink
    d. Pink to tan

108. Most tests in this department are performed on plasma specimens.
    a. Coagulation
    b. Cytology
    c. Hematology
    d. Immunology

109. It is preferable to perform most stat chemistry tests on plasma rather than serum because plasma
    a. can be tested a lot sooner.
    b. gives more accurate results.
    c. is more stable than serum.
    d. tests require less specimen.

110. This is the abbreviation for a test that is always performed on whole blood.
    a. BUN
    b. CBC
    c. LDL
    d. PTT

111. This is the abbreviation for a test that can be done on plasma.
    a. CBC
    b. ESR
    c. Hgb
    d. PTT

112. Serum
    a. can be used for most hematology tests.
    b. contains the clotting factor fibrinogen.
    c. is collected in a nonanticoagulant tube.
    d. normally has a very deep-yellow color.

113. A person with thrombocytosis has abnormally
    a. decreased platelets.
    b. functioning platelets.
    c. increased platelets.
    d. large platelets.

114. A disease that is often characterized by an abnormally low red blood cell count is called
    a. anemia.
    b. leukemia.
    c. neutropenia.
    d. polycythemia.

115. Which of the following is the abbreviation for a test of the formed elements?
    a. ASO
    b. CBC
    c. Lytes
    d. SPEP

116. An abnormal increase in white blood cells is called
    a. leukemia.
    b. leukocytosis.
    c. leukopenia.
    d. leukopoiesis.

117. Which of the following is a diagnostic test for blood cell disorders?
    a. Bilirubin
    b. Creatinine
    c. Ferritin
    d. Glucose

118. The coagulation process plays a role in
    a. hemolysis.
    b. hemopoiesis.
    c. hemostasis.
    d. homeostasis.

119. The ability of platelets to stick to each other is called platelet
    a. aggregation.
    b. adhesion.
    c. cohesion.
    d. inhibition.

120. This ion is essential to the coagulation process.
    a. Calcium
    b. Chloride
    c. Potassium
    d. Sodium

121. The extrinsic or contact activation coagulation pathway is initiated by
    a. activation of plasma coagulation factors.
    b. commencement of platelet aggregation.
    c. tissue factor released from injured tissue.
    d. events occurring within the bloodstream.

122. The first response in the hemostatic process is
    a. fibrin formation.
    b. platelet adhesion
    c. thrombin creation.
    d. vasoconstriction.

123. Platelet plug formation takes place in this phase of the coagulation process.
    a. Amplification
    b. Initiation
    c. Propagation
    d. Termination

124. Platelet activation and blood clotting in general can be inhibited by:
    a. aspirin
    b. antibiotics

    c. sulfates
    d. vitamins

125. A disorder caused most often by lack of factor VIII is
    a. hemophilia.
    b. intravascular coagulation.
    c. thrombocytopenia.
    d. varicose veins.

126. Coagulation problems may result from liver disease because the liver
    a. filters impurities from the blood.
    b. manufactures coagulation factors.
    c. removes damaged red blood cells.
    d. stores and releases calcium ions.

127. Which of the following is an enzyme that plays the major role in coagulation?
    a. Fibrin
    b. Heparin
    c. Plasmin
    d. Thrombin

128. The coagulation process is kept in check by
    a. fibrin degradation.
    b. natural inhibitors.
    c. plasminogen enzymes.
    d. prothrombin activators.

129. This test is used to monitor coumarin therapy.
    a. CBC
    b. DIC
    c. PTT
    d. PT

130. A needle puncture to a vein is normally healed by
    a. activation of factor VIII.
    b. blood clot formation.
    c. platelet plug formation.
    d. vasoconstriction.

131. Obstruction of a blood vessel by an embolus
    a. causes vessel necrosis.
    b. leads to an aneurysm.
    c. results in an embolism.
    d. produces atherosclerosis.

132. Which of the following is a coagulation test?
    a. Digoxin
    b. Hemogram
    c. Myoglobin
    d. Protime

133. Lymph fluid is most like
    a. serum.
    b. plasma.
    c. urine.
    d. whole blood.

134. Lymph fluid originates from excess
    a. blood plasma.
    b. digestive liquid.
    c. tissue fluid.
    d. urinary filtrate.

135. Lymph fluid keeps moving in the right direction because of
    a. functioning of the lymphatic ducts.
    b. lymphatic capillary structure.
    c. pressure from the arterial system.
    d. valves within the lymph vessels.

136. One function of the lymphatic system is to
    a. control all body activities.
    b. make coagulation factors.
    c. remove and destroy bacteria.
    d. secrete regulating hormones.

137. Lymph node tissue has the ability to
    a. create red blood cells.
    b. produce tissue fluid.
    c. remove impurities.
    d. secrete antibodies.

138. Lymphoid tissue is also found in the
    a. heart.
    b. kidneys.
    c. lungs.
    d. thymus.

139. A malignant lymphoid tumor is called
    a. lymphadenopathy.
    b. lymphangitis.
    c. lymphoma.
    d. lymphosarcoma.

140. This test is associated with the lymph system.
    a. Carotene
    b. Cholinesterase
    c. Lipoprotein
    d. Mononucleosis

Answers and Explanations

1. **Answer: d**

WHY: Number 1 points to the superior vena cava, the major vein that returns blood to the heart from the upper part of the body. Number 8 points to the right pulmonary arteries that take blood from the heart to the lungs (Fig. 6-7).

REVIEW: Yes ☐ No ☐

📖 *WORKBOOK Labeling Exercise 6-1 will help you learn the heart structures.*

2. **Answer: b**

WHY: Number 11 points to the left pulmonary veins, which carry oxygen-rich blood from the lungs back to the left atrium of the heart. Number 17 points to the aortic arch, through which oxygenated blood travels from the heart to the systemic system (Fig. 6-7).

REVIEW: Yes ☐ No ☐

3. **Answer: d**

WHY: Number 4 points to the tricuspid valve, also called the right atrioventricular valve, because it is between the right atrium and the right ventricle. Number 15 points to the aortic valve, located at the exit of the left ventricle, where blood is delivered to the aorta (Fig. 6-7).

REVIEW: Yes ☐ No ☐

4. **Answer: d**

WHY: Number 5 points to the right ventricle, which receives blood from the right atrium and delivers it to the pulmonary system. Number 12 points to the left atrium, which receives oxygen-rich blood from the pulmonary system and delivers it to the left ventricle (Fig. 6-7).

REVIEW: Yes ☐ No ☐

5. **Answer: a**

WHY: A major role of the circulatory system is to carry oxygen to the cells and take carbon dioxide away from the cells to the lungs for expiration. The nervous system conveys nerve impulses. Wastes are primarily excreted by the digestive system. Some waste is excreted by sweat glands

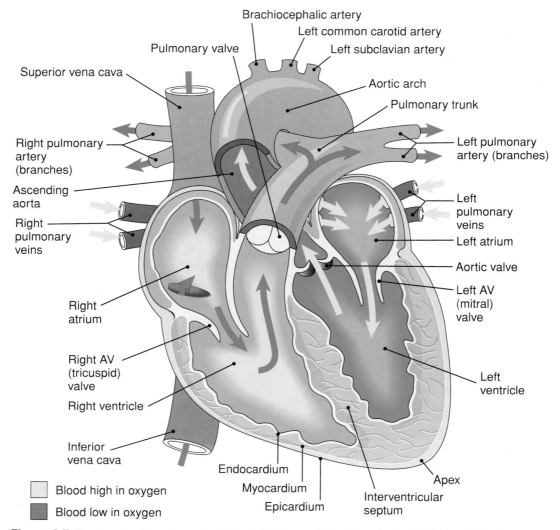

Figure 6-7 The heart and great vessels. (Adapted with permission from Cohen BJ. *Memmler's the Human Body in Health and Disease.* 12th ed. Philadelphia, PA: Lippincott Williams & Wilkins; 2013:318.)

of the skin. The formed elements (blood cells) are produced in the bone marrow of the skeletal system.

REVIEW: Yes ☐ No ☐

6. **Answer: d**

WHY: The pericardium is a double-layered sac enclosing the heart. The space between the layers is filled with fluid, which reduces friction as the heart beats. The endocardium is a thin membrane lining the inside of the heart. The epicardium is the thin outer layer of the heart. The myocardium is the thick muscular middle layer of the heart.

REVIEW: Yes ☐ No ☐

7. **Answer: c**

WHY: The heart (Fig. 6-7) has three layers. The myocardium is the thick muscular middle layer of

the heart. The endocardium, the inner layer, is the thin membrane lining the inside of the heart. The epicardium is the thin outer layer of the heart. The pericardium is the fluid-filled sac surrounding the heart.

REVIEW: Yes ☐ No ☐

8. **Answer: c**

WHY: The human heart (Fig. 6-7) has two sides, a right and a left. Each side has two chambers, an upper and a lower. The right and left upper chambers are called atria (sing., atrium) and the right and left lower chambers are called ventricles.

REVIEW: Yes ☐ No ☐

9. **Answer: b**

WHY: The ventricles, the lower chambers of the heart, are called delivering chambers because they deliver blood to the pulmonary and systemic systems. The left ventricle (Fig. 6-7) delivers oxygen-rich blood through the aortic semilunar valve to the ascending aorta, which is the beginning of the systemic system. The right ventricle delivers deoxygenated blood through the pulmonary semilunar valve to the pulmonary artery. The right and left atria receive blood from the systemic and pulmonary systems, respectively.

REVIEW: Yes ☐   No ☐

10. **Answer: c**

    WHY: The atria (sing., atrium), the upper chambers of the heart (Fig. 6-7), are called receiving chambers because they receive blood from the systemic and pulmonary systems. The right atrium receives blood from the systemic system via the superior (upper) and inferior (lower) venae cavae. The left atrium receives blood from the pulmonary system. The right and left ventricles deliver blood to the pulmonary and systemic systems, respectively.

    REVIEW: Yes ☐   No ☐

11. **Answer: a**

    WHY: The valves at the exits of the ventricles (Fig. 6-7) are called semilunar valves because each flap resembles a half-moon. The pulmonary semilunar valve is located at the exit of the right ventricle and the aortic semilunar valve is located at the exit of the left ventricle. There is no valve between the aortic arch and the aorta. The valves in the veins of the systemic system are similar to semilunar valves but are not called semilunar valves.

    REVIEW: Yes ☐   No ☐

12. **Answer: d**

    WHY: The right atrioventricular (AV) valve, located between the right atrium and the right ventricle (Fig. 6-7), is also called the tricuspid valve because it has three flaps, or cusps. The bicuspid (two cusps) valve, also called the mitral valve, is located between the left atrium and the left ventricle. The pulmonic valve is located at the exit of the right ventricle. The pulmonic valve and the aortic valve, which are located at the exit of the left atrium, are called semilunar valves because they are crescent-shaped, like a half-moon.

    REVIEW: Yes ☐   No ☐

13. **Answer: b**

    WHY: The left atrioventricular (AV) valve (Fig. 6-7) is called the bicuspid valve because it has two

cusps (flaps). It is also called the mitral valve, because the two cusps resemble a miter, the two-sided, pointed hat worn by a bishop.

REVIEW: Yes ☐   No ☐

14. **Answer: c**

    WHY: A wall that divides two cavities is called a septum. The wall that separates the right and left ventricles of the heart is called the interventricular septum (Fig. 6-7). The interatrial septum separates the right and left atria. The walls of the heart, including the septa, have a thick middle layer of muscle called the myocardium. The atrioventricular septum is a small section of septum that separates the right atrium from the left ventricle.

    REVIEW: Yes ☐   No ☐

15. **Answer: b**

    WHY: The heart does not receive oxygen or nourishment from the blood passing through it. The heart receives its blood supply from the right and left coronary arteries, which are the first branches off of the aorta, just beyond the aortic semilunar valve. The carotid arteries carry blood to the brain. The pulmonary arteries carry blood from the right ventricle to the lungs. The pulmonary veins carry blood from the lungs back to the left atrium.

    REVIEW: Yes ☐   No ☐

16. **Answer: a**

    WHY: The atrioventricular valves are attached to the walls of the ventricles by thin threads of tissue called chordae tendineae (Fig. 6-8). These keep the valves from flipping back into the atria, which helps them to close properly so that blood does not flow backward into the atria.

    REVIEW: Yes ☐   No ☐

17. **Answer: d**

    WHY: Partial obstruction of a coronary artery or one of its branches can reduce blood flow to a point where it can no longer meet the oxygen needs of the heart muscle, a condition called myocardial ischemia.

    REVIEW: Yes ☐   No ☐

18. **Answer: b**

    WHY: A heart attack is the death of heart muscle from lack of oxygen. The medical term for this is myocardial infarction (MI). (*Myocardial* means "pertaining to the heart muscle." *Infarction* means "death of tissue resulting from oxygen deprivation.") MI can be caused by complete obstruction

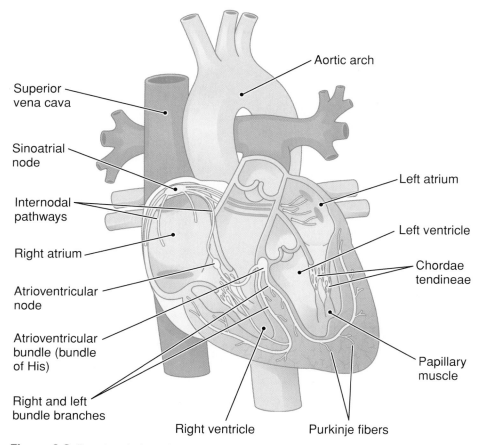

Figure 6-8 The electrical conduction system of the heart. (Adapted with permission from Cohen BJ. *Memmler's the Human Body in Health and Disease.* 12th ed. Philadelphia, PA: Lippincott Williams & Wilkins; 2013:318.)

of a coronary artery or prolonged ischemia (see the answer to question 17). Arrhythmia is an irregularity in the heart rate, rhythm, or beat. *Tachycardia* is the term for a fast heart rate of more than 100 beats per minute.

REVIEW: Yes ☐   No ☐

19. **Answer: d**

WHY: Heart contraction is initiated by an electrical impulse generated by the sinoatrial (SA) node, located in the upper wall of the right atrium (Fig. 6-8). It is called the pacemaker because it influences the rhythm and rate of the heartbeat. The bundle of His is part of the relay system that spreads the electrical impulse throughout the heart muscle. *Chorda tendinea* (pl., *chordae tendineae*) is the name for the thin thread of tissue that keeps an atrioventricular valve from flipping back into the atrium. A papillary muscle is attached to a chorda tendinea and helps open and close it.

REVIEW: Yes ☐   No ☐

20. **Answer: b**

WHY: An electrocardiogram (ECG or EKG) (Fig. 6-9) is the actual record of electrical currents that correspond to each event in heart muscle contraction. Alanine aminotransferase (ALT) is an enzyme associated with liver function. An electroencephalogram (EEG) measures electrical currents from the brain. Troponin T (TnT) is a protein released during muscle damage. Cardiac TnT (cTNT) is specific to heart muscle.

REVIEW: Yes ☐   No ☐

📖 *A list of heart disorders and diagnostic tests can be found in Box 6-1 in the TEXTBOOK.*

21. **Answer: a**

WHY: A cardiac cycle is defined as one complete contraction and relaxation of the heart. Diastole is the relaxing phase of the heart. Cardiac output is the volume of blood pumped by the heart in 1 minute. Systole is the contracting phase of the heart.

REVIEW: Yes ☐   No ☐

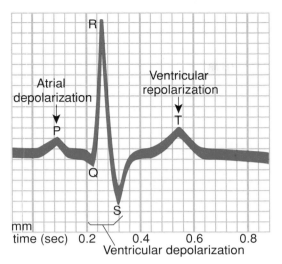

Figure 6-9 A normal ECG tracing showing one cardiac cycle. (Adapted with permission from Cohen BJ. *Memmler's the Human Body in Health and Disease.* 12th ed. Philadelphia, PA: Lippincott Williams & Wilkins; 2013:325.)

22. **Answer: c**

    WHY: The medical term for the contracting phase of the cardiac cycle is *systole*. The closing of the semilunar valves is what creates the second sound of the heartbeat. A cardiac cycle is one complete contraction and subsequent relaxation of the heart. The relaxation phase of the heart is called *diastole*.
    REVIEW: Yes ☐ No ☐

23. **Answer: b**

    WHY: The complete cardiac cycle—involving the simultaneous contraction of both atria pushing the blood into the ventricles, followed by the simultaneous contraction of the ventricles pushing the blood into the exit arteries, and then the relaxation of both—takes approximately 0.8 seconds.
    REVIEW: Yes ☐ No ☐

24. **Answer: a**

    WHY: The P wave on an electrocardiogram tracing (Fig. 6-9) represents the activity of the atria and is usually the first wave seen. The QRS complex (a collection of three waves) along with the T wave represents the activity of ventricles. The atria are called receiving chambers.
    REVIEW: Yes ☐ No ☐

25. **Answer: d**

    WHY: On an electrocardiogram tracing (Fig. 6-9), the QRS complex along with the T wave represents the electrical activity of the ventricles, whereas the P wave by itself represents the activity of the atria.
    REVIEW: Yes ☐ No ☐

26. **Answer: a**

    WHY: The closing of the atrioventricular valves as the ventricles contract results in the first sound of the heartbeat, which is a long, low-pitched sound described as a "lubb." The second sound of the heartbeat comes from the closing of the semilunar valves and is a shorter, sharper sound described as a "dupp."
    REVIEW: Yes ☐ No ☐

27. **Answer: d**

    WHY: Murmurs are abnormal heart sounds, usually caused by faulty valve action. Arrhythmias, extrasystoles, and fibrillations are abnormal contractions, not sounds.
    REVIEW: Yes ☐ No ☐

28. **Answer: b**

    WHY: The heart rate is the number of beats per minute. Average normal heart rate is around 72 beats per minute.
    REVIEW: Yes ☐ No ☐

29. **Answer: d**

    WHY: All of the choices deal with heart rate or rhythm. *Tachycardia* is an abnormally fast rate. *Bradycardia* is an abnormally slow rate. An extrasystole is an extra beat before the normal beat. *Fibrillation* is the term for rapid, uncoordinated contractions.
    REVIEW: Yes ☐ No ☐

30. **Answer: c**

    WHY: The wave of pressure created as the ventricles contract and blood is forced out of the heart and through the arteries creates the throbbing beat known as the pulse.
    REVIEW: Yes ☐ No ☐

31. **Answer: a**

    WHY: *Blood pressure* is defined as the force (pressure) exerted by the blood on the walls of the blood vessels. *Cardiac output* is the volume of blood pumped by the heart in 1 minute. *Heart rhythm* is the regularity of heart action or function. *Pulse rate* is the number of pulses per minute and normally reflects the heart rate, or number of heartbeats per minute.
    REVIEW: Yes ☐ No ☐

32. **Answer: c**

    WHY: *Sphygmomanometer* is the technical term for a blood pressure cuff. An artificial pacemaker is an implanted electrical device that automatically generates electrical impulses to initiate the heartbeat. A machine that records brain waves is used in electroencephalography (EEG). An electrocardiogram (ECG) is a record (tracing) of the electrical currents or waves that correspond to muscle contractions of the heart.

REVIEW: Yes ☐ No ☐

📖 *Practice your ability to define other Chapter 6 terms by doing Matching 6-1 in the WORKBOOK.*

33. **Answer: d**

WHY: Blood pressure is a measure of the pressure exerted on the walls of a blood vessel. It is commonly measured in a large artery, such as the brachial. Blood pressure is expressed in millimeters of mercury and has two components: the systolic pressure, which is the highest pressure reached during ventricular contraction, and the diastolic pressure, which occurs during relaxation of the ventricles. The American Heart Association defines normal blood pressure for the relaxed, sitting adult as a systolic pressure of less than 120 mm Hg and a diastolic pressure of less than 80 mm Hg.

REVIEW: Yes ☐ No ☐

34. **Answer: c**

WHY: Systolic pressure is the pressure in the arteries during contraction of the ventricles. Diastolic pressure is the arterial pressure when the ventricles are relaxed. Because atrial contraction is so very close to ventricular contraction, blood pressure during atrial contraction and relaxation cannot easily be detected and is not normally measured.

REVIEW: Yes ☐ No ☐

35. **Answer: c**

WHY: *Endocarditis* means "inflammation of the endocardium." The endocardium is the thin membrane lining the inner surface of the heart. *Angina pectoris* refers to pain in the area of the heart caused by decreased blood flow to the muscle layer of the heart. *Aortic stenosis* is the term used to describe a narrowing of the aorta or its opening. *Pericarditis* is inflammation of the pericardium, the thin, fluid-filled sac surrounding the heart.

REVIEW: Yes ☐ No ☐

36. **Answer: c**

WHY: Creatine kinase (CK) and lactate dehydrogenase (LDH) are enzymes present in cardiac muscle. They are released during myocardial infarction. Alkaline phosphatase (ALP) and alanine aminotransferase (ALT) are enzymes measured most commonly to determine liver

function. Blood urea nitrogen (BUN) is a kidney function test, and prothrombin time (PT) is a coagulation test used to monitor anticoagulant therapy. A glucose tolerance test (GTT) measures glucose metabolism, and the erythrocyte sedimentation rate (ESR) is a nonspecific indicator of disease, especially inflammatory conditions such as arthritis.

REVIEW: Yes ☐ No ☐

37. **Answer: d**

WHY: Pulmonary circulation carries deoxygenated blood from the right ventricle of the heart to the lungs via the pulmonary artery. It also returns oxygenated blood from the lungs to the left atrium of the heart via the pulmonary vein. The left ventricle pumps the oxygenated blood into the arterial systemic circulation via the aorta. The arterial systemic circulation delivers the blood to the tissues. The venous systemic circulation returns deoxygenated blood to the heart (Figs. 6-7 and 6-10).

REVIEW: Yes ☐ No ☐

38. **Answer: c**

WHY: The femoral vein accompanies the femoral artery in the leg (Fig. 6-11) and is a continuation of the popliteal vein. The brachial, cephalic, and median veins are all found in the arm.

REVIEW: Yes ☐ No ☐

📖 *Check out WORKBOOK Labeling Exercise 6-8 to see how well you can identify all the major leg veins.*

39. **Answer: a**

WHY: Arteries are vessels that carry blood away from the heart. (A way to remember this is to think "AA" for "arteries away.") Veins, such as the vena cava, carry blood to the heart. Capillaries are vessels that connect the ends of the smallest arteries (arterioles) to the smallest veins (venules).

REVIEW: Yes ☐ No ☐

40. **Answer: a**

WHY: The pulmonary vein carries oxygenated (oxygen-rich) blood from the lungs back to the heart (Fig. 6-10). All vessels that return blood to the heart are called veins. All vessels that carry blood away from the heart are called arteries. The general rule of thumb that arteries carry oxygenated blood is true only for the systemic circulation. In the pulmonary circulation, the vessel that carries oxygenated (oxygen-rich) blood from the lungs is called a vein because it is returning the blood to the heart.

REVIEW: Yes ☐ No ☐

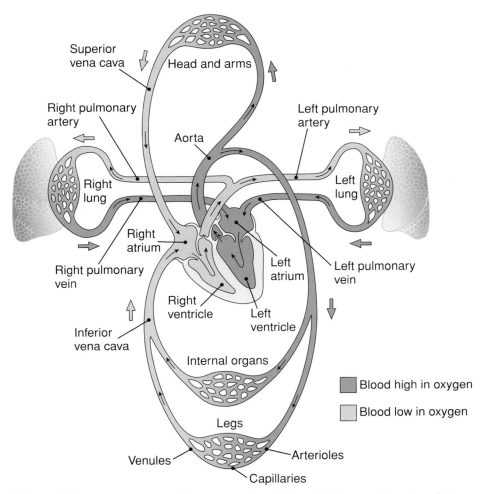

Figure 6-10 A representation of the vascular flow. (Adapted with permission from Cohen BJ. *Memmler's the Human Body in Health and Disease.* 12th ed. Philadelphia, PA: Lippincott Williams & Wilkins; 2013:303.)

41. **Answer: b**

    WHY: Because it is full of oxygen, normal systemic arterial blood is bright red. Normal systemic venous blood is dark red with a bluish tinge. Regardless of what some people think, no one has blue blood.

    REVIEW: Yes ☐   No ☐

42. **Answer: a**

    WHY: The aorta, at the start of the systemic arterial circulation, is almost 1 in wide and is the largest artery in the body. The carotid artery in the neck and the femoral artery in the leg are large arteries but not as large as the aorta. The venae cavae (sing., vena cava) are the largest veins in the body.

    REVIEW: Yes ☐   No ☐

43. **Answer: a**

    WHY: The great saphenous vein runs the entire length of the leg (Fig. 6-11) and is considered the longest vein in the body. The median cubital is a relatively short vein located in the antecubital fossa of the arm. The inferior vena cava, which returns systemic blood to the lower right atrium, is one of the largest veins in the body but not the longest. The right pulmonary vein returns oxygen-rich blood to the heart from the lungs and is nowhere near as long as the great saphenous.

    REVIEW: Yes ☐   No ☐

44. **Answer: d**

    WHY: Unlike the arteries, veins do not have sufficient pressure from the heart's contractions to keep the blood moving through them. Veins rely on movement of nearby skeletal muscles and the opening and closing of the valves within them to keep the blood moving toward the heart (Fig. 6-12). The presence of valves in veins but not arteries is a major structural difference between the arteries and veins.

    REVIEW: Yes ☐   No ☐

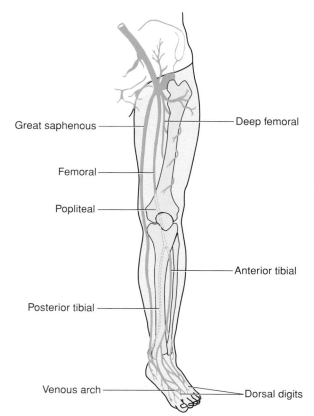

Great saphenous

Femoral

Popliteal

Posterior tibial

Venous arch

Deep femoral

Anterior tibial

Dorsal digits

Figure 6-11 The major veins of the leg and foot. (Adapted with permission from Cohen BJ. *Memmler's the Human Body in Health and Disease*. 11th ed. Philadelphia, PA: Lippincott Williams & Wilkins; 2013:348.)

45. **Answer: d**

WHY: *Venules* is the medical term for the smallest veins. The medical term for the smallest arteries is *arterioles*. Capillaries connect the arterioles (which are the end of the arterial system) to the venules (which are the beginning of venous system). *Lumen* (pl., lumina) is the term for the internal space of any tubular vessel.

REVIEW: Yes ☐ No ☐

46. **Answer: c**

WHY: Capillaries are tiny blood vessels that form the fine network that delivers oxygen and nutrients to the tissues and carries carbon dioxide and other waste products away. They are only one cell thick, which allows gases and nutrients to diffuse through their walls. Arteries, arterioles, and venules have multiple layers and are many cells thick.

REVIEW: Yes ☐ No ☐

47. **Answer: a**

WHY: Blood vessels have three main layers (Fig. 6-13). The tunica adventitia (also called the tunica externa) is the outer layer of an artery or a vein. It is made up of connective tissue and is thicker in arteries than veins. The tunica intima (also called tunica interna) is the inner layer or lining of a blood vessel; it is composed of a single layer of endothelial cells with an underlying basement membrane, a connective tissue layer, and an

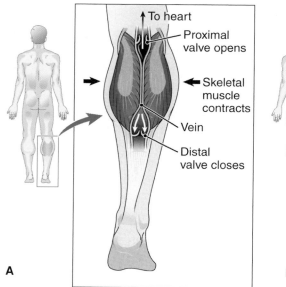

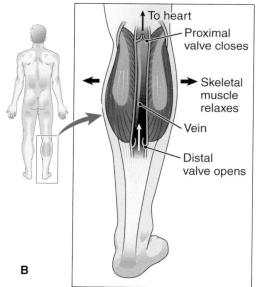

To heart
Proximal valve opens
Skeletal muscle contracts
Vein
Distal valve closes

To heart
Proximal valve closes
Skeletal muscle relaxes
Vein
Distal valve opens

A

B

Figure 6-12 The role of skeletal muscles and valves in blood return. **A:** Contracting skeletal muscle compresses the vein and drives blood forward, opening the proximal valve, whereas the distal valve closes to prevent backflow of blood. **B:** When the muscle relaxes again, the distal valve opens and the proximal valve closes until blood moving in the vein forces it open again. (Adapted with permission from Cohen BJ. *Memmler's the Human Body in Health and Disease*. 11th ed. Philadelphia, PA: Lippincott Williams & Wilkins; 2013:348.)

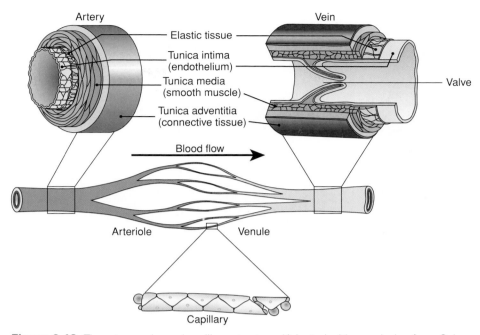

Figure 6-13 The artery, vein, and capillary structure. (Adapted with permission from Cohen BJ. *Memmler's the Human Body in Health and Disease.* 11th ed. Philadelphia, PA: Lippincott Williams & Wilkins; 2013:337.)

elastic membrane. The tunica media is the middle layer, composed of smooth muscle and some elastic fibers. The tunica media is much thicker in arteries than in veins.

REVIEW: Yes ☐ No ☐

48. **Answer: c**

WHY: *Lumen* is the term for the space within a hollow tubular structure such as a blood vessel, intestine, or blood collection needle. *Intima, interna,* and *media* are terms used in identifying blood vessel layers. The tunica intima (also called the tunica interna) is the inner layer of a blood vessel. The tunica media is the middle layer of a blood vessel.

REVIEW: Yes ☐ No ☐

49. **Answer: c**

WHY: The smooth muscle of the tunica media (middle layer) is much thicker in arteries than in veins (Fig. 6-13). The tunica adventitia, or outer layer, is also thicker in arteries. Both veins and arteries are lined with a single layer of endothelial cells. Arteries typically have more elastic tissue than veins.

REVIEW: Yes ☐ No ☐

50. **Answer: c**

WHY: Capillaries (Fig. 6-13) are the smallest blood vessels. They are one cell thick, which allows the exchange of oxygen, carbon dioxide, nutrients, and wastes between the tissue cells and the blood to take place through their walls. Alveoli are thin-walled,

saclike chambers within the lungs, where oxygen and carbon dioxide are exchanged between the air and the blood. Arterioles are tiny arteries that connect with and deliver blood to the capillaries. Venules are tiny veins at the junction where the capillaries merge with the venous circulation.

REVIEW: Yes ☐ No ☐

51. **Answer: d**

WHY: Figure 6-2 is a cross section of an artery and a vein (Fig. 6-14). The structure on the right is a vein. If you look closely, you can see the valve against the wall on the left. Arteries do not have valves. Also, the structure on the left has a very thick middle layer, which is characteristic of arteries. See Figure 6-13 for a comparison diagram of artery, vein, and capillary structure.

REVIEW: Yes ☐ No ☐

52. **Answer: c**

WHY: The right ventricle delivers blood to the pulmonary artery, which takes it to the lungs to pick up oxygen. The left ventricle delivers blood to the aorta by way of the aortic arch. The pulmonary veins carry oxygenated blood from the lungs to the left atrium of the heart (Fig. 6-10).

REVIEW: Yes ☐ No ☐

53. **Answer: b**

WHY: The pulmonary vein, part of the pulmonary circulation, carries oxygenated blood from the

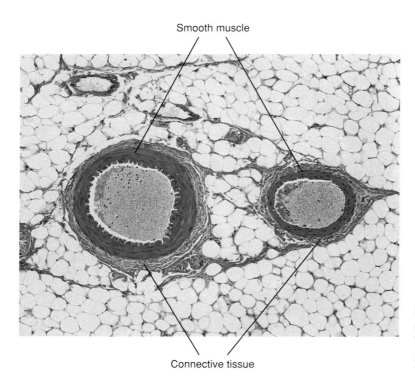

Smooth muscle

Connective tissue

Figure 6-14 A cross-section of an artery and a vein as seen through a microscope. (Reprinted with permission from Cormack DH. *Essential Histology*. 2nd ed. Philadelphia, PA: JB Lippincott; 2001, Plate 11–1.)

lungs to the heart, so that it can be delivered to the systemic circulation. The inferior vena cava delivers deoxygenated blood from the systemic venous circulation to the lower right atrium of the heart. The brachial vein is part of the systemic venous circulation carrying deoxygenated blood. The pulmonary artery carries deoxygenated blood from the heart to the lungs.

REVIEW: Yes ☐   No ☐

54. **Answer: a**

WHY: Blood flows from the heart into the arteries, which branch into smaller and smaller arteries, the smallest of which are called arterioles. Arterioles connect to the capillaries. Capillaries form the bridge between the arterial and venous circulation and are where the exchange of gases, nutrients, and waste products takes place. The opposite ends of the capillaries connect to the smallest veins, which are called venules. Venules merge with larger and larger veins until the blood returns to the heart. Choice "b" is obviously incorrect. In choices "c" and "d," the blood would be traveling in the wrong direction (Fig. 6-10).

REVIEW: Yes ☐   No ☐

55. **Answer: a**

WHY: The antecubital fossa is the area of the arm located in front of (anterior to) the elbow.

REVIEW: Yes ☐   No ☐

56. **Answer: c**

WHY: The median vein (Fig. 6-15) can be found in and below the antecubital (AC) fossa only. Although the basilic, cephalic, and subclavian veins in the arm can be found below the AC crease, they are also prominent in the upper arm.

REVIEW: Yes ☐   No ☐

57. **Answer: b**

WHY: The vein identified by number 1 is the cephalic vein. The vein identified by number 2 is the basilic vein. The vein identified by number 3 is the median cubital vein. (See the H-pattern veins in Fig. 6-16.)

REVIEW: Yes ☐   No ☐

📖 *Do WORKBOOK Labeling Exercises 6-5 and 6-6 to help you learn the names of the AC veins.*

58. **Answer: d**

WHY: The vein identified by number 1 is the median cephalic vein. The vein identified by number 2 is the median basilic vein. The vein identified by number 3 is the median vein. (See the M-pattern veins in Fig. 6-15.)

REVIEW: Yes ☐   No ☐

59. **Answer: a**

WHY: The vein identified by number 1 is the basilic vein. The veins identified by number 2 are

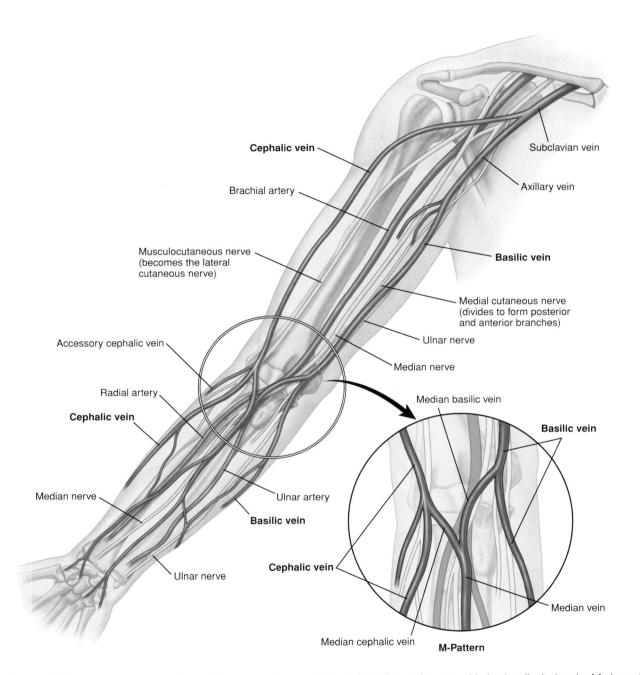

Figure 6-15 The principal veins of the right arm in anatomical position, including major antecubital veins displaying the M-shaped pattern.

the dorsal metacarpal veins. The vein identified by number 3 is the cephalic vein (Fig. 6-17).

REVIEW: Yes ☐   No ☐

60. **Answer: c**

WHY: The basilic vein is normally large, superficial, and easy to palpate. However, it is *not* well anchored, or fixed, within the surrounding tissue. This causes it to roll easily, increasing the possibility of accidental puncture of the median

nerve or the brachial artery, located close to it, and is the major reason it is the last choice for venipuncture.

REVIEW: Yes ☐   No ☐

61. **Answer: d**

WHY: The subclavian vein is in the shoulder area of the arm (Figs. 6-15 and 6-16) and merges with the brachiocephalic vein in the chest (Fig. 6-18). The cephalic vein merges with the subclavian

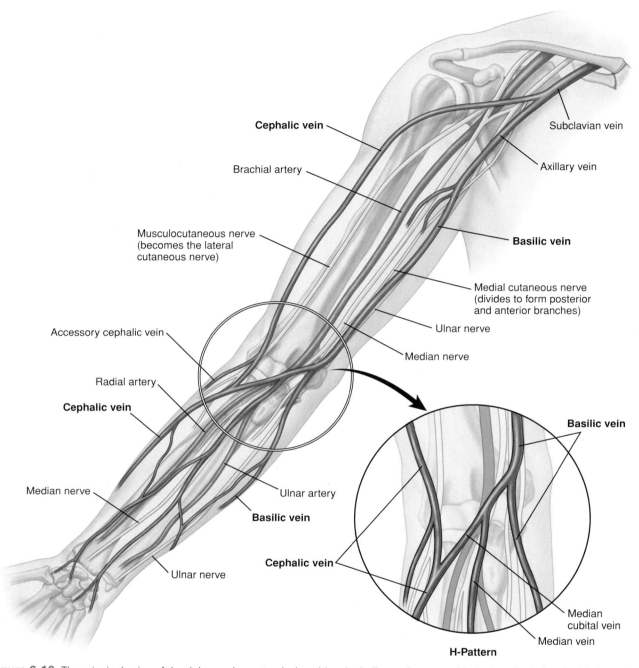

Figure 6-16 The principal veins of the right arm in anatomical position, including major antecubital veins displaying the H-shaped pattern.

vein. The popliteal and saphenous veins are in the leg (Fig. 6-11).

REVIEW: Yes ☐ No ☐

62. **Answer: a**

WHY: Both the anterior and posterior medial cutaneous nerves are very close to the basilic vein and are a major reason this vein is the very last choice for venipuncture (Figs. 6-15 and 6-16).

REVIEW: Yes ☐ No ☐

63. **Answer: d**

WHY: The median cubital, cephalic, and basilic are in the correct order of selection for veins in the H pattern. In choosing the best vein in the H pattern, the first selection is the median cubital because it is large and well anchored and therefore does not bruise easily and is least painful to puncture. The cephalic vein is the next choice because it is fairly well anchored and less painful to puncture than the basilic. The basilic vein

Dorsal Forearm, Wrist, and Hand Veins

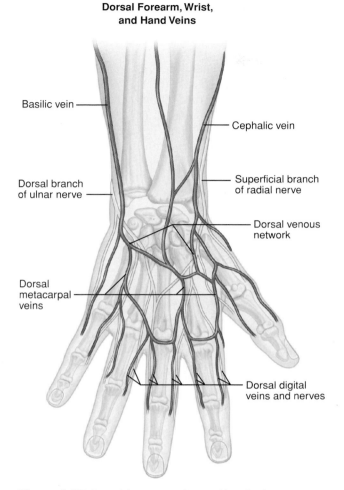

Figure 6-17 Dorsal forearm, wrist, and hand veins.

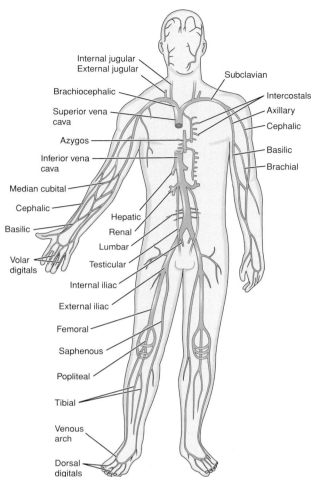

Figure 6-18 The principal veins of the body. (Adapted with permission from Cohen BJ. *Memmler's the Human Body in Health and Disease.* 12th ed. Philadelphia, PA: Lippincott Williams & Wilkins; 2013:343.)

is the last choice because it rolls and bruises easily, is more painful to puncture, and there is the possibility of accidentally hitting the brachial artery and a major nerve when accessing it (Figs. 6-15 and 6-16). According to the CLSI, the basilic vein should not be selected unless the other veins on both arms have been eliminated. The median basilic is an M-pattern vein.

REVIEW: Yes ☐   No ☐

64. **Answer: b**

WHY: When the hand is prone, the palm faces downward, causing the antecubital portion of the cephalic vein to be in line with the little finger. When the arm is in the normal anatomical position, the palm is up and the cephalic vein is on the same side as the thumb.

REVIEW: Yes ☐   No ☐

65. **Answer: b**

WHY: Leg, ankle, and foot veins should *never* be punctured routinely. Serious problems can result

if ankle or foot veins of patients with coagulation problems or poor circulation are used for venipuncture. Test results can also be affected. If no other sites are available, the patient's physician *must* be consulted and permission obtained before performing venipuncture on a leg, ankle, or foot vein of *any* patient.

REVIEW: Yes ☐   No ☐

66. **Answer: d**

WHY: The popliteal vein is located deep in the leg (Fig. 6-11) in the area behind the knee. It is a continuation of the femoral vein.

REVIEW: Yes ☐   No ☐

67. **Answer: c**

WHY: *Embolus* is the medical term for a blood clot or other undissolved matter circulating in the bloodstream. An aneurysm is a bulging or dilation of a blood vessel. An embolism is the obstruction of a blood vessel by an embolus. A thrombus is a stationary blood clot that obstructs or partially obstructs a blood vessel.

REVIEW: Yes ☐ No ☐

68. **Answer: c**

WHY: Phlebitis is the medical term for inflammation of a vein. The term comes from the word root *phleb,* "vein," and the suffix *-itis,* "inflammation." An embolism is the obstruction of a blood vessel by a blood clot or other undissolved foreign matter. Hemostasis is the process of stopping bleeding. Thrombosis is the formation or existence of a blood clot in the vascular system.

REVIEW: Yes ☐ No ☐

69. **Answer: c**

WHY: DIC is the abbreviation for disseminated intravascular coagulation. A DIC test or screen is actually a series of tests used to detect diffuse, uncontrolled coagulation throughout the vascular system. In DIC, continuous generation of thrombin causes depletion of several clotting factors to such an extent that generalized bleeding may occur. Antidiuretic hormone (ADH) is an endocrine system test. A cerebrospinal fluid (CSF) analysis is a nervous system test. Rapid plasma reagin (RPR), a syphilis test, is a reproductive system test.

REVIEW: Yes ☐ No ☐

📖 *A list of vascular system tests can be found in Box 6-3 in the TEXTBOOK.*

70. **Answer: a**

WHY: Atherosclerosis is a form of arteriosclerosis involving changes in the intima of the artery caused by the accumulation of lipid, cholesterol, and calcium material. Cholesterol is a substance produced by the liver; it is also found in animal products such as meat and eggs. It is an essential part of lipid metabolism, but high blood levels increase the risk of developing atherosclerosis. Endocarditis is inflammation of the membrane that lines the inside of the heart. Lipemia is a condition in which there is an abnormal amount of fat in the blood.

REVIEW: Yes ☐ No ☐

71. **Answer: a**

WHY: *Aneurysm* is a medical term for a localized dilation or bulging of a blood vessel, usually an artery. An embolism is the obstruction of a blood vessel by a blood clot or other undissolved foreign matter. Arteriosclerosis is a hardening or thickening and loss of elasticity of the wall of the artery.

Thrombophlebitis is defined as inflammation of the vein in conjunction with the formation of a blood clot.

REVIEW: Yes ☐ No ☐

72. **Answer: c**

WHY: The word root *thromb* means "clot." Phlebitis is inflammation of a vein. The meaning of thrombophlebitis is "inflammation of a vein in conjunction with the formation of a blood clot." Atherosclerosis is a form of arteriosclerosis involving changes in the intima of the artery. Phlebosclerosis is the fibrous hardening of vein walls. *Vasculitis* is a general term meaning "inflammation of blood vessels."

REVIEW: Yes ☐ No ☐

73. **Answer: c**

WHY: The average 154-lb adult has approximately 5 L, or 5.2 quarts, of blood. A more exact blood volume can be calculated on the basis of the fact that the average adult has 70 mL of blood for each kilogram of weight.

REVIEW: Yes ☐ No ☐

74. **Answer: c**

WHY: The normal ratio of plasma to formed elements is approximately 55% plasma and 45% cells. This means that approximately half of a normal blood specimen is serum (in a clot tube) or plasma (in an anticoagulant tube), which is important in determining how much blood to collect for testing purposes.

REVIEW: Yes ☐ No ☐

75. **Answer: b**

WHY: A plasma specimen is obtained by centrifuging blood collected in an anticoagulant tube. Centrifugation separates the cells from the liquid (plasma) portion of the specimen, which is a clear to slightly hazy (due to fibrinogen), pale-yellow fluid that is 91% water and 9% solutes (dissolved substances).

REVIEW: Yes ☐ No ☐

76. **Answer: b**

WHY: Blood is a mixture of fluid and cells. The fluid portion, *plasma,* is approximately 91% water and 9% dissolved substances such as antibodies, nutrients, minerals, and gases. Red blood cells, white blood cells, and platelets make up the cellular portion of blood, referred to as the *formed elements.* Bacteria are not found in the blood under normal circumstances because the immune

Granulocytes

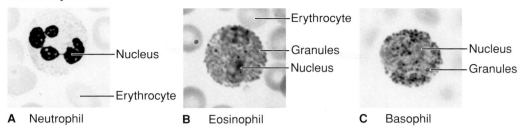

A Neutrophil   B Eosinophil   C Basophil

Figure 6-19 Granulocytes. **A:** Neutrophil. **B:** Eosinophil. **C:** Basophil. (Adapted with permission from Cohen BJ. *Memmler's the Human Body in Health and Disease.* 12th ed. Philadelphia, PA: Lippincott Williams & Wilkins; 2013:292.)

system recognizes them as foreign and destroys them.

REVIEW: Yes ☐ No ☐

77. **Answer: b**

WHY: All leukocytes (white blood cells) contain nuclei. Thrombocytes (platelets) and mature erythrocytes (red blood cells) do not have nuclei. A reticulocyte is an immature red blood cell that contains remnants of nuclear material but not a complete nucleus.

REVIEW: Yes ☐ No ☐

78. **Answer: c**

WHY: Reticulocytes are immature red blood cells that contain remnants of RNA and other material from their nuclear phase in the bone marrow. The remnants can be seen when blood is stained with a special stain used to perform a manual reticulocyte count.

REVIEW: Yes ☐ No ☐

79. **Answer: b**

WHY: An eosinophil (Fig. 6-19B) is a type of granulocytic white blood cell that can ingest and detoxify foreign protein and help turn off immune reactions. Consequently, eosinophils (Eos) increase in numbers during allergic reactions and infestations of parasites such as pinworms.

REVIEW: Yes ☐ No ☐

80. **Answer: b**

WHY: Normal erythrocytes (Fig. 6-20) are described as anuclear biconcave discs that are approximately 7 to 8 microns in diameter.

REVIEW: Yes ☐ No ☐

81. **Answer: a**

WHY: Red blood cells (erythrocytes) are normally the most numerous formed elements in the blood (Figs. 6-20 and 6-21), averaging 4.5 to 5.0 million/mm^3

of blood. Therefore, an erythrocyte count of 4.5 million/mm^3 would be considered normal.

REVIEW: Yes ☐ No ☐

82. **Answer: b**

WHY: The production and development of red blood cells (erythrocytes) occurs in the bone marrow by a process called erythropoiesis.

REVIEW: Yes ☐ No ☐

83. **Answer: d**

WHY: The primary function of red blood cells is to transport oxygen from the lungs to the tissues. A secondary function of red blood cells is to transport carbon dioxide from the tissues to the lungs. Nutrients are dissolved in the plasma, not transported by red blood cells. Certain white blood cells, but not red blood cells, produce antibodies.

REVIEW: Yes ☐ No ☐

84. **Answer: d**

WHY: The medical term for a white blood cell is *leukocyte.* The word root *leuk* means "white," and the suffix *-cyte* means "cell."

REVIEW: Yes ☐ No ☐

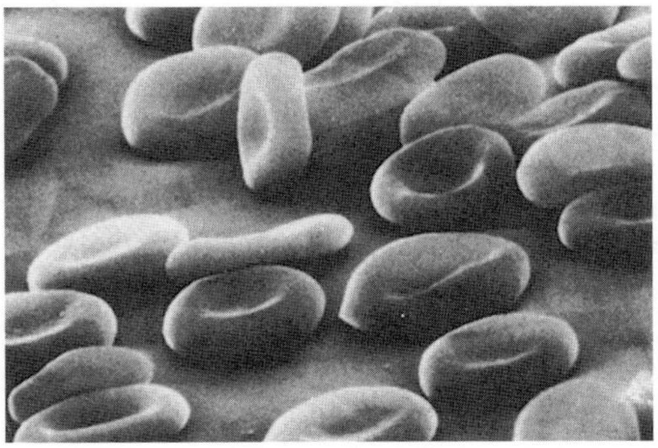

Figure 6-20 Red blood cells as seen under a scanning electron microscope. (Adapted with permission from Cohen BJ. *Memmler's the Human Body in Health and Disease.* 12th ed. Philadelphia, PA: Lippincott Williams & Wilkins; 2013:290.)

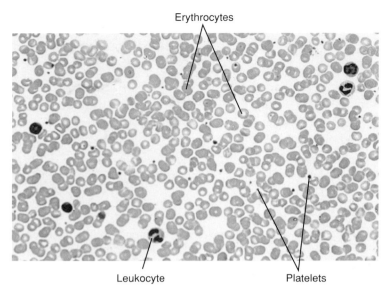

Erythrocytes

Leukocyte

Platelets

Figure 6-21 Blood cells in a stained blood smear as seen under a microscope. (Reprinted with permission from Eroschenko VP. *diFiore's Atlas of Histology.* Philadelphia, PA: Lippincott Williams & Wilkins; 2013:5.)

85. **Answer: b**

WHY: Leukocytes have extravascular function, which means that they do their job outside of the bloodstream. They are able to leave the bloodstream and pass through the spaces between the cells in the walls of blood vessels by a process called diapedesis. Erythrocytes, reticulocytes, and thrombocytes have intravascular function and cannot pass through intact blood vessel walls.

REVIEW: Yes ☐ No ☐

86. **Answer: b**

WHY: The main function of white blood cells (WBCs) is to neutralize or destroy pathogens. Neutrophils (Fig. 6-19A) are a type of WBC that destroys pathogens by phagocytosis, a process in which a pathogen or other foreign matter is surrounded, engulfed, and destroyed by the WBC. This process is also used to remove disintegrated tissue.

REVIEW: Yes ☐ No ☐

87. **Answer: d**

WHY: Neutrophils (Fig. 6-19A) are polymorphonuclear (PMN), which means they have a nucleus that has several lobes connected by thin strands. Another term for this type of nucleus is *segmented.* Consequently, neutrophils are often called polys, PMNs, or segs for short.

REVIEW: Yes ☐ No ☐

88. **Answer: c**

WHY: Injury to a blood vessel exposes protein material in the vessel wall. Contact with this material causes platelets (Fig. 6-22) to degranulate

and stick to one another (platelet aggregation) and to the injured area (platelet adhesion). This results in the formation of a platelet plug that temporarily seals off the injury. If the injury is large, a fibrin clot that includes all of the formed elements (RBCs, WBCs, and platelets) is eventually generated.

REVIEW: Yes ☐ No ☐

89. **Answer: a**

WHY: Erythrocytes (red blood cells) (Figs. 6-20 and 6-21) are described as being anuclear (nonnucleated), biconcave (curved inward on both sides) discs approximately 7 to 8 microns in diameter.

REVIEW: Yes ☐ No ☐

90. **Answer: d**

WHY: Monocytes (Fig. 6-23B) that have left the bloodstream are sometimes referred to as macrophages because they are found in loose connective tissue, where they phagocytize (engulf and

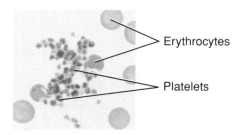

Erythrocytes

Platelets

Platelets

Figure 6-22 Platelets (thrombocytes) in a stained blood smear. (Adapted with permission from Cohen BJ. *Memmler's the Human Body in Health and Disease.* 12th ed. Philadelphia, PA: Lippincott Williams & Wilkins; 2013:294.)

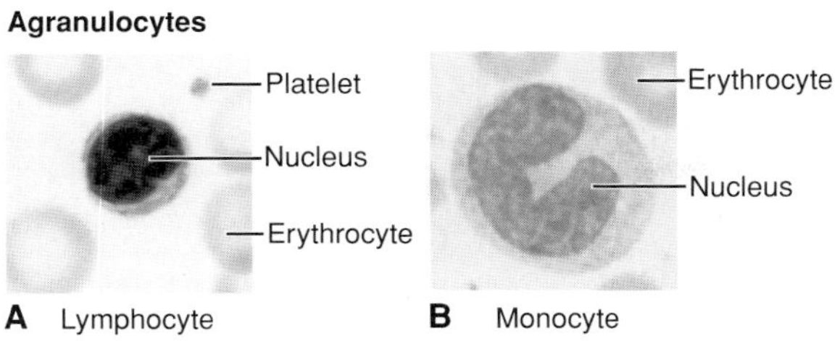

Agranulocytes

Platelet
Nucleus
Erythrocyte

A Lymphocyte

Erythrocyte
Nucleus

B Monocyte

Figure 6-23 Agranulocytes. **A:** Lymphocyte. **B:** Monocyte. (Adapted with permission from Cohen BJ. *Memmler's the Human Body in Health and Disease.* 12th ed. Philadelphia, PA: Lippincott Williams & Wilkins; 2013:292.)

destroy) particles, much like cells of the reticulo-endothelial (RE) system.
REVIEW: Yes ☐ No ☐

91. **Answer: b**
WHY: Lymphocytes (Fig. 6-23A) play a role in immunity and are the second most numerous type of WBC. There are two main types of lymphocytes: T lymphocytes, which directly attack infected cells, and B lymphocytes, which differentiate into plasma cells. Plasma cells produce antibodies that are released into the bloodstream, where they circulate and attack foreign antigens.
REVIEW: Yes ☐ No ☐

92. **Answer: c**
WHY: The number of platelets (Fig. 6-22) in the blood of the average adult is between 150,000 and 400,000 per cubic millimeter (mm^3). Therefore, a platelet count of 300,000/mm^3 is considered normal.
REVIEW: Yes ☐ No ☐

93. **Answer: d**
WHY: *Thromb* means "clotting" and cyte means "cell." *Thrombocyte* is the medical term for platelets, which are cells that function in the clotting process.
REVIEW: Yes ☐ No ☐

📖 *Try your skill at identifying the meaning of other medical terms with WORKBOOK Skills Drill 6-2.*

94. **Answer: c**
WHY: A platelet is not a true cell but a fragment of a large bone marrow cell called a megakaryocyte. When separated into parts (mega-karyo-cyte), this term means "large-nucleated cell."
REVIEW: Yes ☐ No ☐

95. **Answer: b**
WHY: The formed elements are red blood cells, white blood cells, and platelets. The erythrocyte

(red blood cell) is normally the most numerous formed element in the blood, averaging 4.5 to 5.0 million/mm^3 of blood. See Figure 6-21.
REVIEW: Yes ☐ No ☐

96. **Answer: c**
WHY: Human blood type, which is inherited, is determined by the presence or absence of certain types of antigens on the surface of the red blood cells. The ABO blood group system recognizes four blood types based on two antigens called A and B. Type A individuals have the A antigen, type B have the B antigen, type AB have both antigens, and type O have neither A nor B antigen. The Rh system is based on the presence or absence of the Rh antigen. Rh-positive individuals have the Rh antigen, and Rh-negative individuals lack the Rh antigen.
REVIEW: Yes ☐ No ☐

97. **Answer: b**
WHY: Rh sensitization means an Rh-negative individual has been exposed to Rh-positive blood and is thus able to produce antibodies directed against the Rh factor. To prevent sensitization from an Rh-positive fetus, an Rh-negative woman may be given Rh immunoglobulin at certain times during her pregnancy as well as immediately after the baby's birth. Rh immunoglobulin destroys any Rh-positive fetal cells that may have entered her bloodstream, thus preventing sensitization. Only an Rh-negative person can become sensitized to the Rh factor. Carrying an Rh-negative fetus will not cause sensitization.
REVIEW: Yes ☐ No ☐

98. **Answer: a**
WHY: Becoming sensitized means that the individual may produce antibodies against the Rh factor. Rh antibodies produced by the mother and circulating in her bloodstream can cross the placenta into the fetal circulation and cause the agglutination (Fig. 6-24) and destruction of red blood cells in an Rh-positive fetus.
REVIEW: Yes ☐ No ☐

99. **Answer: a**
WHY: The red blood cells of an individual whose blood type is A-negative have the A antigen but lack the Rh antigen. (See the answer to question 96.)
REVIEW: Yes ☐ No ☐

100. **Answer: c**
WHY: Hemolytic disease of the newborn (HDN) is most often the result of an Rh-negative mother

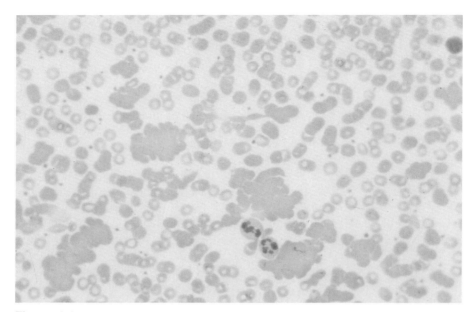

Figure 6-24 Stained blood smear with a number of large clumps of agglutinated red blood cells. (Reprinted with permission from Anderson S, Poulsen K. *Anderson's Atlas of Hematology*. 2nd ed. Philadelphia, PA: Lippincott Williams & Wilkins; 2013.)

being sensitized by a previous Rh-positive fetus, causing her to form Rh antibodies. During a subsequent pregnancy, these antibodies can cross the placenta into the fetal circulation, attack the red blood cells of the fetus, and cause hemolysis.
REVIEW: Yes ☐ No ☐

101. **Answer: c**
WHY: Whole blood, like blood circulating in the bloodstream, consists of liquid called plasma with the formed elements (red blood cells, white blood cells, and platelets) suspended in it. The liquid is called plasma because it still contains fibrinogen and other coagulation factors.
REVIEW: Yes ☐ No ☐

102. **Answer: d**
WHY: A clotted blood specimen is actually made up of two parts, a clotted portion containing cells enmeshed in fibrin and a liquid portion called serum. The liquid portion is called serum because it does not contain fibrinogen. The fibrinogen was used up in the process of clot formation.
REVIEW: Yes ☐ No ☐

103. **Answer: a**
WHY: The buffy coat of a whole-blood specimen is made up of white blood cells and platelets. Therefore, a specimen with an abnormally large buffy coat has either a high white blood cell count or a high platelet count.
REVIEW: Yes ☐ No ☐

104. **Answer: b**
WHY: A whole-blood specimen is collected in an anticoagulant such as EDTA to keep it from clotting. If the specimen is centrifuged or allowed to settle, the clear liquid portion at the top of the specimen is called plasma. Arrow number 1 in Figure 6-6 points to the top portion of the specimen, which is the plasma.
REVIEW: Yes ☐ No ☐

105. **Answer: a**
WHY: Arrow number 2 in Figure 6-6 points to the thin layer of white blood cells and platelets, commonly called the buffy coat, on top of the red blood cells.
REVIEW: Yes ☐ No ☐

106. **Answer: d**
WHY: You cannot visually tell serum from plasma because both serum and plasma are mostly clear, pale-yellow fluids. Plasma is sometimes slightly hazy because of the fibrinogen in it, but serum may also be slightly hazy when fats are present, a condition called lipemia.
REVIEW: Yes ☐ No ☐

107. **Answer: c**
WHY: An eosinophil (Fig. 6-19B) is a type of WBC called a granulocyte because it has granules that are easily visible when viewed on a blood slide stained with a special stain called Wright stain.

Eosinophil granules are large and bead-like and stain bright orange-pink.

REVIEW: Yes ☐   No ☐

108. **Answer: a**

WHY: Coagulation tests are concerned with the blood-clotting process, which involves the activation and interaction of a series of components called coagulation factors. Most coagulation tests (except some point-of-care tests that are performed on whole blood) are performed on plasma because it contains coagulation factors. Serum is obtained from clotted blood and cannot be used for most coagulation tests because the coagulation factors (i.e., fibrinogen) are consumed or partially consumed when blood clots.

REVIEW: Yes ☐   No ☐

109. **Answer: a**

WHY: A fast turnaround time (TAT) is vitally important for stat requests. Serum is ideal for most chemistry tests because nothing has been added to the blood during collection; but to obtain serum, a normal blood specimen must be allowed to clot completely before it can be centrifuged. This can take from 30 to 60 minutes. Blood from patients receiving blood thinners may take even longer. The 30 minutes or more can mean the difference between life and death in a stat situation. With the exception of fibrinogen and other coagulation factors, plasma contains the same analytes as serum. However, because a plasma specimen does not clot, it can be spun (centrifuged) immediately upon reaching the laboratory and therefore tested much sooner.

REVIEW: Yes ☐   No ☐

110. **Answer: b**

WHY: A complete blood count (CBC) is a multipart test that includes erythrocyte, leukocyte, and platelet counts. It is always performed on whole blood because the cells cannot be identified or counted in blood that is clotted. A blood urea nitrogen (BUN) and lactate dehydrogenase (LDL) are chemistry tests that are typically performed on serum. A PTT test is a coagulation test performed on plasma because it contains clotting factors. A PTT can also be performed on whole blood from a fingerstick using a special machine.

REVIEW: Yes ☐   No ☐

111. **Answer: d**

WHY: A partial thromboplastin test (PTT) is a coagulation test performed on plasma because plasma contains clotting factors. A PTT can also be performed on whole blood from a fingerstick using a special machine. A CBC, erythrocyte sedimentation rate (ESR), and hemoglobin (Hgb) are hematology tests that require a whole-blood EDTA specimen.

REVIEW: Yes ☐   No ☐

112. **Answer: c**

WHY: To obtain serum, blood must be allowed to clot. Consequently, serum specimens are collected in tubes that do not contain an anticoagulant. During the clotting process, fibrinogen is split into fibrin, which enmeshes the cells to form the clot. Once the clotting is complete, the specimen is centrifuged; the normally clear, pale-yellow liquid obtained is called serum. Serum does not contain fibrinogen because it was used up in the clotting process. Most hematology tests are performed on whole-blood specimens collected in EDTA tubes, not on serum.

REVIEW: Yes ☐   No ☐

113. **Answer: c**

WHY: *Thromb, cyt,* and *osis* mean "clotting," "cell," and "condition," respectively. Thrombocytosis is a condition in which the clotting cells (platelets) are abnormally increased.

REVIEW: Yes ☐   No ☐

114. **Answer: a**

WHY: Anemia is a blood disorder usually characterized by an abnormal reduction in the number of red blood cells in the circulating blood. Leukemia is a disorder characterized by an abnormal increase in white blood cell (WBC) numbers along with an increase in abnormal forms of WBCs. Polycythemia is overproduction of red blood cells. Thrombocytopenia is abnormally decreased platelets.

REVIEW: Yes ☐   No ☐

115. **Answer: b**

WHY: The formed elements are red blood cells, white blood cells, and platelets. Assessing the formed elements is part of a hematology test called a complete blood count (CBC). The antistreptolysin (ASO) test checks for the antibody against streptolysin O, a red blood cell–destroying substance produced by a certain type of streptococcus. Electrolytes ("lytes") is a panel of chemistry tests that measure ions in the blood, most commonly sodium, potassium, chloride, and bicarbonate. Serum protein electrophoresis (SPEP) is a chemistry test that identifies various protein components in a serum specimen.

REVIEW: Yes ☐   No ☐

116. **Answer: b**

   WHY: When broken into parts, *leuko-cyt-osis* means "white cell condition." The term is used to describe an abnormal increase of white blood cells. Leukemia is a disorder characterized by an abnormal increase in WBC numbers along with an increase in abnormal WBC forms. Leukopenia is an abnormal decrease in WBC numbers. Leukopoiesis is leukocyte production.

   REVIEW: Yes ☐   No ☐

117. **Answer: c**

   WHY: Ferritin, the form in which iron is stored in the tissues, is a whole-blood chemistry test that is also used in the diagnosis of blood disorders. Creatinine is a kidney function test performed in the chemistry department. Bilirubin is a chemistry test used to diagnose or monitor liver function. Glucose is a chemistry test used in the diagnosis of diabetes, hypoglycemia, and other disorders of carbohydrate metabolism.

   REVIEW: Yes ☐   No ☐

118. **Answer: c**

   WHY: *Hemostasis* means "stopping or controlling the flow of blood." Coagulation plays a major role in hemostasis. Hemolysis is the destruction of red blood cells. Hemopoiesis is the production and maturation of red blood cells. Homeostasis is the state of equilibrium or balance the body strives to maintain.

   REVIEW: Yes ☐   No ☐

119. **Answer: a**

   WHY: *Platelet aggregation* is the term used to describe the ability of platelets to stick to each other. Platelet adhesion is the ability of platelets to stick to surfaces. The property of adhering is called cohesion. Inhibition is the stopping or suppression of a function.

   REVIEW: Yes ☐   No ☐

120. **Answer: a**

   WHY: Ions are particles that carry an electrical charge. The coagulation process requires the presence of calcium ions, which have a positive charge, for proper function. Chloride, sodium, and potassium are also ions. They function in other body processes, however.

   REVIEW: Yes ☐   No ☐

121. **Answer: c**

   WHY: The word *extrinsic* means "originating outside." The extrinsic/contact activation coagulation pathway is initiated by cell-based tissue factor

(TF). TF is normally outside the bloodstream but is exposed to the blood as a result of tissue injury. Platelet aggregation is part of platelet plug formation, which occurs as a result of TF initiation of the coagulation process.

   REVIEW: Yes ☐   No ☐

122. **Answer: d**

   WHY: The first response in the hemostatic process (Fig. 6-25) is the constriction of blood vessels (vasoconstriction) to slow down blood loss. Platelet adhesion, thrombin generation, and the conversion of fibrinogen to fibrin occur during the second response, which is platelet plug formation. Thrombin generation and fibrin formation also take place during the third response, which is hemostatic plug formation. The fourth response is fibrinolysis, the process that dissolves (i.e., degrades) the fibrin clot after the site heals.

   REVIEW: Yes ☐   No ☐

123. **Answer: b**

   WHY: Platelet adhesion and aggregation take place in the initiation phase of the coagulation process, which results in the formation of the platelet plug. The amplification and propagation phases involve the formation of the stable blood clot called the hemostatic plug. Termination of coagulation is the end result of the propagation phase and also the work of natural inhibitors.

   REVIEW: Yes ☐   No ☐

   📖 *Find the latest information on the coagulation process in Chapter 6 of the TEXTBOOK.*

124. **Answer: a**

   WHY: Aspirin (salicylic acid) inhibits platelet activation (and blood clotting in general) and is often prescribed as a "blood *thinner*" or "*antiplatelet agent*" to those at risk of heart attack or stroke.

   REVIEW: Yes ☐   No ☐

125. **Answer: a**

   WHY: Hemophilia is a hereditary blood disorder characterized by very long bleeding times. The most common type of hemophilia is caused by the lack of clotting factor VIII. Disseminated intravascular coagulation (DIC) is a pathological form of diffuse rather than local coagulation in which coagulation factors are consumed to such an extent that bleeding occurs. Thrombocytopenia is an abnormally decreased number of platelets. Varicose veins—swollen, knotted veins—are not a coagulation disorder.

   REVIEW: Yes ☐   No ☐

The Hemostatic Process

Vasoconstriction

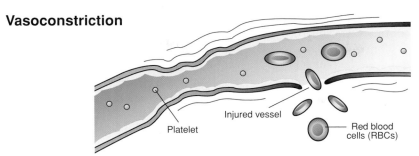

Primary Platelet Plug Formation

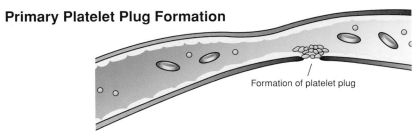

Secondary Hemostatic Plug Formation

Fibrinolysis

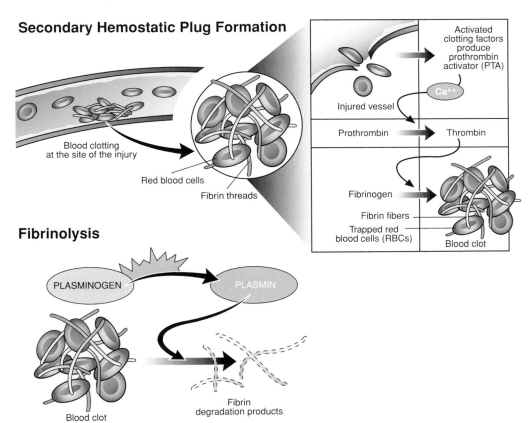

Figure 6-25 The hemostastatic process.

126. Answer: b

WHY: The liver plays a major role in coagulation. It manufactures the clotting factors fibrinogen and prothrombin and is the source of heparin, a naturally formed anticoagulant found in the bloodstream.

REVIEW: Yes ☐ No ☐

127. Answer: d

WHY: Thrombin functions throughout the coagulation process. Its major role is to convert fibrinogen to soluble fibrin, but it also intensifies coagulation, supports platelet plug formation, activates protein C to stop its formation, and initiates the breakdown of the fibrin clot by its role in plasmin production. Plasmin is an enzyme that causes clot lysis in the last hemostatic response to injury, fibrinolysis. Heparin is a natural anticoagulant. Fibrin is an elastic, threadlike protein that reinforces the platelet plug and the blood clot.

REVIEW: Yes ☐ No ☐

128. **Answer: b**

WHY: Substances called natural inhibitors circulate in the plasma along with the coagulation factors. They normally keep the coagulation process in check and limited to local sites by binding with activated coagulation factors that escape the clotting site.

REVIEW: Yes ☐ No ☐

129. **Answer: d**

WHY: The protime (PT) test evaluates extrinsic pathway function and is used to monitor coumarin therapy. A complete blood count (CBC) is a hematology test that evaluates the formed elements. DIC stands for disseminated intravascular coagulation, which is evaluated with a test called a DIC screen. The test for the activated partial thromboplastin time (APTT or PTT) evaluates the intrinsic coagulation pathway and is used to monitor heparin therapy.

REVIEW: Yes ☐ No ☐

130. **Answer: c**

WHY: For some injuries such as a needle puncture to a vein, platelet plug formation in the initiation phase of the coagulation process is enough to seal the site until healing occurs, in which case the coagulation process goes no further. For larger injuries, the process continues to hemostatic plug (blood clot) formation, which involves activation of a series of coagulation factors (including factor VIII). Vasoconstriction plays a role in reducing blood flow in the immediate area of injury to prevent blood from escaping the vessel but by itself is not enough to seal an injury.

REVIEW: Yes ☐ No ☐

131. **Answer: c**

WHY: A circulating blood clot, part of a clot, or other mass of undissolved matter is called an embolus. The sudden obstruction of a blood vessel by an embolus is called an embolism.

REVIEW: Yes ☐ No ☐

132. **Answer: d**

WHY: A protime (PT), also called a prothrombin time, is a coagulation test. Digoxin is a chemistry test for a drug of the same name that is used in patients with certain heart problems. A hemogram is a type of hematology report that lists the results of a complete blood count. Myoglobin is an oxygen-binding protein found in cardiac and skeletal muscle.

REVIEW: Yes ☐ No ☐

133. **Answer: b**

WHY: Lymph fluid is similar to plasma but is 95% water instead of 90%. Plasma is unlike serum because it contains fibrinogen and serum does not. The composition of lymph fluid is very different from the composition of whole blood and urine.

REVIEW: Yes ☐ No ☐

134. **Answer: c**

WHY: Body cells are bathed in tissue fluid acquired from the bloodstream. Much of the fluid diffuses back into the capillaries along with waste products of metabolism. Excess tissue fluid filters into lymphatic capillaries, where it is called lymph.

REVIEW: Yes ☐ No ☐

135. **Answer: d**

WHY: Lymph fluid moves through lymph vessels primarily by skeletal muscle contraction, much as blood moves through the veins. Like veins, the lymph vessels have valves to keep the lymph flowing in the right direction.

REVIEW: Yes ☐ No ☐

136. **Answer: c**

WHY: The lymphatic system (Fig. 6-26) returns tissue fluid to the bloodstream, protects the body by removing microorganisms and impurities, processes lymphocytes, and delivers fats absorbed from the small intestine to the bloodstream. The lymphatic system *does not* control all body activities, make coagulation factors, or secrete regulating hormones.

REVIEW: Yes ☐ No ☐

137. **Answer: c**

WHY: Lymph node tissue (*lymphoid tissue*) is a special kind of tissue that is able to trap microorganisms, remove impurities, and process lymphocytes. It does *not* have the ability to create red blood cells, produce tissue fluid, or secrete antibodies.

REVIEW: Yes ☐ No ☐

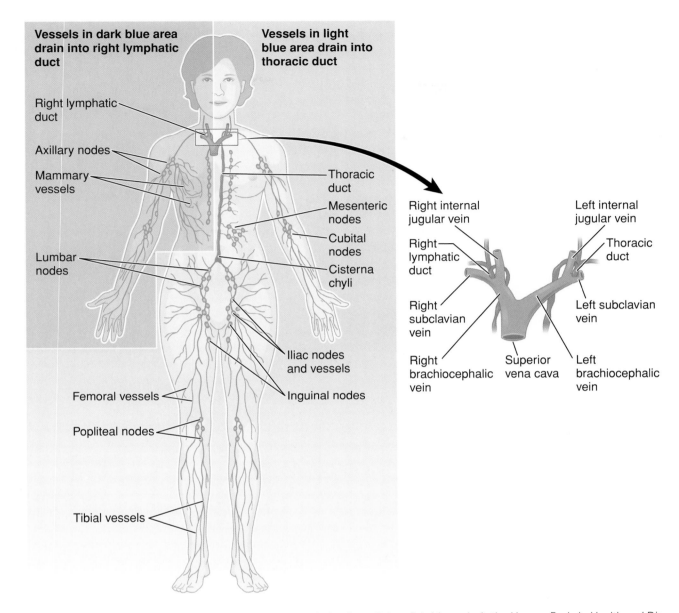

Figure 6-26 The lymphatic system. (Adapted with permission from Cohen BJ. *Memmler's the Human Body in Health and Disease.* 12th ed. Philadelphia, PA: Lippincott Williams & Wilkins; 2013:366.)

138. Answer: d

WHY: Lymphoid tissue is also found in other areas of the body, including the thymus, tonsils, gastro-intestinal tract, and spleen. It is not found in the heart, lungs, or kidneys.

REVIEW: Yes ☐ No ☐

📖 *Find out more about the lymphatic system in Chapter 6 of the TEXTBOOK.*

139. Answer: d

WHY: *Lymphosarcoma* is the medical term for a malignant lymphoid tumor. The word parts

lympho-sarc-oma combine to mean "lymphoid fleshy malignant tumor."

REVIEW: Yes ☐ No ☐

140. Answer: d

WHY: Mononucleosis is an acute infectious disease that primarily affects lymphoid tissue. The mononucleosis (mono) test is the most common test associated with the lymph system.

REVIEW: Yes ☐ No ☐

Chapter 7

Blood Collection Equipment, Additives, and Order of Draw

Study Tips

- Complete the activities in the companion WORKBOOK.

- Find an example of each tube and put them in a ziplock bag to carry with you. Arrange them according to additives and then according to order of draw. Underline each expiration date. Write on the tube whether the sample will be whole blood or clotted blood.

- Go over the cautions and key points in the TEXTBOOK.

- Identify ETS and syringe system components and parts of components by name, memorize the gauges, and lengths of needles used in blood collection.

- List tube stopper colors in the order of draw on the left side of a sheet of paper. List the additives associated with each stopper color down the center of the paper. List the departments that use that color of tube stopper on the right side of the paper. Fold the paper in thirds and quiz yourself by first naming the additive associated with each stopper color. Then quiz yourself on the departments that use that type of tube.

- Make a list of the various blood collection devices on a sheet of paper, with the situations when they are used on the back. Find a partner and quiz each other on the situations that require the use of each device.

- Practice the memory jogger for the order of draw until it is committed to memory.

Overview

The primary duty of the phlebotomist is to collect blood specimens for laboratory testing. Blood is collected by several methods, including arterial puncture, capillary puncture, and venipuncture. This chapter assesses knowledge of general blood collection equipment and supplies commonly needed regardless of the method of collection, equipment and supplies specific to venipuncture, additives used in blood collection, and the order of draw for collecting or filling blood specimen tubes. A phlebotomist must be familiar with all the types of equipment in order to select appropriate collection devices for the type and condition of the patient's vein and the type and amount of specimen required for the test. Choosing the appropriate tools and using them correctly helps assure the safe collection of quality blood specimens. (Knowledge of equipment specific to capillary puncture and arterial puncture is assessed in Chapters 10 and 14, respectively.)

Review Questions

Choose the BEST answer.

1. Which blood specimen additive can inhibit the metabolism of glucose by the cells?
   a. EDTA
   b. Heparin
   c. NaF
   d. Oxalate

2. Which of the following items is unnecessary when performing a routine venipuncture?
   a. Disinfectant
   b. Evacuated tubes
   c. Safety needle
   d. Tourniquet

3. A serum specimen is requested. Which of the following evacuated tubes can be used to collect it?
   a. EDTA
   b. PPT
   c. PST
   d. SST

4. Which of the following are all anticoagulants that remove calcium from the specimen by forming insoluble calcium salts and therefore prevent coagulation?
   a. EDTA, lithium heparin, citrate
   b. NaF, sodium heparin, EDTA
   c. Oxalate, SPS, sodium heparin
   d. Sodium citrate, EDTA, oxalate

5. In a successful venipuncture, evacuated tubes fill automatically as soon as the tube stopper is pierced because of
   a. equal pressure in the vein and tube.
   b. premeasured vacuum in each tube.
   c. pressure from the arterial system.
   d. tourniquet pressure on the vein.

6. Lavender stopper tubes are most commonly used to collect
   a. chemistry tests.
   b. coagulation tests.
   c. hematology tests.
   d. immunology tests.

7. Which of the following is one reason the evacuated tube system (ETS) is the preferred blood collection system?
   a. Exposure of the blood to contaminants is avoided.
   b. Needles used with the ETS have a smaller lumen.
   c. The collector's exposure to blood is eliminated.
   d. Using a syringe can collapse a vein more easily.

8. Lithium heparin is a suitable anticoagulant for which of the following tests?
   a. CBC
   b. Lytes
   c. Lithium
   d. Protime

9. Which one of the following additives can be found in a royal blue–top collection tube?
   a. Citrate
   b. EDTA
   c. Fluoride
   d. Oxalate

10. Measurement of copper, a trace element, requires blood collection in a tube with a
    a. green top.
    b. lavender top.
    c. light blue top.
    d. royal blue top.

11. The blood to additive ratio is most critical for a specimen collected in this tube.
    a. Lavender top
    b. Light blue top
    c. Light green top
    d. Royal blue top

12. If phlebotomists have dermatitis, they should
    a. change their gloves more frequently.
    b. see if wearing glove liners will help.
    c. use sanitizer instead of soap and water.
    d. wash their hands thoroughly and often.

13. Decontamination of hands after glove removal is essential because
    a. decontamination is needed to quickly restore normal flora.
    b. gloves cause pathogens to multiply on surface of the skin.
    c. hand contamination might not be visible to the naked eye.
    d. All of the above.

14. Which of the following is a disinfectant?
    a. Benzalkonium chloride
    b. Chlorhexidine gluconate
    c. Household bleach
    d. Hydrogen peroxide

15. Which disinfectant is preferred by the HICPAC for use on surfaces and instruments?
    a. CDC-approved solution of 2% phenol
    b. Commercial brand of Lysol disinfectant
    c. Manufactured povidone–iodine dilution
    d. EPA-registered sodium hypochlorite product

16. After a blood spill, a disinfectant is applied and must have at least _____ minutes of contact time for cleanup to be effective.
    a. 2 minutes
    b. 5 minutes
    c. 10 minutes
    d. 30 minutes

17. If hands are heavily contaminated with organic material and a sink is not available, the phlebotomist should clean them with
    a. alcohol-based hand cleaner and sterile gauze pads.
    b. detergent-containing wipes followed by a sanitizer.
    c. hydrogen peroxide followed by a hand sanitizer.
    d. three separate 70% isopropyl swabs used in a row.

18. The purpose of a transillumination device is to
    a. input patient ID information.
    b. locate veins for venipuncture.
    c. transfer blood from a syringe.
    d. All of the above.

19. Which statement is incorrect? A properly applied tourniquet should
    a. distend or inflate the veins of choice.
    b. make veins larger and easier to find.
    c. restrict venous and arterial blood flow.
    d. stretch vein walls so they are thinner.

20. This needle gauge is used for autologous blood collection.
    a. 15 to 17
    b. 18 to 21
    c. 21 to 23
    d. 23 to 25

21. Needle safety features work by
    a. covering or shielding the needle.
    b. retracting the needle after use.
    c. using a device to blunt the needle.
    d. All of the above.

22. OSHA regulations require that after use
    a. needles be automatically ejected into the sharps container.
    b. needles be removed from the tube holders before disposal.
    c. tube holders be sanitized soon after the needle is removed.
    d. tube holders with needle attached be disposed of as a unit.

23. The headspace in an evacuated tube is
    a. a consistent amount of air space left when a tube is filled properly.
    b. due to premature depletion of tube vacuum when a vein is missed.
    c. room left in a tube if the tube is not completely filled with blood.
    d. space inside a colored tube stopper that should not touch the blood.

24. Tubes designed by the manufacturer to be "short draw" are
    a. bad for coagulation testing.
    b. made to fill only partially.
    c. smaller than regular tubes.
    d. tubes without anticoagulants.

25. Types of ETS tube additives include
    a. anticoagulants.
    b. clot activators.
    c. separator gels.
    d. All of the above.

26. Plastic red–top tubes used to collect blood specimens contain
    a. anticoagulants.
    b. clot activators.
    c. no additives.
    d. preservatives.

27. Improper handling or storage of evacuated tubes can affect
    a. additive integrity.
    b. shape of the tube.
    c. vacuum of a tube.
    d. All of the above.

28. This would be the best tube for collecting a STAT test that must be performed on serum.
    a. PPT
    b. PST
    c. RST
    d. SST

29. Which additive is used to collect donor units of blood?
    a. ACD
    b. CPD
    c. SPS
    d. All of the above

30. A specimen collected in this type of additive will separate if allowed to stand.
    a. Citrate
    b. Heparin
    c. Oxalate
    d. All of the above

31. What is the advantage of collecting STAT chemistries in a green-top tube?
    a. Plasma specimens can be centrifuged right away
    b. The turnaround time for results is much shorter
    c. Whole blood tests can be performed right away
    d. All of the above

32. This antiseptic has been traditionally used to obtain the high degree of skin antisepsis required when collecting blood cultures.
    a. 70% ethyl alcohol
    b. 70% isopropanol
    c. Hydrogen peroxide
    d. Povidone–iodine

33. Which of the following is the *preferred* solution to use to clean up blood spills?
    a. 5.25% sodium hypochlorite
    b. An EPA-approved bleach product
    c. Fresh solution of soap and water
    d. Undiluted 70% isopropyl alcohol

34. Antiseptics are
    a. corrosive chemical compounds.
    b. safe for use on human skin.
    c. used on surfaces and instruments.
    d. used to kill pathogenic microbes.

35. A solution used to clean the site before routine venipuncture is
    a. 5.25% sodium hypochlorite.
    b. 70% isopropyl alcohol.
    c. 70% methanol.
    d. Povidone–iodine.

36. Why are gauze pads a better choice than cotton balls for covering the site and holding pressure following venipuncture?
    a. Cotton balls are not very absorbent
    b. Cotton ball fibers can stick to the site
    c. Gauze pads are a more sterile choice
    d. Gauze pads deliver more pressure

37. CLSI standards advise against using these on infants and children younger than 2 years of age.
    a. Adhesive bandages.
    b. Evacuated tubes.
    c. Isopropyl alcohol.
    d. Vinyl tourniquets.

38. Which of the following should be deleted from a list of required characteristic of a sharps container?
    a. Leak proof
    b. Lid that locks
    c. Puncture resistant
    d. Red in color

39. It is best if tourniquets are
    a. cleaned daily with bleach.
    b. thrown away when soiled.
    c. used once and then discarded.
    d. wiped with alcohol after use.

40. Wearing gloves during phlebotomy procedures is mandated by the following agency:
    a. CDC
    b. FDA
    c. HICPAC
    d. OSHA

41. What criterion is used to decide which needle gauge to use for venipuncture?
    a. Depth of the selected vein
    b. Size and condition of the vein
    c. Type of test being collected
    d. Your personal preference

42. To what does the "gauge" of a needle relate?
    a. Diameter
    b. Length
    c. Strength
    d. Volume

43. Which needle gauge has the largest bore or lumen?
    a. 18
    b. 20
    c. 21
    d. 22

44. Multisample needles are typically available in these gauges.
    a. 16 to 18
    b. 18 to 20
    c. 20 to 22
    d. 22 to 24

45. The slanted tip of a needle is called the
    a. bevel.
    b. hub.
    c. lumen.
    d. shaft.

46. The purpose of the rubber sleeve that covers the tube end of a multiple-sample needle is to
    a. enable smooth tube placement and removal.
    b. maintain the sterile condition of the sample.
    c. prevent leakage of blood during tube changes.
    d. protect the needle and help keep it sharp.

47. A phlebotomy needle that does *not* have a safety feature
    a. cannot be used for any venipuncture procedure.
    b. must be used with a holder that has a safety feature.
    c. requires immediate recapping after venipuncture.
    d. should be removed from the holder before disposal.

48. Which of the following plays no role in deciding what size tubes to use for ETS blood collection?
    a. Age and weight of the patient.
    b. Patient's allergy to antiseptics.
    c. Sample size needed for testing.
    d. Size and condition of the veins.

49. Mixing additive tubes involves
    a. gently shaking them up and down.
    b. slowly rocking them back and forth.
    c. turning the wrist 90 degrees and back.
    d. turning the wrist 180 degrees and back.

50. Which of the following stopper colors identifies a tube used for coagulation testing?
    a. Green
    b. Lavender
    c. Light blue
    d. Red

51. Which of the following tubes will yield a serum sample?
    a. Green top
    b. Lavender top
    c. Light blue top
    d. Red top

52. The cleaning agent in hand sanitizers used in healthcare is
    a. alcohol based.
    b. phenol based.
    c. sodium hypochlorite.
    d. zephiran chloride.

53. Which of the following tube stopper colors indicates something other than the presence (or absence) and type of additive in the tube?
    a. Green
    b. Lavender
    c. Light blue
    d. Royal blue

54. Heparin prevents blood from clotting by
    a. activating calcium.
    b. binding calcium.
    c. chelating thrombin.
    d. inhibiting thrombin.

55. Which department would most likely perform the test on a specimen collected in an SPS tube?
    a. Chemistry
    b. Coagulation
    c. Hematology
    d. Microbiology

56. A royal blue–top tube with green color coding on the label contains
    a. EDTA.
    b. heparin.
    c. no additive.
    d. sodium citrate.

57. Which one of the following substances is an anticoagulant?
    a. Oxalate
    b. Phosphate
    c. Silica
    d. Thrombin

58. It is important to fill oxalate tubes to the stated fill capacity because excess oxalate
    a. causes hemolysis of blood specimens.
    b. changes WBC staining characteristics.
    c. erroneously increases potassium levels.
    d. leads to the formation of microclots.

59. Which of the following substances is contained in a serum separator tube?
    a. K₃EDTA
    b. Lithium heparin
    c. Sodium citrate
    d. Thixotropic gel

60. What is the purpose of an antiglycolytic agent?
    a. Enhance the clotting process
    b. Inhibit electrolyte breakdown
    c. Preserve glucose
    d. Prevent clotting

61. Glass particles present in serum separator tubes
    a. activate clotting.
    b. deter clotting.
    c. inhibit glycolysis.
    d. prevent hemolysis.

62. Which is the *best* tube for collecting an ETOH (ethanol) specimen?
    a. Gray top
    b. Green top
    c. Lavender top
    d. Light blue top

63. Identify the tubes needed to collect a CBC, PTT, and STAT potassium by color and in the proper order of collection for a multiple tube draw.
    a. Gold top, yellow top, light blue top
    b. Lavender top, SST royal blue top
    c. Light blue top, green top, lavender top
    d. Red top, gray top, light blue top

64. During venipuncture the tourniquet should not be left on longer than
    a. 30 seconds.
    b. 1 minute.
    c. 2 minutes.
    d. 5 minutes.

65. Which one of the following tubes is filled first when multiple tubes are filled from a syringe?
    a. Blood culture tube
    b. Complete blood count tube
    c. Nonadditive tube
    d. STAT potassium tube

66. This test is collected in a light blue–top tube.
    a. Glucose
    b. Platelet count
    c. Prothrombin time
    d. Red blood count

67. Which of the following STAT tests is typically collected in a lithium heparin tube?
    a. Blood type and screen
    b. Complete blood count
    c. Electrolyte panel
    d. Prothrombin time

68. This tube stopper color indicates that the tube contains EDTA.
    a. Green
    b. Lavender
    c. Light blue
    d. Royal blue

69. What anticoagulant is contained in a PST?
    a. ACD
    b. Citrate
    c. Heparin
    d. Oxalate

70. The purpose of sodium citrate in specimen collection is to
    a. accelerate coagulation.
    b. inhibit glucose breakdown.
    c. preserve glucose values.
    d. protect coagulation factors.

71. The part of a syringe that shows measurements in cc or mL is called the
    a. adapter.
    b. barrel.
    c. hub.
    d. plunger.

72. This part of the evacuated tube holder is meant to aid in smooth tube removal.
    a. Barrel
    b. Flange
    c. Hub
    d. Sleeve

73. The *best* choice of equipment for drawing difficult veins is a
    a. butterfly and ETS holder.
    b. lancet and microtainer.
    c. needle and ETS holder.
    d. needle and 10-cc syringe.

74. Mixing equipment from different manufacturers can result in
    a. carryover of an additive
    b. improper fit of the needle.
    c. wrong choices of additives.
    d. All of the above.

75. You are *most* likely to increase the chance of hemolyzing a specimen if you use a
    a. 21-gauge needle and ETS tube to collect a specimen from a median vein.
    b. 22-gauge needle and syringe to collect a specimen from a difficult vein.
    c. 23-gauge butterfly needle to collect a specimen from a hand vein.
    d. 25-gauge butterfly needle to collect a specimen from a small child.

76. The purpose of a tourniquet in the venipuncture procedure is to
    a. block the flow of arterial blood into the area.
    b. enlarge veins so they are easier to find and enter.
    c. obstruct blood flow to concentrate the analyte.
    d. redirect more blood flow to the venipuncture site.

77. If a blood pressure cuff is used for venipuncture in place of a tourniquet, the pressure used must be
    a. below the patient's diastolic pressure.
    b. between the diastolic and the systolic pressure.
    c. equal to the patient's systolic pressure.
    d. equal to the patient's venous pressure.

78. In general, an anticoagulant is unable to
    a. bind calcium or inhibit thrombin.
    b. inhibit the metabolism of glucose.
    c. keep the blood in its natural state.
    d. prevent the specimen from clotting.

79. Needle safety devices must
    a. allow the phlebotomist to safely activate it using both hands.
    b. create a barrier between a user's hand and the needle after use.
    c. provide temporary containment of the used venipuncture needle.
    d. All of the above.

80. This gel separator tube contains EDTA.
    a. EST
    b. PPT
    c. PST
    d. SST

81. Which additive contains a substance that inhibits phagocytosis of bacteria by white blood cells?
    a. Silica (glass) clot activator
    b. Sodium or lithium heparin
    c. Sodium polyanethol sulfonate
    d. Thixotropic silicon barrier gel

82. Which type of test can potentially be affected by tissue thromboplastin contamination?
    a. Chemistry
    b. Coagulation
    c. Microbiology
    d. Serology

83. Which of the following tests would be most affected by carryover of K_2EDTA?
    a. BUN
    b. Glucose
    c. Potassium
    d. Sodium

84. Carryover from this tube has a greater potential to negatively affect the specimen in the next tube drawn.
    a. Half full nonadditive tube
    b. Overfilled gray–top tube
    c. Underfilled EDTA tube
    d. All of the above

85. A trace-element specimen tube should be collected
    a. after any other tubes.
    b. before any other tubes.
    c. separately or by syringe.
    d. with a 21-gauge butterfly.

86. A pink-top tube containing EDTA is primarily used for
    a. blood bank tests.
    b. chemistry tests.
    c. coagulation tests.
    d. microbiology tests.

87. The blood collection equipment shown in Figure 7-1 can be used
    a. as a syringe.
    b. as an ETS.
    c. with a butterfly.
    d. in all of the above ways.

88. Identify the tubes needed to collect a PT, STAT lytes, and BC in the proper order of collection.
    a. Gold, yellow, light blue
    b. Light blue, lavender, yellow
    c. SST, yellow, light blue
    d. Yellow, light blue, PST

89. Which one of the following tubes is additive free?
    a. BD clear/red
    b. BD green/gray
    c. Vacuette blue
    d. Vacuette red

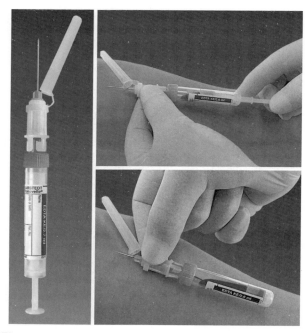

Figure 7-1 S-Monovette Blood Collection System. (Courtesy of Sarstedt, Inc., Newton, NC.)

90. Which chemistry tube could contain either of two different forms of an anticoagulant because both have the same stopper color?
    a. Blue
    b. Gray
    c. Green
    d. Tan

91. Which additive can be found in four separate tubes with different stopper colors?
    a. EDTA
    b. Heparin
    c. Potassium oxalate
    d. Sodium citrate

92. Which stopper color is the same for two completely different types of additives used by two different departments?
    a. Blue
    b. Green
    c. Tan
    d. Yellow

93. Due to allergenic reactions, which type of glove is not recommended to be used in healthcare facilities?
    a. Latex
    b. Neoprene
    c. Polyethylene
    d. Vinyl

94. Which of the following additives is most commonly used for chemistry tests?
    a. ACD
    b. Citrate
    c. Heparin
    d. SPS

95. An ETS holder and a syringe transfer device look very similar. What is the difference between the two?
    a. The hub on the transfer device attaches to a multisample needle or syringe barrel
    b. The transfer device is smaller in size than the regular holder and has no flanges
    c. There is a permanently attached needle with a sleeve inside the transfer device
    d. There is no difference between the ETS holder and the syringe transfer device

96. A prothrombin time (PT) and platelet count are ordered on an 80-year-old female patient. Deciding to use a butterfly and "short draw" evacuated tubes on the tiny cephalic vein on the dorsal side of her right arm, the phlebotomist collects one light blue–top tube and then a lavender top. Why would you suspect that the PT test results might be incorrect and the platelet count unaffected?
    a. No tube was drawn to remove air in the butterfly tubing.
    b. PTs should never be collected using "short draw" tubes.
    c. The tubes were drawn in the wrong collection sequence.
    d. Venipuncture of the tiny vein led to specimen hemolysis.

97. A home care phlebotomist had a requisition to collect a CBC, plasma K, PTT, and PT. He collected the tubes from the client, who was lying on the sofa with her arm elevated above her shoulder on a table next to the sofa. As he collected the tests in the following order: CBC, K, and finally the PT and PTT, he was careful to invert the tubes as specified. Later that day, the lab called the phlebotomist to say that three of the tests would have to be redrawn. Which three tests most likely had questionable results and needed to be redrawn?
    a. CBC, PT, and potassium
    b. Potassium, PTT, and PT
    c. PTT, potassium, and CBC
    d. PTT, PT, and CBC

98. While collecting a STAT blood culture and electrolytes on a child in the emergency room, the physician asked the phlebotomist to get an extra tube of blood to check for metal poisoning. Which one of the following tubes would the phlebotomist add to the ones already being collected?
    a. Gold
    b. Gray
    c. Pink
    d. Royal blue

99. Which one of the following tubes/additives would be used to collect a DNA test?
    a. Gold/clot activator
    b. Light green/heparin
    c. Yellow/ACD
    d. Yellow/SPS

100. Electrolytes should never be collected in a
    a. gold top.
    b. gray top.
    c. light green top.
    d. red/gold top.

Answers and Explanations

1. **Answer: c**

   WHY: A substance that prevents glycolysis, the breakdown, or metabolism of glucose (blood sugar) by blood cells, is called a glycolytic inhibitor or an antiglycolytic agent. The most common antiglycolytic agent is sodium fluoride (NaF). It preserves glucose for up to 3 days and also inhibits the growth of bacteria.
   REVIEW: Yes ☐ No ☐

2. **Answer: a**

   WHY: Antiseptics, not disinfectants, are routinely used when performing venipuncture. Disinfectants are chemical substances or solutions that are used to remove or kill microorganisms on surfaces and instruments. They are typically corrosive and not safe for use on human skin.
   REVIEW: Yes ☐ No ☐

3. **Answer: d**

   WHY: SST stands for serum separator tube, a gel-barrier tube from Becton Dickinson (BD). This tube does not contain an anticoagulant, so blood collected in it will yield serum. The gel in the tube prevents glycolysis after the tube has been centrifuged. The EDTA tube and plasma preparation tube (PPT) both contain the anticoagulant EDTA. The plasma separator tube (PST) contains the anticoagulant heparin. Anticoagulants prevent the blood from clotting; consequently, they yield plasma when centrifuged.
   REVIEW: Yes ☐ No ☐

4. **Answer: d**

   WHY: Sodium citrate, oxalate, and EDTA are all anticoagulants that prevent blood from clotting by chelating (binding) or precipitating calcium so it is not available to the coagulation process. Sodium polyanethol sulfonate (SPS) also binds calcium, however lithium and sodium heparin prevent clotting by inhibiting the formation of thrombin needed to convert fibrinogen to fibrin in the coagulation process. Sodium fluoride (NaF) is an antiglycolytic agent, not an anticoagulant.
   REVIEW: Yes ☐ No ☐

5. **Answer: b**

   WHY: Evacuated tubes fill with blood automatically because there is a vacuum (negative pressure) in them. The vacuum is premeasured by the manufacturer so that the tube will draw the precise volume of blood indicated.
   REVIEW: Yes ☐ No ☐

6. **Answer: c**

   WHY: EDTA prevents coagulation and is primarily used to provide whole blood specimens for hematology tests because it preserves cell morphology and inhibits platelet aggregation or clumping.
   REVIEW: Yes ☐ No ☐

7. **Answer: a**

   WHY: The most common, efficient, and CLSI-preferred system for collecting blood samples is the ETS. Because it is a closed system in which the patient's blood flows directly into a collection tube, it offers many benefits. For example, blood can be collected without being exposed to air or outside contaminants. Blood collected in a syringe is exposed to air and there is possibility of outside contamination. In addition, the needle must be removed from a syringe to attach a transfer device used to fill the tubes. This can expose the user to the patient's blood. The ETS minimizes the collector's exposure to blood, but does not eliminate it as there is often a small amount of blood on the stopper where the needle entered the tube. The ETS system can collapse a fragile vein more easily than a syringe. A syringe is often used in difficult draw situations because the vacuum pull can be adjusted to minimize the chance of vein collapse.

Syringe needles are available in the same gauges as ETS needles so an equivalent gauge ETS needle would have the same size lumen as a syringe needle.

REVIEW: Yes ☐   No ☐

8. **Answer: b**

WHY: Lithium heparin causes the least interference in chemistry testing and is the most widely used anticoagulant for plasma and whole-blood chemistry tests. Heparinized plasma is often used for STAT chemistry tests and other rapid-response situations when a fast turnaround time (TAT) for chemistry tests is needed.

REVIEW: Yes ☐   No ☐

9. **Answer: b**

WHY: Royal blue–top tubes contain EDTA, heparin, or no additive to meet various test requirements. Tube labels are typically color coded to indicate the type of additive, if any, in the tube.

REVIEW: Yes ☐   No ☐

10. **Answer: d**

WHY: Royal blue–top tubes are made of materials that are as free of trace-element contamination as possible and are used for trace-element tests, such as copper.

REVIEW: Yes ☐   No ☐

11. **Answer: b**

WHY: Coagulation tests are collected in light blue–top sodium citrate tubes. For accurate results coagulation tests require there a 9:1 ratio of blood to additive. If tubes are not filled to within 90% of their stated volume dilution of the blood results, the results can be falsely elevated. Some tubes have arrows to show fill levels from minimum to maximum (Fig. 7-2).

REVIEW: Yes ☐   No ☐

12. **Answer: b**

WHY: Dermatitis is a condition that can be caused by wearing gloves, required frequent hand washing, and drying effects of alcohol-based hand sanitizers. Since frequent hand decontamination

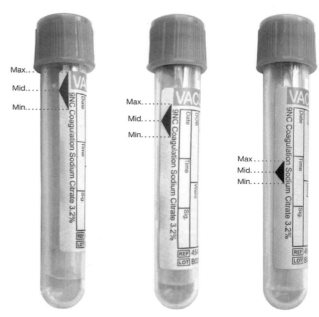

Figure 7-2 Guide showing fill levels for Vacuette sodium citrate tubes. (Courtesy of Greiner Bio-One International AG, Kremsmünster, Austria.)

is necessary wearing glove liners (Fig. 7-3) might help prevent skin irritation.

REVIEW: Yes ☐   No ☐

13. **Answer: c**

WHY: Any type of glove may contain defects and contamination is not always visible. Consequently, decontamination of hands after glove removal is essential and made very convenient, for instance, by wall-mounted hand sanitizer dispensers, such as shown in Figure 7-4.

REVIEW: Yes ☐   No ☐

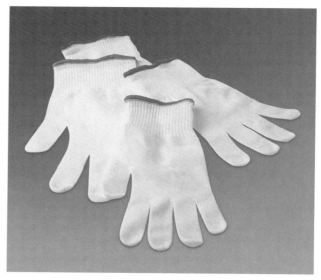

Figure 7-3 UltraFIT glove liners. (Courtesy of Erie Scientific Co., Portsmouth, NH.)

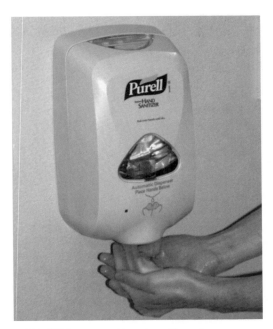

Figure 7-4 Wall-mounted hand sanitizer dispenser.

14. **Answer: c**

WHY: Household bleach, or 5.25% sodium hypochlorite, is an effective disinfectant. The other choices are antiseptics. Antiseptics are substances used to prevent sepsis that are safe to use on skin (Box 7-1).

REVIEW: Yes ☐   No ☐

15. **Answer: d**

WHY: According to CDC and HICPAC *Guidelines for Environmental Infection Control in Healthcare Facilities,* use of EPA-registered sodium hypochlorite products for disinfecting surfaces and instruments is preferred.

REVIEW: Yes ☐   No ☐

Box 7-1

Antiseptics Used in Blood Collection

- 70% Ethyl alcohol
- 70% Isopropyl alcohol (isopropanol)
- Benzalkonium chloride (e.g., Zephiran chloride)
- Chlorhexidine gluconate
- Hydrogen peroxide
- Povidone–iodine (0.1–1% available iodine)
- Tincture of iodine

16. **Answer: c**

WHY: A spill involving large amounts of blood or other body fluids requires at least 10 minutes of contact time with a disinfectant for the cleanup to be considered effective.

REVIEW: Yes ☐   No ☐

17. **Answer: b**

WHY: When hands are heavily contaminated with organic material and a sink is not available, it is recommended that hands be cleaned with detergent-containing wipes followed by the use of an alcohol-based hand cleaner or sanitizer.

REVIEW: Yes ☐   No ☐

18. **Answer: b**

WHY: Transillumination is the inspection of an organ by passing light through its walls. Transillumination devices can be used to locate veins. They work by shining a high-intensity light through the patient's subcutaneous tissue, this highlights the veins, which absorb the light rather than reflecting it and stand out as dark lines (Fig. 7-5).

REVIEW: Yes ☐   No ☐

19. **Answer: c**

WHY: A properly applied tourniquet is tight enough to restrict venous flow out of the area,

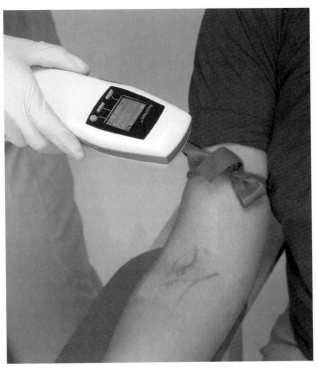

Figure 7-5 AccuVein AV300 being used to locate veins on a patient's arm. (Courtesy of AccuVein LLC, Huntington, NY.)

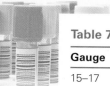

Table 7-1: Common Venipuncture Needle Gauges with Needle Type and Typical Use

Gauge	Needle Type	Typical Use
15–17	Special needle attached to collection bag	Collection of donor units, autologous blood donation, and therapeutic phlebotomy
20 20	Multisample Hypodermic	Sometimes used when large-volume tubes are collected or large-volume syringes are used on patients with normal-size veins
21 21	Multisample Hypodermic	Considered the standard venipuncture needle for routine venipuncture on patients with normal veins or syringe blood culture collection
22 22	Multisample Hypodermic	Used on older children and adult patients with small veins or syringe draws on difficult veins
23	Butterfly	Veins of infants and children and difficult or hand veins of adults

but not so tight as to restrict arterial flow into the area. Restriction of venous flow distends or inflates the veins, making them larger and easier to find and stretches the vein walls, making them thinner and easier to pierce with a needle.

REVIEW: Yes ☐ No ☐

20. **Answer: a**

WHY: 15- to 17-gauge needles are used for autologous blood donation, collection of donor units of blood, and for therapeutic phlebotomy (Table 7-1).

REVIEW: Yes ☐ No ☐

21. **Answer: d**

WHY: Needle safety features include resheathing devices such as shields that cover the needle after use (Fig. 7-6), blunting devices, and equipment with devices that retract the needle after the use.

REVIEW: Yes ☐ No ☐

22. **Answer: d**

WHY: OSHA regulations require that the tube holder with needle attached be disposed of as a unit in the sharps container after use. OSHA guidelines state that holders should not be reused and the needle should not be removed from the tube holder.

REVIEW: Yes ☐ No ☐

23. **Answer: a**

WHY: Evacuated tubes fill with blood automatically because there is a vacuum. The vacuum is premeasured by the manufacturer so that the tube will draw the precise volume of blood indicated. Tubes do not fill with blood all the way to the stopper. When filled properly, there is always a consistent amount of headspace between the level of blood in the tube and the tube stopper.

REVIEW: Yes ☐ No ☐

24. **Answer: b**

WHY: Some manufacturers offer special "short draw" (Fig. 7-7) tubes designed to partially fill without compromising test results. These tubes are used in situations in which it is difficult or inadvisable to draw larger quantities of blood. They are typically the same size as regular-fill

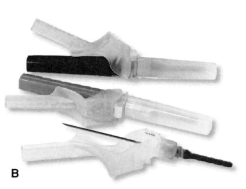

A **B**

Figure 7-6 A: BD Vacutainer® Passive Shielding Blood Collection Needle. (Courtesy of Becton Dickinson, Franklin Lakes, New Jersey.) **B:** BD Eclipse multisample safety needles, **(top)** black 22 gauge, **(Center)** green 21 gauge. (Courtesy of Becton Dickinson, Franklin Lakes, NJ.)

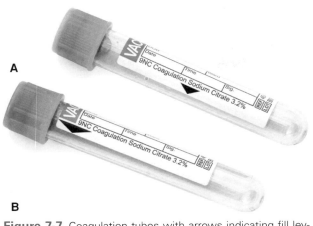

A

B

Figure 7-7 Coagulation tubes with arrows indicating fill levels. **A:** Regular draw tube. **B:** Short draw tube.

tubes but contain adjusted amounts of additive. The "short draw" tubes can be used for any of the tests for which regular tubes are used.

REVIEW: Yes ☐   No ☐

25. **Answer: d**

WHY: Most ETS tubes contain some type of additive. An additive is any substance placed within a tube other than the tube stopper or the coating of the tube. Additives include anticoagulants, clot activators, preservatives, and separator gels.

REVIEW: Yes ☐   No ☐

26. **Answer: b**

WHY: Plastic red–top tubes are for collecting serum specimens and contain a clot activator. With the advent of plastic tubes, very few tubes are additive free anymore. Even serum tubes have an additive if they are plastic because plastic is so slick that platelet aggregation and adhesion is inhibited unless the tube contains a clot activator.

REVIEW: Yes ☐   No ☐

27. **Answer: d**

WHY: Improper handling or storage may affect additive integrity and tube vacuum, which can lead to compromised test results or improper filling, respectively. If plastic tubes are not stored properly, heat will cause them to melt and become disfigured.

REVIEW: Yes ☐   No ☐

28. **Answer: c**

WHY: A rapid serum tube (RST) contains thrombin, which normally clots the blood in 5 minutes. A plasma preparation tube (PPT) contains EDTA and a plasma separation tube (PST) provide

plasma for testing, not serum. A serum separator tube provides serum, but can take up to 30 minutes to clot.

REVIEW: Yes ☐   No ☐

29. **Answer: b**

WHY: CPD stands for citrate phosphate dextrose, which is used to collect units of blood for transfusion. Acid citrate dextrose (ACD) is used in immunohematology for tests such as HLA phenotyping. Sodium polyanethol sulfate (SPS) is found in tubes used to collect blood cultures.

REVIEW: Yes ☐   No ☐

30. **Answer: d**

WHY: Citrates, heparin, and oxalates are all anticoagulants so the cells will be free flowing and not clotted. That means they will separate from the plasma if allowed to stand for an extended amount of time or if the specimen is centrifuged.

REVIEW: Yes ☐   No ☐

31. **Answer: d**

WHY: Green-top tubes contain heparin. The big advantage of performing STAT chemistry tests on heparinized specimens relates to a faster turnaround time (TAT) for test results than when serum is used for the test. Heparinized specimens for plasma tests can be centrifuged right away, whereas serum specimens must be clotted which can take up to 30 minutes or more. Whole blood chemistry tests can be performed right away.

REVIEW: Yes ☐   No ☐

32. **Answer: d**

WHY: Collection of some specimens, such as blood cultures, requires a higher degree of skin antisepsis than obtained by using isopropyl alcohol. Povidone–iodine, in the form of swabsticks or sponge pads, has been the traditional skin antiseptic used to collect these specimens. The use of an alcohol-based preparation for these procedures is increasing, however, because many patients are allergic to povidone–iodine. Antiseptics used in blood collection are listed in Box 7-1.

REVIEW: Yes ☐   No ☐

33. **Answer: b**

WHY: According to CDC and HICPAC *Guidelines for Environmental Infection Control in Healthcare Facilities,* use of EPA-registered or approved sodium hypochlorite products is preferred, but solutions made from 5.25% sodium hypochlorite (household bleach) may be used. A 1:100 dilution is recommended for decontaminating nonporous

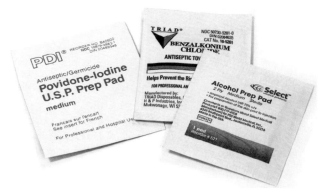

Figure 7-8 Examples of antiseptic prep pads.

surfaces after cleaning up blood or other body fluid spills in patient care settings.

REVIEW: Yes ☐   No ☐

34. **Answer: b**

WHY: Disinfectants are corrosive chemical compounds that are bactericidal (kill bacteria). Some also kill viruses such as human immunodeficiency virus and hepatitis. Disinfectants are used on surfaces and instruments to kill potential pathogens, but are *not* safe for use on human skin. Antiseptics *are* safe for use on human skin.

REVIEW: Yes ☐   No ☐

35. **Answer: b**

WHY: The most common antiseptic used for routine blood collection is 70% isopropyl alcohol (isopropanol) in the form of individually wrapped prep pads (Fig. 7-8). Bleach (5.25% sodium hypochlorite) is a disinfectant and is not safe to use on human skin. Methanol can be toxic when absorbed through the skin and is not used as a skin antiseptic. Povidone–iodine is sometimes used for collection of sterile specimens such as blood cultures.

REVIEW: Yes ☐   No ☐

36. **Answer: b**

WHY: Gauze or gauzelike pads are preferred for holding pressure over a venipuncture site because the fibers from cotton, Dacron, or rayon balls tend to stick to the site and reinitiate bleeding when removed because they dislodge the platelet plug.

REVIEW: Yes ☐   No ☐

37. **Answer: a**

WHY: Adhesive bandages should not be used on infants and children younger than 2 years of age because of the danger of aspiration and suffocation if they are accidentally removed from the site.

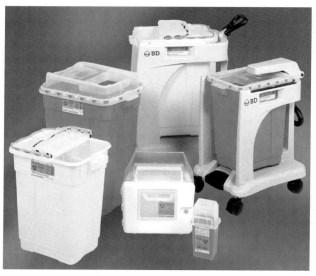

Figure 7-9 Several styles of sharps containers. (Courtesy of Becton Dickinson, Franklin Lakes, NJ.)

They can also tear the delicate skin of infants, especially newborns.

REVIEW: Yes ☐   No ☐

38. **Answer: d**

WHY: The Occupational Safety and Health Administration (OSHA) requires that sharps containers (Fig. 7-9) be rigid, leak proof, puncture resistant, and disposable and have locking lids that can be easily sealed when the container is filled to its stated capacity. OSHA also requires that they be marked with a biohazard symbol, but they do not require that all of the containers be red in color.

REVIEW: Yes ☐   No ☐

39. **Answer: c**

WHY: Although presently there is no regulatory requirement to dispose of tourniquets after a single use, a number of studies have shown that reusable tourniquets have the potential to transmit bacteria, including methicillin-resistant *Staphylococcus aureus* (MRSA). Consequently the best infection control measure is to use a new tourniquet for each patient. Bleach disintegrates latex and makes it gummy. Alcohol is an antiseptic and would not necessarily destroy bloodborne pathogens. Disposable tourniquets should be discarded when soiled, but microorganism contamination is invisible, which is why it is best not to reuse them in the first place.

REVIEW: Yes ☐   No ☐

40. **Answer: d**

WHY: OSHA's Bloodborne Pathogen Standard is a federal law that mandates wearing of gloves during most phlebotomy procedures. The CDC and HICPAC provide guidelines for wearing gloves, but the guidelines are not federal laws. The FDA regulates glove quality.

REVIEW: Yes ☐   No ☐

41. **Answer: b**

WHY: The needle gauge for venipuncture is selected according to the size and condition of the patient's vein, the type of procedure, and the equipment being used. Personal preference and the depth of the vein influence the length of needle used, rather than the gauge. The type of test being collected does not normally influence selection of the needle gauge or length.

REVIEW: Yes ☐   No ☐

42. **Answer: a**

WHY: The gauge of a needle is a number that is inversely related to the diameter of the lumen or internal space of the needle. It is an indication of the size of the needle; the larger the number, the smaller its diameter, and vice versa. Most needles are color coded according to gauge; however, color coding varies by manufacturer. Multisample needles typically have color-coded caps. Several manufacturers use yellow for 20-gauge, green for 21-gauge, and black for 22-gauge needles (Figs. 7-6 and 7-10).

REVIEW: Yes ☐   No ☐

43. **Answer: a**

WHY: "Bore" is a term used to describe the diameter of a needle and the size of the hole it makes. There is an inverse relationship between the gauge number and the bore or diameter of the lumen of a needle. Therefore, the needle gauge with the largest bore or lumen is the one with the smallest number.

REVIEW: Yes ☐   No ☐

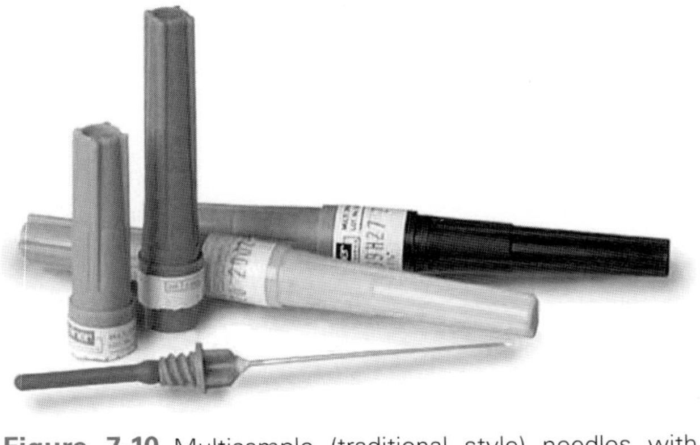

Figure 7-10 Multisample (traditional style) needles with color-coded caps. **Left:** Green 21 gauge. **Center:** Yellow 20 gauge. **Right:** Black 22 gauge. (Courtesy of Greiner Bio-One, Kremsmünster, Austria.)

44. **Answer: c**

WHY: ETS multisample needles (Figs. 7-6 and 7-10) are generally available in 20-, 21-, and 22-gauge. A 21-gauge needle is considered the standard needle for routine venipuncture. Syringe needles and butterfly needles are available in smaller-size gauges for difficult draw situations.

REVIEW: Yes ☐   No ☐

45. **Answer: a**

WHY: The end of the needle that is inserted into the vein is called the bevel because it is cut on a slant or "beveled" to allow the needle to penetrate the vein easily and prevent coring (removal of a portion of the skin or vein). The hub of a needle is the end that attaches to a syringe or tube holder. The lumen of a needle is the internal space of the needle. The shaft is the long cylindrical part of the needle. ETS needle parts are shown in Figure 7-11.

REVIEW: Yes ☐   No ☐

46. **Answer: c**

WHY: The rubber sleeve (Fig. 7-11) of a multiple-sample needle retracts as the needle is inserted into the tube, allowing the tube to fill with blood, and recovers the needle as the tube is removed, preventing leakage of blood into the tube holder. It is not possible to maintain a sterile sample unless the sample is collected in a sterile manner. The flanges on the holder were designed to enable smooth tube placement and removal.

REVIEW: Yes ☐   No ☐

47. **Answer: b**

WHY: A needle without a safety feature (Fig. 7-10) can be used for blood collection. However, according to OSHA regulations, it must be used with a tube holder that has a safety feature (Fig. 7-12). In addition, a needle must never be recapped or removed from its holder after use unless it has been demonstrated that it is specifically required by a medical procedure or there is no feasible alternative. In such instances, a mechanical device or some method other than a two-handed procedure must be used.

REVIEW: Yes ☐   No ☐

48. **Answer: b**

WHY: The size and condition of the patient's vein and sample volume required for testing play a major role when selecting the size of tubes to use for venipuncture. Age and weight play a role when drawing infants and young children so as not to deplete their blood volumes. Age is also a

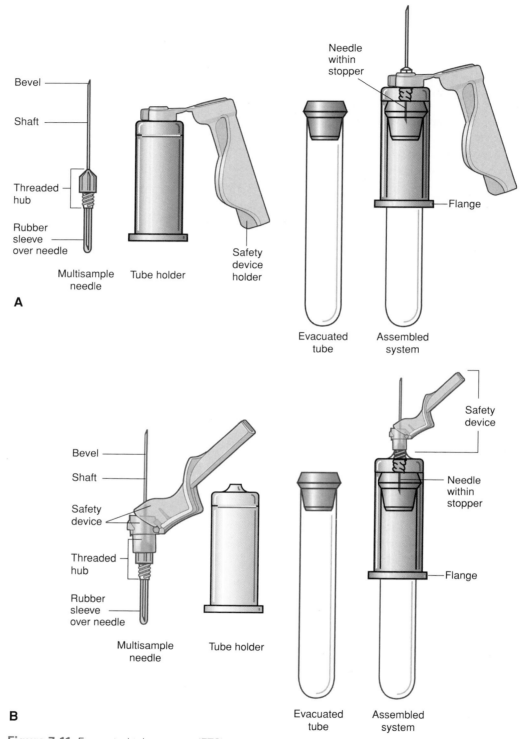

Figure 7-11 Evacuated tube system (ETS) components. **A:** Traditional needle and safety tube holder. **B:** Safety needle and traditional tube holder.

consideration when drawing elderly patients with fragile veins. Allergies play a role in selecting the antiseptic to use, not tube size.

REVIEW: Yes ☐ No ☐

49. **Answer: b**

WHY: Additive tubes require mixing by inversion. The number of inversions depends upon the type of additive and manufacturer instructions. One

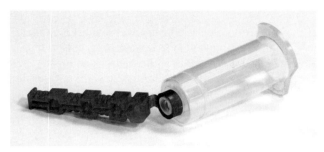

Figure 7-12 Tube holder with needle resheathing device.

inversion is defined by tube manufacturer Becton Dickinson (BD) as a turn of the wrist of 180 degrees and back again.

REVIEW: Yes ☐ No ☐

50. **Answer: c**

WHY: A light blue–top tube typically contains the anticoagulant sodium citrate as the additive. Sodium citrate prevents coagulation by binding calcium. It is used for coagulation specimens because it does the best job of preserving the coagulation factors and adding calcium back to the specimen during testing easily reverses its binding effects. The most common use of green tops is to collect plasma for chemistry tests. Lavender tops are most commonly used to collect whole blood for hematology tests. Red tops are most often used for chemistry, serology, and blood bank tests.

REVIEW: Yes ☐ No ☐

51. **Answer: d**

WHY: There are two types of red-top tubes, glass and plastic. Blood collected in either of these tubes will clot and when centrifuged, a clear fluid called serum separates from the clotted cells. Green, lavender, and light blue–top tubes contain anticoagulants. Specimens that are collected in anticoagulant tubes are prevented from clotting and yield whole blood specimens. When blood in anticoagulant tubes is centrifuged, clear fluid separates from the cells and is called plasma. Green-top tubes are typically centrifuged to yield plasma for certain chemistry tests. The most common use of light blue tops is to provide plasma for coagulation tests.

REVIEW: Yes ☐ No ☐

52. **Answer: a**

WHY: The CDC *Guideline for Hand Hygiene in Healthcare Settings* recommends the use of alcohol-based hand sanitizers as a substitute for hand washing, provided the hands are not visibly soiled.

REVIEW: Yes ☐ No ☐

53. **Answer: d**

WHY: Most tube stopper colors indicate the presence (or absence) and type of additive in a tube. A green stopper indicates heparin, a lavender stopper indicates EDTA, and light blue normally indicates sodium citrate. A royal blue stopper, however, indicates that the tube and stopper are virtually trace element–free. A royal blue top can contain no additive, potassium EDTA, or sodium heparin. Additive color coding of a royal blue–top tube is typically indicated on the label.

REVIEW: Yes ☐ No ☐

54. **Answer: d**

WHY: Heparin prevents coagulation by inhibiting thrombin during the coagulation process. Thrombin is necessary for the formation of fibrin from fibrinogen. Without thrombin, a fibrin clot cannot form.

REVIEW: Yes ☐ No ☐

55. **Answer: d**

WHY: Sodium polyanethol sulfonate (SPS) tubes are used to collect blood cultures, which are performed in the microbiology department. SPS is an anticoagulant with special properties that inhibit proteins that destroy bacteria, prevent phagocytosis of bacteria by white blood cells, and reduce the activity of some antibiotics.

REVIEW: Yes ☐ No ☐

56. **Answer: b**

WHY: A royal blue stopper signifies that the tube and stopper contain the lowest levels of trace elements available (i.e., they are virtually trace element–free). Royal blue–top tubes are available with EDTA, heparin, no additive (glass tube), or clot activator (plastic tube). Color coding on the label indicates what additive, if any, is in the tube. Green color coding on the label of a royal blue top indicates that it contains heparin.

REVIEW: Yes ☐ No ☐

57. **Answer: a**

WHY: Oxalate is an anticoagulant that prevents coagulation by precipitating calcium and the form most widely used is potassium oxalate. Thromboplastin is found in tissue fluid and activates the extrinsic clotting pathway. Silica is used as a clot activator in ETS clotting tubes. Phosphate is an additive found in the special anticoagulants, ACD and CPD.

REVIEW: Yes ☐ No ☐

58. **Answer: a**

    WHY: Excess oxalate causes hemolysis, the destruction of red blood cells and the liberation of hemoglobin into the plasma. Hemolysis will increase potassium levels, but the gray-top tube containing potassium oxalate as the anticoagulant cannot be used to collect potassium specimens for obvious reasons. Microclot formation can result from too little anticoagulant, rather than too much. Hematology tests, such as evaluating stained WBCs, are collected in EDTA tubes not oxalate.

    REVIEW: Yes ☐ No ☐

59. **Answer: d**

    WHY: Thixotropic gel is an inert (nonreacting) synthetic substance that forms a physical barrier between the cellular portion of a specimen and the serum or plasma portion after the specimen has been centrifuged. The gel is normally found in or near the bottom of the tube. When used in a serum tube it is called serum separator, and the tube is referred to as a serum separator tube (SST) or a gel-barrier tube. When used in a tube that contains heparin, it is called plasma separator and the tube is referred to as a plasma separator tube (PST). If it is used in a tube that contains EDTA, the tube is called a plasma preparation tube (PPT). At this time, there is no gel tube that contains sodium citrate. Gel can be seen in the second and fourth tubes from the left in Figure 7-13.

    REVIEW: Yes ☐ No ☐

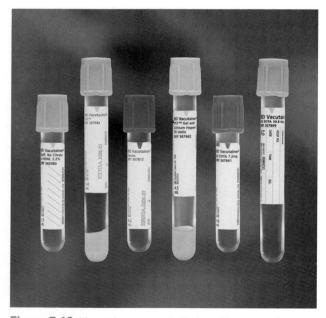

Figure 7-13 Vacutainer evacuated tubes. (Courtesy of Becton Dickinson, Franklin Lakes, NJ.)

60. **Answer: c**

    WHY: An antiglycolytic agent is a substance that inhibits or prevents glycolysis (metabolism of glucose) by the cells of the blood. The most common glycolytic inhibitors are sodium fluoride and lithium iodoacetate.

    REVIEW: Yes ☐ No ☐

61. **Answer: a**

    WHY: Glass (silica) particles are called clot activators and are present in serum separator tubes to make the blood clot faster. Glass particles enhance or accelerate clotting by providing increased surface for platelet activation, aggregation, and adhesion. Other substances that function as clot activators in other types of tubes include inert clays such as siliceous earth, kaolin, and celite, and the clotting components thromboplastin and thrombin.

    REVIEW: Yes ☐ No ☐

62. **Answer: a**

    WHY: A gray-top tube typically contains sodium fluoride, which prevents glycolysis. It is used for alcohol determinations and glucose tests. Alcohol values are stable because glycolysis (the metabolism of glucose or sugar in the form of alcohol) is prevented. Sodium fluoride also inhibits growth of bacteria and protects the specimen from an increase in alcohol resulting from fermentation by bacteria.

    REVIEW: Yes ☐ No ☐

63. **Answer: c**

    WHY: A CBC is a hematology test collected in a lavender-top tube. A PTT is a coagulation test collected in a light blue–top tube. A STAT potassium is a chemistry test collected in a green-top tube. The proper order of draw for these tubes is light blue first, green next, and lavender last (Table 7-2).

    REVIEW: Yes ☐ No ☐

64. **Answer: b**

    WHY: Proper tourniquet application allows arterial blood flow into the area below the tourniquet but obstructs venous flow away from the area. This causes the veins to enlarge and makes them easier to find and pierce with a needle. However, the obstruction of blood flow can change blood components if the tourniquet is left in place for more than 1 minute.

    REVIEW: Yes ☐ No ☐

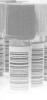

Table 7-2: Order of Draw, Stopper Colors, and Rationale for Collection Order

Order of Draw	Tube Stopper Color	Rationale for Collection Order
Blood cultures (sterile collections)	Yellow SPS Sterile media bottles	Minimizes chance of microbial contamination
Coagulation tubes	Light blue	The first additive tube in the order because all other additive tubes affect coagulation test
Glass nonadditive tubes	Red	Prevents contamination by additives in other tubes
Plastic clot activator tubes Serum separator tubes (SSTs)	Red Red and gray rubber Gold plastic	Filled after coagulation tests because silica particles activate clotting and affect coagulation tests (carryover of silica into subsequent tubes can be overridden by anticoagulant in them)
Plasma separator tubes (PSTs) Heparin tubes	Green and gray rubber Light green plastic Green	Heparin affects coagulation tests and interferes in collection of serum specimens; causes the least interference in tests other than coagulation tests
EDTA tubes Plasma preparation tubes (PPTs)	Lavender, Pink Pearl top	Responsible for more carryover problems than any other additive: elevates Na and K levels, chelates and decreases calcium and iron levels, elevates PT and PTT results
Oxalate/fluoride tubes	Gray	Sodium fluoride and potassium oxalate affect sodium and potassium levels, respectively. Filled after hematology tubes because oxalate damages cell membranes and causes abnormal RBC morphology. Oxalate interferes in enzyme reactions

65. **Answer: a**

    WHY: Tubes or containers for specimens such as blood cultures that must be collected in a sterile manner are always collected first in the order of draw for both the syringe and ETS system of venipuncture (Table 7-2).
    REVIEW: Yes ☐   No ☐

66. **Answer: c**

    WHY: A prothrombin time (PT) is a coagulation test and is collected in a light blue–top tube containing sodium citrate. The best tube for collecting a glucose specimen is a gray top containing an antiglycolytic agent such as sodium fluoride. A platelet count is sometimes ordered to assess coagulation, but it is a hematology test collected in a lavender-top tube. A red blood count is a hematology test and is collected in a lavender-top tube.
    REVIEW: Yes ☐   No ☐

67. **Answer: c**

    WHY: Most chemistry tests have been traditionally performed on serum, but to save the time it takes for a serum specimen to clot before it can be tested, STAT electrolytes and other STAT chemistry tests are often performed on plasma specimens collected in lithium heparin tubes. (Sodium heparin tubes must not be used for STAT electrolytes because sodium is one of the

electrolytes measured.) In addition, heparinized plasma may be the best specimen for all potassium tests because cells release potassium when they clot, which can artificially elevate serum results. Regardless of whether serum or plasma is used, the type of specimen should be consistent for any additional potassium tests on the same patient.
    REVIEW: Yes ☐   No ☐

68. **Answer: b**

    WHY: A lavender (or purple) top indicates that the tube contains EDTA. Most hematology tests are collected in lavender-top tubes. A green stopper indicates a heparin-containing tube, and a light blue stopper indicates the presence of sodium citrate unless it has a special yellow label. A royal blue stopper indicates that the tube and stopper are as free of trace elements as possible. A royal blue stopper sometimes contains EDTA, but only if it has lavender color coding on the label or EDTA is written on the label. Figure 7-13 shows a variety of tubes that have different colors of stoppers.
    REVIEW: Yes ☐   No ☐

69. **Answer: c**

    WHY: A plasma separator tube (PST) contains heparin. Some gel-barrier tubes, such as the plasma preparation tube (PPT), contain EDTA. Serum separator tubes (SSTs) are gel-barrier tubes, but they do not contain anticoagulant. Anticoagulants are used to obtain either whole blood or plasma specimens. In the separator tubes, the plasma can be removed from the cells so that the integrity of the specimen is maintained.

REVIEW: Yes ☐   No ☐

70. **Answer: d**

WHY: Sodium citrate is the anticoagulant contained in light blue–top tubes used to collect plasma for coagulation tests. It is used for coagulation tests because it does the best job of protecting the coagulation factors. The ratio of blood to anticoagulant is critical in coagulation testing, so it is important for sodium citrate tubes to be filled to their stated capacity.

REVIEW: Yes ☐   No ☐

71. **Answer: b**

WHY: The barrel of a syringe holds the fluid being aspirated or administered and is measured in cubic centimeters (cc) or milliliters (mL). The plunger is a rodlike device that fits tightly into the barrel. Pulling on the plunger creates the vacuum that allows the barrel to fill with the fluid being aspirated. The hub is where the needle attaches to the syringe. Syringe components are shown in Figure 7-14.

REVIEW: Yes ☐   No ☐

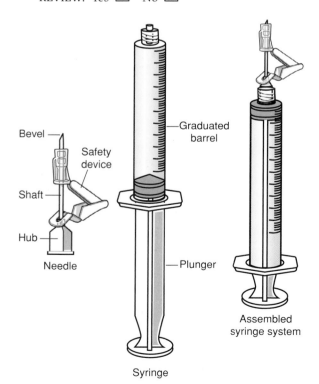

Figure 7-14 Syringe system components.

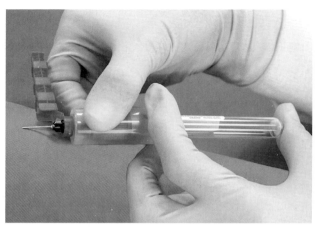

Figure 7-15 Proper placement of fingers and thumb when advancing a tube in an ETS holder.

72. **Answer: b**

WHY: The flanges or extensions on the sides of the tube end of the holder are there to aid in tube placement and removal. Figure 7-15 shows proper placement of fingers and thumb when advancing a tube in an ETS holder.

REVIEW: Yes ☐   No ☐

73. **Answer: a**

WHY: A butterfly needle (Fig. 7-16) is an indispensable tool for collecting blood from small or difficult veins because it allows much more flexibility and precision than either a regular needle and evacuated tube holder or needle and syringe. A lancet and microtainer can be used to collect some specimens by skin puncture, but there are several tests that cannot be collected by this method.

REVIEW: Yes ☐   No ☐

74. **Answer: b**

WHY: Although evacuated tube collection system components from different manufacturers are similar, they are not necessarily interchangeable. Mixing components from different manufacturers can lead to problems such as improper needle fit and

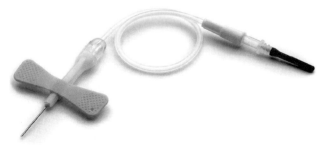

Figure 7-16 Vacuette safety butterfly blood collection system. (Courtesy of Greiner Bio-One, Kremsmünster, Austria.)

needles coming unscrewed, or tubes popping off of the needle during venipuncture procedures. Color coding of tube tops is generally universal, with only a few minor variations in each company's product, so selecting the proper additive tube is not normally an issue. Carryover of additive is typically related to errors in specimen collection technique.

REVIEW: Yes ☐ No ☐

75. **Answer: d**

WHY: The 25-gauge butterfly needles are sometimes successfully used to collect blood specimens from infants and others with difficult veins. However, any time a needle smaller than 23 gauge is used to collect blood, the chance of trauma to the red blood cells and resulting hemolysis is increased.

REVIEW: Yes ☐ No ☐

76. **Answer: b**

WHY: The purpose of a tourniquet in the venipuncture procedure is to block the venous flow, not the arterial flow, so that blood flows freely into the area but not out. This causes the veins to enlarge, making them easier to find and penetrate with a needle. The tourniquet does not redirect blood flow but does change the volume of the flow. The tourniquet must not be left on for longer than 1 minute because obstruction of blood flow changes the concentration of some analytes, leading to erroneous test results.

REVIEW: Yes ☐ No ☐

77. **Answer: a**

WHY: A blood pressure cuff may be used in place of a tourniquet by those familiar with its operation. The patient's blood pressure is taken, and the pressure is then maintained below the patient's diastolic pressure. In the absence of a blood pressure reading the cuff pressure should not exceed 40 mm Hg.

REVIEW: Yes ☐ No ☐

78. **Answer: b**

WHY: An anticoagulant prevents coagulation or clotting of the blood either by binding calcium and making it unavailable to the coagulation process, or by inhibiting thrombin formation, which is needed in the coagulation process. A specimen that is not allowed to clot because of the addition of an anticoagulant remains as it was in the body and is called a whole blood sample. Anticoagulants do not inhibit glucose metabolism.

REVIEW: Yes ☐ No ☐

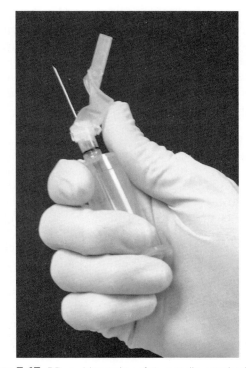

Figure 7-17 BD multisample safety needle attached to traditional tube holder. (Becton Dickinson, Franklin Lakes, NJ.)

79. **Answer: b**

WHY: A needle safety device (Fig. 7-17) should allow the user's hand to remain behind the needle at all times, create a barrier between the hands of the user and the needle after use, be activated using a one-handed technique, and provide permanent (not temporary) containment of the needle. A needle safety feature should never be a temporary measure.

REVIEW: Yes ☐ No ☐

80. **Answer: b**

WHY: An EDTA tube that contains a separator gel is called a plasma preparation tube, or PPT. A plasma separator tube (PST) contains heparin and gel. A serum separator tube (SST) contains silica particles or clot activator and gel. There is no separator gel tube called an EST.

REVIEW: Yes ☐ No ☐

81. **Answer: c**

WHY: Sodium polyanethol sulfonate (SPS) is used in tubes for blood culture collection because in addition to being an anticoagulant, this additive is formulated to inhibit phagocytosis of bacteria by white blood cells. SPS reduces the action of a protein called complement that destroys bacteria, slows down phagocytosis (ingestion of bacteria by leukocytes), and reduces the activity of certain antibiotics. Heparin inhibits thrombin. Silica activates or enhances clotting. When a specimen is centrifuged, thixotropic gel becomes a physical barrier between the serum or plasma and the cells to prevent the cells from metabolizing substances in the serum or plasma.

REVIEW: Yes ☐ No ☐

82. **Answer: b**

WHY: Tissue thromboplastin affects coagulation tests the most because it is a substance found in tissue that activates the extrinsic coagulation pathway. Tissue thromboplastin is picked up by the needle as it penetrates the skin during venipuncture and is flushed into the first tube filled during ETS collection, or mixed with blood collected in a syringe. Although it is no longer considered a significant problem for prothrombin time (PT) and partial thromboplastin time (PTT) tests unless the draw is difficult or involves a lot of needle manipulation, it may compromise results of other coagulation tests. Therefore, any time a coagulation test other than PT or PTT is the first or only tube collected, a few milliliters of blood should be drawn into a "discard" tube.

REVIEW: Yes ☐ No ☐

83. **Answer: c**

WHY: K_2EDTA contains potassium. (K is the chemical symbol for potassium, and K_2EDTA is an abbreviation for dipotassium EDTA.) Carryover of potassium EDTA formulations into tubes for potassium testing have been known to significantly increase potassium levels in the specimen, causing erroneously elevated test results.

REVIEW: Yes ☐ No ☐

84. **Answer: c**

WHY: Lavender stoppers contain the anticoagulant EDTA. According to the Clinical and Laboratory Standards Institute (CLSI), carry over from an underfilled additive tube has a greater potential to negatively affect the test results in a subsequent tube. Carryover from a nonadditive tube would not affect the next tube. A gray-top tube is drawn last so there is no subsequent tube to affect.

REVIEW: Yes ☐ No ☐

85. **Answer: c**

WHY: A needle can pick up contaminants going through tube stoppers. Trace elements are measured in such small quantities that these contaminants could affect test rests. Consequently, a trace-element tube should be collected separately, or to prevent another stick if other tests are

ordered, a syringe can be used and the trace-element tube filled last after changing to a new transfer device.

REVIEW: Yes ☐ No ☐

86. **Answer: a**

WHY: A pink-top EDTA tube typically has a special label for ID information and is used primarily for blood bank tests.

REVIEW: Yes ☐ No ☐

87. **Answer: d**

WHY: The S-Monovette Blood Collection System shown in Figure 7-1 is a complete system for blood collection in which the blood collection tube and collection apparatus are combined in a single unit. The unit allows the specimen to be collected by either an evacuated tube system (ETS) or syringe system technique. The units are available with regular or butterfly-style needles.

REVIEW: Yes ☐ No ☐

88. **Answer: d**

WHY: A prothrombin time (PT) is collected in a light blue–top tube, STAT electrolytes (lytes) require a green top or a PST, and a blood culture (BC), although usually collected in special bottles, is sometimes collected in a yellow-top SPS tube. The BC (yellow) is collected first because it requires a sterile collection site. The PT (light blue) is collected next, and the lytes (green or PST) are collected last.

REVIEW: Yes ☐ No ☐

89. **Answer: a**

WHY: A BD clear top or glass red–top tube has no additive. A plastic red–top tube has a clot activator. A plasma separator tube (PST) contains heparin and barrier gel. A serum separator tube (SST) has clot activator and barrier gel (Table 7-3).

REVIEW: Yes ☐ No ☐

90. **Answer: c**

WHY: Green stopper color means the additive in the tube is heparin. Heparin is an anticoagulant that is available in ETS tubes in two forms, lithium heparin and sodium heparin. Each form has its own tube; however, both lithium heparin and sodium heparin tubes have green stoppers (Table 7-3). Consequently, the phlebotomist must be careful in selecting the right tube for the ordered test because the two forms of heparin are not normally interchangeable.

REVIEW: Yes ☐ No ☐

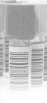

Table 7-3: Common Stopper Colors, Additives, and Departments

Stopper Color(s)	Additive	Department(s)
Light blue	Sodium citrate	Coagulation
Red (glass)	None	Chemistry, blood bank, serology/immunology
Red (plastic)	Clot activator	Chemistry
Red/light gray Clear	Nonadditive	NA (Discard tube only)
Red/black (tiger) Gold	Clot activator and gel separator	Chemistry
Green/gray Light green	Lithium heparin and gel separator	Chemistry
Green	Lithium heparin Sodium heparin	Chemistry
Lavender (purple)	EDTA	Hematology
Pink	EDTA	Blood bank
Gray	Sodium fluoride and potassium oxalate Sodium fluoride and EDTA Sodium fluoride	Chemistry
Orange Gray/yellow	Thrombin	Chemistry
Royal blue	None (red label) EDTA (lavender label) Sodium heparin (green label)	Chemistry
Tan	EDTA	Chemistry
Yellow	Sodium polyanethol sulfonate (SPS)	Microbiology
Yellow	Acid citrate dextrose (ACD)	Blood bank/immunohematology

91. **Answer: a**
    WHY: Lavender, pink, royal blue (lavender label), and BD tan stopper tubes all contain the anticoagulant EDTA (Table 7-3).
    REVIEW: Yes ☐ No ☐

92. **Answer: d**
    WHY: The sodium polyanethol sulfonate (SPS) tube that is processed in the microbiology department has a yellow stopper, as does the tube containing acid citrate dextrose (ACD) that is used by the immunohematology department for DNA testing (Table 7-3).
    REVIEW: Yes ☐ No ☐

93. **Answer: a**
    WHY: Because of the prevalence of latex allergies in glove users and patients, latex gloves and other items made of latex (e.g., tourniquets) are not recommended for use in healthcare facilities. Gloves and other items made of alternative materials are available.
    REVIEW: Yes ☐ No ☐

94. **Answer: c**
    WHY: Both lithium and sodium heparin are used by the chemistry department (Table 7-3). Acid citrate dextrose (ACD) is used for certain immunohematology tests. Sodium citrate is most commonly used for coagulation tests. Sodium polyanethol sulfonate (SPS) is used for blood cultures which are microbiology tests.
    REVIEW: Yes ☐ No ☐

95. **Answer: c**
    WHY: A syringe transfer device (Fig. 7-18A) is similar to an ETS tube holder but has a permanently attached needle inside the holder. The needle with sleeve is the same as you would find on a multisample ETS needle. This allows the transfer device holder to be attached to a syringe and ETS tubes inserted, pierced by the needle inside the holder, and filled from the syringe (Fig. 7-18B).
    REVIEW: Yes ☐ No ☐

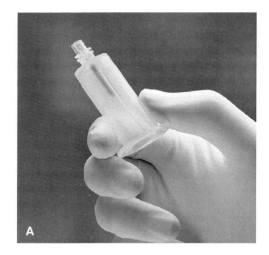

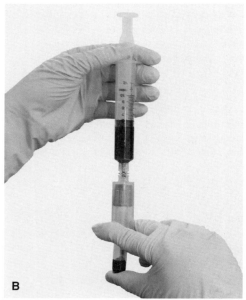

Figure 7-18 Syringe transfer devices. **A:** BD transfer device. (Courtesy of Becton Dickinson, Franklin Lakes, NJ.) **B:** Greiner transfer device attached to a syringe.

96. **Answer: a**

WHY: The first tube collected with a butterfly will underfill because of air in the tubing. If the tube contains an additive, underfilling will affect the blood-to-additive ratio. If a citrate tube is the first tube to be collected, it is important to draw a few milliliters of blood into a nonadditive tube or another additive tube of the same type, and discard it before collecting the first tube. This practice is referred to as collecting a "clear" or discard tube (Fig. 7-19) and is especially critical when collecting coagulation tests with a butterfly.

REVIEW: Yes ☐ No ☐

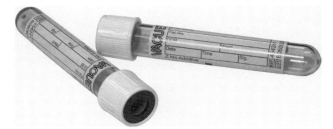

Figure 7-19 Nonadditive tubes used as discard or "clear" tubes.

97. **Answer: b**

WHY: Tubes were drawn in the wrong order, and the position of the patient's arm during the venipuncture most likely allowed them to fill from the stopper end first. This allows blood in the tube to be in contact with the needle so that carryover of additive from one tube to the next can occur. Since the lab asked for three of the tests to be redrawn, it is probable that there was carryover of potassium EDTA from the lavender CBC tube to the potassium (K) tube which was filled after it. Potassium is collected in a heparin tube. Heparin most likely carried from potassium tube into the PT and PTT tube. Consequently, the potassium, PT and PTT would all be affected and need to be recollected.

REVIEW: Yes ☐ No ☐

98. **Answer: d**

WHY: The royal blue–top tubes are used for toxicology studies, which would include metal poisoning. Royal blue stoppers indicate trace element–free tubes. These tubes are used for substances present in such small quantities that trace-element contamination commonly found in other tubes may leach into the specimen and falsely elevate test results. A trace-element tube should be collected separately or a syringe used for the draw and the transfer device changed before filling the royal blue top. This minimizes the chance of contamination picked up by the transfer needle from the stoppers of other tubes filled before it.

REVIEW: Yes ☐ No ☐

99. **Answer: c**

WHY: The yellow topped tube containing ACD solution is available in two formulations (solution A and solution B) for immunohematology tests such as DNA testing used in paternity evaluation. The acid citrate prevents coagulation by binding calcium, with little effect on cells and platelets. Dextrose acts as a red blood cell nutrient and preservative by maintaining red cell viability.

REVIEW: Yes ☐ No ☐

100. **Answer: b**

WHY: The most common electrolytes tested are sodium and potassium. A gray-top tube typically contains sodium fluoride and potassium oxalate that would greatly increase sodium and potassium results. A tube with a light green top contains lithium heparin, which is the preferred additive for electrolyte testing. Tubes with gold or red and black tops are serum separator tubes. Although recent studies suggest plasma is the preferred specimen for electrolytes testing, many labs still use serum specimens.

REVIEW: Yes ☐   No ☐

Venipuncture Procedures

Study Tips

- Complete the activities in Chapter 8 of the companion WORKBOOK.

- Grab a partner and role-play proper identification including how to handle ID discrepancies and other problems.

- Get together with several others and practice arm positioning, tourniquet application and release, and vein selection procedures on one another.

- Identify how to handle ASAP, stat, timed, and fasting tests.

- Make a list of venipuncture steps, cut out each step, scramble them, and then put them back in the correct order.

- Role-play how to handle issues associated with drawing blood from children and geriatric patients.

- Use a protractor to create 10-, 15-, and 30-degree angles.

Overview

Venipuncture is the process of collecting or "drawing" blood from a patient's vein and the most common way to collect blood specimens for laboratory testing. It is the most frequent procedure performed by a phlebotomist, and the most important step in this procedure is patient identification. This chapter addresses how to correctly identify all types of patients and how to safely obtain high-quality blood specimens from them. Venipuncture techniques covered in this chapter include ETS, butterfly, and syringe procedures on arm and hand veins. This chapter also addresses challenges and unique issues associated with pediatric, geriatric, dialysis, long-term care, home care, and hospice patients.

Review Questions

Choose the BEST answer.

1. When properly anchoring a vein, the
   a. index and middle fingers are pulling the skin parallel to the arm just below the site.
   b. index finger is pulling the skin above the site and thumb is pulling toward the wrist.
   c. thumb is 1 to 2 in below the intended site and is pulling the skin toward the wrist.
   d. thumb is next to the intended vein and pressing heavily downward into the tissue.

2. Which of the following actions is unlikely to help a phlebotomist gain a patient's trust?
   a. Acting confident and assured in bedside manner
   b. Being professional in dress and personal appearance
   c. Collecting a specimen before the requested time
   d. Labeling the blood specimen while at the bedside

3. It is unlikely that misidentifying a patient specimen would result in
   a. a civil action malpractice lawsuit.
   b. being dismissed from the facility.
   c. no reprimand if no one was hurt.
   d. temporary suspension of duties.

4. Needle phobia is defined as a/an
   a. anxiety about admission to the hospital.
   b. inability to watch while others are drawn.
   c. intense fear of needles and being stuck.
   d. personal preference for smaller needles.

5. Symptoms of needle phobia can include
   a. arrhythmia.
   b. fainting.
   c. light-headedness.
   d. all of the above.

6. A basic step that can be taken to minimize any trauma associated with a venipuncture is to
   a. allow the patient to sit in the waiting room for half an hour before collection.
   b. choose the most skilled phlebotomist available to perform the venipuncture.
   c. have the patient wear an eye mask or close his or her eyes during the procedure.
   d. thoroughly explain every detail of the draw before doing the venipuncture.

7. Proper use of a hand sanitizer includes
   a. allowing the alcohol to evaporate completely.
   b. rubbing it in between and around the fingers.
   c. using a very generous amount of the sanitizer.
   d. all of the above.

8. To examine by touch or feel is to
   a. ambulate.
   b. anchor.
   c. palpate.
   d. pronate.
   📖 *Have some fun by finding this term in the scrambled words activity in the WORKBOOK.*

9. In most cases, needle insertion should be performed
   a. at a 45-degree angle to the surface of the arm.
   b. using a smooth, steady motion forward.
   c. with a deliberate and rapid forward jab.
   d. with the bevel of the needle face down.

10. To "seat" the needle in the vein means to
    a. anchor the vein while inserting the needle.
    b. increase the angle needed to enter the vein.
    c. redirect the needle to gain entry to the vein.
    d. thread part of the needle within the lumen.

11. Going without food or drink except water for 8 to 12 hours is defined as
    a. fasting.
    b. NPO.
    c. routine.
    d. TDM.

12. The reason a test is ordered "timed" is to
    a. assess a patient's condition after surgery.
    b. determine patient suitability for surgery.
    c. draw it at the best time for accurate results.
    d. establish a clinical diagnosis or prognosis.

13. Examples of timed tests include
    a. basic metabolic panel, potassium, and glucose.
    b. blood cultures, cardiac enzymes, and cortisol.
    c. calcium, ferritin, and complete blood count.
    d. creatinine, lactic acid, and reticulocyte count.

14. A test is ordered "fasting" to
    a. assess a patient after outpatient surgery.
    b. eliminate the effects of diet on test results.
    c. determine patient eligibility for surgery.
    d. standardize test results on critical patients.

15. Bending the arm up to apply pressure to the site after venipuncture has not been shown to
    a. disrupt the platelet plug when the arm is eventually lowered.
    b. enable the site to quickly stop bleeding after needle removal.
    c. increase the possibility of bruising and hematoma formation.
    d. keep the wound open, especially if it is at the side of the arm.

16. The unique number assigned to a specimen request is called the
    a. accession number.
    b. health facility number.
    c. patient date of birth.
    d. patient ID number.

17. Failure of the patient to follow required diet restrictions before specimen collection could lead to
    a. compromised patient care and treatment.
    b. erroneous and meaningless test results.
    c. misinterpreted test results by the physician.
    d. all of the above.

18. Which of the following individuals has legal authority to authorize patient testing?
    a. Laboratory director
    b. Patient's nurse
    c. Patient's physician
    d. Phlebotomist

19. Test requisition information must include the
    a. ordering physician.
    b. patient's diagnosis.
    c. patient's location.
    d. prior draw times.

20. A type of care for patients who are terminally ill is
    a. elder care.
    b. home care.
    c. hospice care.
    d. long-term care.

21. Using information from the computer requisition (Fig. 8-1), identify the number that points to the type of tube to be drawn.
    a. 1
    b. 2
    c. 3
    d. 4

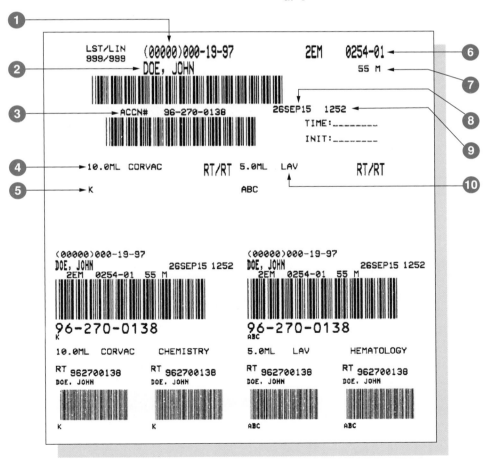

Figure 8-1 A computer requisition with bar code.

22. Using information from the computer requisition (Fig. 8-1), identify the number that points to the patient's age.
    a. 1
    b. 6
    c. 7
    d. 9

23. Using information from the computer requisition (Fig. 8-1), identify the number that points to the accession number.
    a. 1
    b. 3
    c. 6
    d. 7

24. Information represented by a patient ID bar code typically includes the patient's
    a. credit information and employer.
    b. health status and lab test results.
    c. medical record number and name.
    d. all of the above

25. If a patient is known to be combative and you are asked to collect a blood specimen from him, what should you do?
    a. Enlist another person's assistance if necessary.
    b. Make certain there is an unobstructed exit route.
    c. Place your equipment out of the patient's reach.
    d. All of the above.

26. When received by the laboratory, inpatient requisitions are typically sorted according to
    a. alphabetical order by name and then by test requested.
    b. collection priority, date and time, and patient location.
    c. difficulty of draw and type of equipment needed.
    d. proximity of the patient's room to the laboratory.

27. Steps taken to unmistakably connect a specimen and the accompanying paperwork to a specific individual are called
    a. accessioning the specimen.
    b. bar-coding specimen labels.
    c. collection verification.
    d. patient identification.

28. Which priority does a timed test typically have?
    a. First
    b. Second
    c. Third
    d. Fourth

29. A test that is ordered stat should be collected
    a. as soon as it is possible to do so.
    b. immediately, without any hesitation.
    c. on the next closest scheduled sweep.
    d. within 1 hour of the test request.

30. Which of the following tests is commonly ordered stat?
    a. Creat
    b. Diff
    c. Lytes
    d. RAST

31. If a test is ordered stat, it may mean that the patient is in
    a. critical condition.
    b. fragile condition.
    c. rehabilitation.
    d. transition status.

32. When a test is ordered ASAP, it means that
    a. the patient is in critical condition and needs the results now.
    b. the patient requires a test that the timing of collection is critical.
    c. results are needed soon for an appropriate response.
    d. results from blood work are needed for medication. Next medication dosage is based on the test result.

33. A preop patient
    a. has been admitted to the hospital.
    b. is an ambulatory outpatient.
    c. is being assessed after surgery.
    d. will soon be going to surgery.

34. Tests are classified as routine if they are ordered
    a. for collection at a specific time and place.
    b. in the course of establishing a diagnosis.
    c. to assess a patient's condition after surgery.
    d. to specifically eliminate the effects of diet.

35. This term means the same as stat.
    a. Fasting
    b. Med emerg
    c. Postop
    d. Timed

36. A patient who is NPO
    a. cannot have any food or drink.
    b. cannot have anything but water.
    c. is in critical but stable condition.
    d. is recovering from minor surgery.

37. An example of a test that is commonly ordered fasting is
    a. BUN.
    b. cortisol.
    c. glucose.
    d. PTT.

38. Which liquid is acceptable to drink when one is fasting?
    a. Black coffee
    b. Diet soda
    c. Plain water
    d. Sugarless tea

39. Which is a common postop test?
    a. CBC
    b. ESR
    c. H&H
    d. PTT

40. You arrive to draw a specimen on an inpatient. The patient's door is closed. What do you do?
    a. Knock lightly, open the door slowly, and ask whether it is all right to enter.
    b. Knock softly and wait for someone in the room to come to the door.
    c. Leave to draw another patient in the same area and come back later.
    d. Open the door, announce yourself, and quickly proceed into the room.

41. There is a sign above the patient's bed that reads, "No blood pressures or venipuncture, right arm," as seen in Figure 8-2. The patient has an intravenous (IV) line in the left forearm. You have a request to collect a complete blood count (CBC) on the patient. How should you proceed?
    a. Ask the patient's nurse to collect the specimen from the IV.

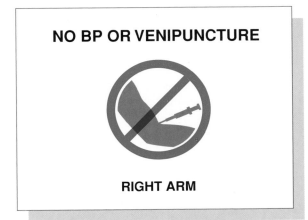

NO BP OR VENIPUNCTURE

RIGHT ARM

Figure 8-2 A warning sign indicating "No blood pressures or venipuncture in right arm."

b. Ask the patient's nurse what to do when the sign is posted.
    c. Collect a CBC from the right arm without using a tourniquet.
    d. Collect the specimen from the left hand by finger puncture.

42. A code is a way to
    a. convey important information without alarming the public.
    b. transmit messages over the facility's public address system.
    c. use numbers or words to represent important information.
    d. all of the above.

43. DNR means
    a. do not alert the nurse.
    b. do not call 911.
    c. do not call relatives.
    d. do not resuscitate.

📖 *Take a look at the Matching Exercise 8-1 in the WORKBOOK to see if you can define other key terms.*

44. You greet your patient in the following manner: "Hello, my name is Jean and I am here to collect a blood specimen. Is that all right with you?" The patient responds by saying, "OK, but I would rather not." How do you proceed?
    a. Ask another phlebotomist to draw the specimen.
    b. Come back at a later time to collect the specimen.
    c. Determine what the problem is before proceeding.
    d. Go ahead and draw the specimen without comment.

45. Which one of the following tests is used to identify protein disorders that lead to nerve damage?
    a. ANA
    b. ESR
    c. PTT
    d. SPEP

46. Your inpatient is asleep when you arrive to draw blood. What do you do?
    a. Call out the patient's name softly and shake the bed gently.
    b. Cancel the test and ask the nurse to resubmit the requisition.
    c. Check back every 15 minutes until the patient has awakened.
    d. Fill out a form stating that the specimen was not obtained and why.

47. Laboratory results can be negatively affected if the phlebotomist
    a. awakens a sleeping patient and raises the head of the patient's bed.
    b. collects a specimen in dim lighting conditions in the patient's room.
    c. draws a specimen from an unconscious patient without assistance.
    d. while preparing to collect a specimen, startles a patient who is asleep.

48. In collecting a blood specimen from an unconscious patient, it is unnecessary to
    a. have someone assist you just in case the patient moves.
    b. identify yourself and inform the patient of your intent.
    c. move the patient to a special phlebotomy collection area.
    d. talk to the patient as you would to a patient who is alert.

49. What do you do if a physician is with the patient and the specimen is ordered stat?
    a. Ask the patient's nurse to collect the stat specimen immediately.
    b. Come back later when you know the physician is no longer there.
    c. Introduce yourself and ask for permission to draw the specimen.
    d. Say "excuse me" to both and proceed to collect the specimen.

50. What is the best thing to do if family or visitors are with a patient?
    a. Ask them to wait outside of the room until you are finished.
    b. Come back later to collect the specimen when they have left.
    c. Have the patient's nurse tell everyone that they should leave.
    d. Tell them to quietly watch from the opposite side of the bed.

51. Your patient is not in the room when you arrive to collect a timed specimen. The patient's nurse states that the patient will be unavailable for several hours. What should you do?
    a. Ask the nurse to have the patient brought to the lab when the patient is available.
    b. Fill out a delay slip stating you were unable to collect the specimen.
    c. Report the situation to a supervisor and tell him or her to cancel the request.
    d. Return to the lab and put the request in the stack for the next sweep.

52. Misidentification of a specimen for this test is *most* likely to have fatal consequences.
    a. Blood culture
    b. Cold agglutinin
    c. Platelet count
    d. Type and screen

53. You arrive to collect a specimen on a patient named John Doe in 302B. How do you verify that the patient in 302B is indeed John Doe?
    a. Ask him, "Are you John Doe?" If he says yes, collect the specimen.
    b. Ask him for his name and date of birth and match it to the requisition.
    c. Check his ID band. If it matches the requisition, draw the specimen.
    d. Have the nurse verify the patient's name after you check his ID band.

54. Which requisition information *must* match information on the patient's ID band?
    a. Medical record number
    b. Name of the physician
    c. Room and bed number
    d. Test collection priority

55. The medical record number on the ID band matches the number on your requisition, but the patient's name is spelled differently than the one on your requisition. What should you do?
    a. Collect the specimen and report the error to the patient's nurse.
    b. Do not collect the specimen until the difference is resolved.
    c. Draw the specimen because the medical record number matches.
    d. Make the correction on the requisition and draw the specimen.

56. An unconscious inpatient does not have an ID band. The name on an envelope on the patient's nightstand matches with the requisition. What should you do?
    a. Ask the nurse to verify the patient's ID and collect the specimen.
    b. Complete the required procedure and then file an incident report.
    c. Do not start any procedure until the nurse attaches an ID bracelet.
    d. Make a computer entry to will alert other phlebotomists of the issue.

57. What would be the system of choice to identify laboratory specimens from an unconscious woman in the ER?
    a. Assign a name to the patient, such as Jane Doe.
    b. Assign a number to the patient until she is admitted.
    c. Use a three-part identification band with special tube labels.
    d. Wait to process the specimens until the patient can be identified.

58. Which type of inpatient is most likely to have more than one ID band?
    a. Adult
    b. Child
    c. Newborn
    d. Outpatient

59. What is the most critical error a phlebotomist can make?
    a. Collect a timed specimen late
    b. Fail to obtain the desired specimen
    c. Misidentify the patient's specimen
    d. Unknowingly give a patient a bruise

60. Your patient is not wearing an ID band. You see that the ID band is taped to the nightstand. The information matches your requisition. What do you do?
    a. Ask the patient to state her name; if it matches the requisition, continue.
    b. Ask the patient's nurse to attach an ID band and proceed when it is attached.
    c. Go to the nurses' station, get an ID bracelet, attach it, and then proceed.
    d. Tell the nurse that you will not collect the specimen and return to the lab.

61. Which one of the following types of patients is *least* likely to need his or her identity confirmed by the patient's nurse or a relative?
    a. A grouchy, geriatric patient
    b. A crying, 3-year-old child
    c. A mentally incompetent patient
    d. A non-English-speaking patient

62. The laboratory receptionist finishes checking a patient in and hands you the test request. The request is for a patient named Mary Smith. You call the name, and a woman who was just checked in responds. She is also the only patient in the waiting room. How do you verify that she is the correct patient?
    a. Ask the woman to state her complete name and date of birth to confirm her identity.
    b. Assume that you do not have to verify her identity because the receptionist already did.
    c. Conclude that she must be the right one because she is the only one in the waiting room.
    d. Decide that she must be right one because she answered you when you called the name.

63. A cheerful, pleasant bedside manner and exchange of small talk are unlikely to
    a. divert attention from any discomfort associated with the draw.
    b. increase the patient's confidence in the phlebotomist's abilities.
    c. keep the patient from fainting during the venipuncture procedure.
    d. redirect the patient's thoughts away from what is going to happen.

64. Your patient is cranky and rude to you. What do you do?
    a. Ask the patient's nurse to draw the specimen as you stand by to assist.
    b. Be as professional as you can and collect the specimen in a normal way.
    c. Do not speak to the patient; just get the necessary blood work and leave.
    d. Refuse to draw blood from the patient and leave the request for another phlebotomist.

65. Which of the following is part of informed consent for specimen collection?
    a. Advising the patient of his or her prognosis
    b. Explaining what disorders the test can detect
    c. Informing the patient that you are a student
    d. Notifying the patient of future venipunctures

66. The patient asks if the test you are about to draw is for diabetes. How do you answer?
    a. Explain that it is best to discuss the test with the physician.
    b. If the test is for glucose say, "Yes, it is" but do not elaborate.
    c. Say, "HIPAA confidentiality rules won't let me tell you."
    d. Tell the patient that it is not for a glucose test even if it is.

67. An inpatient vehemently refuses to allow you to collect a blood specimen. What should you do?
    a. Convince the patient to cooperate and collect the sample anyway.
    b. Have the nurse physically restrain the patient and draw the specimen.
    c. Notify the patient's nurse and document the patient's refusal.
    d. Return to the lab, cancel the test request, and inform the physician.

68. You arrive to draw a fasting specimen. The patient is just finishing breakfast. What do you do?
    a. Check with the patient's nurse to see if the specimen should be collected or the draw rescheduled.
    b. Collect the specimen, but write "nonfasting" on the lab slip and the specimen.
    c. Do not draw the blood, fill out an incident slip, and leave a copy for the nurse.
    d. Proceed to collect the specimen, since the patient had not quite finished eating.

69. If you assemble equipment after selecting and cleaning the blood collection site, you will
    a. be more apt to allow sufficient time for the alcohol to dry.
    b. have a better idea of what equipment you will need to use.
    c. waste less equipment by knowing exactly what is needed.
    d. all of the above.

70. When performing a venipuncture, hand decontamination is required
    a. after drawing your last patient.
    b. before and after each patient.
    c. only after drawing the patient.
    d. only before putting on gloves.

71. Which of the following is the best thing to do if your hands are visibly contaminated?
    a. Clean them with a hand sanitizer.
    b. Cover them up with clean gloves.
    c. Wash them with soap and water.
    d. Wipe them with an alcohol pad.

72. You must collect a specimen on a 6-year-old. The child is a little fearful. What do you do?
    a. Explain what you are going to do to the child in simple terms.
    b. Restrain the child and draw the specimen without explanation.
    c. Tell the child that you will give him a treat if he does not cry.
    d. Tell the child to relax and not to worry because it will not hurt.

73. If the patient asks whether the procedure will hurt, you should say that it
    a. could hurt if you watch, so look the other way.
    b. is painless and will be over before you know it.
    c. might hurt just a little, but only for a short time.
    d. hurts only if the phlebotomist is inexperienced.

74. What is the proper arm position for routine venipuncture?
    a. Downward in a straight line from shoulder to wrist, palm up
    b. Extended straight forward at about waist height and palm up
    c. Held out at an angle, bent at the elbow, and the palm up
    d. Straight down to the elbow, parallel elbow to wrist, palm up

75. Outpatients who have previously fainted during a blood draw should be
    a. allowed to sit up in order to carefully watch the draw.
    b. asked to lie down, or sit in a reclining drawing chair.
    c. drawn in a separate room that has first-aid equipment.
    d. permitted to sit in a chair if accompanied by an adult.

76. Which of the following acts can lead to liability issues?
    a. Asking visitors to leave the room while you draw a specimen.
    b. Drawing a patient who is lying in bed talking on a cell phone.
    c. Lowering a bed rail to make access to the patient's arm easier.
    d. Pulling the curtain between the beds while drawing a specimen.

77. Never leave a tourniquet on for more than
    a. 30 seconds.
    b. 1 minute.
    c. 2 minutes.
    d. 3 minutes.

78. Where is the best place to apply the tourniquet?
    a. About 3 to 4 in above the venipuncture site
    b. Distal to the venipuncture site on the forearm
    c. Distal to the wrist bone if drawing a hand vein
    d. Immediately above the venipuncture site

79. If the tourniquet is too tight
    a. arterial flow below it may be stopped.
    b. blood below it may hemoconcentrate.
    c. the pressure can cause the arm to ache.
    d. all of the above.

80. All of the following actions are acceptable during the vein selection process EXCEPT:
    a. Having a patient pump his or her fist
    b. Lowering the arm alongside the chair
    c. Palpating the antecubital area firmly
    d. Using warmth to increase blood flow

81. In selecting a venipuncture site, how can you tell a vein from an artery?
    a. A vein has a lot less resilience.
    b. A vein pulses and feels larger.
    c. An artery has a distinct pulse.
    d. An artery is more superficial.

82. What does a sclerosed vein feel like?
    a. Bouncy and resilient
    b. Hard and cord-like
    c. Pulsating and firm
    d. Soft and pliable

83. It is acceptable to use an ankle vein if
    a. coagulation tests are requested.
    b. the patient is partially paralyzed.
    c. the physician gives permission.
    d. there are no other suitable sites.

84. Which of the following will help you avoid inadvertently puncturing an artery during venipuncture?
    a. Avoid drawing the basilic vein in the antecubital area.
    b. Do not select a site that is near where you feel a pulse.
    c. Do not select a vein that overlies or is close to an artery.
    d. All of the above.

85. You must collect a light blue–top tube for a special coagulation test from a patient who has an intravenous (IV) line in the left wrist area and dermatitis all over the right arm and hand. The veins on the right arm and hand are not readily visible. What is the best way to proceed?
    a. Apply a tourniquet on the right arm over a towel and do the draw.
    b. Ask the patient's nurse to collect the specimen from the IV line.
    c. Collect from the left antecubital area without using a tourniquet.
    d. Collect the specimen by capillary puncture from the left hand.

86. What is the *best* thing to do if the vein can be felt but not seen, even with the tourniquet on?
    a. Insert the needle where you think it is and probe until you find it.
    b. Keep the tourniquet on while cleaning the site and during the draw.
    c. Look for visual clues on the skin to remind you where the vein is.
    d. Mark the spot using a felt-tipped pen and clean it off when finished.

87. Release the tourniquet as soon as blood flow is established to
    a. allow arterial blood flow to return to normal.
    b. decrease hemoconcentration of the specimen.
    c. increase the venous flow to the vein selected.
    d. all of the above.

88. What is the latest CLSI-recommended way to clean a venipuncture site?
    a. Cleanse the area thoroughly with disinfectant using concentric circles.
    b. Cleanse with a circular motion from the center to the periphery.
    c. Use friction to clean an area 2-3 inches in diameter in the selected area.
    d. Wipe using a scrubbing motion from the outside area to the center.

89. Which of the following is the least important reason to wait 30 seconds for the alcohol to dry before needle insertion?
    a. It allows the process of evaporation to help destroy any microbes.
    b. It avoids a stinging sensation when the needle penetrates the skin.
    c. It gives the phlebotomist time to prepare equipment and supplies.
    d. It prevents hemolysis of the specimen from alcohol in the needle.

90. What happens if you advance the tube past the guideline on the holder before needle insertion?
    a. The ETS tube will fail to fill with blood because of loss of tube vacuum.
    b. Nothing; the line is actually a fill guideline for all evacuated tubes.
    c. The needle sleeve stops penetration of the tube until fully advanced.
    d. There will be transfer of the tube additive to the needle at that point.

91. Visual inspection of the needle tip before inserting it in a patient's vein would be unable to detect
    a. the presence of external contamination.
    b. flaws that could damage a vein.
    c. proper positioning of the bevel.
    d. that the needle is out of date.

92. Which of the following steps are in the right order for the venipuncture procedure?
    a. Clean the site, prepare equipment, sanitize hands, apply tourniquet.
    b. Sanitize hands, put on gloves, select the vein, release tourniquet.
    c. Select the site, apply the tourniquet, prepare equipment, clean the site.
    d. Select the vein, clean the site, position the patient, put on the gloves.

93. You are about to draw blood from a patient. You touch the needle to the skin but change your mind and pull the needle away. What do you do next?
    a. Clean the site and try again using the same needle.
    b. Stop and obtain a new needle before trying again.
    c. Try it again immediately using that same needle.
    d. Wipe the needle across an alcohol pad and retry.

94. What is the best angle to use for needle insertion during routine venipuncture?
    a. Less than 15 degrees
    b. 30 degrees or less
    c. 35 to 45 degrees
    d. 45 to 60 degrees

95. In performing venipuncture, the needle is inserted
    a. as you prefer.
    b. bevel facing up.
    c. bevel side down.
    d. bevel sideways.

96. How can you tell when the needle is in the vein as you insert it into the patient's arm?
    a. Blood will enter the ETS tube.
    b. The needle will start to vibrate.
    c. You will feel a slight "give."
    d. You will hear a hissing sound.

97. When is the best time to release the tourniquet during venipuncture?
    a. After the last tube has been filled completely
    b. After the needle is withdrawn and covered
    c. As soon as blood begins to flow into the tube
    d. As soon as the needle penetrates the skin

98. Which of the following analytes is least affected by prolonged tourniquet application?
    a. Potassium
    b. Prothrombin
    c. Red cell count
    d. Total protein

99. Which of the following would be considered improper specimen collection technique?
    a. Collect sterile specimens before all other specimens.
    b. Draw a "clear" tube before special coagulation tests.
    c. Fill each tube until the normal vacuum is exhausted.
    d. Position the arm so tubes fill from stopper end first.

100. It is important to fill anticoagulant tubes to the proper level to ensure that
    a. the specimen yields enough serum for the required tests.
    b. there is a proper ratio of blood to anticoagulant additive.
    c. there is an adequate amount of blood to perform the test.
    d. tissue fluid contamination of the specimen is minimized.

101. It is important to mix anticoagulant tubes immediately after filling them to
    a. avoid microclot formation.
    b. encourage coagulation.
    c. inhibit hemoconcentration.
    d. minimize hemolysis.

102. You are in the middle of drawing a blood specimen using the evacuated-tube method when you realize that you just filled an EDTA tube and still have a green-top tube to collect. What do you do?
    a. Do not collect the green tube until the next collection sweep.
    b. Draw several milliliters into a discard tube, then fill the green one.
    c. Draw the green one next and hope that there is no carryover.
    d. It is acceptable to draw the EDTA before the green stopper.

103. How many times do you mix nonadditive tubes?
    a. 2 or 3
    b. 5 to 10
    c. 8 to12
    d. None

104. What may happen if you mix tubes too vigorously?
    a. Hemolysis
    b. Jaundice
    c. Lipemia
    d. No effect

105. Use several layers of gauze during needle removal so that
    a. blood will not contaminate your gloved hand.
    b. it will not hurt when you pull out the needle.
    c. pressure is adequate and bruising is prevented.
    d. the patient does not see you pull out the needle.

106. It is better to use gauze and not cotton balls for pressure over the site because cotton balls
    a. are not sufficiently porous to soak up all of the blood at the site.
    b. attract more airborne contaminants and are therefore less sterile.
    c. can irritate a patient's skin because they have loose cotton fibers.
    d. may pull the platelet plug away from the puncture site upon removal.

107. Applying pressure on the gauze as the needle is removed can cause the
    a. needle to bend.
    b. patient to faint.
    c. skin to be slit.
    d. All the above.

108. A needle safety feature that is not activated in the vein or automatically, should be activated
    a. after some pressure has been applied to the site.
    b. as you are dropping the needle in the sharps container.
    c. immediately after the needle is withdrawn.
    d. while the tube is still engaged in the holder.

109. Which of these steps are in the right venipuncture procedure order?
    a. Establish blood flow, release tourniquet, fill and mix tubes, remove needle
    b. Fill and mix all the tubes, release tourniquet, remove needle, apply pressure
    c. Fill the tubes, remove needle, release tourniquet, mix tubes, apply pressure
    d. Release tourniquet, fill tubes, remove needle, apply pressure, mix all tubes

110. Proper needle disposal involves
    a. disposing of the needle and tube holder in the sharps container as one unit.
    b. ejecting the needle from the tube holder so that the holder can be reused.
    c. removing the needle from the holder after engaging the needle safety device.
    d. unscrewing the needle from the holder by using a slot in the sharps container.

111. Labeling of routine inpatient blood specimens should take place
    a. at the bedside immediately after collection.
    b. before the blood specimens are collected.
    c. in the lab processing area after collection.
    d. outside the patient's room after collection.

112. Which of the following information on a specimen label would be considered optional?
    a. Patient's room number and bed
    b. Patient's first and last name
    c. Phlebotomist's initials or ID
    d. The date and time of the draw

113. The patient's identification number is included on specimen tube labels to
    a. avoid confusing multiple specimens from the same patient.
    b. avoid confusing specimens from patients with the same name.
    c. be used for an accession number in processing the specimen.
    d. be used for insurance identification and payment purposes.

114. The following precautionary information was given to an outpatient after venipuncture. No other tests were scheduled. Which information was unnecessary?
    a. Do not carry a heavy bag or large purse on that arm.
    b. Do not drink or eat for 2 hours after collection.
    c. Do not lift any heavy objects for at least 1 hour.
    d. Leave the bandage on for a minimum of 15 minutes.

115. Which of the following specimens requires routine (normal) handling?
    a. Ammonia
    b. Bilirubin
    c. Cholesterol
    d. Cryoglobulin

116. Which of the following is not a valid reason for failure to obtain a blood specimen?
    a. The patient adamantly refuses to have blood taken.
    b. The patient was unavailable at the designated time.
    c. You made an attempt but were unable to obtain the blood.
    d. You did not have the right equipment on your tray.

117. You have just made two unsuccessful attempts to collect a fasting blood specimen from an outpatient. The patient rotates his arm, and you note a large vein that you had not seen before. How do you proceed?

    a. Ask another phlebotomist to collect the fasting specimen.
    b. Ask the patient to come back later so that you can try again.
    c. Call the supervisor for permission to make a third attempt.
    d. Make a third attempt on the newly discovered large vein.

118. A patient has difficult veins and you decide to use a butterfly for the draw. *Butterfly* is another name for a

    a. hypodermic needle.
    b. multisample needle.
    c. needle safety feature.
    d. winged infusion set.

119. What is the advantage of using a butterfly?

    a. Blood flows faster than with ETS needles.
    b. Butterflies are less expensive than other needles.
    c. Butterflies make it easier to draw difficult veins.
    d. There is a greater choice in butterfly needle size.

120. Although the evacuated tube system (ETS) is the preferred method of blood collection, it may be necessary to use a syringe when

    a. a large amount of blood is needed.
    b. the patient's veins are very fragile.
    c. there are no butterfly needles left.
    d. you need the blood to flow faster.

121. How can you tell that you are in a vein when you are using a syringe?

    a. A "flash" of blood will appear in the hub of the needle.
    b. Blood will automatically pump into the syringe barrel.
    c. There will be a very slight vibration in the needle.
    d. You cannot tell when you are in a vein with a syringe.

122. Success of pediatric blood collection is most dependent on

    a. aseptic technique.
    b. correct order of draw.
    c. patient immobilization.
    d. tourniquet application.

123. Doing this before obtaining a blood specimen from a child is a bad idea.

    a. Establishing rapport with the child
    b. Greeting the parents and the child
    c. Telling the child it will not hurt
    d. Telling the child what to expect

124. A butterfly and 23-gauge needle is the best choice to use for venipuncture on a young child because

    a. children like the idea of using a butterfly.
    b. children's veins are often very sclerosed.
    c. flexible tubing allows for arm movement.
    d. it eliminates excessive bleeding.

125. In transferring blood from a syringe to evacuated tubes, which is the proper technique?

    a. Force the blood through the needle into the tubes by pushing the syringe plunger.
    b. Hold the tube steady in your hand while the syringe needle penetrates the stopper.
    c. Place the evacuated tube in a rack before penetrating stopper with the needle.
    d. Use a specially designed engineering device called a syringe transfer device.

126. In drawing blood from an older child, the most important consideration is

    a. assuring the child that it won't be painful.
    b. explaining all of the tests being collected.
    c. explaining the importance of holding still.
    d. offering the child a reward for not crying.

127. An additive should be mixed

    a. after the next tube is placed in the tube holder.
    b. as soon as it is removed from the tube holder.
    c. when all the other tubes have been collected.
    d. while the very next tube is being collected.

128. Tremors associated with this disease can make blood collection difficult

    a. Alzheimer's
    b. Arthritis
    c. Diabetes
    d. Parkinson's

129. A diabetic outpatient has had a mastectomy on her right side and cannot straighten her left arm because of arthritis. The best place to collect a blood specimen is

    a. an ankle or foot vein on either of her legs.
    b. the left forearm or hand, using a butterfly.
    c. the right arm below the antecubital fossa.
    d. the right hand, using a capillary puncture.

130. The most common reason a patient must undergo dialysis treatment is
    a. end stages of renal disease.
    b. Parkinson's disease effects.

    c. problems with coagulation.
    d. rheumatoid arthritis effects.

Answers and Explanations

1. **Answer: c**

   WHY: To anchor or pull the vein taut (Fig. 8-3), place the thumb a minimum of 1 to 2 in below and slightly to the side of the intended venipuncture site and pull the skin toward the wrist in line with the vein.

   REVIEW: Yes ☐ No ☐

2. **Answer: c**

   WHY: The manner in which you present yourself and interact with the patient sets the stage for whether or not you will gain the patient's trust. A phlebotomist with a professional bedside manner and appearance will more easily gain a patient's trust. An assured phlebotomist will convey that confidence to patients and help them feel at ease. Collecting a specimen earlier than the assigned time of collection could affect the results of the test and undermine the patient's confidence and trust in your knowledge and abilities.

   REVIEW: Yes ☐ No ☐

3. **Answer: c**

   WHY: Obtaining a specimen from the wrong patient can have serious, even fatal, consequences, especially specimens for type and crossmatch before blood transfusion. Misidentifying a patient or specimen can be grounds for dismissal of the person responsible and can even lead to a malpractice lawsuit (civil action) against that person. Even if no one was hurt by the misidentification, it is a serious error and would, at the least, result in a reprimand and thorough documentation of the incident.

   REVIEW: Yes ☐ No ☐

4. **Answer: c**

   WHY: Needle phobia is defined as intense fear of needles. The signs by the patient that suggest this phobia, such as extreme fear or apprehension in advance of venipuncture, should not be taken lightly. Although a patient may be anxious about being admitted to the hospital or have a needle

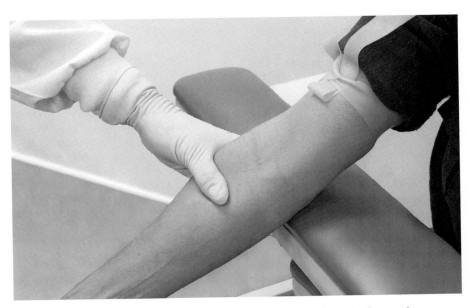

Figure 8-3 Proper placement of thumb and fingers in anchoring a vein.

preference for the venipuncture procedure, these do not constitute needle phobias.

REVIEW: Yes ☐ No ☐

5. **Answer: d**

WHY: Symptoms of needle phobia include pallor (paleness), profuse sweating, light-headedness, nausea, and fainting. In severe cases, patients have been known to suffer arrhythmia and even cardiac arrest.

REVIEW: Yes ☐ No ☐

6. **Answer: b**

WHY: Basic steps that can be taken to minimize any trauma associated with the venipuncture include the following: (1) having the patient lie down; (2) applying an ice pack to the site for 10 to 15 minutes before the venipuncture; and (3) having the most experienced and skilled phlebotomist perform the venipuncture. Explaining every little detail of the procedure, having patients close or cover their eyes, or having them wait outside the blood-drawing room to calm down simply increases the trauma of this experience.

REVIEW: Yes ☐ No ☐

7. **Answer: d**

WHY: When using hand sanitizers, it is important to use a generous amount and allow the alcohol to evaporate to achieve proper antisepsis. As shown in Figure 8-4, the sanitizer must be rubbed between and on the back of the fingers as well as the palms.

REVIEW: Yes ☐ No ☐

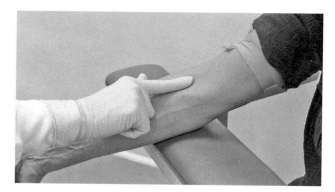

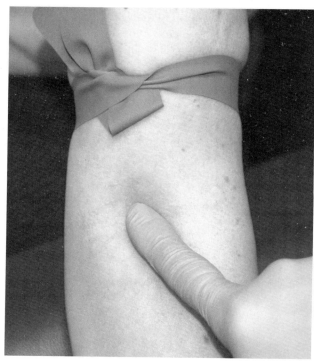

Figure 8-5 A phlebotomist palpating the antecubital area for a vein.

8. **Answer: c**

WHY: To examine by touch or feel is the definition of palpate, which is a chapter key term. Some veins are easily visible; others have to be located by feel, which is called palpating. Palpating involves pushing down on the skin with the tip of the index finger (Fig. 8-5). Palpating also helps determine the vein's patency, the size and depth, and the direction or the path that it follows.

REVIEW: Yes ☐ No ☐

📖 *Do Matching 8-1 in the WORKBOOK to see how well you know the definitions of all the Chapter 8 key terms.*

9. **Answer: b**

WHY: For antecubital-site venipunctures, insert the needle into the skin at an angle of 30 degrees

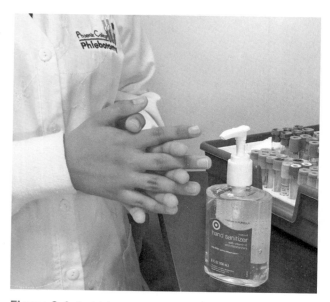

Figure 8-4 A phlebotomist applying hand sanitizer.

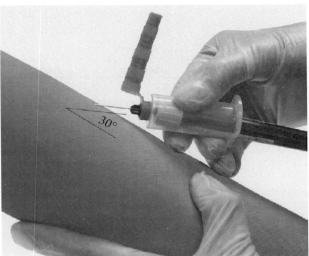

Figure 8-6 An illustration of a 30-degree angle of needle insertion.

or less (Fig. 8-6), depending on the depth of the vein. Use one smooth, steady, forward motion to penetrate first the skin and then the vein. Advancing the needle too slowly prolongs any discomfort. A rapid jab can result in missing the vein or going all the way through it. The needle bevel should be face up, not down.
REVIEW: Yes ☐ No ☐

10. **Answer: d**
WHY: A needle is seated in a vein by carefully threading it within the lumen or the central area of the vein. This may mean changing the angle of the needle slightly to accommodate the vein's path.
REVIEW: Yes ☐ No ☐

11. **Answer: a**
WHY: Some tests are affected by the patient's diet. To eliminate the effects of diet, these tests are typically ordered fasting. This means that the patient must go without food or drink except water for 8 to 12 hours before the specimen is to be collected. NPO (*nil per os*) means that the patient is not allowed to have anything by mouth, including water. Patients are NPO before surgical procedures, not blood tests (Table 8-1).
REVIEW: Yes ☐ No ☐

12. **Answer: c**
WHY: A "timed" test means that the test is collected at a specific time because the results will be the most accurate at that specific moment (Table 8-1).
REVIEW: Yes ☐ No ☐

📖 *Test your knowledge of other test status designations with WORKBOOK Knowledge Drill 8-4.*

13. **Answer: b**
WHY: Blood cultures, cardiac enzymes, and cortisol levels are timed tests (Table 8-1). It is critical to collect timed tests as close as possible to the requested time because that is when the information gained from results is most useful to the physician.
REVIEW: Yes ☐ No ☐

14. **Answer: b**
WHY: Fasting means "to go without food or drink except water for 8 to 12 hours." Fasting eliminates the effects food or drink may have on the results (see Table 8-1).
REVIEW: Yes ☐ No ☐

15. **Answer: b**
WHY: Studies show that folding the arm back at the elbow to hold pressure or keep the gauze in place after a blood draw actually increases the chance of bruising by keeping the wound open. This is especially true if the puncture site is to the side of the arm. The chance of disrupting the platelet plug is also increased when the arm is lowered.
REVIEW: Yes ☐ No ☐

16. **Answer: a**
WHY: The term accession means "the process of recording in the order received." To accession a specimen means "to take steps to unmistakably connect the specimen and the accompanying paperwork with a specific individual." To do this, each specimen request is given a unique number called the "accession number," which is different from the patient ID number, date of birth, or the health facility's number assigned to that patient at admission.
REVIEW: Yes ☐ No ☐

17. **Answer: d**
WHY: If required diet restrictions for a test are not met before the specimen is collected, the results can be erroneous and meaningless. The test results can also be misinterpreted by the physician, which leads to compromised patient care and treatment. The phlebotomist should always verify the patient's diet status before collecting the specimen.
REVIEW: Yes ☐ No ☐

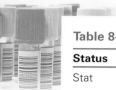

Table 8-1: Common Test Status Designations

Status	Meaning	When Used	Conditions	Examples	Priority
Stat	Immediately (from Latin *statim*)	Test results are urgently needed on critical patients	Immediately collect, test, and report results. Alert lab staff when delivered. ER stats typically have priority over other stats	Glucose H&H Electrolytes Cardiac enzymes	First
Med	Medical. Same as stat Emergency	Same as stat Emergency	Same as stat (replaces stat)	Same as stat	
Timed	Collect at a specific time	Tests for which timing is critical for accurate results	Collect as close as possible to requested time. Record actual time collected	2-hour PP GTT, cortisol Cardiac enzymes TDM blood cultures	Second
ASAP	As soon as possible	Test results are needed soon to respond to a serious situation, but patient is not critical	Follow hospital protocol for type of test	Electrolytes Glucose H&H	Second or third depending on test
Fasting	No food or drink except water for 8–12 hours prior to specimen	To eliminate diet effects on test results collection	Verify patient has fasted. If patient has not fasted, check to see if specimen should still be collected	Glucose Cholesterol Triglycerides	Fourth
NPO	Nothing by mouth (from Latin *nil per os*)	Prior to surgery or other anesthesia procedures	Do not give patient food or water. Refer requests to physician or nurse	N/A	N/A
Preop	Before an operation	To determine patient eligibility for surgery	Collect before the patient goes to surgery	CBC PTT Platelet function studies	Same as ASAP
Postop	After an operation	Assess patient condition after surgery	Collect when patient is out of surgery	H&H	Same as ASAP
Routine	Relating to established procedure	Used to establish a diagnosis or monitor a patient's progress	Collect in a timely manner but no urgency involved. Typically collected on morning sweeps or the next scheduled sweep	CBC Chem profile	None

18. Answer: c

WHY: Typically, a physician or other qualified healthcare professional requests laboratory testing. Exceptions are certain rapid tests that can be purchased and performed at home by consumers or blood specimens requested by law enforcement officials and used as evidence. A few states have legalized "Direct Access Testing" (DAT), in which patients are allowed to request certain blood tests themselves. So far, DAT is not widespread and the number of tests that can be requested is limited.

REVIEW: Yes ☐   No ☐

19. Answer: a

WHY: Test requisitions require specific information to ensure that the right patient is tested, the

physician's orders are met, the correct tests are performed at the proper time under the required conditions, and the patient is billed correctly. The patient's location is generally given on inpatient requisitions only. There is no need for the patient's diagnosis, if known, to be on the request for blood work. By the Health Insurance Portability and Accountability Act (HIPAA), release of such information is limited to those with a valid need to know. Prior draw times are not normal requisition information.

REVIEW: Yes ☐   No ☐

20. Answer: c

WHY: Hospice is a type of care designed for patients who are dying or terminally ill. Most hospice patients have incurable forms of cancer. Hospice care allows terminally ill patients to spend their last days in a peaceful, supportive atmosphere that emphasizes pain management to help keep them comfortable.

REVIEW: Yes ☐ No ☐

21. **Answer: d**

WHY: On the sample requisition in Figure 8-1, the type of tube to be collected appears as a mnemonic code with the volume of tube requested preceding the type of tube requested. In the example, the type of tube requested is a 10-mL Corvac (type of serum separator tube). A 5.0-mL lavender-top tube is also requested.

REVIEW: Yes ☐ No ☐

22. **Answer: c**

WHY: On the sample requisition in Figure 8-1, the patient's age is signified by the number "55" followed by the letter "M," which means that the patient is a 55-year-old male.

REVIEW: Yes ☐ No ☐

23. **Answer: b**

WHY: A computer requisition has an accession number given to the patient's sample during the data-entry phase. On the sample requisition in Figure 8-1, arrow number 3 points to the accession number.

REVIEW: Yes ☐ No ☐

24. **Answer: c**

WHY: A bar code is a series of black stripes and white spaces of varying widths that correspond to letters and numbers. The stripes can be grouped together to represent information such as medical record numbers, laboratory tests, and patient names.

REVIEW: Yes ☐ No ☐

25. **Answer: d**

WHY: If a patient exhibits unpredictable behaviors it is essential for an additional person or employee to be enlisted to assist if necessary. In addition, make certain you have an obstructed exit route in case it is needed. Also be mindful of where you place equipment and keep it out of the reach of the patient. As with any patient always have a gauze pad ready and be prepared to release the tourniquet quickly in case the patient pulls the needle out, or suddenly jerks causing the needle to either come out or go deep into the arm.

REVIEW: Yes ☐ No ☐

26. **Answer: b**

WHY: After the laboratory receives them, requisitions are sorted according to priority of collection, date and time of collection, and location of the patient.

REVIEW: Yes ☐ No ☐

27. **Answer: a**

WHY: The steps taken to unmistakably connect a specimen and the accompanying paperwork to a specific individual is called accessioning the specimen. The accession number is automatically assigned when the request is entered into the computer.

REVIEW: Yes ☐ No ☐

28. **Answer: b**

WHY: A timed test typically has second priority. It must be collected as close to the required time as possible, but a stat test would have priority over it.

REVIEW: Yes ☐ No ☐

29. **Answer: b**

WHY: *Stat* comes from the Latin word *statim*, which means "immediately." A test that is ordered stat should be collected immediately, without hesitation (Table 8-1).

REVIEW: Yes ☐ No ☐

30. **Answer: c**

WHY: Abnormal electrolyte levels can lead to death; consequently electrolyte tests are often ordered stat (Table 8-1).

REVIEW: Yes ☐ No ☐

31. **Answer: a**

WHY: When a test is ordered stat, it means that the results on a patient in critical condition are urgently needed (Table 8-1). A patient who is in critical condition is in a life-or-death situation.

REVIEW: Yes ☐ No ☐

32. **Answer: c**

WHY: ASAP means "as soon as possible." If a test is ordered ASAP, it means that test results are needed soon to respond appropriately to an unexpected situation but the patient is not in critical condition or in immediate danger of dying (Table 8-1).

REVIEW: Yes ☐ No ☐

33. **Answer: d**

WHY: *Preop* means "before an operation" and indicates that the patient will soon be going to surgery (Table 8-1).

REVIEW: Yes ☐ No ☐

34. **Answer: b**

    WHY: Routine tests are those that are typically ordered in the course of establishing a diagnosis or monitoring a patient's care (Table 8-1).

    REVIEW: Yes ☐   No ☐

35. **Answer: b**

    WHY: *Medical emergency* (med emerg) means the same as stat (Table 8-1). It has replaced stat in some institutions to identify specimens whose results are needed immediately to respond to critical situations.

    REVIEW: Yes ☐   No ☐

36. **Answer: a**

    WHY: NPO comes from Latin (*nil per os*) and means nothing by mouth. Patients who are NPO cannot have food or drink, not even water (Table 8-1). Patients are typically NPO before surgery, not after.

    REVIEW: Yes ☐   No ☐

37. **Answer: c**

    WHY: Glucose levels normally rise with the intake of food and return to normal fasting levels within 2 hours if no more food is eaten. Glucose levels are ordered fasting to see if glucose is being metabolized properly (Table 8-1). If glucose is not being metabolized properly, fasting levels will not be normal.

    REVIEW: Yes ☐   No ☐

38. **Answer: c**

    WHY: The only liquid that it is acceptable to drink when fasting is water (Table 8-1).

    REVIEW: Yes ☐   No ☐

39. **Answer: c**

    WHY: *Postop* means "after an operation" (Table 8-1). Both hemoglobin and hematocrit are indications of the RBC count. H&H levels are a common postop test to monitor blood levels after surgery.

    REVIEW: Yes ☐   No ☐

40. **Answer: a**

    WHY: If the door to the room is closed, you should knock lightly and proceed with caution. Even if the door is open, it is a good idea to knock lightly to make occupants aware that you are about to enter and to get their attention so that you can ask if it is all right to enter.

    REVIEW: Yes ☐   No ☐

41. **Answer: d**

    WHY: Because the specimen is a complete blood count (CBC), it can easily be collected by finger stick from the left hand. The right arm should not be used. Collecting the CBC from the IV is not worth the risk when it can easily be collected by capillary puncture. A competent phlebotomist should be able to decide what to do in this situation without having to ask the nurse.

    REVIEW: Yes ☐   No ☐

42. **Answer: d**

    WHY: Codes are one of the ways healthcare institutions convey important information over a public address system to those who need to know without alarming the general public. Codes use numbers or words to convey information. For example, code "blue" typically means that someone has stopped breathing.

    REVIEW: Yes ☐   No ☐

43. **Answer: d**

    WHY: *DNR* means "do not resuscitate." It means that no code should be called or heroic measures taken if the patient stops breathing. It is sometimes used when patients are terminally ill.

    REVIEW: Yes ☐   No ☐

44. **Answer: c**

    WHY: When you ask if it is all right to draw a patient's blood and the patient replies, "Yes, but I would rather not," or something similar, he or she has given permission and taken it back in the same breath. You should not draw blood from the patient until you are certain that you have permission.

    REVIEW: Yes ☐   No ☐

45. **Answer: d**

    WHY: One of the tests used to identify protein or immune globulin disorders that lead to nerve damage is serum protein electrophoresis (SPEP). See Table 8-2 for more tests commonly ordered for geriatric patients and the indications for ordering.

    REVIEW: Yes ☐   No ☐

46. **Answer: a**

    WHY: It is acceptable procedure to wake a patient for a blood draw. If an inpatient is asleep, call out his or her name softly and shake the bed gently. Do not shake the patient because you may startle him or her, which can affect test results. Never attempt to collect a blood specimen from a sleeping patient. Besides not having consent for the draw, such an attempt can also startle the patient, and you or the patient may be injured.

    REVIEW: Yes ☐   No ☐

Table 8-2: Tests Commonly Ordered on Geriatric Patients

Test	Typical Indications for Ordering
ANA, RA, or RF	Diagnose lupus and rheumatoid arthritis, which can affect nervous system function
CBC	Determine hemoglobin levels, detect infection, and identify blood disorders
BUN/creatinine	Diagnose kidney function disorders that may be responsible for problems such as confusion, coma, seizures, and tremors
Calcium/magnesium	Identify abnormal levels associated with seizures and muscle problems
Electrolytes	Determine sodium and potassium levels, critical to proper nervous system function
ESR	Detect inflammation, identify collagen vascular (i.e., connective tissue) diseases
Glucose	Detect and monitor diabetes; abnormal levels can cause confusion, seizures, or coma or lead to peripheral neuropathy
PT/PTT	Monitor blood-thinning medications, important in heart conditions, coagulation problems, and stroke management
SPEP, IPEP	Identify protein or immune globulin disorders that lead to nerve damage
VDRL/FTA	Diagnose or rule out syphilis, which can cause nerve damage and dementia

47. Answer: d

WHY: A startle reflex can affect test results and should be avoided. Collecting the specimen in dim lighting or collecting a specimen from an unconscious patient should not affect test results provided that the specimen is collected properly. When a phlebotomist awakens a patient and elevates the head of the patient's bed before collecting the specimen, there should be no negative effect on the specimen.

REVIEW: Yes ☐ No ☐

48. Answer: c

WHY: Some patients can hear what is going on around them despite being considered unconscious. Identify yourself and inform the patient of your intent, talking to him or her as you would an alert the patient. In addition, an unconscious patient may be able to feel pain and may move during a blood draw, so it is important to have someone assist you by holding the patient's arm still. The patient's blood may be drawn in the bed where he or she is. No special collection area is necessary.

REVIEW: Yes ☐ No ☐

49. Answer: c

WHY: If a physician is with the patient and the test is ordered stat, it is generally acceptable procedure to politely introduce yourself, explain why you are there, and ask permission to collect the specimen. The physician may or may not give you permission. If permission is not given, the stat will have to wait until the physician leaves.

REVIEW: Yes ☐ No ☐

50. Answer: a

WHY: It is acceptable and in the best interest of all to ask family or visitors to step out of the room temporarily while you collect a blood specimen. Most will be more than willing to do so.

REVIEW: Yes ☐ No ☐

51. Answer: b

WHY: All specimens and test requests must be accounted for. Generally, if a patient is unavailable for testing, a delay slip is filled out stating why you were unable to collect the specimen. The original is left at the nurses' station, and a copy goes back to the laboratory. It is then up to the patient's nurse to notify the lab when the patient is available for testing and the phlebotomist can return.

REVIEW: Yes ☐ No ☐

52. Answer: d

WHY: Misidentification of a type and screen could lead to a patient getting the wrong type of blood and a possible fatal transfusion reaction.

REVIEW: Yes ☐ No ☐

📖 *Review required identification information in Chapter 8 of the TEXTBOOK.*

53. Answer: b.

WHY: Proper patient identification involves asking the patient to state his or her name and date of birth. (CLSI now recommends also having the patient spell the last name.) Information on the ID band is then matched with requisition. Verbal statement of identity is important. An ill or hard-of-hearing patient may answer "yes" to almost anything. It is not unheard of for a patient to be wearing an ID band with incorrect information.

REVIEW: Yes ☐ No ☐

54. **Answer: a**

WHY: It is important that certain information on the ID band match the information on the requisition exactly. The medical record number is mandatory information and should match exactly. The room number may change during a patient's stay in the hospital and should not be relied on as proper identification. In addition, the physician may change or the patient may have more than one physician ordering tests. Test status and collection priority may change with each order and is not information that is found on the ID band.

REVIEW: Yes ☐ No ☐

55. **Answer: b**

WHY: Any discrepancy in the patient's name, date of birth, or medical record number between the requisition and the patient's ID band should be addressed and resolved before a specimen is collected.

REVIEW: Yes ☐ No ☐

56. **Answer: c**

WHY: Patient identification should never be based on information that is not attached to the patient. If the patient is not wearing an ID band, ask the patient's nurse to make positive identification and attach an ID band before the specimen is drawn.

REVIEW: Yes ☐ No ☐

57. **Answer: c**

WHY: It is not uncommon for an emergency room to receive an unconscious patient with no identification. Specimens should not be collected without some way to positively connect the specimen with the patient. In many institutions, a special three-part ID band will be attached to the unidentified patient's wrist. The special ID band has a unique number. The same number is on labels that are placed on specimens collected from that patient.

REVIEW: Yes ☐ No ☐

58. **Answer: c**

WHY: A newborn may have more than one ID band: one with the infant's information and one with the mother's.

REVIEW: Yes ☐ No ☐

📖 *Review newborn infant identification protocol in Chapter 8 of the TEXTBOOK.*

59. **Answer: c**

WHY: The most critical error a phlebotomist can make is misidentifying a patient specimen. A

misidentified specimen can have serious or even fatal consequences for the patient, especially if the specimen is for a type and screen for a blood transfusion. Misidentification of a patient's specimen can be grounds for dismissal of the person responsible and can even lead to a malpractice lawsuit against that person.

REVIEW: Yes ☐ No ☐

60. **Answer: b**

WHY: Identification should never be verified from an ID band that is not attached to the patient. An ID band on the nightstand could belong to a patient who previously occupied that bed. Even if the ID band and the requisition match, it is not adequate as proper identification of the patient. If an ID band is not attached to the patient, you must ask the patient's nurse to attach an ID band before you can collect the specimen.

REVIEW: Yes ☐ No ☐

61. **Answer: a**

WHY: The patient's nurse or other caregiver, or a relative, may be needed to confirm the identity of a patient who is a very young child or someone who is mentally incompetent or cannot speak English. The term geriatric means "relating to old age"; it does not mean senile or fragile. One would expect that this type of patient could identify himself or herself correctly.

REVIEW: Yes ☐ No ☐

62. **Answer: a**

WHY: Never make assumptions about a person's identity and do not rely on others to identify patients for you. Always verify patient identification yourself by asking the patient to state his or her name and date of birth.

REVIEW: Yes ☐ No ☐

63. **Answer: c**

WHY: A cheerful, pleasant bedside manner and exchange of small talk puts both you and the patient at ease, helps you gain the patient's trust and confidence, and helps divert attention from any discomfort associated with the blood draw. What it may not affect is the tendency for a patient to faint—a vasovagal response to venipuncture or needles.

REVIEW: Yes ☐ No ☐

64. **Answer: b**

WHY: Most patients understand that blood tests are needed in the course of their treatment. However, illness can be quite stressful and occasionally a patient who is tired of being "poked" will be cranky and rude. It is important to remain polite and professional and draw the specimen in your normal way. You may discover that the patient will actually apologize to you by the time you have finished.

REVIEW: Yes ☐ No ☐

65. **Answer: c**

WHY: Advising a patient of his or her prognosis or explaining what disorders the test can detect is a physician's responsibility. It is not a phlebotomist's duty and is not necessary to informed consent. Informing a patient that you are a student is important to informed consent. A patient has a right to refuse to have blood drawn by a student. Knowing that you are going to draw a blood specimen is necessary to informed consent. Many patients request to know the name of the test before consenting to a blood draw.

REVIEW: Yes ☐ No ☐

66. **Answer: a**

WHY: There are many reasons why a physician will order certain tests. Any attempt to explain why a test was ordered may mislead the patient. For example, a glucose test may be ordered because the patient is taking medication that can affect glucose levels, not because diabetes is suspected. Usually such inquiries are handled by explaining that the doctor has ordered the tests as part of the patient's care and that he or she will be happy to explain the tests if asked. The Health Insurance Portability and Accountability Act (HIPAA) clearly states that patient confidentiality must be protected. This does not apply to inquiries by patients about their own tests.

REVIEW: Yes ☐ No ☐

67. **Answer: c**

WHY: When it has been determined that a patient truly refuses to cooperate, you should write on the requisition that the patient has refused to have blood drawn. You should also notify the patient's nurse and the phlebotomy supervisor that the specimen was not obtained because of patient refusal. Some institutions have a special form on which you state that you were unable to collect the specimen and the reason why. The original form is left at the nurse's station and a copy goes to the lab.

REVIEW: Yes ☐ No ☐

68. **Answer: a**

WHY: If you determine that the patient has not been fasting, notify the patient's nurse so that a

determination can be made regarding whether to proceed with the test. If you are told to proceed with collection, write "nonfasting" on the requisition and specimen label so that testing personnel know the status of the patient.

REVIEW: Yes ☐ No ☐

69. **Answer: d**

WHY: If you wait to assemble equipment after selecting the collection site, you will have a better idea of what equipment to use and will ultimately waste less equipment. For example, if you have a multisample needle and holder ready before you select the site, it will have to be thrown away if you later decide to use a butterfly instead. However, if you had waited until after selecting the site to select equipment, you would know to select the butterfly equipment. There is plenty of time to get equipment ready while you are waiting for the alcohol to dry after cleaning the site, and you will be more apt to allow sufficient time for the alcohol to dry.

REVIEW: Yes ☐ No ☐

📖 *Do WORKBOOK Skills Drill 8-3 to see how well you know all the steps of the venipuncture procedure.*

70. **Answer: b**

WHY: In performing a routine blood draw, the hands must be decontaminated before glove application at the beginning of the procedure and at the end after glove removal, before proceeding to the next patient.

REVIEW: Yes ☐ No ☐

71. **Answer: c**

WHY: According to CDC guidelines, hands that are visibly dirty or contaminated with blood or other body fluids must be washed with soap and water. If hand-washing facilities are not available, the hands should be cleaned with detergent-containing wipes followed by an alcohol-based hand cleaner.

REVIEW: Yes ☐ No ☐

72. **Answer: a**

WHY: Do everything you can to establish a rapport with the child and his or her parents. Even young children can sense when you are not being honest with them. Tell the child that the procedure may be slightly uncomfortable without being overly blunt. Never tell a child it will not hurt. Offering a child a treat is a temporary distraction but does nothing to instill trust in the phlebotomist and the procedure. In addition, any treat, sticker, or

toy should be a reward just for going through the procedure, not for being brave enough to not cry.
REVIEW: Yes ☐   No ☐

73. **Answer: c**

WHY: You should never tell a patient that a venipuncture will not hurt, nor should you suggest that it will hurt a great deal. Some patients are more sensitive to pain than others. Tell the patient that it may hurt a little, but only for a short time. You should warn patients just before you slip the needle into the vein to help them prepare for it. You can suggest to a fearful patient that he or she look away as the needle goes in, but do not imply that looking away will keep it from hurting.
REVIEW: Yes ☐   No ☐

74. **Answer: a**

WHY: Proper arm position is important for successful venipuncture. An arm in proper position for routine venipuncture is supported firmly and extended downward in a straight line from shoulder to wrist (Fig. 8-3) with the palm up. It should not be bent at the elbow. Be aware of the angle of the arm when you are collecting your samples. If the arm is straight forward, the tubes will not fill from the bottom up. The hand may be turned palm-down when you are accessing the cephalic vein or hand veins.
REVIEW: Yes ☐   No ☐

75. **Answer: b**

WHY: Patients rarely faint when they are lying down. An outpatient who has previously fainted during a blood draw should be asked to lie down, or the drawing chair should be reclined if possible. Sitting upright poses the danger of injury should the patient faint and fall, so no exceptions should be made. In addition, a person who has fainted may be difficult to revive if he or she is not in a supine position.
REVIEW: Yes ☐   No ☐

76. **Answer: c**

WHY: It is acceptable to lower a bedrail to make blood collection easier; however, you can be held liable if you forget to raise it again after you are finished and the patient falls out of bed and is injured.
REVIEW: Yes ☐   No ☐

77. **Answer: b**

WHY: Blockage of blood flow (stasis) by the tourniquet causes hemoconcentration, which affects specimen composition and leads to erroneous test results. To minimize these effects, the tourniquet should never be left in place longer than 1 minute.
REVIEW: Yes ☐   No ☐

78. **Answer: a**

WHY: The best place to apply the tourniquet is 3 to 4 in above the intended venipuncture site (Fig. 8-7). If it is too close to the collection site, the vein may collapse as blood is withdrawn; if it is too far away, it may be ineffective. Applying a tourniquet distal to or below a venipuncture site would prevent blood flow into the area and result in vein collapse and unsuccessful venipuncture. In drawing blood from a hand vein, the tourniquet is applied proximal to the wrist bone, not distal.
REVIEW: Yes ☐   No ☐

79. **Answer: d**

WHY: A tourniquet that is too tight may prevent arterial blood flow into the area, resulting in failure to obtain blood. A tourniquet that is too tight increases the effects of hemoconcentration and contributes to erroneous results on the sample. A tourniquet that is too tight can also pinch and hurt the patient, cause the arm to ache, and cause it to turn red or purple.
REVIEW: Yes ☐   No ☐

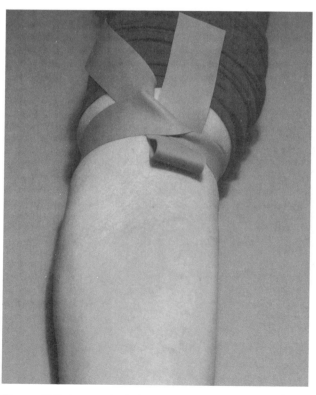

Figure 8-7 A properly tied tourniquet with ends pointing toward the shoulder.

📖 *Answer the questions in WORKBOOK Knowledge Drill 8-5 to see if you need to enhance your knowledge of tourniquet application.*

80. **Answer: a**

WHY: To enhance vein selection, you are encouraged to palpate the antecubital area, lower the arm, or use a warm towel to increase blood flow. It is not a good idea to have a patient pump (repeatedly open and close) his or her fist because this may cause erroneous results for some tests, most notably potassium levels, as a result of hemoconcentration.

REVIEW: Yes ☐ No ☐

81. **Answer: c**

WHY: You can easily tell an artery from a vein because an artery has a pulse; a vein does not. Veins are normally more superficial and more resilient than arteries and may feel larger for that reason.

REVIEW: Yes ☐ No ☐

82. **Answer: b**

WHY: A normal vein feels bouncy and resilient; a sclerosed vein feels hard and cord-like and lacks resiliency. A sclerosed vein is difficult to penetrate, rolls easily, and should not be used for venipuncture.

REVIEW: Yes ☐ No ☐

83. **Answer: c**

WHY: Ankle veins are sometimes used as a last resort, but only after obtaining permission from the patient's physician.

REVIEW: Yes ☐ No ☐

84. **Answer: d**

WHY: To avoid inadvertently puncturing an artery, never select a vein that overlies or is close to an artery or near where you feel a pulse. Avoid drawing from the basilic vein because it is in the area of the brachial artery.

REVIEW: Yes ☐ No ☐

85. **Answer: a**

WHY: When a person has dermatitis and there is no other site available, it is acceptable to apply the tourniquet over a towel or washcloth placed over the patient's arm. A coagulation test should not be collected from an IV, and a coagulation tube cannot be collected by fingerstick. The area above an IV must not be used regardless of whether you use a tourniquet.

REVIEW: Yes ☐ No ☐

86. **Answer: c**

WHY: If the vein can be felt but not seen, try to mentally visualize its location. It often helps to note the position of the vein in reference to a mole, hair, or skin crease. Never insert the needle blindly or probe to find a vein because damage to nerves and tissue may result. Never leave the tourniquet on for more than 1 minute because hemoconcentration of the specimen may result. Marking the site with a felt-tipped pen could contaminate the specimen or transfer disease from patient to patient.

REVIEW: Yes ☐ No ☐

87. **Answer: b**

WHY: The CLSI guidelines recommend that the tourniquet be released as soon as blood flow is established. This avoids hemoconcentration of the specimen and helps to ensure accurate test results. Arterial flow should not be affected by the tourniquet if the pressure is correct. Venous flow should return to normal, not increase, when the tourniquet is released.

REVIEW: Yes ☐ No ☐

88. **Answer: c**

WHY: CLSI standards recommend cleaning the site with antiseptic using friction to clean an area 2 to 3 inches in diameter around the selected site of needle entry. Although previous CLSI standards recommended using a circular motion, starting at the point of expected needle entry, and moving outward in ever-widening concentric circles, this is no longer considered necessary. If the site is especially dirty, clean it again using a new alcohol-soaked gauze or alcohol prep pad (Fig. 8-8).

REVIEW: Yes ☐ No ☐

89. **Answer: c**

WHY: Alcohol takes around 30 seconds to evaporate completely. The evaporation process helps destroy microbes. Allowing the alcohol to dry before venipuncture also prevents hemolysis of the specimen and a stinging sensation when the needle is inserted. This is a desirable time to prepare equipment, but it is not a reason why you wait for the alcohol to dry.

REVIEW: Yes ☐ No ☐

90. **Answer: a**

WHY: When the tube is advanced past the guideline on the holder, the stopper is penetrated, causing the tube to lose its vacuum. A tube that has lost its vacuum will fail to fill with blood, which means that you will have to replace it with a new tube.

REVIEW: Yes ☐ No ☐

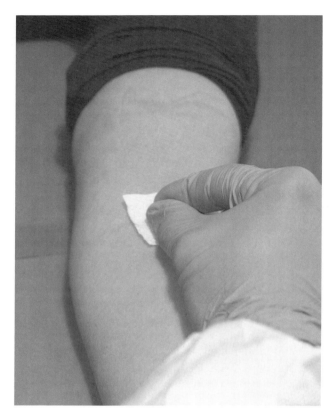

Figure 8-8 Cleaning a venipuncture site.

91. **Answer: d**

WHY: Visually inspecting the needle tip before insertion not only ensures that you are entering with the bevel up but also prevents damage and unnecessary pain during the procedure should the point or beveled edges have imperfections. Needles are sterile when first opened as long as they are not allowed to touch anything, and they should not have any external contamination. However, they should be checked nonetheless because contaminants have been observed on rare occasions. You cannot tell that a needle is outdated by inspecting the tip. The expiration date is typically printed on the label that covers the twist-apart shields or on the packaging, as in the case of butterfly needles. Outdated needles must be discarded during regular inventory of the stock.

REVIEW: Yes ☐ No ☐

92. **Answer: b**

WHY: The correct order for the venipuncture procedure would be to sanitize the hands, put on the gloves, select the vein, and then release the tourniquet. Gloves are required by OSHA to protect the phlebotomist from potential exposure to bloodborne pathogens. Due to infection control

issues, most healthcare facilities require phlebotomists to put on gloves immediately after hand sanitization, before touching the patient. Diet restrictions should be verified and positioning of the patient should take place before vein selection has begun.

REVIEW: Yes ☐ No ☐

📖 *Refer to Procedure 8-2 in the TEXTBOOK for the correct order of all the venipuncture procedure steps.*

93. **Answer: b**

WHY: If the needle touches the skin and then is withdrawn before piercing the tissue, the needle is considered contaminated and a new needle should be used for the draw to avoid a possible infection. Always be aware of any contamination to the needle to prevent using it to penetrate the skin and possibly taking bacteria into a patient's vascular system.

REVIEW: Yes ☐ No ☐

94. **Answer: b**

WHY: Under normal circumstances the best angle for routine antecubital venipunctures depends on the depth of the vein but should be less than 30 degrees (Fig. 8-6). When you are using a butterfly, the angle will normally be less than 10 degrees, as seen in Figure 8-9.

REVIEW: Yes ☐ No ☐

95. **Answer: b**

WHY: A venipuncture needle is always inserted with the bevel up.

REVIEW: Yes ☐ No ☐

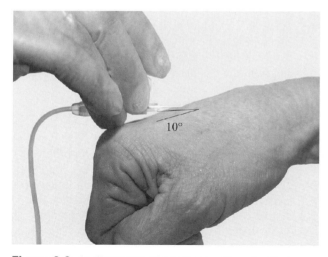

Figure 8-9 An illustration of needle insertion at a 10-degree angle.

96. **Answer: c**

    WHY: When the needle enters the vein, you will feel a slight "give," or decrease in resistance. Some phlebotomists describe this as a "pop." If the needle hisses, the vacuum of the tube is drawing in air, which means that the needle bevel is partially or totally out of the vein and not completely under the skin. If you can feel the needle vibrate, the needle bevel is against the vein wall or a valve, causing flapping of tissue against the needle opening. When you are using the ETS, blood does not flow until the tube is fully engaged after the needle is in the vein.

    REVIEW: Yes ☐ No ☐

97. **Answer: c**

    WHY: According to the CLSI guidelines, the best time to release the tourniquet is as soon as blood begins to flow into the first tube. Releasing the tourniquet as well as having the patient release the fist minimizes the effects of stasis and hemoconcentration on the specimen. A tourniquet should not remain in place longer than 1 minute.

    REVIEW: Yes ☐ No ☐

98. **Answer: b**

    WHY: Prolonged tourniquet application or vigorous fist pumping lead to hemoconcentration of the specimen, notably affecting potassium, protein levels, and cell counts.

    REVIEW: Yes ☐ No ☐

99. **Answer: d**

    WHY: The arm should be in a downward position during venipuncture so that tubes fill from the bottom up and not from the stopper end first. This keeps blood in the tube from coming in contact with the needle, preventing reflux of tube contents into the patient's vein and minimizing the chance of additive carryover between tubes. Collecting sterile specimens before filling tubes for other specimens, clearing for special coagulation tests, and filling tubes until the normal vacuum is exhausted are all part of proper venipuncture technique.

    REVIEW: Yes ☐ No ☐

100. **Answer: b**

    WHY: It is important to fill additive tubes to the proper fill level to ensure a proper ratio of additive to blood. The proper fill level is attained by allowing the tube to fill until the normal vacuum is exhausted and blood ceases to flow into the tube. Tubes will not fill completely because there is always dead space at the top. Blood in an anticoagulant tube does not clot. A partially filled tube would likely yield enough specimen to perform the test; however, the results would be inaccurate. Tissue thromboplastin is a problem for some tests, particularly special coagulation tests collected in tubes with light-blue tops. However, contamination can be minimized by first collecting a discard tube to flush the tissue thromboplastin out of the needle.

    REVIEW: Yes ☐ No ☐

101. **Answer: a**

    WHY: Lack of or inadequate mixing immediately after filling anticoagulant tubes can lead to microclot formation. Adequate mixing requires inversion of the tube, as shown in Figure 8-10. Anticoagulant tubes are not supposed to clot, so coagulation would definitely not be encouraged. Hemoconcentration is related to dehydration of the patient, fist pumping, and prolonged tourniquet application, not mixing of the tube. Hemolysis can be caused by mixing tubes too vigorously. Nonadditive tubes do not require mixing.

    REVIEW: Yes ☐ No ☐

102. **Answer: b**

    WHY: To avoid EDTA contamination of the green-top tube, draw a few milliliters of blood into a plain red-top discard tube. Penetrating the stopper

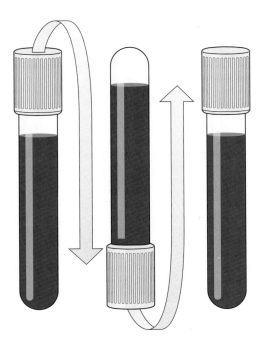

= One inversion

Figure 8-10 Illustration showing one complete tube inversion.

of the red-top tube should help clear contamination from the outside of the needle. Drawing a few milliliters of blood into the discard tube should flush any contamination from inside the needle. If the error had been discovered after the green-top tube had started to fill, that green-top tube could be considered the discard tube and another green top collected after it.

REVIEW: Yes ☐ No ☐

103. **Answer: d**

WHY: Nonadditive tubes should not be mixed. In fact, mixing may cause hemolysis if the sample has already begun to clot.

REVIEW: Yes ☐ No ☐

104. **Answer: a**

WHY: Vigorous mixing or shaking of the tube can cause hemolysis because red cells are fragile and can rupture easily.

REVIEW: Yes ☐ No ☐

105. **Answer: a**

WHY: Using several layers of gauze helps create adequate pressure to stop the bleeding and keeps the blood from soaking through and contaminating your glove. The purpose of using gauze as the needle is pulled out has nothing to do with whether the patient sees the needle come out or not. Whether or not it hurts when you pull the needle out depends on your technique, not the amount of gauze used. You could use several layers of gauze and still have bruising if you did not apply adequate pressure to the site.

REVIEW: Yes ☐ No ☐

106. **Answer: d**

WHY: Gauze pads are preferred for applying pressure to the puncture site because the loose cotton fibers of cotton balls tend to stick to the site, pulling platelets with them when the cotton ball is removed. This disrupts the platelet plug and reinitiates bleeding.

REVIEW: Yes ☐ No ☐

107. **Answer: c**

WHY: The gauze should be held lightly in place by the fingers until the needle exits the vein; then pressure should be applied. Applying pressure to the gauze while the needle is still in the arm can cause the needle to slit the skin, producing pain. The pressure applied should not bend the needle bevel or cause the patient to faint, however.

REVIEW: Yes ☐ No ☐

108. **Answer: c**

WHY: An uncovered, used needle is a danger to the phlebotomist. A needle safety feature should be engaged immediately after needle removal (Fig. 8-11). Any delay increases the risk of accidental needle injury to the phlebotomist.

REVIEW: Yes ☐ No ☐

109. **Answer: a**

WHY: According to the CLSI, the tourniquet should be released as soon as blood flow is established so as to minimize the effects of hemoconcentration. Additive tubes should be mixed as soon as they are removed from the tube holder for proper additive function, including the prevention of microclot formation in anticoagulant tubes. Pressure should be applied immediately after the needle is removed from the arm or hand.

REVIEW: Yes ☐ No ☐

110. **Answer: a**

WHY: According to the regulations of the Occupational Safety and Health Administration (OSHA), a needle and holder are to be disposed of as a single unit, as shown in Figure 8-12. Removing the needle from the holder either by ejecting or unscrewing it subjects the user to needlestick

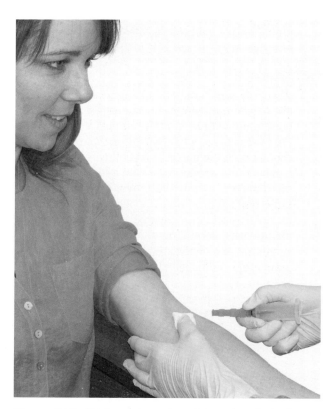

Figure 8-11 Phlebotomist activated the safety device immediately after removing the needle.

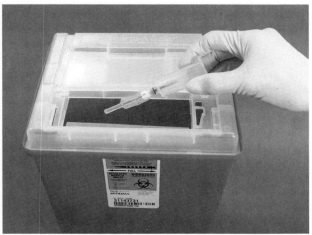

Figure 8-12 Discarding a needle and tube holder as a unit.

hazards posed by the exposed rubber sleeve end of the needle.

REVIEW: Yes ☐ No ☐

111. **Answer: a**

WHY: Inpatient blood specimens should be labeled at the bedside immediately following collection (Fig. 8-13). If tubes are labeled before collection and one of the tubes is not used at that time, another patient's blood could end up in that labeled tube. If tubes are labeled away from the bedside, the specimen can be misidentified.

REVIEW: Yes ☐ No ☐

112. **Answer: a**

WHY: The patient's first and last name, hospital or medical record number, date of birth, date and time of the draw, and the phlebotomist's initials are mandatory information on a specimen label. The room number and bed may be found on the label if it was generated by a computer, but this is considered optional information.

REVIEW: Yes ☐ No ☐

113. **Answer: b**

WHY: The patient's ID number is included on the specimen label to avoid confusing samples. It is not unusual to have patients with the same or similar names in the hospital at the same time, but two patients will not have the same hospital or medical record number.

REVIEW: Yes ☐ No ☐

114. **Answer: b**

WHY: Carrying a bag or purse on the venipuncture arm, lifting heavy objects with that arm, or removing the bandage prematurely can all disturb

the healing process, reinitiate bleeding, and lead to bruising of the site. The dietary restrictions may be necessary before the venipuncture but not afterward.

REVIEW: Yes ☐ No ☐

115. **Answer: c**

WHY: An ammonia specimen is transported on ice, a bilirubin specimen must be protected from light, and a cryoglobulin specimen must be transported at body temperature (37°C). A cholesterol specimen, however, does not require special handling.

REVIEW: Yes ☐ No ☐

116. **Answer: d**

WHY: Patient refusal, unavailability, or the fact that you tried but were unsuccessful are all valid reasons for failure to obtain a specimen. Not having the right equipment to collect a specimen makes a phlebotomist appear disorganized and unprofessional and is not an acceptable reason for failure to collect a specimen. You should check to see that you have the proper equipment for the test before leaving to collect the specimen.

REVIEW: Yes ☐ No ☐

117. **Answer: a**

WHY: After two unsuccessful attempts at blood collection, *do not* try a third time. Ask another phlebotomist to take over. Unsuccessful venipuncture attempts are frustrating to the patient and the phlebotomist. With the exception of stat and other priority specimens, if the second phlebotomist is also unsuccessful, it is a good idea to give the patient a rest and come back at a later time. An outpatient may be given the option of returning another day, after consultation with his or her physician.

REVIEW: Yes ☐ No ☐

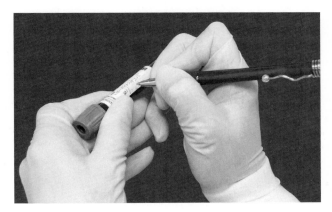

Figure 8-13 Labeling a tube.

118. **Answer: d**

    WHY: A winged infusion set is called a butterfly because it resembles one. A phlebotomist using a butterfly in a hand vein is shown in Figures 8-14 and 8-15.

    REVIEW: Yes ☐ No ☐

    📖 *See Procedure 8-3 in the TEXTBOOK for correct hand-vein venipuncture procedure.*

119. **Answer: c**

    WHY: The small size of the needle and flexibility afforded by the tubing makes a butterfly a good choice for drawing small, difficult, or hand veins.

    REVIEW: Yes ☐ No ☐

120. **Answer: b**

    WHY: A needle and syringe or butterfly and syringe may be used if the patient has small, fragile, or weak veins that collapse easily. The vacuum pressure of the evacuated tube may be too great for such veins. When a syringe is used, the pressure can be controlled by pulling slowly on the syringe plunger.

    REVIEW: Yes ☐ No ☐

121. **Answer: a**

    WHY: When a syringe needle is inserted in a vein, a "flash" of blood will usually appear in the hub of the needle.

    REVIEW: Yes ☐ No ☐

    📖 *To review syringe venipuncture, refer to Procedure 8-4 in the TEXTBOOK.*

122. **Answer: c**

    WHY: A big factor in successful blood collection from pediatric patients is proper immobilization.

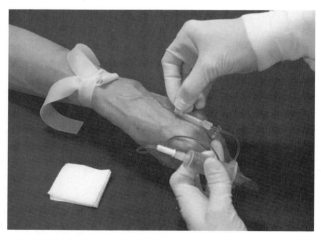

Figure 8-14 A phlebotomist drawing a hand vein with a tourniquet applied on the forearm just proximal to the wrist bone.

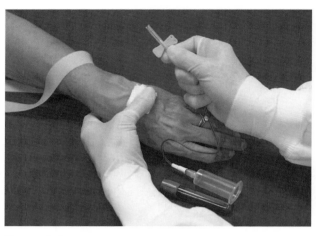

Figure 8-15 A phlebotomist preparing to remove a butterfly needle after using it to collect a specimen from a hand vein.

Preventing excessive movement makes the process quicker and safer for both the patient and the phlebotomist.

REVIEW: Yes ☐ No ☐

123. **Answer: c**

    WHY: It is important to greet the parents and child and try to establish rapport with each of them. Explain what you are going to do in terms the child can understand so that he or she will know what to expect. Answer questions honestly. *Never* tell a child that it won't hurt, because chances are that it will, even if just a little.

    REVIEW: Yes ☐ No ☐

124. **Answer: c**

    WHY: Small children seldom hold still for blood collection. The flexibility of the butterfly tubing enables successful blood collection despite some movement by the child. Children do like the idea of the butterfly, but it is not the reason it is used.

    REVIEW: Yes ☐ No ☐

125. **Answer: d**

    WHY: The safest and proper way to transfer blood from a syringe into evacuated tubes is to use a syringe transfer device, as shown in Figure 8-16. If a transfer device is not available, the second best way is to place the tube in a rack before penetrating the tube stopper with the needle. Holding the tube with your hand is dangerous because the needle may slip and stick your hand. Never force the blood into the tube by pushing on the syringe plunger; let the vacuum of the tube draw the blood into it. Pushing on the plunger and forcing blood into the tube can hemolyze the specimen and can also allow blood to spurt out around the needle and contaminate you.

REVIEW: Yes ☐ No ☐

126. **Answer: c**

WHY: Older children appreciate honesty and will be more cooperative if you explain what you are going to do and stress the importance of holding still. However, it is unnecessary to explain all of the tests being collected. Never tell the child that it won't hurt, because chances are that it will, even if just a little. It is all right to offer the child a reward for being brave, but *do not* put conditions on receiving the reward, such as "You can only have the reward if you don't cry." Some crying is to be anticipated, and it is important to let the child know that it is all right to cry.

REVIEW: Yes ☐ No ☐

127. **Answer: b**

WHY: The CLSI standards state that additive tubes should be mixed immediately after they are drawn, which requires them to be mixed as soon as they are removed from the tube holder (Fig. 8-17).

REVIEW: Yes ☐ No ☐

128. **Answer: d**

WHY: Parkinson's disease is a neurological disorder that causes the patient to have resting

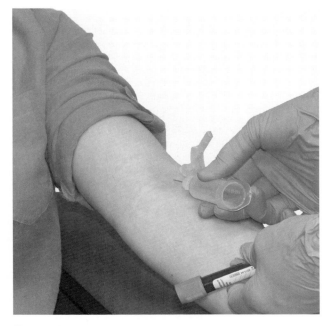

Figure 8-17 Phlebotomist immediately mixing the heparin tube before adding another tube or ending the draw.

tremors. Resting tremors are involuntary rhythmic movements typically confined to the forearms and hands. They occur when the arms are relaxed. Such tremors can make blood collection difficult.

REVIEW: Yes ☐ No ☐

129. **Answer: b**

WHY: In this scenario it is best to draw the specimen from the left arm in a position that the patient chooses. *Never* use force to extend a patient's arm. A butterfly offers the flexibility needed to access veins from an awkward angle. Diabetes can affect circulation and healing in the lower extremities and generally makes venipuncture of leg, ankle, and foot veins off limits. A blood draw should not be performed on the same side as a mastectomy without approval of the patient's physician.

REVIEW: Yes ☐ No ☐

130. **Answer: a**

WHY: The most common reason a patient must undergo dialysis is end-stage renal disease (ESRD), a serious condition in which the kidneys have deteriorated to a point at which they fail (no longer function). The most common cause of ESRD is diabetes, and the second most common cause is high blood pressure. Patients with ESRD require ongoing dialysis treatments or a kidney transplant.

REVIEW: Yes ☐ No ☐

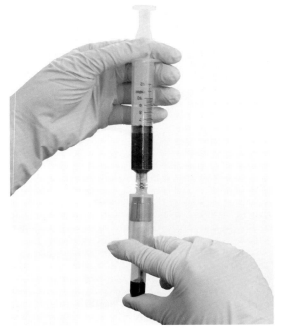

Figure 8-16 Filling an ETS tube using a syringe transfer device.

Chapter 9
Preanalytical Considerations

Study Tips

- List physiological preanalytical variables on the left half of a sheet of paper. Write lab tests affected by each one on the right half. Fold the paper in half; variable side up. Quiz yourself by naming tests affected by each variable listed. Turn the paper over and quiz yourself by naming variables that affect the test listed.

- Study the key points and cautions in the corresponding chapter of the textbook. Describe a theme they all indicate. Place a P next to caution statements that address a patient safety issue. Place an S next to those that address specimen quality issues. Use a P and an S for statements that address both issues.

- List problem sites that may be encountered when collecting blood specimens and describe how each one should be handled. Then have someone quiz you on how to handle each problem site listed. Do the same thing with patient complications and procedural errors.

- Identify five things that can result in specimen contamination.

- Draw two parallel lines resembling a vein. Use a pencil or pen as a needle and show various needle positions that result in failed venipuncture.

- Complete the activities in Chapter 9 of the companion workbook.

Overview The preanalytical (before analysis) phase of the testing process begins when a test is ordered and ends when testing begins. Numerous factors associated with this phase of the testing process, if not properly addressed, can lead to errors that can compromise specimen quality, jeopardize the health and safety of the patient, and ultimately increase the cost of medical care. Since each blood collection situation is unique, a phlebotomist have—in addition to possessing the technical skills needed to perform a blood draw—the ability to recognize preanalytical factors and address them if applicable, to avoid or reduce any negative impact. This chapter addresses physiological variables, problem venipuncture sites, various types of vascular access devices (VADs), patient complications and conditions, procedural errors, specimen quality issues, and how to troubleshoot failed venipuncture.

Review Questions

Choose the BEST answer.

1. The preanalytical phase of the testing process begins when a
   a. blood or body fluid specimen is collected.
   b. patient is admitted to a healthcare facility.
   c. specimen is submitted for processing.
   d. test is ordered by a patient's physician.

2. Most reference ranges are based on normal laboratory test values for
   a. fasting patients.
   b. healthy people.
   c. ill individuals.
   d. treated patients.

3. Diurnal variations associated with some blood components are
   a. abnormal changes that occur once a day.
   b. changes that follow a monthly cycle.
   c. normal fluctuations throughout the day.
   d. variations that occur on an hourly basis.

4. A patient's arm is swollen. The term used to describe this condition is
   a. cyanotic.
   b. edematous.
   c. sclerosed.
   d. thrombosed.

5. Lipemia results from
   a. high fat content of the blood.
   b. improper specimen handling.
   c. increased number of platelets.
   d. specimen hemoconcentration.

6. A patient with a high degree of jaundice typically has
   a. bruising and petechiae.
   b. edematous extremities.
   c. hemolyzed specimens.
   d. yellow skin and sclera.

7. Lymphostasis is
   a. impaired secretion of lymph fluid.
   b. obstruction of the flow of lymph.
   c. reduced lymphocyte production.
   d. stoppage of lymphoid functions.

8. This is the medical term for a nervous system response to abrupt pain, stress, or trauma.
   a. Circadian response
   b. Iatrogenic reflux
   c. Vasovagal syncope
   d. Venous stagnation

9. Small nonraised red or purple spots appear on the patient's skin below where the tourniquet has just been tied. What are they and what causes them?
   a. A rash from tying the tourniquet too tightly
   b. Bilirubin spots as a result of a diseased liver
   c. Dermatitis from an allergy to the tourniquet
   d. Petechiae due to capillary or platelet defects

10. Venous stasis is
    a. backflow of tissue fluid into a vein.
    b. stage 1 of the coagulation process.
    c. stoppage of the normal blood flow.
    d. vein collapse from excess pressure.

11. A hematoma is a
    a. blood clot inside of a vein.
    b. pool of fluid from an IV.
    c. swelling or mass of blood.
    d. symptom of nerve injury.

12. Mastectomy is the medical term for breast
    a. biopsy.
    b. reduction.
    c. removal.
    d. surgery.

13. Exsanguination is
    a. autologous donation of blood.
    b. iatrogenic depletion of blood.
    c. life-threatening loss of blood.
    d. therapeutic removal of blood.

14. Which of the following is a product of the breakdown of red blood cells?
    a. Bilirubin
    b. Creatinine
    c. Glucagon
    d. Lipid (fat)

15. A vein that is thrombosed is
    a. clotted.
    b. patent.
    c. scarred.
    d. swollen.

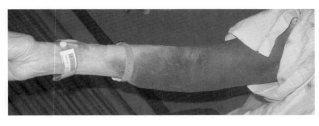

Figure 9-1 Appearance of a patient's arm after a venipuncture. (Photo courtesy of Sue Kucera.)

16. A patient experiences a momentary loss of consciousness or a miniseizure while you are drawing his blood. The last tube has just started to fill. Which of the following is the *wrong* thing to do?
    a. Complete the draw as quickly as you can.
    b. Immediately discontinue the blood draw.
    c. Notify the appropriate first aid personnel.
    d. Prevent the patient from injuring himself.

17. The patient has an IV in the left forearm and a large hematoma in the antecubital area of the right arm. The *best* place to collect a specimen by venipuncture is the
    a. left arm above the IV entry point.
    b. left arm below the IV entry point.
    c. right arm distal to the hematoma.
    d. right arm in the antecubital area.

18. Which of the following conclusions is probable? Figure 9-1 shows an arm with
    a. bruising that was most likely caused by a reflux reaction.
    b. discoloration from prolonged application of a tourniquet.
    c. evidence of partial exsanguination of the antecubital area.
    d. the results of hematoma blood moving after venipuncture.

19. Hemoconcentration from prolonged tourniquet application increases
    a. blood plasma volume.
    b. nonfilterable analytes.
    c. pH and oxygen levels.
    d. specimen hemolysis.

20. Which of the following is the medical term for fainting?
    a. Sclerose
    b. Stasis
    c. Supine
    d. Syncope

21. In which instance is the patient closest to basal state? The patient who
    a. arrived at the lab at 0800 and had not eaten since dinner the prior night.
    b. came straight to the lab after working all night, but was fasting at work.
    c. has been awake but lying down quietly resting for the last several hours.
    d. is awakened for a blood draw at 0600 after fasting since 0800 last night.

22. The *best* specimens to use for establishing inpatient reference ranges for blood tests are
    a. basal state specimens.
    b. fasting specimens.
    c. postprandial specimens.
    d. steady-state specimens.

23. Which test requires the patient's age when calculating results?
    a. Cold agglutinin titer
    b. C-reactive protein
    c. Creatine kinase MB
    d. Creatinine clearance

24. Which of the following tests is most affected by altitude?
    a. Cholesterol
    b. Electrolytes
    c. Magnesium
    d. RBC count

25. Persistent diarrhea in the absence of fluid replacement may cause
    a. hemoconcentration.
    b. iatrogenic anemia.
    c. petechiae formation.
    d. red cell destruction.

26. You must collect a protime specimen from a patient with IVs in both arms. The *best* place to collect the specimen is
    a. above one of the IVs.
    b. below one of the IVs.
    c. from an ankle vein.
    d. from one of the IVs.

27. A lipemic specimen is a clue that the patient was probably
    a. basal state
    b. dehydrated.
    c. jaundiced.
    d. not fasting.

28. A 12-hour fast is normally required when testing for this analyte.
    a. Bilirubin
    b. Calcium
    c. Electrolytes
    d. Triglycerides

29. This blood component exhibits diurnal variation, with peak levels occurring in the morning.
    a. Cortisol
    b. Creatinine
    c. Glucose
    d. Phosphate

30. Tests influenced by diurnal variation are typically ordered
    a. fasting.
    b. pre-op.
    c. STAT.
    d. timed.

31. A drug known to interfere with a blood test should be discontinued for how many hours before the test specimen is collected?
    a. 1 to 3
    b. 4 to 24
    c. 25 to 30
    d. 48 to 72

32. When a patient is on drug therapy, a test result can be a false positive if
    a. a prescribed drug acts to enhance the desired test reaction.
    b. an analyte and the drug compete for the reaction test sites.
    c. anticoagulant reflux occurred during specimen collection.
    d. serum used for the test came from a partially filled tube.

33. Which of the following analytes can remain elevated for 24 hours or more after exercise?
    a. CK
    b. CO_2
    c. K^+
    d. pH

34. Which hormone is most affected by the presence of a fever?
    a. Insulin
    b. Melatonin
    c. Testosterone
    d. Thyroxine

35. Which analyte has a higher reference range for males than for females?
    a. Cholesterol
    b. Hematocrit
    c. Magnesium
    d. Potassium

36. An icteric blood specimen indicates
    a. bilirubin test results could be elevated.
    b. it probably was not a fasting specimen.
    c. the collection procedure was incorrect.
    d. the blood could be hemoconcentrated.

37. What changes occur in the bloodstream when a patient goes from supine to standing?
    a. Nonfilterable elements increase
    b. Red blood cell counts decrease
    c. The level of calcium decreases
    d. Volume of plasma is increased

38. Why do pregnant patients have lower reference ranges for red blood cell (RBC) counts?
    a. Frequent bouts of nausea lead to hemoconcentration.
    b. Increased body fluids result in dilution of the RBCs.
    c. Poor appetite results in a temporary form of anemia.
    d. The growing fetus uses up the mother's iron reserves.

39. Which of the following analytes is typically increased in chronic smokers?
    a. Bicarbonate
    b. Hemoglobin
    c. O_2 saturation
    d. Vitamin B_{12}

40. When selecting a venipuncture site do not use an arm with
    a. a very strong basilic pulse.
    b. an active AV graft or fistula.
    c. evidence of a recent draw.
    d. tattoos from elbow to wrist.

41. Of the following factors known to affect basal state, which is automatically accounted for when reference ranges are established?
    a. Diurnal variation
    b. Drug interferences
    c. Effects of exercise
    d. Geographic locale

42. Temperature and humidity control in a laboratory is important because it
    a. ensures the test results will be normal.
    b. maintains the integrity of specimens.
    c. prevents hemolysis of the specimens.
    d. reduces any interference from drugs.

43. Scarred or burned areas should be avoided as blood collection sites because
    a. analytes are diluted in such areas.
    b. circulation is possibly impaired.
    c. specimens tend to be hemolyzed.
    d. veins are most likely thrombosed.

44. A vein that feels hard, cordlike, and lacks resiliency is most likely
    a. an artery.
    b. collapsed.
    c. sclerosed.
    d. superficial.

45. Drawing blood from an edematous extremity may cause
    a. erroneous specimen results.
    b. hemolysis of the specimen.
    c. premature specimen clotting.
    d. rapid formation of petechiae.

46. If you have no choice but to collect a specimen from an arm with a hematoma, collect the specimen
    a. above it.
    b. beside it.
    c. distal to it.
    d. through it.

47. When a blood specimen is collected from a saline lock, it is important to draw
    a. a 5-mL discard tube before the specimen tubes.
    b. coagulation specimens before other specimens.
    c. extra tubes in case other tests are ordered later.
    d. two tubes per test in case one is contaminated.

48. Which of the following veins is often the easiest to feel on obese patients?
    a. Basilic
    b. Brachial
    c. Cephalic
    d. Median

49. The serum or plasma of a lipemic specimen appears
    a. cloudy white.
    b. dark yellow.
    c. foamy pink.
    d. pink to red.

50. A phlebotomist must collect a hemoglobin specimen from a patient in ICU. There is an IV in the patient's left wrist. There is no suitable antecubital vein or hand vein in the right arm. What should the phlebotomist do?
    a. Ask another phlebotomist to collect it.
    b. Collect it from a leg, ankle, or foot vein.

c. Draw it from a hand vein below the IV.
d. Perform a finger stick on the right hand.

51. It is *not* a good idea to collect a CBC from a screaming infant because the
    a. chance of hemolysis is increased.
    b. platelets are more likely to clump.
    c. specimen may be hemoconcentrated.
    d. WBCs may be temporarily elevated.

52. A type of line commonly used to monitor blood pressure and collect blood gas specimens.
    a. A-line
    b. CVC
    c. IV
    d. PICC

53. A vascular access pathway that is surgically created to provide access for dialysis.
    a. AV shunt
    b. CVC
    c. Saline lock
    d. PICC

54. Collecting blood specimens from an arm on the same side as a mastectomy without permission from the patient's physician is prohibited because
    a. results on that arm will be elevated.
    b. that arm is susceptible to infection.
    c. there is a lot less feeling in that arm.
    d. veins in that arm will collapse easily.

55. Figure 9-2 is an illustration of a/an
    a. A-line.
    b. CVC.
    c. fistula.
    d. PICC.

56. A subcutaneous vascular access device consisting of a small chamber attached to an indwelling line that is implanted under the skin and located by palpating the skin.
    a. Groshong CVC
    b. Implanted port
    c. PICC line
    d. Saline lock

57. The way to bandage a venipuncture site when the patient is allergic to the glue in adhesive bandages is to
    a. apply a bandage that is latex-free.
    b. wait 5 minutes to apply a bandage.
    c. wrap a warm wash cloth around it.
    d. wrap it with self-adhering material.

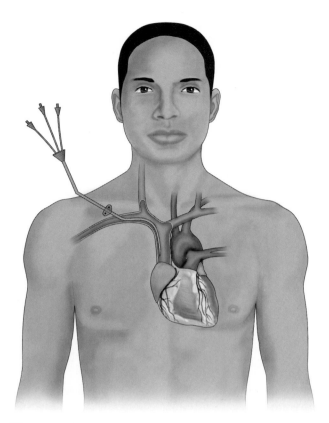

Figure 9-2 (Reprinted with permission from Taylor CR, Lillis C, LeMone P, Lynn P. *Fundamentals of Nursing: The Art and Science of Nursing Care.* 6th ed. Philadelphia, PA: Lippincott Williams & Wilkins; 2008.)

58. You may have to be careful about what type of equipment is brought into the room if a patient is severely allergic to

   a. adhesive.
   b. iodine.
   c. latex.
   d. perfume.

59. What is the best thing to do if a venipuncture site continues to bleed after 5 minutes?

   a. Have the patient hold pressure until it stops.
   b. Make a note of the problem on the lab slip.
   c. Report it to the patient's physician or nurse.
   d. Wrap the site with a tight pressure bandage.

60. Which patient should be asked to lie down during a blood draw? A patient with a

   a. central venous catheter.
   b. coagulation disorder.
   c. history of syncope.
   d. severe latex allergy.

61. During a blood draw a patient says he feels faint. What should the phlebotomist do?

   a. Ask him if it is OK to continue the draw.
   b. Discontinue the draw and lower his head.
   c. Keep him upright and complete the draw.
   d. Use an ammonia inhalant to revive him.

62. An outpatient becomes weak and pale after a blood draw. What should the phlebotomist do?

   a. Accompany the patient to his or her car.
   b. Have the patient lie down until recovered.
   c. Offer the patient a glass of water to drink.
   d. Tell the patient to go get something to eat.

63. If an outpatient tells you before a blood draw that she is feeling nauseated, you should

   a. advise her to begin slow, deep breathing.
   b. draw the specimen; watching her closely.
   c. have her lie down until she feels better.
   d. suggest that she come back another day.

64. Pain associated with venipuncture can be minimized by

   a. desensitizing the site by rubbing hard with alcohol.
   b. putting the patient at ease with a little small talk.
   c. tying the tourniquet tight enough to numb the arm.
   d. warning the patient that the draw might hurt a lot.

65. A site could potentially be used for venipuncture even if

   a. petechiae appear below the tourniquet.
   b. scarring from a deep burn is present.
   c. the arm appears slightly edematous.
   d. the only vein feels hard and cordlike.

66. Which of the following situations is *least* likely to cause contamination of the specimen?

   a. Cleaning a finger stick site with isopropyl alcohol.
   b. Drawing from the median vein with an IV in the hand.
   c. Touching the filter paper while collecting a PKU.
   d. Using povidone-iodine to clean a heel puncture site.

67. A phlebotomist has tried twice to collect a light blue top tube on a patient with difficult veins. Both times the phlebotomist has been able to collect only a partial tube. What should the phlebotomist do?

   a. Collect the specimen by a skin puncture.
   b. Have someone else collect the specimen.

c. Pour the two tubes together and mix well.

d. Send one to the lab marked "difficult draw".

68. The ratio of blood to anticoagulant is *most* critical for which of the following tests?

    a. Alkaline phosphatase

    b. Complete blood count

    c. Glycohemoglobin

    d. Prothrombin time

69. Which of the following is the *best* indication that you have accidentally punctured an artery?

    a. A hematoma starts to form.

    b. Blood obtained is dark red.

    c. Blood pulses into the tube.

    d. There isn't any way to tell.

70. A term used to describe anemia brought on by withdrawal of blood for testing purposes is

    a. hemolytic.

    b. iatrogenic.

    c. icteric.

    d. neutropenic.

71. If you suspect that you have accidentally collected an arterial specimen instead of a venous specimen

    a. apply a pressure bandage to the venipuncture site.

    b. ask another phlebotomist to recollect the specimen.

    c. discard it and collect a new one from another site.

    d. keep it, but label it as a possible arterial specimen.

72. Infection of a venipuncture site can result from

    a. following the wrong order of draw.

    b. leaving the tourniquet on too long.

    c. touching the site after cleaning it.

    d. using an unsterile ETS tube holder.

73. Blind or deep probing for a vein can result in

    a. an arterial puncture.

    b. greater vein patency.

    c. loss of tube vacuum.

    d. tube additive reflux.

74. A patient complains of marked pain when you insert the needle. The pain radiates down his arm and does not subside. What should you do?

    a. Ask him if he wants you to stop the draw.

    b. Collect the specimen as quickly as you can.

c. Discontinue the venipuncture immediately.

d. Say "Hold on or I'll have to stick you again".

75. A stinging sensation when the needle is first inserted is *most* likely the result of

    a. an imperfection in the needle bevel.

    b. not letting the alcohol dry thoroughly.

    c. tying the tourniquet excessively tight.

    d. pushing down during needle insertion.

76. Which is the *best* way to avoid reflux?

    a. Draw the specimen while the patient is supine.

    b. Follow correct order of draw when filling tubes.

    c. Keep the tourniquet on until the last tube is full.

    d. Make certain that tubes fill from the bottom up.

77. Which of the following is *least* likely to impair vein patency?

    a. Improperly redirecting the needle

    b. Leaving a tourniquet on too long

    c. Multiple draws to the same vein

    d. Probing to locate a missed vein

78. Prolonged tourniquet application can affect blood composition because it causes

    a. delayed hemostasis.

    b. dilution of plasma.

    c. hemoconcentration.

    d. specimen hemolysis.

79. The serum or plasma of a hemolyzed specimen appears

    a. clear yellow.

    b. cloudy white.

    c. greenish yellow.

    d. pink or reddish.

80. Which action is *least* likely to cause specimen hemolysis?

    a. Drawing a large tube using a small needle

    b. Mixing a blood specimen too vigorously

    c. Pulling back a syringe plunger too quickly

    d. Using a transfer device for a syringe draw

81. Which of the following can cause a hematoma to form as a result of a blood draw?

    a. Entering the lumen of the vein without hesitation.

    b. Failing to apply adequate pressure after the draw.

    c. Mixing the first tube while collecting the second.

    d. Removing the tourniquet as the first tube is filling.

82. You are in the process of collecting a blood specimen on a patient with difficult veins. You had to redirect the needle but it is now in the vein, and the first tube has just started to fill. The blood is filling the tube slowly. The skin around the venipuncture site starts to swell. You have several more tubes to fill. What should you do?

    a. Ask the patient if it hurts; if not, continue the draw.
    b. Continue the draw after pushing the needle in deeper.
    c. Pull back on the needle slightly and finish the draw.
    d. Stop the draw at once and apply pressure to the site.

83. A vein with walls that have temporarily drawn together and shut off blood flow during venipuncture is called a

    a. blown vessel.
    b. collapsed vein.
    c. reflux reaction.
    d. inactive fistula.

84. You are collecting a blood specimen. The needle is in the vein and blood flow has been established. As the tube is filling, you hear a hissing sound, there is a spurt of blood into the tube, and blood flow stops. What *most* likely happened is the

    a. bevel came out of the skin and the tube vacuum escaped.
    b. needle went all the way through the back wall of the vein.
    c. patient had a sudden and dramatic drop in blood pressure.
    d. tube had a crack in it and there was no more vacuum left.

85. A needle that has gone through the back wall of the vein may cause

    a. a hissing sound when you engage the tube.
    b. blood to enter the tube slowly or not at all.
    c. reflux of specimen into surrounding tissue.
    d. the tube to fill with air that is in the tissues.

86. When a vein rolls, the needle typically

    a. ends up in the lumen of the vein.
    b. goes all the way through the vein.
    c. lands against an inside vein wall.
    d. slips beside instead of in the vein.

87. You are in the process of collecting a blood specimen. The needle is inserted but the tube is filling very slowly. A hematoma starts forming rapidly. What has *most* likely happened is the

    a. needle is only partly in the vein.
    b. needle is up against a vein wall.

    c. patient has a clotting disorder.
    d. tube is slowly loosing vacuum.

88. You are performing a multitube blood draw. You collect the first tube without a problem. The second tube fails to fill with blood. You pull the needle back and nothing happens. You push the needle a little deeper and nothing happens. You remove the tube, pull back the needle a little, rotate the bevel, and reset the tube. Still nothing happens. Which of the following actions should you take next?

    a. Discontinue the draw and try at another site.
    b. Let someone else take over and give it a try.
    c. Redirect the needle until you get blood flow.
    d. Try a new tube in case it is a vacuum issue.

89. You insert the needle during a venipuncture. You engage the tube in the tube holder, but do not get blood flow. You determine that the needle is beside the vein. You redirect it two times and still do not get blood flow, even after trying a new tube. What should you do next?

    a. Anchor the vein and redirect the needle again.
    b. Ask a coworker to redirect the needle for you.
    c. Discontinue the draw and try again at a new site.
    d. Try pushing the needle deeper and then redirect.

90. Which of the following is most apt to be the cause of vein collapse during venipuncture?

    a. Several large-volume tubes have been collected.
    b. Tourniquet application has exceeded 1 minute.
    c. Tourniquet pressure is below diastolic pressure.
    d. Tube vacuum is too much for the size of the vein.

91. A bariatric tourniquet is used for

    a. ABG collection.
    b. difficult draws.
    b. obese patients.
    c. all the above.

92. An injury referred to as "Claw hand" can be caused by

    a. arterial thrombosis.
    b. infection of a vein.
    c. ulnar nerve injury.
    d. vasovagal syncope.

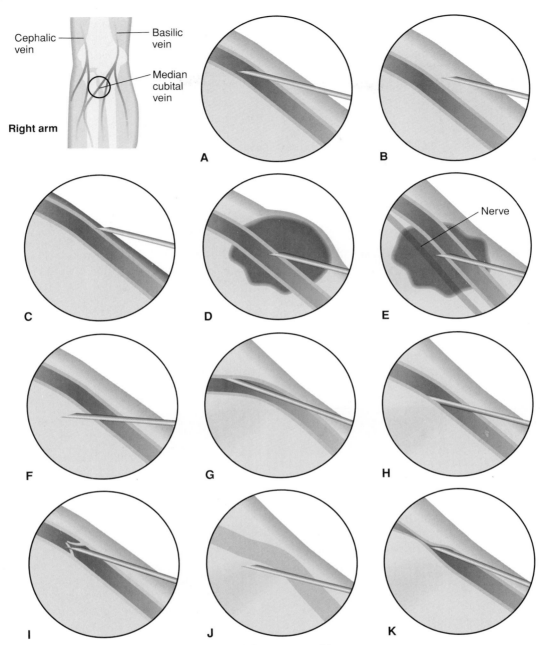

Figure 9-3 Needle positions.

93. A quadriplegic patient
    a. can feel pain if there is no sensory damage.
    b. cannot speak due to upper body paralysis.
    c. is paralyzed only from the waist down.
    d. must have blood drawn by a physician.

Use Figure 9-3, Needle Position, to answer questions 94 to 100.

94. The phlebotomist is quite certain the needle is in the vein, but there is no blood flowing to the tube. He can sense a slight needle vibration or quiver which reminds him of another time this happened. Which illustration shows what has happened?
    a. A
    b. G
    c. H
    d. I

95. Which illustration shows what can happen if the vacuum draw of a tube is too much for the vein being used for the venipuncture?
    a. D
    b. G
    c. H
    d. K

96. Which illustration depicts what can happen if the vein is not anchored well?
    a. A
    b. H
    c. I
    d. J

97. This illustration is an example of a situation that is most likely to lead to legal issues.
    a. C
    b. E
    c. G
    d. J

98. Correcting the situation in this illustration involves slowly pulling back the needle until blood flow is established.
    a. B
    b. G
    c. I
    d. J

99. If what this illustration depicts starts to happen, the venipuncture should be terminated immediately.
    a. D
    b. F
    c. H
    d. I

100. This illustrated situation would cause the tube to make a hissing sound and it would fail to fill with blood.
    a. B
    b. C
    c. E
    d. F

Answers and Explanations

1. **Answer: d**

   WHY: Preanalytical means "prior to analysis." The preanalytical phase of the testing process includes all of the steps taken before a specimen is analyzed. Consequently, it begins when the test is ordered and ends when testing begins.

   REVIEW: Yes ☐   No ☐

2. **Answer: b**

   WHY: Most tests are performed to screen for, diagnose, or monitor disease. To be properly evaluated, test results need to be compared with test result values expected of healthy individuals. Therefore, values for most tests are established using specimens from healthy individuals. Because results vary somewhat from person to person, the results used for comparison become a range of values with high and low limits, commonly called a reference range. Most reference ranges are given for fasting patients, established using specimens from healthy, fasting individuals. Fasting patients, however, are not always healthy individuals. Some tests do have reference ranges for patients who are ill or are being treated for certain disorders, such as diabetes, but these reference ranges are less common.

   REVIEW: Yes ☐   No ☐

3. **Answer: c**

   WHY: Diurnal means "happening daily." The levels of many blood components exhibit diurnal variations, or normal fluctuations or changes throughout the day. These normal variations are typically greatest between early morning and late afternoon.

   REVIEW: Yes ☐   No ☐

4. **Answer: b**

   WHY: Edema is the accumulation of fluid in the tissues, characterized by swelling. An extremity with edema is described as being edematous. Cyanotic means "marked by cyanosis, or bluish in color from lack of oxygen." Sclerosed means "hardened." Thrombosed means "clotted." Sclerosed and thrombosed are terms used to describe damaged veins.

   REVIEW: Yes ☐   No ☐

5. **Answer: a**

   WHY: The term "lipemia" comes from the word root "lip," which means "fat." Lipemia is the presence of increased fats (lipids) in the blood. Lipids do not dissolve in water and thus high levels of lipids are visible in the serum or plasma causing it to look cloudy or milky white.

   REVIEW: Yes ☐ No ☐

6. **Answer: d**

   WHY: Jaundice, also called icterus, is a condition characterized by increased bilirubin (a product of the breakdown of red blood cells) in the blood, leading to deposits of yellow bile pigment in the skin, mucous membranes, and sclera (whites of the eyes), giving the patient a yellow appearance.

   REVIEW: Yes ☐ No ☐

7. **Answer: b**

   WHY: Stasis means "stopping, controlling, or standing." Lymphostasis is defined as the obstruction or stoppage of the flow of lymph (lymph fluid).

   REVIEW: Yes ☐ No ☐

8. **Answer: c**

   WHY: Vasovagal means "relating to vagus nerve action on blood vessels." Syncope is the medical term for fainting. Vasovagal syncope is sudden faintness or loss of consciousness resulting from a nervous system response to abrupt pain, stress, or trauma. Circadian means "having a 24-hour cycle." Iatrogenic means "an adverse condition brought on by the effects of treatment," and reflux means "backflow," as in the backflow of blood into a patient's vein during venipuncture. Venous stagnation or stasis is the stoppage of normal venous blood flow.

   REVIEW: Yes ☐ No ☐

9. **Answer: d**

   WHY: Petechiae (Fig. 9-4) are small, nonraised red-, purple-, or brownish-colored spots that appear on a patient's skin when a tourniquet is applied. The spots are due to a defect in the capillary walls allowing blood to leak into the skin. Some of the causes for petechiae are certain medications like aspirin, prolonged straining of the capillaries when vomiting or prolonged tourniqueting, and even some infectious diseases, such as strep throat.

   REVIEW: Yes ☐ No ☐

10. **Answer: c**

    WHY: Venous stasis (also called venostasis) is a condition in which the normal flow of blood

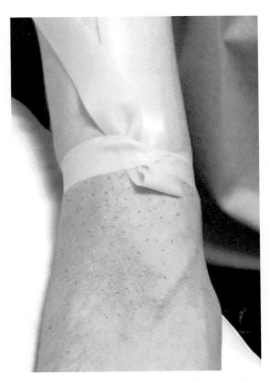

Figure 9-4 Petechiae (Photo courtesy of medtraining. org. Used with permission.)

through a vein is stopped or slowed. Stasis means "stopping, controlling, or standing." Venous means "relating to a vein."

REVIEW: Yes ☐ No ☐

11. **Answer: c**

    WHY: Hematoma (Fig. 9-1) is the medical term for a swelling or mass of blood under the skin caused by leakage of blood from a blood vessel. A hematoma can occur during or after venipuncture or arterial puncture, often as a result of poor technique. A blood clot within a vein is called a thrombus. A pool of fluid from an IV would cause localized edema. A hematoma is not a symptom of nerve injury, but pressure from the pooling of blood in the tissue could injure a nerve.

    REVIEW: Yes ☐ No ☐

    📖 **To see more situations that can trigger hematoma formation see Box 9-1 in the TEXTBOOK.**

12. **Answer: c**

    WHY: The surgical removal of a breast, which is sometimes done in the treatment of breast cancer, for example, is called a mastectomy. It is derived from the Greek word *mastos* which means "breast." The suffix *-tomy* means "incision or cutting."

    REVIEW: Yes ☐ No ☐

13. **Answer: c**

WHY: Exsanguination is massive blood loss or removal of blood to a point where life cannot be sustained. Autologous donation of blood is giving blood for one's own use. Iatrogenic is an adjective used to describe an adverse condition brought on as a result of treatment. Blood depletion because of blood being removed for testing is called iatrogenic blood loss. Life may be threatened if more than 10% of a patient's blood volume is removed at one time or over a short period of time. Blood is sometimes removed for therapeutic purposes, such as, when treating polycythemia, but not in quantities that would cause exsanguination.

REVIEW: Yes ☐ No ☐

14. **Answer: a**

WHY: Bilirubin is a yellowish pigment that is the product of the breakdown of red blood cells by the body. High levels of bilirubin in the blood lead to deposits of the pigment in the skin, mucous membranes, and sclera (whites of the eyes), a condition called jaundice.

REVIEW: Yes ☐ No ☐

15. **Answer: a**

WHY: Thrombosed means "clotted." A thrombosed vein is not necessarily scarred or swollen. A patent vein is a vein that is freely open, not clotted.

REVIEW: Yes ☐ No ☐

📖 *Have fun learning the meaning of this and other words by doing the crossword in Chapter 9 of the WORKBOOK.*

16. **Answer: a**

WHY: *Do not* attempt to complete the draw on a patient who has a seizure or even a miniseizure during venipuncture. Continuing the draw is dangerous and could result in injury to the patient. In addition, you could receive an accidental needlestick. Discontinue the draw immediately and remove, shield, and discard the needle as soon as possible. Try to prevent the patient from injuring himself or herself and notify the appropriate first aid personnel as soon as possible.

REVIEW: Yes ☐ No ☐

17. **Answer: c**

WHY: When one arm has an IV it is preferred that the specimen be collected from the other arm if possible. Never collect a blood specimen above an IV or a hematoma. When there is no alternative site, perform the venipuncture below or distal to the hematoma. Venipuncture through or close to a hematoma is painful to the patient and can result in collection of blood from outside the vein that is hemolyzed or contaminated by the IV, and unsuitable for testing. Going below (distal) to the hematoma ensures collection of blood that is free-flowing and unaltered by the effects of the clotting and hemolysis in the area.

REVIEW: Yes ☐ No ☐

18. **Answer: d**

WHY: A hematoma is a swelling or mass of blood that can be caused by blood leaking from a blood vessel during or immediately after a venipuncture. A bruise eventually spreads into the surrounding area. The bruising in Figure 9-1 most likely resulted from a very large hematoma that formed during a venipuncture. After the venipuncture the pool of blood apparently migrated to low areas of the arm while the patient was in a resting position in the hospital bed.

REVIEW: Yes ☐ No ☐

19. **Answer: b**

WHY: Hemoconcentration is a condition in which plasma and small, filterable components of the blood pass through the walls of the blood vessels into the tissues, *decreasing* blood plasma volume and concentrating and therefore increasing nonfilterable or suspended blood components such as red blood cells. Oxygen and pH are usually tested on arterial blood and a tourniquet is not used in collection. Hemoconcentration does not cause specimen hemolysis.

REVIEW: Yes ☐ No ☐

20. **Answer: d**

WHY: Syncope is the temporary loss of consciousness and the ability to maintain an upright position as a result of inadequate blood flow to the brain, and is the medical term for fainting. Sclerose means "to harden." Stasis is stagnation of blood or other fluids. Supine means "lying on the back, face up."

REVIEW: Yes ☐ No ☐

21. **Answer: d**

WHY: Basal state refers to the condition of the body early in the morning when a patient is still at rest and fasting (approximately 12 hours after the last intake of food). The patient who has just awakened at 0600 hours (6 AM) and has not eaten since the previous evening meal is closest to basal state.

REVIEW: Yes ☐ No ☐

22. **Answer: a**

    WHY: Inpatient reference ranges for laboratory tests are typically established using basal state specimens to eliminate the effects of diet, exercise, and other factors on results.

    REVIEW: Yes ☐ No ☐

23. **Answer: d**

    WHY: Some physiological functions, such as kidney function, normally decrease with age. Creatinine is removed (cleared) from the blood plasma by the kidneys. The amount removed is measured by the creatinine clearance test. Since kidney function declines with age, the patient's age is required when calculating the results of the creatinine clearance test.

    REVIEW: Yes ☐ No ☐

24. **Answer: d**

    WHY: Red blood cells carry oxygen to the tissue cells. The oxygen content of the air decreases as the altitude increases. The decrease in oxygen content at higher altitudes causes the body to produce more red blood cells in order to fulfill the body's oxygen requirements.

    REVIEW: Yes ☐ No ☐

25. **Answer: a**

    WHY: Persistent diarrhea without fluid replacement leads to dehydration, which is a decrease in total body fluid, including blood plasma. Blood components become concentrated in the smaller plasma volume, a condition called hemoconcentration.

    REVIEW: Yes ☐ No ☐

26. **Answer: b**

    WHY: It is preferred that blood specimens not be drawn from an arm with an intravenous (IV) line (Fig. 9-5). However, according to CLSI, a specimen can be drawn *below* an IV after it has been shut off for a minimum of 2 minutes. (A phlebotomist should *never* shut off an IV. It must be shut off by the patient's nurse.) It should be noted on the requisition that the specimen was drawn below an IV after it was shut off. The type of IV fluid should also be noted. Never draw above an IV because the specimen may be contaminated with IV fluid. Drawing blood specimens from ankle veins requires permission from the patient's physician and is not recommended for protimes or other coagulation specimens, or patients who have coagulation problems. Only nurses and other specially trained personnel are allowed to collect specimens from an IV.

    REVIEW: Yes ☐ No ☐

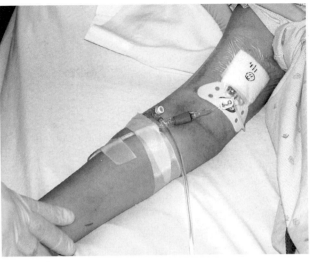

Figure 9-5 Patient's arm with an intravenous (IV) line.

27. **Answer: d**

    WHY: Fasting serum or plasma is normally clear yellow. The serum or plasma of a lipemic specimen is milky (cloudy white) because of high fat (lipid) content. Presence of fats is an indication that the patient may not have been fasting prior to specimen collection. A 12-hour fast is generally required to remove the effects of lipids from the blood. The presence of lipemia in a truly fasting specimen is not that common.

    REVIEW: Yes ☐ No ☐

    📖 *Have some fun with the WORKBOOK exercise, Knowledge Drill 9-7 as you explore how many colors serum can be.*

28. **Answer: d**

    WHY: Triglycerides are a type of lipid. A 12-hour fast is required to remove the effects of food ingestion on the triglyceride content of the blood (see answers to questions 26 and 27).

    REVIEW: Yes ☐ No ☐

29. **Answer: a**

    WHY: Diurnal variations are normal fluctuations throughout the day. Cortisol levels exhibit diurnal variation with highest levels occurring in the morning. Creatinine, glucose, and phosphate also exhibit diurnal variation; however, blood levels of these analytes are *lowest* in the morning.

    REVIEW: Yes ☐ No ☐

30. **Answer: d**

    WHY: For consistency in evaluating or comparing results, tests that exhibit diurnal variation or fluctuations throughout the day are often ordered for a specific time of day. The requested time of collection is typically a time when the highest level of the analyte is expected.

REVIEW: Yes ☐ No ☐

31. **Answer: b**

WHY: According to College of American Pathologists (CAP) guidelines, drugs known to interfere with blood tests should be stopped or avoided for 4 to 24 hours (depending on the drug) before specimens for the affected tests are collected. Drugs that interfere with urine tests should be stopped 48 to 72 hours before specimen collection.

REVIEW: Yes ☐ No ☐

32. **Answer: a**

WHY: When a prescribed drug acts to enhance the desired test reaction, the results will be falsely elevated. If the substance tested (analyte) is competing for the same test sites in the testing process as the drug, the results will be falsely decreased. Reflux of anticoagulant during specimen collection may cause an adverse patient reaction, but does not affect the specimen being collected. Testing serum obtained from a partially filled red top should not affect test results as long as there is enough specimen to perform the test.

REVIEW: Yes ☐ No ☐

33. **Answer: a**

WHY: Exercise elevates blood levels of a number of components, including skeletal enzymes such as creatine kinase (CK) and lactate dehydrogenase (LDH), which may stay elevated for 24 hours or more. CO_2 and pH levels decrease with exercise. Potassium (K^+) levels increase with exercise, but usually return to normal levels after several minutes of rest.

REVIEW: Yes ☐ No ☐

34. **Answer: a**

WHY: Hypoglycemia caused by fever increases insulin levels followed by a rise in glucagon levels. Melatonin levels are affected by light, increasing at night when it is dark and decreasing during daylight hours. Testosterone exhibits diurnal variation with highest levels occurring in the morning. Thyroxine is a hormone that is secreted by the thyroid and increases the metabolic rate.

REVIEW: Yes ☐ No ☐

35. **Answer: b**

WHY: A patient's sex has a determining effect on the concentration of a number of blood

components. These differences are reflected in separate male and female reference ranges for certain analytes. For example, males tend to have greater muscle mass and normally have higher red blood cell counts to supply the muscles with oxygen. Consequently red blood cell counts and related tests such as hematocrit and hemoglobin have higher reference ranges for males. The hematocrit is a measure of the percentage of a specimen that is red blood cells.

REVIEW: Yes ☐ No ☐

36. **Answer: a**

WHY: Icterus (also called jaundice) is a condition characterized by increased bilirubin in the blood and other body fluids and deposits of the yellow pigment in the skin, mucous membranes, and sclera (whites of the eyes), giving the patient a yellow appearance. Body fluid specimens with high bilirubin levels have an abnormal deep yellow to yellow-brown color, and are described as being icteric. The presence of icterus is not related to a patient's fasting state, the collection procedure, or hemoconcentration.

REVIEW: Yes ☐ No ☐

37. **Answer: a**

WHY: When a patient stands up after being supine (lying down), blood plasma filters into the tissues, *decreasing* plasma volume and *increasing* nonfilterable or suspended elements such as calcium, iron, proteins, and red blood cells.

REVIEW: Yes ☐ No ☐

38. **Answer: b**

WHY: Normal body fluid increases in pregnancy include an increase in blood plasma levels. The increased volume of plasma has a dilution effect on the red blood cells (RBCs), reducing RBC count results. Consequently, the reference ranges for RBC counts on pregnant women are lower than for women who are not pregnant. Hemoconcentration would elevate RBC counts. Anemia from poor appetite or inadequate iron reserves represent situations that typically result in abnormal patient results that are lower than reference ranges.

REVIEW: Yes ☐ No ☐

39. **Answer: b**

WHY: Chronic smokers have impaired ability to transport oxygen to the cells because as much as 10% of their hemoglobin is bound to carbon monoxide acquired from cigarette smoke. The body compensates for this by increasing the number of

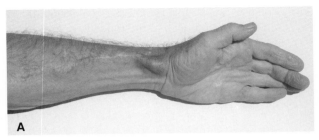 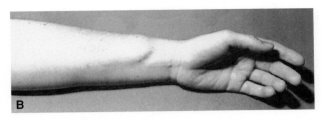

Figure 9-6 Arms with arteriovenous (AV) shunts. **A:** Fistula. **B:** Graft.

red blood cells. Consequently hemoglobin, which is a component of red blood cells, typically increases also. Bicarbonate, O_2 saturation, and vitamin B_{12} levels are usually decreased in chronic smokers.

REVIEW: Yes ☐   No ☐

40. **Answer: b**

WHY: An arm with an AV shunt (Fig. 9-6) should be avoided as a blood collection site. Fistulas and grafts are types of AV shunts. An arm where venipuncture was performed recently is not ruled out as a current venipuncture site, although it is best to alternate arms if possible, when venipuncture times are close together. Tattoos do not rule out using the arm for blood collection unless the tattoo is fresh. The basilic vein is always a last choice for venipuncture, because it lies near the basilic artery and a major nerve. However, the presence of a strong basilic artery pulse in the arm is not an issue as long as the specimen is not collected from the basilic vein.

REVIEW: Yes ☐   No ☐

📖 *Review unusual venipuncture sites and problems with each in the WORKBOOK Exercise Matching 9-3.*

41. **Answer: d**

WHY: Reference ranges for specimens are established using basal state specimens. Environmental factors associated with geographic location do affect basal state. However, because all the specimens used to calculate reference ranges come from individuals in that particular location, geographical factors are usually automatically reflected in the reference range values.

REVIEW: Yes ☐   No ☐

42. **Answer: b**

WHY: Temperature and humidity are known to affect test values. Closely controlling these environmental factors in a clinical laboratory standardizes the test environment, and helps ensure specimen integrity and proper functioning of equipment. Controlling temperature and

humidity can help ensure accuracy of test results. It does not ensure that test results will be normal or lessen drug interference in testing. Hemolysis usually results from improper specimen collection or handling technique before the specimen gets to the lab.

REVIEW: Yes ☐   No ☐

43. **Answer: b**

WHY: Scarred and burned areas should be avoided as blood collection sites because circulation in these areas could be impaired. This can result in hemoconcentration, which can concentrate, not dilute analytes. Veins do not normally become sclerosed or thrombosed due to scarring or burns. Hemolyzed specimens typically result from collection errors, not from scars or burns on the arm.

REVIEW: Yes ☐   No ☐

44. **Answer: c**

WHY: The word root *scler* means hard. A vein that feels hard, cordlike, and lacks resiliency is said to be sclerosed. An artery has a pulse that can be felt, which easily distinguishes it from a vein since a vein has no pulse. A collapsed vein typically cannot be felt at all even if it is superficial which means close to the surface of the skin.

REVIEW: Yes ☐   No ☐

45. **Answer: a**

WHY: Edema is swelling caused by the abnormal accumulation of fluid in the tissues. Specimens collected from edematous areas may yield erroneous test results due to contamination with the fluid in the tissue or altered blood composition related to the swelling and impaired circulation in the area.

REVIEW: Yes ☐   No ☐

46. **Answer: c**

WHY: If you have no other choice, it is acceptable to collect a blood specimen distal, or below a hematoma, where blood flow is least affected by it. A venipuncture in the area of a hematoma,

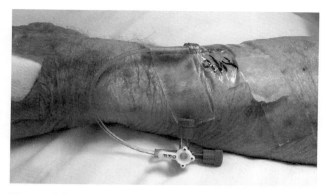

Figure 9-7 Saline lock with needleless entry stopcock.

including above, beside, or through it, is painful to the patient, and can yield erroneous results related to the obstruction of blood flow by the hematoma. It can also result in collection of contaminated and possibly hemolyzed blood from the hematoma, instead of blood from the vein.

REVIEW: Yes ☐ No ☐

47. **Answer: a**

WHY: When a blood specimen is collected from a saline lock (Fig. 9-7), a 5-mL discard tube must be drawn first to eliminate residual saline or heparin used to flush the device and keep it from clotting. The only extra tube collected is the clear tube. Drawing coagulation specimens from a saline lock is not recommended. Only nurses and specially trained personnel draw from such devices.

REVIEW: Yes ☐ No ☐

48. **Answer: c**

WHY: Veins on obese patients can be deep and difficult to find. The cephalic vein is sometimes the easiest vein to palpate. To locate it, rotate the patient's arm so that the hand is prone. In this position, the weight of excess tissue often pulls downward, making the cephalic vein easier to feel and penetrate with a needle.

REVIEW: Yes ☐ No ☐

49. **Answer: a**

WHY: An abnormally high concentration of lipids (fatty substances) in the blood is called *lipemia*. Lipemia can persist for up to 12 hours. Because lipids are insoluble in water they make serum or plasma look milky (cloudy white) or turbid and the specimen is described as being *lipemic*.

REVIEW: Yes ☐ No ☐

50. **Answer: d**

WHY: The most expedient thing to do in this situation is to collect the specimen by finger

stick. A capillary specimen can be collected and on its way to the lab in the time it would take to call another phlebotomist to come and collect the specimen, the IV to be shut off for 2 minutes to collect the specimen below it, or permission obtained to collect the specimen from a leg, ankle, or foot vein.

REVIEW: Yes ☐ No ☐

51. **Answer: d**

WHY: Studies performed on crying infants have demonstrated significant increases in white blood cell (WBC) counts, which are a part of a complete blood count (CBC). Counts returned to normal within 1 hour after crying stopped. For this reason, it is best if CBCs or WBC specimens are obtained after the infant has been sleeping or resting quietly for at least 30 minutes. Because an infant usually cries during blood collection, the specimens should be collected as quickly as possible. If a specimen must be collected while an infant is crying, it should be noted on the report.

REVIEW: Yes ☐ No ☐

52. **Answer: a**

WHY: An arterial line (A-line) (Fig. 9-8) or catheter is most commonly located in the radial artery and is used to provide continuous measurement of a patient's blood pressure. It is also commonly used for collection of blood gas specimens.

REVIEW: Yes ☐ No ☐

53. **Answer: a**

WHY: The surgically created connection of an artery and a vein in the forearm is called an AV shunt (Fig. 9-6) and is most commonly created to provide access for dialysis. A dialysis shunt created by direct permanent fusion of the artery and vein is called a **fistula** (Fig. 9-6A)

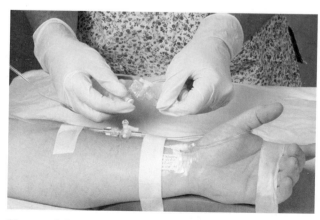

Figure 9-8 Nurse working with a patient's arterial line (A-line).

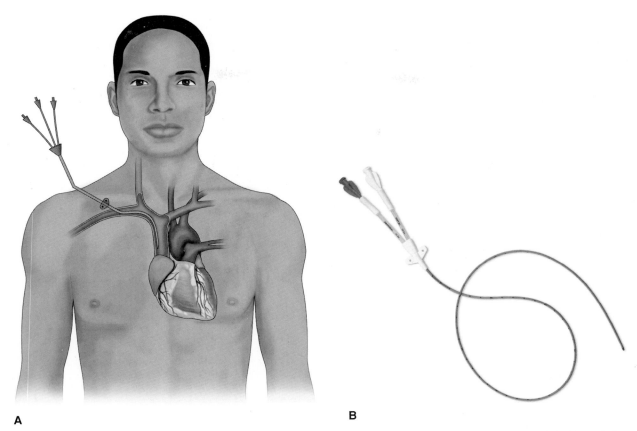

Figure 9-9 A: Central venous catheter (CVC) placement. (Reprinted with permission from Taylor CR, Lillis C, LeMone P, Lynn P. *Fundamentals of Nursing: The Art and Science of Nursing Care.* 6th ed. Philadelphia, PA: Lippincott Williams & Wilkins; 2008.) **B:** Groshong® CVC. (Courtesy of Bard Access Systems, Inc., Salt Lake City, UT.)

and is visible as a large bulging section of vein. If the shunt was created using a piece of vein or tubing to form a loop from the artery to the vein that can be seen under the skin it is called a **graft** (Fig. 9-6B). A central venous catheter (CVC) is a line inserted into a large vein and advanced into the superior vena cava proximal to the right atrium (Fig. 9-9). It is used to administer medications and sometimes draw blood specimens. A saline lock (Fig. 9-7) is a special winged needle set or cannula that can be left in a patient's arm for up to 48 hours and used to administer medications and draw blood. A peripherally inserted central catheter (PICC) (Fig. 9-10) is inserted into the peripheral venous system (veins of the extremities) and threaded into the central venous system (main veins leading to the heart).
REVIEW: Yes ☐   No ☐

54. **Answer: b**
WHY: Blood should never be collected from an arm on the same side as a mastectomy (breast removal) without first consulting the patient's

physician. Lymphostasis (stoppage of lymph flow) that can occur when lymph nodes have been removed leaves the area susceptible to infection. It is thought that test results could be affected by lymphedema due to lymphostasis, but not necessarily elevated. The patient won't necessarily have less feeling in that arm. Veins in that arm do not necessarily collapse readily.
REVIEW: Yes ☐   No ☐

📖 *A case study concerning this topic can be found at the end of Chapter 9 of the TEXTBOOK.*

55. **Answer: b**
WHY: A central venous catheter or CVC (Fig. 9-9) is an indwelling line inserted into a main vein, such as the subclavian, and advanced into the vena cava. The exit end is surgically tunneled under the skin to a site several inches away in the chest. One or more short lengths of capped tubing protrude from the exit site (Fig. 9-9A), which is normally covered with a transparent dressing. There are a number of different types of CVCs, including Broviac®, Groshong®, and Hickman®. An A-line is an arterial line and is usually located

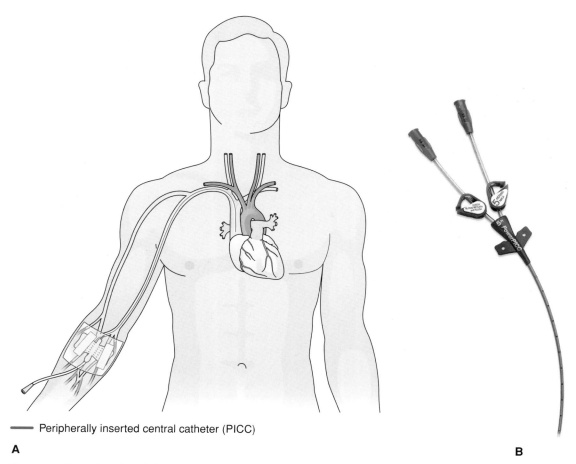

Peripherally inserted central catheter (PICC)

A

B

Figure 9-10 A: Peripherally inserted central catheter (PICC) placement. (Reprinted with permission from Taylor CR, Lillis C, LeMone P, Lynn P. *Fundamentals of Nursing: The Art and Science of Nursing Care.* 6th ed. Philadelphia, PA: Lippincott Williams & Wilkins; 2008.) **B:** Power PICC® (Courtesy of Bard Access Systems, Inc., Salt Lake City, UT.)

on the underside of the wrist. A fistula (Fig. 9-6A) is a fused artery and vein in the underside of the lower arm that is used for the purpose of hemodialysis. See the answer to question number 53 for a description of a PICC (Fig. 9-10).

REVIEW: Yes ☐   No ☐

threaded into a main vein leading to the heart. A saline lock (Fig. 9-7) is explained in the answer to question 53.

REVIEW: Yes ☐   No ☐

📖 *The WORKBOOK Matching Exercise 9-4, gives you a chance to compare VADs and scenarios.*

56. **Answer: b**

WHY: A subcutaneous vascular access device (SVAD), also called an implanted port (Fig. 9-11), is a small chamber that is attached to an indwelling line. The chamber is surgically implanted under the skin in the upper chest or arm. It is located by palpating the skin, and access is gained by inserting a special noncoring needle through the skin into the self-sealing septum (wall) of the chamber. Groshong is a trade name of CVC (Fig. 9-9). (See explanation of question 55 for a description of a CVC.) A peripherally inserted central catheter (PICC) (Fig. 9-10) is a type of line inserted into a peripheral vein and

57. **Answer: d**

WHY: Some patients are allergic to the glue used in adhesive bandages. Using a latex-free bandage is not an option because the patient is allergic to the adhesive used for the bandage, not necessarily latex. A good option is to cover the site with a clean folded gauze square and wrap it with bandaging material such as Coban that sticks to itself, not the skin. Another option if the patient is alert and competent is to ask him or her to hold pressure over the site until bleeding stops in lieu of bandaging. Waiting 5 minutes before applying a bandage does not correct the adhesive allergy issue. Wrapping the site with a warm wash cloth

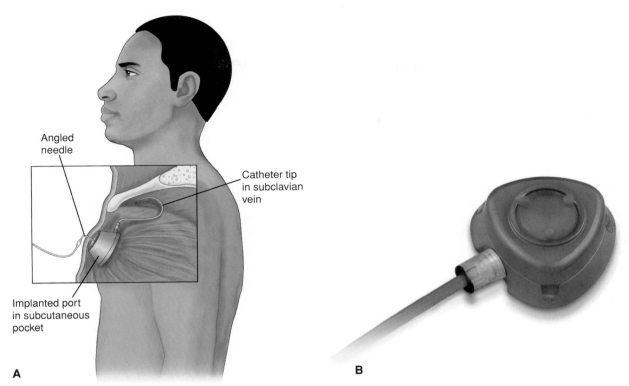

Angled
needle

Catheter tip
in subclavian
vein

Implanted port
in subcutaneous
pocket

A

B

Figure 9-11 A: Implanted port placement. (Reprinted with permission from Taylor CR, Lillis C, LeMone P, Lynn P. *Fundamentals of Nursing: The Art and Science of Nursing Care.* 6th ed. Philadelphia, PA: Lippincott Williams & Wilkins; 2008.)
B: PowerPort® implanted port. (Courtesy of Bard Access Systems, Inc., Salt Lake City, UT.)

would increase blood flow and could make the site take longer to stop bleeding.

REVIEW: Yes ☐   No ☐

58. **Answer: c**

WHY: Increasing numbers of individuals are developing allergies to latex. Some allergies are so severe that being in the same room where latex materials are used can set off a life-threatening reaction. If an inpatient is known to have a severe allergy to latex, there is typically a warning sign on the door to the room. It is important that no items made of latex be brought into the room. Fortunately, manufacturers have come up with latex-free alternatives to many items commonly used in healthcare, but other items still contain latex parts and many nonmedical items such as balloons, rubber bands, and even the soles of shoes may have latex in them.

REVIEW: Yes ☐   No ☐

59. **Answer: c**

WHY: A site that continues to bleed 5 minutes after venipuncture is not normal. The patient's nurse or physician must be notified so the situation can be addressed. Continue to apply pressure

and do not dismiss an outpatient or leave an inpatient until bleeding has stopped or the appropriate personnel have taken charge of the situation. Never wrap a pressure bandage around a site in lieu of holding pressure. Always check the site before applying a bandage. Otherwise you will not know if bleeding has stopped.

REVIEW: Yes ☐   No ☐

60. **Answer: c**

WHY: Syncope means "fainting." A patient with a history of fainting during blood collection should be asked to lie down during a blood draw.

REVIEW: Yes ☐   No ☐

61. **Answer: b**

WHY: If an outpatient feels faint during blood collection, discontinue the draw immediately and lower his or her head. Do not ask the patient if you should continue. You should not continue the draw, even if the patient wants you to do so. The use of ammonia inhalants is not recommended as they can have adverse side effects such as respiratory distress in asthmatic individuals.

REVIEW: Yes ☐   No ☐

62. **Answer: b**

    WHY: An outpatient who becomes weak and pale following a draw may faint and should be asked to lie down until he or she recovers. If the patient cannot be moved from the chair, lower his or her head and apply a cold compress or wet washcloth to the back of the neck. Do not allow the patient to leave until 15 minutes after recovery. The patient should not drive for at least 30 minutes.

    REVIEW: Yes ☐   No ☐

63. **Answer: a**

    WHY: A feeling of nausea often precedes vomiting, so it is a good idea to give the patient an emesis basin to hold as a precaution. Apply a cold, damp washcloth or other cold compress to the patient's forehead and ask him or her to breathe slowly and deeply. Do not attempt blood collection until the nausea subsides. Drawing the specimen regardless of her nausea may stimulate her to vomit. The nausea will not necessarily subside if you have her lie down. Coming back another day will not solve the problem if this is a reaction to the thought of having blood drawn. In addition, returning another day may be an imposition to the patient, especially if she is from out of town or has otherwise traveled some distance to get to the lab. It may also delay any treatment if the physician is waiting for results to decide on a course of action.

    REVIEW: Yes ☐   No ☐

64. **Answer: b**

    WHY: Engaging in small talk before venipuncture can put patients at ease and help them relax. A relaxed patient is less likely to feel as much pain associated with the draw as someone who is anxious and tense. Rubbing with alcohol can abrade the skin and can be painful rather than desensitizing. Tying the tourniquet too tight can make the arm feel numb, but numbness is a sign of nerve compression and is never recommended. A venipuncture should not "hurt a lot." Telling patients that the draw might be painful can increase their anxiety and actually make them more tense. The patient should be warned just before the needle enters the arm, however, to prevent a startle reflex.

    REVIEW: Yes ☐   No ☐

65. **Answer: a**

    WHY: Petechiae (Fig. 9-4) are small red, purple, or brownish, nonraised spots that appear with tourniquet application on some patients with platelet or capillary defects. They do not compromise test

results and may not be avoidable because they will probably occur at any site that is chosen. Sites with massive scarring, or edema, and veins that feel hard and cordlike should be avoided.

    REVIEW: Yes ☐   No ☐

66. **Answer: a**

    WHY: Cleaning a skin puncture site with isopropyl alcohol is accepted technique. Collecting blood from the median vein above an IV may contaminate or dilute the specimen with IV fluid. Touching the filter paper while collecting a phenylketonuria (PKU) specimen can be a source of contamination that leads to erroneous results. Povidone-iodine should not be used to clean skin puncture sites because it interferes with phosphorus, potassium, and uric acid test results.

    REVIEW: Yes ☐   No ☐

67. **Answer: b**

    WHY: There is no skin puncture container for collecting plasma specimens for coagulation tests because, except for those who can be performed with special point-of-care instruments, coagulation tests cannot be performed by skin puncture. Partially filled coagulation tubes have an incorrect blood-to-additive ratio and are unacceptable for testing. Pouring two partially filled tubes together also results in an improper ratio of blood to additive and is unacceptable. A phlebotomist should never make more than two attempts at venipuncture on a patient at one time. After the second attempt, another phlebotomist should be asked to collect the specimen.

    REVIEW: Yes ☐   No ☐

68. **Answer: d**

    WHY: A prothrombin time is a coagulation test. The ratio of blood to anticoagulant is *most* critical for coagulation tests because a ratio of nine parts blood to one part anticoagulant must be maintained for accurate test results. The excess anticoagulant in a tube that does not fill to the correct level dilutes the plasma portion of the specimen used for testing, causing falsely prolonged test results.

    REVIEW: Yes ☐   No ☐

69. **Answer: c**

    WHY: Blood pulsing or spurting into the tube is an indication that you may have accidentally hit an artery. A hematoma will not necessarily form when you hit an artery instead of a vein if the needle bevel is completely within the artery and adequate pressure is held over the site after the needle is removed from it. Color is not a good way to identify arterial blood. Normal venous blood is typically dark red. Arterial blood in normal individuals is bright red, but it may look as dark as venous blood if the patient has a pulmonary problem.

REVIEW: Yes ☐ No ☐

70. **Answer: b**

WHY: Iatrogenic is an adjective used to describe an adverse condition brought on by the effects of treatment. Blood loss as a result of removal for testing purposes is called iatrogenic blood loss. Removal of blood on a regular basis or in large quantities can lead to anemia in some patients, especially infants.

REVIEW: Yes ☐ No ☐

71. **Answer: d**

WHY: An inadvertently collected arterial specimen can usually be submitted for testing, rather than redrawing the patient. However, the specimen should be labeled as arterial because some test values are different for arterial specimens. If you suspect that you have accidentally punctured an artery, you must hold pressure over the site for 3 to 5 minutes. Do not have the patient hold pressure or apply a pressure bandage in lieu of holding pressure.

REVIEW: Yes ☐ No ☐

72. **Answer: c**

WHY: Infection at the site following venipuncture is rare but not unheard of. Using proper aseptic technique, including not touching the site after it has been cleaned, minimizing the time between removing the needle cap and venipuncture, not opening adhesive bandages ahead of time, and reminding the patient to keep the bandage on for at least 15 minutes after specimen collection, should minimize the risk of infection. The wrong order of draw or leaving a tourniquet on too long can affect the specimen but does not cause infection of the site. ETS tube holders are not normally sterile because they should not come in contact with the venipuncture site.

REVIEW: Yes ☐ No ☐

73. **Answer: a**

WHY: Blind or deep probing during venipuncture is usually painful and can result in the accidental piercing of nerves and arteries and the possibility of permanent damage. Lawsuits have been filed over permanent nerve injuries caused directly by needles or indirectly by compression of the nerves

by hematomas that resulted from inadvertent arterial sticks. Patency is the state of being freely open. Rather than causing vein patency, probing can damage veins and make them less patent. Probing does not cause reflux or loss of tube vacuum.

REVIEW: Yes ☐ No ☐

74. **Answer: c**

WHY: Marked (extreme or significant) pain, numbness of the arm, and pain that radiates up or down the arm are signs of nerve involvement and any one of them requires immediate removal of the needle. A patient may not understand the significance of the symptoms or may be stoic in an effort to not appear weak. It is up to the phlebotomist to recognize the signs of nerve injury and discontinue the venipuncture immediately. Continuing the draw can worsen the damage.

REVIEW: Yes ☐ No ☐

📖 *The cautions in Chapter 9 of the TEXTBOOK deal with this and other important topics. WORKBOOK Knowledge Drill 9-1 will help you learn them.*

75. **Answer: b**

WHY: Performing venipuncture before the alcohol has dried completely is the most common cause of a stinging sensation to the patient. Blood collection needles are used only once and are not likely to be dull or flawed, but they should be examined when first opened to detect defects that could cause pain or injure the patient. Pushing down on the needle as it is inserted can be painful but does not normally produce a stinging sensation. A tourniquet that is tied too tightly is typically described as a pinching sensation.

REVIEW: Yes ☐ No ☐

76. **Answer: d**

WHY: "Reflux" is a term used to describe the backflow of blood from a collection tube into a patient's vein during venipuncture. Reflux can happen if there is a pressure change in the vein that occurs normally or when the tourniquet is released. It can only occur if blood in the tube is in contact with the needle during venipuncture. Reflux of blood mixed with an additive such as EDTA can cause an adverse patient reaction. Keeping the arm in a downward position so that tubes fill from the bottom up (Fig. 9-12), and avoiding back-and-forth movement of tube contents during blood collection, prevents blood in the tube from being in contact with the tube holder end of the needle and therefore prevents reflux.

REVIEW: Yes ☐ No ☐

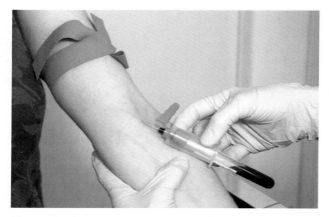

Figure 9-12 Tube positioned to avoid reflux.

77. **Answer: b**

    WHY: Leaving the tourniquet on too long is not likely to impair vein patency (state of being freely open). It may, however, lead to erroneous test results caused by hemoconcentration brought on by prolonged blockage of blood flow. Improperly redirecting the needle, probing for deep veins, and performing numerous venipunctures in the same area are all actions that can damage veins and impair vein patency.

    REVIEW: Yes ☐   No ☐

78. **Answer: c**

    WHY: Prolonged tourniquet application causes stagnation of blood flow (venous stasis), which causes the plasma portion of the blood to filter into the tissues. This decreases blood plasma volume and increases nonfilterable blood components, a condition called hemoconcentration. To minimize the effects of hemoconcentration, the tourniquet should be released within 1 minute of application and the patient should not be allowed to continuously make and release (or pump) a fist.

    REVIEW: Yes ☐   No ☐

79. **Answer: d**

    WHY: Hemolysis is the destruction of red blood cells and the liberation of hemoglobin into the serum or plasma portion of the specimen, causing it to appear pink to reddish depending on the degree of hemolysis. The specimen is described as being hemolyzed.

    REVIEW: Yes ☐   No ☐

80. **Answer: d**

    WHY: Mixing tubes vigorously instead of gently inverting them, pulling blood into a syringe too quickly, and using a small-bore needle to collect blood into a large-volume tube can all result in hemolysis of the specimen. Transferring blood

from a syringe to a tube using a transfer device should *not* cause hemolysis if done correctly.

REVIEW: Yes ☐   No ☐

81. **Answer: b**

    WHY: Hematoma formation can be caused by several different errors in phlebotomy technique, including failure to apply adequate pressure to the site after a blood draw, leakage of blood from a vein because the needle is only partly inserted in the vein (Fig. 9-13D), and leakage of blood from a hole made by a needle that penetrated through the back wall of the vein (Fig. 9-13F) during needle entry or the collection process. A needle bevel that enters the lumen of the vein is right where it should be (Fig. 9-13A) and would not be the cause of hematoma formation. Mixing one tube while filling another, and removing the tourniquet as the first tube is filling are accepted procedures and would not cause a hematoma.

    REVIEW: Yes ☐   No ☐

82. **Answer: d**

    WHY: Blood filling the tube slowly is a sign that the needle bevel is not completely within the vein (Fig. 9-13D,E), which allows blood to leak into the tissues. A hematoma, the most common venipuncture complication, is caused by blood leaking into the tissues and identified by swelling at or near the venipuncture site. It is painful to the patient, results in unsightly bruising (Fig. 9-1), and can cause compression injuries to nerves and lead to lawsuits. If a hematoma starts to form during blood collection, immediately release the tourniquet, withdraw and discard the needle, and hold pressure over the site for a minimum of 2 minutes.

    REVIEW: Yes ☐   No ☐

83. **Answer: b**

    WHY: A vein is said to be collapsed (Fig. 9-13K) when its walls temporarily retract, cutting off blood flow. A vein can collapse if the tube being drawn has too much vacuum, a syringe plunger is pulled back too quickly, or the tourniquet is tied too tightly or too close to the site. It can also collapse when the tourniquet is removed during the draw, especially if the tourniquet was too tight and inflated the vein excessively. A blown vein results from a small tear or enlarged hole at the site of needle entry that causes blood to escape quickly and the vein to collapse as a result. A reflux reaction is a patient reaction to the backflow of a tube additive into his or her vein during venipuncture. The type of fistula of importance to phlebotomists is the artificial connection between

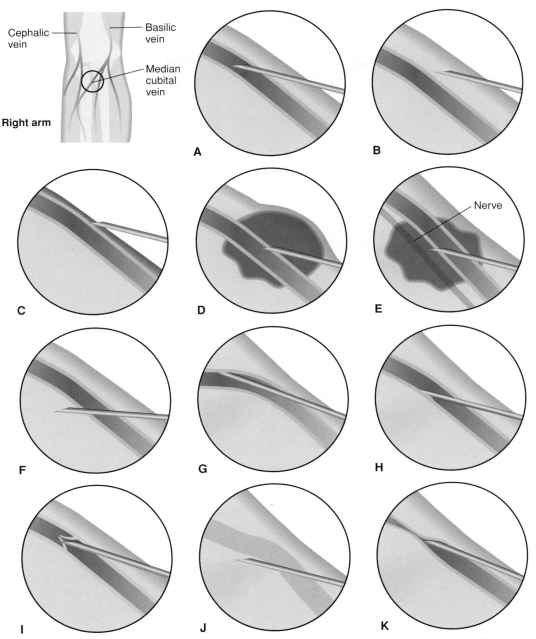

Figure 9-13 Needle position. **A:** Correct needle position; blood can flow freely into the needle. **B:** Needle not inserted far enough; needle does not enter vein. **C:** Needle bevel partially out of the skin; tube vacuum will be lost. **D:** Needle bevel partially into the vein; causes blood leakage into tissue. **E:** Needle bevel partially through the vein; causes blood leakage into tissue. **F:** Needle bevel completely through the vein; no blood flow obtained. **G:** Needle bevel against the upper vein wall prevents blood flow. **H:** Needle bevel against the lower vein wall prevents blood flow. **I:** Needle bevel penetrating a valve prevents blood flow. **J:** Needle beside the vein; caused when a vein rolls to the side. **K:** Collapsed vein prevents blood flow despite correct needle position.

an artery and a vein. An AV fistula can last for many years, but occasionally they get plugged or clotted and will not function. If not fixable, a new one will be created and the old one will become inactive, and may be left in place.

REVIEW: Yes ☐　No ☐

84. **Answer: a**

WHY: When the vacuum escapes from an evacuated tube during blood collection, it typically makes a hissing sound. This can happen if the needle bevel backs out of the skin even slightly (Fig. 9-13C), allowing the tube to draw air instead of blood. If the needle penetrates all the way through a vein, the tube will not draw blood but the vacuum will still be intact because the bevel is under the skin. A drop in a patient's blood pressure would not cause a hissing sound. A tube with a crack in it and no vacuum would not draw blood or make a hissing sound because the vacuum was gone before the draw was even started.

REVIEW: Yes ☐ No ☐

85. **Answer: b**

WHY: If the needle penetrates part way through the bottom wall of the vein (Fig. 9-13E), blood will enter the tube more slowly than usual because it is leaking into the tissues at the same time. If the needle bevel has penetrated all the way through the bottom wall (Fig. 9-13F), there may be no blood flow at all. Pulling back on the needle slightly is necessary to establish proper flow. A hissing sound indicates that the vacuum escaped from the tube, which can happen if the needle bevel backs out of the skin slightly, not when it goes through the vein. A needle penetrating through the back wall of a vein is not known to cause reflux of specimen into the tissues nor does it cause the tube to fill with air.

REVIEW: Yes ☐ No ☐

86. **Answer: d**

WHY: Healthy vein walls are sturdy. If a vein is not anchored well, it may roll (move away) slightly and the needle may slip beside the vein (Fig. 9-13J) instead of going into it. The lumen of a vein is the hollow portion through which the blood flows. A needle bevel should end up in the lumen of the vein during venipuncture (Fig. 9-13A). A needle can go through a vein (Fig. 9-13E,F) if it is inserted too quickly or deeply, and if the tube holder is not held securely during the draw (e.g., when pushing a tube onto the needle). The needle bevel can end up against an inside wall of the vein if the needle enters it at an angle that is too shallow, if there is a bend in the vein (Fig. 9-13G), or if the bevel is down (Fig. 9-13H) instead of up when it enters the vein.

REVIEW: Yes ☐ No ☐

📖 *WORKBOOK Labeling Exercise 9-1 will help you learn to troubleshoot other venipuncture problems.*

87. **Answer: a**

WHY: If the needle bevel is only partially inserted in the vein during blood collection (Fig. 9-13D), the tube will fill very slowly and blood will

leak into the tissue around the vein, causing a hematoma.

REVIEW: Yes ☐ No ☐

88. **Answer: d**

WHY: Failure to achieve blood flow in a second tube after the first tube filled without a problem initially suggests that the needle position could have changed slightly when the tube was removed and replaced. If this had been the case, however, blood flow would have been reestablished with slight manipulation of the needle. This suggests there could be a problem with the tube. Always try a new tube before giving up on a blood draw. Further redirections of the needle amount to probing and should not be done.

REVIEW: Yes ☐ No ☐

89. **Answer: c**

WHY: Multiple redirections of the needle while attempting venipuncture amount to probing, which is dangerous and should not be done, even if a second phlebotomist takes over the draw for you. If you cannot obtain blood flow with one or two redirections of the needle, discontinue the draw and try again at a new site.

REVIEW: Yes ☐ No ☐

90. **Answer: d**

WHY: A vein may collapse (Fig. 9-13K) if the tube being drawn has too much vacuum for the size of the vein. Tourniquet application exceeding a minute is not good for the specimen, but does not normally cause the vein to collapse. Tourniquet pressure is not usually measured, but when a blood pressure cuff is used as a tourniquet it should be maintained below diastolic blood pressure. Filling several large volume tubes should not cause a normal vein to collapse if proper procedures were followed for equipment selection and vein selection.

REVIEW: Yes ☐ No ☐

91. **Answer: c**

WHY: Bariatric means *pertaining to the treatment of obesity,* but the term is also used as a polite way to refer to individuals and items for individuals who are extremely overweight whether or not they are actually being treated for obesity. Consequently a bariatric tourniquet is an extra large size tourniquet designed for use on obese patients. A tourniquet is not used for arterial blood gas (ABGs) or any other arterial specimens. Obese patients may be difficult draws but not all difficult draws are obese patients.

REVIEW: Yes ☐ No ☐

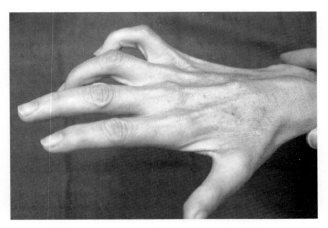

Figure 9-14 Abnormal hand position called "Claw hand" caused by ulnar nerve injury.

92. **Answer: c**

    WHY: Nerve injury is a serious phlebotomy complication that can result in permanent damage to motor or sensory nerve function of the arm or hand. The condition referred to as "Claw hand" (Fig. 9-14) can be caused by a direct or compression injury to the ulnar nerve. Nerve compression injuries can occur from blood pooling and clotting beneath the vein as a result of accidental arterial puncture or blood leaking from the vein because the needle went all the way through it on initial needle entry.

    REVIEW: Yes ☐   No ☐

93. **Answer: a**

    WHY: A person who is paralyzed in both arms and legs is called a quadriplegic. Paralysis is the loss of muscle function. A person who is paralyzed can feel pain if there is no sensory damage. Quadriplegics can speak if the paralysis is only from the neck down. Phlebotomists can draw quadriplegic patients although the loss of muscle function can result in stagnation of blood flow and an increased chance of vein thrombosis that is magnified by venipuncture. Consequently strict venipuncture procedures must be followed (e.g., no probing or lateral needle redirection) and firm pressure must be held over the site after the draw until it is certain that blood flow has ceased.

    REVIEW: Yes ☐   No ☐

94. **Answer: d**

    WHY: This illustration shows that the needle has become stuck in one of the valves in the vein (Fig. 9-13I). Valves can cause an unusual problem for the phlebotomist if, in fact, the needle should pierce the valve tissue in the middle of the lumen.

    REVIEW: Yes ☐   No ☐

95. **Answer: d**

    WHY: This illustration shows a collapsed vein in front of the needle (Fig. 9-13K). This happens if the vein is so fragile or weak that it cannot withstand the vacuum pressure once the tube is inserted in holder.

    REVIEW: Yes ☐   No ☐

96. **Answer: c**

    WHY: If a vein is not firmly fixed in the tissue or anchored well by the phlebotomist, the needle could slip to the side of the vein instead of into it (Fig. 9-13J).

    REVIEW: Yes ☐   No ☐

97. **Answer: b**

    WHY: This illustration shows a needle that has passed partway through the vein (Fig. 9-13E) and is allowing a hematoma to form beneath the vein. The nerve below the vein could be hit, which means there would be a sharp pain felt by the patient and the venipuncture would have to be immediately discontinued. Even if the underlying nerve is not hit by the needle, the blood pooling beneath the vein could cause a compression injury to the nerve. Both situations, if not handled appropriately, could lead to injury of the patient and possible legal action.

    REVIEW: Yes ☐   No ☐

98. **Answer: b**

    WHY: The veins in our arms are not predictably straight. This illustration shows the needle bevel up against an unexpected curve in the vein (Fig. 9-13G). (In this case the needle bevel could also end up slightly in the vein wall). This means that there may be very little or no blood entering the needle. The phlebotomist must first release the tube so there is no vacuum pull on the vein that could damage it. Then slowly pull back the needle until the bevel is in the center of the vein and blood flow is established.

    REVIEW: Yes ☐   No ☐

99. **Answer: a**

    WHY: A swelling or lump on the outside of the arm around the needle indicates that the needle is not all the way in the vein and a hematoma is forming (Fig. 9-13D). This means that the needle must come out immediately, pressure applied, and the hematoma treated.

    REVIEW: Yes ☐   No ☐

100. **Answer: b**

     WHY: This illustration shows that the needle has not penetrated the skin all the way (Fig. 9-13C) and consequently is not seated in the lumen of the vein where it should be. A characteristic "hissing" sound should tell the phlebotomist immediately that the vacuum is pulling air into the tube, which means the vacuum pull of the tube will be lost. The corrective action is to push the needle into the vein and exchange the tube for a new one with vacuum.

     REVIEW: Yes ☐   No ☐

Chapter 10

Capillary Puncture Equipment and Procedures

Study Tips

- Complete the activities in Chapter 10 of the companion WORKBOOK.

- Draw an infant heel and mark proper puncture sites.

- Go over the cautions and key points in the TEXTBOOK.

- Identify correct finger puncture sites on your hand.

- List four circumstances when capillary puncture is appropriate.

- Quiz yourself on the meanings of key terms and abbreviations.

- Study infant capillary precautions and then see how many you can list in 1 minute.

Overview Drops of blood for testing can be obtained by puncturing or making an incision in the capillary bed in the dermal layer of the skin with a lancet, other sharp device, or laser. Terms typically used to describe this technique include capillary, dermal, or skin puncture, regardless of the actual type of device or method used to penetrate the skin, and the specimens obtained are respectively referred to as capillary, dermal, or skin puncture specimens. (To best reflect the nature and source of the specimen, and for simplification and consistency, the terms capillary specimen and capillary puncture are used in this chapter.) With the advent of laboratory instrumentation capable of testing small sample volumes, specimens for many laboratory tests can now be collected in this manner. This chapter covers capillary equipment, principles, collection sites, and procedures. Although steps may differ slightly, procedures in this chapter were written to conform to CLSI standards.

Review Questions

Choose the BEST answer.

1. "Arterialized" means
   a. arterial content has been increased.
   b. composition is the same as arterial.
   c. oxygen levels equal arterial levels.
   d. venous blood flow has increased.

2. A blood smear is
   a. blood collected on a special filter paper.
   b. blood spread out on a microscope slide.
   c. blood made from a heparinized specimen.
   d. blood used to identify the types of bacteria.

3. The calcaneus is a bone located in the
   a. earlobe.
   b. finger.
   c. heel.
   d. thumb.

4. This is the abbreviation for a pulmonary function test
   a. AFP
   b. CBG
   c. PKU
   d. TSH

5. A cyanotic extremity would
   a. appear jaundiced.
   b. be bluish in color.
   c. exhibit erythema.
   d. look pale yellow.

6. A differential test is unable to determine
   a. a platelet estimate.
   b. packed cell volume.
   c. red cell morphology.
   d. WBC characteristics.

7. "Feather" is a term used to describe the appearance of
   a. a newborn screening blood spot.
   b. blood in a thick malaria smear.
   c. lipemia in a bilirubin specimen.
   d. the thinnest area of a blood film.

8. Fluid in the spaces between the cells is called
   a. interstitial fluid.
   b. intracellular fluid.
   c. lymphatic fluid.
   d. peritoneal fluid.

9. This is the name of a sharp-pointed device used today to make capillary punctures.
   a. Bullet
   b. Fleam
   c. Lancet
   d. Scalpel

10. Which of the following statements most accurately describes capillary puncture blood?
    a. A mix of venous, arterial, and capillary blood
    b. Mostly tissue fluid mixed with arterial blood
    c. Mostly venous blood mixed with tissue fluid
    d. Nearly identical to a venous blood specimen

11. Which statement concerning microhematocrit tubes is incorrect?
    a. They are coated with lithium heparin
    b. They are filled using capillary action
    c. They are narrow-bore capillary tubes
    d. They are used for PCV determination

12. Referring to Figure 10-1, identify the letters of the fingers that are recommended as sites for capillary puncture.
    a. A and B
    b. B and C
    c. C and D
    d. D and E

13. Osteochondritis is
    a. abnormal bone formation and growth.
    b. an inherited bone metabolism disorder.
    c. infection of the bone and bone marrow.
    d. inflammation of the bone and cartilage.

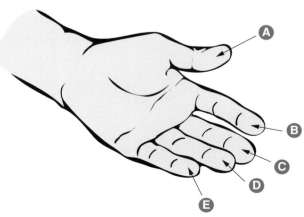

Figure 10-1 An adult hand.

14. This is a term for the bottom surface of the heel.

    a. Distal
    b. Dorsal
    c. Lateral
    d. Plantar

15. Whorls as related to capillary puncture are

    a. blebs created during skin tests.
    b. formations seen in blood films.
    c. newborn screening blood spots.
    d. spiral patterns of fingerprints.

16. The temperature of heel warming devices should never exceed

    a. 37°C.
    b. 42°C.
    c. 98°F.
    d. 112°F.

17. Which of the following is the medical term for a finger bone?

    a. Calcaneus
    b. Clavicle
    c. Patella
    d. Phalanx

18. CBG specimens are collected in

    a. amber syringe–style devices.
    b. bullets with heparin in them.
    c. circles on special filter paper.
    d. narrow-bore capillary tubes.

19. Capillary specimens contain

    a. arterial blood.
    b. tissue fluids.
    c. venous blood.
    d. all of the above.

20. Which numbered arrows on the diagram of an infant's foot in Figure 10-2 point toward the safest areas for capillary puncture?

    a. 1 and 4
    b. 2 and 3
    c. 3 and 5
    d. 4 and 5

21. Which of the following are required characteristics of capillary puncture lancets?

    a. A controlled depth of puncture
    b. Blades or points that are sterile
    c. Permanently retractable blades
    d. All of the above

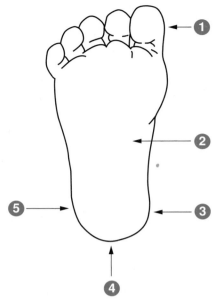

Figure 10-2 An infant foot.

22. Which of the following equipment is used to collect a manual packed cell volume test?

    a. Circles on filter paper
    b. Glass microscope slide
    c. Microhematocrit tube
    d. Mixing bar and magnet

23. Which of the following equipment should be deleted from a list of capillary blood gas equipment?

    a. Caps for both tube ends
    b. Filter paper for blotting
    c. Magnet and metal bar
    d. All of the above

24. Which capillary specimen should be collected separately?

    a. Bilirubin
    b. CBGs
    c. NBS
    d. Potassium

25. Which of the following is an indication for capillary puncture?

    a. The patient is badly burned except for his feet.
    b. The person is receiving IVs for chemotherapy.
    c. The physician requested capillary draws only.
    d. All of the above.

26. The composition of blood obtained by capillary puncture more closely resembles

    a. arterial blood.
    b. lymph fluid.
    c. tissue fluid.
    d. venous blood.

27. If venous blood is placed in a microtube, it is important to

    a. label it as a venous specimen.
    b. shield the specimen from light.
    c. transport it to the laboratory ASAP.
    d. vigorously mix the specimen.

28. A laboratory report form should state that a specimen has been collected by capillary puncture

    a. for equipment inventory control purposes.
    b. because results can vary by specimen source.
    c. so other tests will be capillary collections.
    d. to satisfy liability insurance requirements.

29. Blood collected by puncturing the skin is called capillary blood because

    a. it is collected with capillary tubes.
    b. it is from the dermal capillary bed.
    c. microtubes fill by capillary action.
    d. small drops of blood are collected.

30. This test is typically performed on capillary blood.

    a. CBC
    b. GTT
    c. PKU
    d. PTT

31. Reference values for this test are higher for capillary specimens.

    a. Calcium
    b. Glucose
    c. Phosphorus
    d. Total protein

32. You need to collect blood cultures, and green, light blue, and purple top tubes on an adult with difficult veins. Which of these can be collected by skin puncture?

    a. Blood cultures and green top
    b. Blood cultures and purple top
    c. Green top and purple top
    d. Light blue and purple top

33. If collected by capillary puncture, which of the following specimens should be collected in an amber microtube (Fig. 10-3)?

    a. Bilirubin
    b. Glucose
    c. Lead
    d. PKU

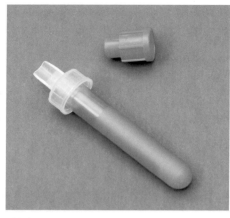

Figure 10-3 An amber-colored microcollection container used to protect a specimen from effects of ultraviolet light.

34. Situations that require a venipuncture instead of capillary puncture include when a

    a. bilirubin is ordered on a 1-year-old.
    b. glucose is ordered on a diabetic patient.
    c. K+ test using i-STAT is ordered in ER.
    d. plasma protime specimen is ordered.

35. Which of the following patient conditions would make capillary puncture a good choice for specimen collection?

    a. Acute dehydration
    b. Iatrogenic anemia
    c. Poor circulation
    d. State of shock

36. Which of the following is normally a proper site for finger puncture on an adult?

    a. Distal segment of the middle finger
    b. End segment of either of the thumbs
    c. Medial segment of the index finger
    d. Proximal phalanx of the ring finger

37. Which of the following would be excluded from a list of reasons why capillary puncture is the preferred method to obtain blood from infants and children?

    a. Restraining used for venipuncture can cause injury.
    b. Results on capillary specimens are more accurate.
    c. They have small blood volumes compared with adults.
    d. Venipuncture can damage their veins and tissues.

38. Which of the following sites would normally be eliminated as a capillary puncture site?
    a. Index finger of a woman
    b. Infant lateral plantar heel
    c. Middle finger of an adult
    d. Ring finger on an IV arm

39. It is necessary to control the depth of lancet insertion during heel puncture to avoid
    a. damage to the tendons.
    b. injuring the calcaneus.
    c. puncturing an artery.
    d. unnecessary bleeding.

40. According to CLSI, depth of heel puncture should not exceed
    a. 1.5 mm.
    b. 2.0 mm.
    c. 2.4 mm.
    d. 4.9 mm.

41. Which of the following can be a complication of a heel puncture that is too deep?
    a. Osteoarthritis
    b. Osteoporosis
    c. Osteomyelitis
    d. Osteosarcoma

42. Which of the following is the safest area of an infant's foot for capillary puncture?
    a. Any area of the arch
    b. Center of the big toe
    c. Medial plantar heel
    d. Posterior curvature

43. A recommended capillary puncture site on children 2 years of age or older is on the
    a. bottom of an earlobe.
    b. fleshy side of a thumb.
    c. pad of a middle finger.
    d. medial or lateral heel.

44. In which of the following areas does capillary specimen collection differ from routine venipuncture for tests that can be collected either way?
    a. Additives used
    b. Antiseptic used
    c. ID procedures
    d. Order of draw

45. The distance between the skin surface and the bone in the end segment of a finger is
    a. shortest at the side and the tip.
    b. equal throughout the fingertip.
    c. thickest of all in the fifth finger.
    d. thinnest in the middle finger.

46. The major blood vessels of the skin are located
    a. at the dermal–subcutaneous junction.
    b. between the epidermis and the dermis.
    c. in the epidermis and the subcutaneous.
    d. within the epidermis and the dermis.

47. A capillary puncture that parallels the whorls of the fingerprint will
    a. allow blood to run down the finger.
    b. cause blood to form in round drops.
    c. continue to bleed for a lot longer.
    d. make specimen collection easier.

48. A list of capillary puncture equipment would exclude
    a. blood culture bottles.
    b. various lancet types.
    c. microcollection tubes.
    d. skin warming devices.

49. Which color-coded microtube would be used to collect a CBC?
    a. Gray
    b. Green
    c. Lavender
    d. Yellow

50. If the following tests are collected from a patient by capillary puncture, which test specimen is collected first?
    a. Bilirubin
    b. CBC
    c. Lytes
    d. Glucose

51. What is the purpose of warming the site before capillary puncture?
    a. Enhance visibility of veins
    b. Increase the flow of blood
    c. Prevent sample hemolysis
    d. Relax and comfort patients

52. For accurate results, the heel *must* be warmed before collecting a capillary specimen for this test.
    a. CBG
    b. Lytes
    c. PKU
    d. WBC

53. The recommended antiseptic for cleaning capillary puncture sites is
    a. 70% isopropanol.
    b. povidone–iodine.
    c. soap and water.
    d. tincture of iodine.

54. The antiseptic must be completely dried before performing capillary puncture to avoid
    a. hematoma formation.
    b. hemoconcentration.
    c. premature clotting.
    d. specimen hemolysis.

55. Tests affected by povidone–iodine contamination of a capillary specimen include
    a. phosphorus.
    b. potassium.
    c. uric acid.
    d. all of the above.

56. Errors in capillary glucose results have been attributed to
    a. excessive depth of the capillary puncture.
    b. failure to collect the initial drop of blood.
    c. isopropanol contamination of the specimen.
    d. warming of the site before capillary puncture.

57. Proper finger puncture technique would exclude
    a. choosing a middle or ring finger site.
    b. puncturing parallel to the fingerprint.
    c. trying not to squeeze or milk the site.
    d. warming the site before puncturing.

58. Hemolysis of a capillary specimen can erroneously elevate results for this test.
    a. Cholesterol
    b. Hemoglobin
    c. Potassium
    d. RBC count

59. One purpose of wiping away the first drop of blood (Fig. 10-4) during capillary specimen collection is to
    a. avoid contamination with bacteria.
    b. reduce tissue fluid contamination.
    c. improve blood flow to the site.
    d. minimize platelet aggregation.

60. Which of the following actions taken while filling microcollection tubes would be considered incorrect technique?
    a. Letting blood run down the tube's inside wall
    b. Scooping up blood as it runs down the finger
    c. Tapping the tube gently to settle the specimen
    d. Touching the tube's scoop to each blood drop

61. Which of the following would be *least* likely to introduce excess tissue fluid into a capillary puncture specimen?
    a. Collecting the first drop
    b. Pressing hard on the site
    c. Squeezing the puncture
    d. Wiping the alcohol dry

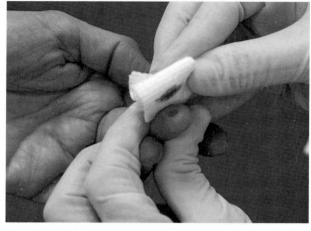

Figure 10-4 Wiping the first blood drop with gauze.

62. Which of the following can result in microclot formation in a specimen collected in an anti-coagulant microtube?
    a. Mixing it too soon
    b. Mixing it forcefully
    c. Overfilling the tube
    d. Underfilling the tube

63. During multisample capillary specimen collection, blood smears and EDTA specimens are obtained before other specimens to minimize
    a. effects of platelet aggregation.
    b. hemolysis of red blood cells.
    c. specimen hemoconcentration.
    d. tissue fluid contamination.

64. A blood smear is required for this test.
    a. Manual differential
    b. Neonatal bilirubin
    c. Newborn screening
    d. Packed cell volume

65. An acceptable routine blood smear
    a. covers the entire slide.
    b. forms a bullet shape.
    c. has a feathered edge.
    d. looks short and thick.

66. A blood smear prepared from an EDTA specimen should be made
    a. after the blood cells settle in the tube.
    b. at the time the specimen is collected.
    c. before the specimen has been mixed.
    d. within 1 hour of specimen collection.

67. When making a blood smear by hand using two glass slides, the typical angle required of the spreader slide is
    a. 15 degrees.
    b. 20 degrees.
    c. 30 degrees.
    d. 45 degrees.

68. If the phlebotomist makes a blood smear that is too short, he or she should try again and
    a. decrease the angle of the spreader slide.
    b. increase the angle of the spreader slide.
    c. place a smaller blood drop on the slide.
    d. put more pressure on the spreader slide.

69. It is unlikely that holes in a blood smear would be caused by
    a. low hemoglobin.
    b. dirt on the slide.
    c. high lipid level.
    d. smudged slide.

70. Collection of a thick blood smear may be requested to detect
    a. elevated bilirubin.
    b. hypothyroidism.
    c. malaria microbes.
    d. phenylketonuria.

71. A premature baby weighing 2.1 kg needs to have blood drawn for special laboratory tests. What percentage of the total blood volume of an infant that size is represented by 10 mL?
    a. 2.5%
    b. 4.0%
    c. 5.5%
    d. 9.0%

72. Which statement concerning capillary blood gases is untrue?
    a. They are less dangerous to collect than ABGs.
    b. Results are much more accurate than ABGs.
    c. Specimens contain venous and arterial blood.
    d. Collection exposes the blood specimen to air.

73. An infant may require a blood transfusion if blood levels of this substance exceed 18 mg/dL.
    a. Bilirubin
    b. Carnitine
    c. Galactose
    d. Thyroxine

74. Phenylketonuria is a
    a. disorder caused by excessive phenylalanine ingestion.
    b. contagious condition caused by lack of phenylalanine.
    c. genetic disorder involving phenylalanine metabolism.
    d. temporary condition caused by lack of phenylalanine.

75. Which of the following is a newborn screening test?
    a. Bilirubin
    b. GALT
    c. H & H
    d. WBC

76. Falsely decreased bilirubin results can be caused by
    a. collecting the specimen 5 minutes late.
    b. failing to protect the specimen from light.
    c. puncturing the heel close to the calcaneus.
    d. using isopropyl alcohol to clean the site.

77. Which of the following is least likely to contaminate a PKU test?
    a. Neglecting to discard the first blood drop.
    b. Touching the inside of a filter paper circle.
    c. Stacking specimen slips while wet or dry.
    d. Using isopropyl alcohol to clean the site.

78. Correct newborn screening test collection or handling includes
    a. applying blood drops to both sides of the filter paper.
    b. hanging a specimen slip to dry in a vertical position.
    c. layering successive blood drops in a collection circle.
    d. using one large drop to entirely fill a collection circle.

79. Neonatal screening for this disorder is required by law in the United States.
    a. Diabetes
    b. HDN
    c. HBV
    d. PKU

80. Jaundice in a newborn is associated with high levels of
    a. bilirubin.
    b. glucose.
    c. ketones.
    d. thyroxine.

81. It is inappropriate to apply a bandage to a capillary puncture site on an infant or child younger than 2 years of age because it can
    a. irritate an infant's tender skin.
    b. pull off and be a choking hazard.
    c. tear delicate skin when removed.
    d. all of the above.

82. Which of the following action words associated with capillary puncture procedure steps are in the correct order?
    a. Clean, puncture, warm, wipe, collect
    b. Clean, warm, puncture, collect, wipe
    c. Warm, clean, puncture, wipe, collect
    d. Warm, puncture, clean, wipe, collect

83. The best way to mix blood in an additive microtube is to
    a. invert it gently.
    b. shake it briskly.
    c. roll it in the hands.
    d. tap it sharply.

84. Strong repetitive pressure, such as squeezing or milking a site during capillary specimen collection
    a. is necessary to obtain adequate blood flow.
    b. can hemolyze and contaminate specimens.
    c. improves the accuracy of CBC test results.
    d. increases venous blood flow into the area.

85. Which of the following collection devices fill by capillary action?
    a. Amber microtubes
    b. Filter paper circles
    c. Hematocrit tubes
    d. Lavender bullets

86. Capillary puncture is preferred for infants because
    a. all infant laboratory tests require capillary collection.
    b. capillary blood results are more accurate.
    c. it is less painful to infants than a venipuncture.
    d. venipuncture can damage the veins of infants.

87. Lancets with permanently retractable blades are disposed of in the
    a. autoclave waste.
    b. biohazard trash.
    c. sharps container.
    d. regular trash can.

88. Capillary puncture is a poor choice for specimen collection if the patient is
    a. comatose.
    b. dehydrated.
    c. jaundiced.
    d. nauseated.

89. Which of the following steps should be omitted from infant heel puncture?
    a. Apply bandage.
    b. Clean the site.
    c. ID the patient.
    d. Warm the site.

90. After making a blood smear
    a. blow on it until dry.
    b. let it dry naturally.
    c. place it in alcohol.
    d. wave it until dry.

91. All of the following tests can be collected by capillary puncture EXCEPT
    a. blood culture.
    b. electrolytes.
    c. hemoglobin.
    d. lithium level.

92. Neonatal screening is the testing of
    a. babies for contagious diseases.
    b. infants with certain symptoms.
    c. newborns for certain disorders.
    d. pregnant women for diseases.

93. Microhematocrit tubes with a red band on one end contain
    a. EDTA.
    b. heparin.
    c. nothing.
    d. silica.

94. In an infant's heel, the area of the vascular bed that is rich in capillary loops is located
    a. between 0.35 and 0.82 mm deep.
    b. from 1.00 mm to 2.00 mm deep.
    c. in the top layer of the epidermis.
    d. starting at around 2.4 mm deep.

95. Which of the following capillary puncture techniques is incorrect?
    a. Discard equipment packaging in the regular trash
    b. Position the site downward to promote blood flow
    c. Press the lancet down into the skin so it does not slip
    d. Tap microtubes gently to settle blood to the bottom

96. Pain fibers increase in abundance below
    a. 0.8 mm.
    b. 1.2 mm.
    c. 2.0 mm.
    d. 2.4 mm.

97. Neonatal screening for this disorder is required by law in all 50 states.
    a. Galactosemia
    b. Hypothyroidism
    c. Phenylketonuria
    d. All of the above

98. Capillary action is a term used to describe how
    a. arterial blood enters the capillaries.
    b. blood fills a microhematocrit tube.
    c. cells spread across a blood smear.
    d. warming can increase blood flow.

99. This is an inherited amino acid metabolism disorder.
    a. GALT
    b. Hb SS
    c. MSUD
    d. All of the above

100. Applying gentle pressure during a capillary puncture
    a. can hemolyze red cells.
    b. helps blood flow freely.
    c. is incorrect procedure.
    d. removes alcohol residue.

Answers and Explanations

1. **Answer: a**
   WHY: "Arterialized" is a term used to describe a capillary blood specimen in which the arterial content has been increased by warming the site before collection. Warming changes the composition of a specimen because it increases blood flow into the area from the arteries. Although this specimen more closely resembles arterial blood than one that has not been warmed, oxygen levels and other components would not be exactly the same.
   REVIEW: Yes ☐   No ☐

2. **Answer: b**
   WHY: A blood smear or film is a drop of blood spread on a glass microscope slide. Blood smears can be made from fresh blood or blood collected in EDTA, depending on the test requested. A manual differential is the most common reason a blood smear is made. A differential is used to identify and count the different types of cells in a blood smear. Blood collected on a special type of filter paper is required for most newborn screening tests.
   REVIEW: Yes ☐   No ☐

3. **Answer: c**
   WHY: "Calcaneus" is the medical term for the heel bone. Finger bones, including the thumb, are

called phalanges (singular, phalanx). The earlobe is cartilage, not bone.
   REVIEW: Yes ☐   No ☐
   📖 **WORKBOOK Labeling Exercise 10-2 will help you identify the areas of the infant foot that are safe for capillary puncture.**

4. **Answer: b**
   WHY: Capillary blood gases (CBGs) are collected to assess levels of blood components, such as oxygen, carbon dioxide, and pH, which are measures of pulmonary function.
   REVIEW: Yes ☐   No ☐

5. **Answer: b**
   WHY: Cyanotic means "marked by cyanosis or bluish in color from lack of oxygen"; consequently, a cyanotic extremity looks bluish in color. Jaundiced skin would be a deep yellow color and erythema indicates redness in the skin.
   REVIEW: Yes ☐   No ☐

6. **Answer: b**
   WHY: A differential determines the type and characteristics of WBCs, RBC morphology, and an estimate of the platelet count. Packed cell volume (PCV) is another name for hematocrit (HCT), which is part of a complete blood count (CBC), but not part of a differential.
   REVIEW: Yes ☐   No ☐

7. **Answer: d**

   WHY: A properly made routine blood film or smear shows a smooth transition from thick to thin. The thinnest area of the film is only one cell thick and is called the feather because of its appearance when held up to the light. The feather is the area where a manual differential is performed.

   REVIEW: Yes ☐ No ☐

   📖 *Procedure 10-5 in the TEXTBOOK demonstrates how to make a proper routine blood smear.*

8. **Answer: a**

   WHY: Interstitial means "pertaining to spaces between tissues"; consequently, fluid in the spaces between the cells is called interstitial fluid. Intracellular fluid is the fluid within cells. Fluid in the lymphatic system is called lymph. Lymph is derived from excess tissue fluid, and is similar to, but not the same as, interstitial fluid. Peritoneal fluid is found in the abdominal cavity.

   REVIEW: Yes ☐ No ☐

9. **Answer: c**

   WHY: The typical lancet is a sterile, disposable, sharp-pointed, or bladed device used to puncture or make an incision in the skin to obtain a capillary blood specimen. A microcollection container is sometimes called a bullet because it resembles one. A fleam is the name for the early day lancet. A scalpel should never be used for capillary puncture because puncture depth cannot be controlled.

   REVIEW: Yes ☐ No ☐

10. **Answer: a**

    WHY: Capillary puncture blood is a mixture of arterial blood (from arterioles), venous blood (from venules), and capillary blood, along with interstitial and intracellular fluids from the surrounding tissues.

    REVIEW: Yes ☐ No ☐

11. **Answer: a**

    WHY: Microhematocrit tubes are thin, narrow-bore, disposable plastic or plastic-clad glass tubes that fill by capillary action. They are most commonly used to collect and perform manual hematocrit (HCT) tests. An HCT is also called a packed cell volume (PCV) test. Some microhematocrit tubes are coated with ammonium heparin, not lithium heparin.

    REVIEW: Yes ☐ No ☐

12. **Answer: c**

    WHY: The fingers identified by letters C and D in Figure 10-1 are the middle and ring fingers, which are the recommended fingers to use for capillary puncture (Fig. 10-5).

    REVIEW: Yes ☐ No ☐

13. **Answer: d**

    WHY: Osteochondritis means "inflammation of the bone and cartilage." It can be the result of capillary punctures that are too deep.

    REVIEW: Yes ☐ No ☐

    📖 *WORKBOOK Skills Drill 10-2 will give you an opportunity to identify medical terminology word parts and define medical terms.*

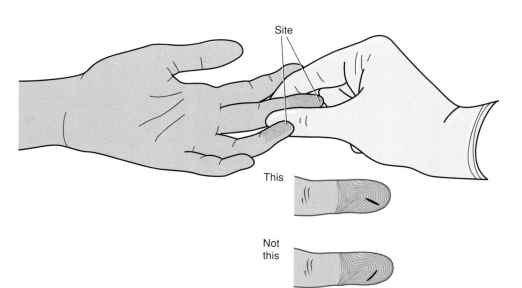

Figure 10-5 The recommended site and direction of finger puncture.

14. **Answer: d**

    WHY: Plantar means "concerning the sole or bottom of the foot." Distal means "farthest from the center of the body, origin, or point of attachment." Dorsal means "to the back of the body." Lateral means "toward the side of the body."
    REVIEW: Yes ☐ No ☐

15. **Answer: d**

    WHY: Whorls are circular or spiral patterns formed by the lines of the fingerprint.
    REVIEW: Yes ☐ No ☐

16. **Answer: b**

    WHY: To prevent burning the patient, heel warmers and other materials used to warm the collection site before capillary puncture should provide a uniform temperature that does not exceed 42°C.
    REVIEW: Yes ☐ No ☐

17. **Answer: d**

    WHY: The medical term for a finger or toe bone is phalanx (plural, phalanges). "Calcaneus" is the medical term for heel bone. "Clavicle" is the medical term for the shoulder bone. "Patella" is the medical term for the kneecap.
    REVIEW: Yes ☐ No ☐

18. **Answer: d**

    WHY: Capillary blood gas (CBG) specimens are collected in special long, thin, narrow-bore plastic capillary tubes. They are generally 100 mm long with a capacity of 100 μL. They typically contain sodium heparin and are color-coded with a green band. Other equipment required includes a device to warm the site, stirrers, and a magnet for mixing the specimen, and caps for both ends of the capillary tube so that the anaerobic condition of the specimen can be maintained. Capillary blood gas equipment is shown in Figure 10-6.
    REVIEW: Yes ☐ No ☐

19. **Answer: d**

    WHY: Capillary specimens are a mixture of arterial and venous blood and tissue fluids that include interstitial fluid from the tissue spaces between the cells and intracellular fluid from within the cells.
    REVIEW: Yes ☐ No ☐

20. **Answer: c**

    WHY: According to Clinical and Laboratory Standards Institute (CLSI) standards, the safest areas

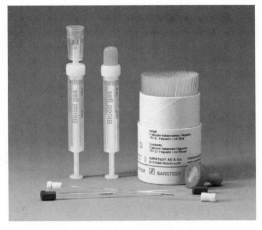

Figure 10-6 Capillary blood gas collection equipment displayed with arterial blood gas syringes. (Courtesy of Sarstedt, Inc., Newton, NC.)

for heel puncture are on the plantar surface of the heel, medial to an imaginary line extending from the middle of the great toe to the heel, or lateral to an imaginary line extending from between the fourth and fifth toes to the heel (Fig. 10-7). Punctures in other areas of an infant's foot risk bone, nerve, tendon, and cartilage injury.
REVIEW: Yes ☐ No ☐

21. **Answer: d**

    WHY: Capillary puncture lancets should be sterile and disposable after a single use. They should also have puncture depths that are controlled, and blades or points that are permanently retractable for safety.
    REVIEW: Yes ☐ No ☐

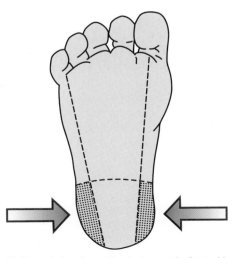

Figure 10-7 An infant foot. Shaded areas indicated by arrows represent recommended safe areas for heel puncture.

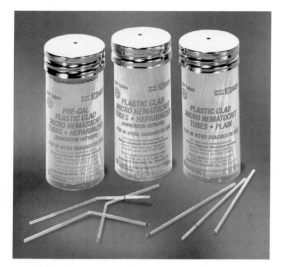

Figure 10-8 Plastic clad microhematocrit tubes. (Courtesy of Becton-Dickinson, Franklin Lakes, NJ.)

22. **Answer: c**

WHY: A plastic or plastic-clad glass microhematocrit tube (Fig. 10-8) is used to collect and perform a manual hematocrit (packed cell volume) test.

REVIEW: Yes ☐ No ☐

23. **Answer: b**

WHY: Capillary blood gas equipment (Fig. 10-6) typically includes a special long, thin capillary tube, a magnet, and a small metal bar to aid in mixing the specimen, and caps for sealing both ends of the tube. Blotting with filter paper is not part of the procedure.

REVIEW: Yes ☐ No ☐

24. **Answer: c**

WHY: According to CLSI standards, newborn screening (NBS) specimens should be collected separately. With the exception of NBS specimens, bilirubin, CBGs, and potassium specimens can be collected at the same time as other capillary specimens provided the capillary order of collection is followed. The order of collection for capillary specimens is capillary blood gases (CBGs), EDTA specimens, other additive specimens, and specimens requiring serum.

REVIEW: Yes ☐ No ☐

25. **Answer: d**

WHY: Indications for capillary collection are varied, and may be an appropriate choice for adults and older children. Physicians may request that their patients have only capillary draws and a physician's orders must be followed. If a person is badly burned and the only available choice

for blood collection is somewhere on the feet, capillary puncture on the toes will save the foot veins for other uses. Sometimes all available veins are fragile and when the patient is having some sort of IV therapy, they should be saved for that reason.

REVIEW: Yes ☐ No ☐

26. **Answer: a**

WHY: Capillaries contain both venous and arterial blood. The percentage of arterial blood is higher, however, because arterial blood enters the capillaries under pressure. Consequently, the composition of blood obtained by capillary puncture more closely resembles arterial blood than venous blood. This is especially true if the area has been warmed, because warming increases arterial flow into the area.

REVIEW: Yes ☐ No ☐

27. **Answer: a**

WHY: Sometimes venous blood obtained by syringe during difficult draw situations is put into microcollection containers. When this is done, it is important to label the specimen as venous. Otherwise, it will be assumed to be a skin puncture specimen, which may have different normal values.

REVIEW: Yes ☐ No ☐

28. **Answer: b**

WHY: Test results can vary depending on the source of the specimen. A laboratory report form should indicate that a specimen was collected by skin puncture, because skin puncture blood differs in composition from venous blood and may have different reference ranges for some tests.

REVIEW: Yes ☐ No ☐

29. **Answer: b**

WHY: Blood obtained by puncturing the skin with a lancet is called capillary blood because it comes from the area of the dermis that is rich in capillaries and referred to as the vascular or capillary bed.

REVIEW: Yes ☐ No ☐

30. **Answer: c**

WHY: Phenylketonuria (PKU) is a newborn screening test. PKU and most other newborn screening tests were designed to be performed on capillary blood and are typically performed on capillary specimens collected by heel puncture. CBCs can be performed on capillary specimens but are most commonly performed on venipuncture

specimens. Glucose tolerance tests (GTTs) are rarely performed on capillary specimens. PTTs are typically performed on venous specimens and are only performed on capillary specimens by using special point-of-care testing instruments.
REVIEW: Yes ☐ No ☐

31. **Answer: b**
WHY: Reference values for glucose tests are higher for capillary puncture specimens. They are lower for calcium, phosphorus, and total protein.
REVIEW: Yes ☐ No ☐

32. **Answer: c**
WHY: Blood cultures cannot be collected by capillary puncture because of the volume of blood required for testing and contamination issues. The light blue top tube cannot be collected by capillary puncture because coagulation tests are greatly affected by tissue thromboplastin. Green top and purple top microtubes are available.
REVIEW: Yes ☐ No ☐

33. **Answer: a**
WHY: Infant bilirubin specimens are collected in amber microcollection containers (Fig. 10-3) to help protect them from light. Light breaks down bilirubin and leads to false low values.
REVIEW: Yes ☐ No ☐
📖 *WORKBOOK Case Study Exercise 10-1 will give you a chance to review issues that arise when drawing blood from a newborn in the nursery.*

34. **Answer: d**
WHY: Light blue top tubes cannot be collected by capillary puncture for coagulation tests that are performed later in the laboratory. Light blue top capillary tubes are available from some manufacturers, but are to be used for venous blood only (e.g., in difficult draw situations when only a small amount of blood is collected by syringe). There are, however, some point-of-care instruments that directly perform coagulation tests from capillary blood that is immediately placed in the instrument and tested.
REVIEW: Yes ☐ No ☐

35. **Answer: b**
WHY: Capillary puncture is generally *not* appropriate for patients who are dehydrated or have poor circulation to the extremities from other causes, such as a state of shock, because specimens may be hard to obtain and may not be representative of blood elsewhere in the body. Capillary puncture

is actually a good choice for a patient with iatrogenic anemia, so that as little blood as possible is removed.
REVIEW: Yes ☐ No ☐

36. **Answer: a**
WHY: The palmar surface of the distal or end segment of the middle or ring finger (Fig. 10-5) is the recommended site for routine skin puncture on an adult.
REVIEW: Yes ☐ No ☐
📖 *WORKBOOK Skills Drill 10-3 is a good review of the important CLSI guidelines associated with the fingerstick procedure.*

37. **Answer: b**
WHY: Capillary puncture is the preferred method to obtain blood from infants and children for several reasons. Restraining methods used during venipuncture can injure infants and children. They have such small blood volumes that removing larger quantities of blood typical of venipuncture can lead to anemia. Removal of more than 10% of an infant's blood volume at one time can lead to cardiac arrest. In addition, venipuncture in infants and children is difficult and may damage veins and surrounding tissues. Test results on capillary specimens are *not* more accurate than results on venous specimens.
REVIEW: Yes ☐ No ☐

38. **Answer: a**
WHY: Under normal circumstances, capillary puncture should not be performed on an index finger. The index finger is usually more calloused and harder to poke. It is also more sensitive so the puncture can be more painful, and because typically that finger is used more, a patient may notice the pain longer. Like venipuncture, a capillary puncture can be performed below an IV. The lateral plantar surface of an infant's heel and the middle or ring finger of an adult are recommended capillary puncture sites.
REVIEW: Yes ☐ No ☐
📖 *See Table 10-2 in the TEXTBOOK for a list of finger puncture precautions.*

39. **Answer: b**
WHY: The depth of lancet insertion must be controlled to avoid injuring the heel bone. The medical term for the heel bone is "calcaneus." Puncturing an artery or damaging tendons is avoided by puncturing in a recommended area. A deep puncture does not necessarily produce more bleeding.
REVIEW: Yes ☐ No ☐

40. **Answer: b**

    WHY: Studies have shown that heel punctures deeper than 2.0 mm risk injuring the calcaneus, or heel bone. For this reason, the latest Clinical and Laboratory Standards Institute (CLSI) capillary puncture standard states that heel puncture depth should not exceed 2.0 mm.

    REVIEW: Yes ☐ No ☐

41. **Answer: c**

    WHY: A deep heel puncture can penetrate the calcaneus (heel bone), leading to painful osteo-myelitis (inflammation of the bone including the marrow) or osteochondritis (inflammation of the bone and cartilage).

    REVIEW: Yes ☐ No ☐

    📖 *The crossword in Chapter 10 is a fun way to review many words associated with Capillary Collection.*

42. **Answer: c**

    WHY: According to the CLSI, the safest areas for performing heel puncture are on the plantar surface of the heel, medial to an imaginary line extending from the middle of the great (big) toe to the heel, or lateral to an imaginary line extending from between the fourth and fifth toes to the heel (Fig. 10-7). Thus, safe areas are on the medial or lateral plantar surface of the heel. Punctures should not be performed in the central portion of the heel or the posterior curvature of the heel because bone and cartilage injury can occur. All areas of the arch should be avoided because nerves and tendons can be injured. The big toe should not be punctured because it has an artery that could inadvertently be punctured.

    REVIEW: Yes ☐ No ☐

43. **Answer: c**

    WHY: The recommended site for capillary punc-ture in older children and adults (Fig. 10-5) is the pad (fleshy portion) of the palmar surface of the distal or end segment of a middle or ring finger.

    REVIEW: Yes ☐ No ☐

44. **Answer: d**

    WHY: Capillary puncture releases tissue thrombo-plastin, which activates the coagulation process and leads to platelet clumping and microclot formation in specimens that are not collected quickly. This affects hematology specimens the most; consequently, they are collected first. Serum specimens are collected last because they are supposed to clot. In the order of draw for venipuncture, which was designed to minimize

problems caused by additive carryover between tubes, serum specimens are collected before hematology specimens. Carryover is not an issue with capillary collection. Isopropyl alcohol is the recommended antiseptic for capillary puncture and routine venipuncture. Patient identification is the same regardless of the specimen collection method. Additives in microcollection tubes and stopper colors correspond to those of evacuated tubes.

    REVIEW: Yes ☐ No ☐

45. **Answer: a**

    WHY: The distance between the skin surface and the bone in the end segment of the finger varies. It is less at the side and tip of the finger than at the center. It is thinnest in the fifth, or little, finger.

    REVIEW: Yes ☐ No ☐

46. **Answer: a**

    WHY: The major blood vessels of the skin are located at the dermal–subcutaneous junction, which in a newborn's heel is located between 0.35 and 1.6 mm below the surface of the skin (Fig. 10-9).

    REVIEW: Yes ☐ No ☐

47. **Answer: a**

    WHY: If a capillary puncture is made parallel to the whorls of the fingerprint (Fig. 10-5), blood will run down the grooves of the fingerprint rather than forming round drops that are easy to collect. It will not bleed longer.

    REVIEW: Yes ☐ No ☐

48. **Answer: a**

    WHY: Blood cultures cannot be collected by capillary puncture because of the large volume of blood required. In addition, capillary blood is exposed to the skin and the air during collection, which increases the possibility of contamination.

    REVIEW: Yes ☐ No ☐

49. **Answer: c**

    WHY: A bullet with a lavender stopper contains EDTA, which is the additive used to collect com-plete blood counts (CBCs).

    REVIEW: Yes ☐ No ☐

50. **Answer: b**

    WHY: A complete blood count (CBC) is a hema-tology test. When collected by capillary puncture, slides, platelet counts, and other hematology tests are collected first to avoid the effects of platelet aggregation (clumping) and microclot formation.

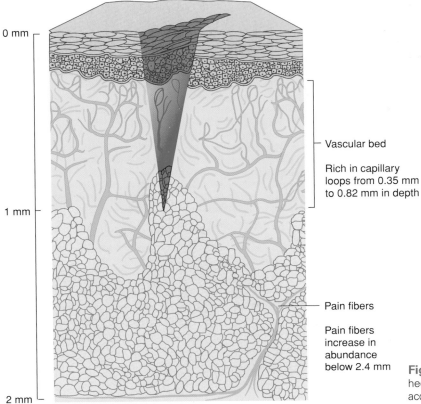

0 mm

1 mm

2 mm

Vascular bed

Rich in capillary
loops from 0.35 mm
to 0.82 mm in depth

Pain fibers

Pain fibers
increase in
abundance
below 2.4 mm

Figure 10-9 A cross-section of full-term infant's heel showing lancet penetration depth needed to access the capillary bed.

Other anticoagulant containers are collected next, and serum specimens are collected last.

REVIEW: Yes ☐ No ☐

📖 *WORKBOOK Case Study 10-2 is a good way to remember how important order of draw is in capillary collection.*

51. **Answer: b**

WHY: Warming the site before capillary puncture increases blood flow up to seven times. Warming is said to *arterialize* the specimen because it increases arterial blood flow into the area. Enhancing visibility of veins is *not* necessary for capillary puncture. Hemolysis is mainly caused by squeezing the site, puncturing before the alcohol is dry, or using the first drop of blood instead of wiping it away; it can happen regardless of whether or not the site was warmed.

REVIEW: Yes ☐ No ☐

52. **Answer: a**

WHY: Warming the site for 5 to 10 minutes to increase arterial blood flow into the area is an important step in the collection of capillary blood gas (CBG) specimens. This arterializes the specimen, which means it increases the arterial content and makes it more similar to arterial blood. A towel or diaper dampened with warm

tap water can be used to warm the site; however, care must be taken not to get the water too hot, or the patient may be scalded. Special warming devices (Fig. 10-10) that provide a uniform temperature that does not exceed 42°C are available. Warming the site before collecting other specimens is done to make collection easier, not for accuracy of results.

REVIEW: Yes ☐ No ☐

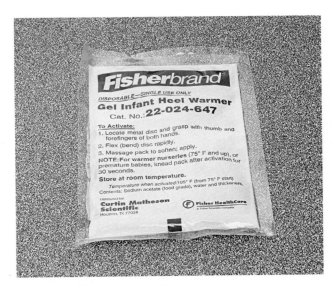

Figure 10-10 An infant heel warmer.

53. **Answer: a**

    WHY: The Clinical and Laboratory Standards Institute (CLSI) recommends using 70% isopropyl alcohol (isopropanol or ETOH) to cleaning capillary puncture sites.

    REVIEW: Yes ☐ No ☐

54. **Answer: d**

    WHY: The antiseptic used to clean a capillary puncture site is isopropyl alcohol. If the site is not completely dry before capillary puncture, alcohol residue can cause hemolysis of the specimen and lead to erroneous test results.

    REVIEW: Yes ☐ No ☐

55. **Answer: d**

    WHY: Povidone–iodine contamination of capillary puncture blood has been shown to cause erroneous results for bilirubin, uric acid, phosphorus, and potassium tests.

    REVIEW: Yes ☐ No ☐

    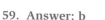 *A memory jogger in Chapter 10 of the TEXTBOOK will show you a fun way to remember this fact.*

56. **Answer: c**

    WHY: Errors in glucose results have been attributed to isopropyl alcohol (isopropanol) contamination of the specimen. Deep punctures can injure bone but do not affect test results. The first drop of blood should be wiped away (Fig. 10-4) to eliminate alcohol residue and tissue fluid contamination. Errors in glucose results have not been attributed to warming the site.

    REVIEW: Yes ☐ No ☐

57. **Answer: b**

    WHY: Finger sticks should be made perpendicular to the whorls or grooves of the fingerprint (Fig. 10-5) so that the blood forms round drops (Fig. 10-11) that can be collected easily. A puncture parallel to the whorls allows the blood to run down the finger and makes collection difficult.

    REVIEW: Yes ☐ No ☐

58. **Answer: c**

    WHY: Blood cells contain potassium. Residual alcohol can hemolyze blood cells, releasing potassium into the liquid portion of the specimen, erroneously elevating potassium results.

    REVIEW: Yes ☐ No ☐

59. **Answer: b**

    WHY: It is important to wipe away the first drop of blood during capillary puncture (Fig. 10-4)

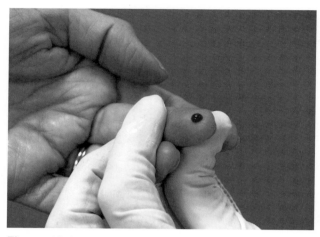

Figure 10-11 A round blood drop forming at the puncture site.

because excess tissue fluid that is typically found in the first drop can affect test results. Omitting the first drop from the sample also eliminates alcohol residue that can keep the blood from forming well-rounded drops, and also hemolyze the specimen.

REVIEW: Yes ☐ No ☐

60. **Answer: b**

    WHY: Scooping or scraping up blood that runs down the finger is *not* a proper technique because it introduces contamination, activates platelets, and can cause hemolysis of the specimen. Correct technique includes touching the tube's scoop to the drop of blood (Fig. 10-12) and letting the blood run down the inside of the tube. An occasional tap of the tube may be necessary to settle the blood to the bottom of the tube.

    REVIEW: Yes ☐ No ☐

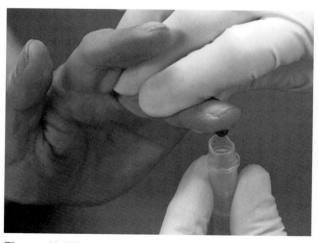

Figure 10-12 Touching the scoop of a microtube to a drop of blood.

61. Answer: d

WHY: Collecting the first drop instead of wiping it away, pressing hard on the site, and squeezing the site can all introduce excess tissue fluid into the specimen and affect test results, and can also cause hemolysis. Wiping the alcohol dry can contaminate the site and is *not* a recommended technique but does *not* affect the tissue fluid level in the specimen.

REVIEW: Yes ☐ No ☐

62. Answer: c

WHY: Microtubes contain a proper amount of anticoagulant for the recommended fill level. If a microtube is overfilled, there is not enough anticoagulant for the increased volume of blood, which can result in the formation of microclots, or complete clotting of the specimen. A specimen should be mixed as soon as possible after collection. Mixing a specimen forcefully can cause hemolysis. Underfilling a tube can result in excess anticoagulant for the volume of blood, which can cause distortion of the cells.

REVIEW: Yes ☐ No ☐

63. Answer: a

WHY: Blood smears and EDTA specimens are obtained before other specimens to minimize the effects of platelet aggregation (clumping). When tissue is disrupted by skin puncture, the coagulation process is set in motion and platelets start to aggregate (stick or clump together) and adhere to the site to seal off the injury. This can lead to erroneously low platelet counts. Platelets are evaluated and their numbers estimated as part of a differential performed on a blood smear. A platelet count is part of a complete blood count performed on an EDTA specimen.

REVIEW: Yes ☐ No ☐

64. Answer: a

WHY: A manual differential is performed on a stained blood smear. A neonatal bilirubin test is typically performed on serum collected in an amber microtube or bullet. Most newborn screening tests involve the collection of blood in circles on special filter paper. A manual packed cell volume (PCV) or hematocrit (HCT) is collected in a microhematocrit tube.

REVIEW: Yes ☐ No ☐

65. Answer: c

WHY: An acceptable smear (Fig. 10-13) will cover about one-half to three-fourths of the surface of the slide and have the appearance of a feather,

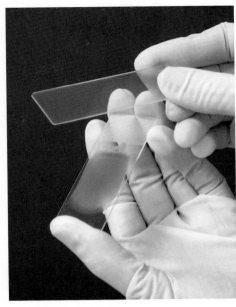

Figure 10-13 A completed blood smear.

in that there will be a smooth gradient from thick to thin when held up to the light. The thinnest area of a properly made smear, often referred to as the "feather," is one cell thick and is the most important area because that is where a differential is performed.

REVIEW: Yes ☐ No ☐

66. Answer: d

WHY: A blood smear prepared from an EDTA specimen should be made within 1 hour of collection to prevent cell distortion caused by prolonged contact with the anticoagulant.

REVIEW: Yes ☐ No ☐

67. Answer: c

WHY: When a blood smear is prepared using the two-slide method, one slide holds the drop used to make the smear and a second slide, placed on the first slide at an angle of approximately 30 degrees (Fig. 10-14), is used to spread the drop of blood across the slide and create the blood film.

REVIEW: Yes ☐ No ☐

68. Answer: a

WHY: Blood smears that are too long or too short are not acceptable. The length of a blood smear can be controlled by adjusting the angle of the spreader slide or the size of the drop of blood. If a smear is too short, decreasing the angle of the spreader slide or using a larger drop of blood on the next attempt should result in a longer smear.

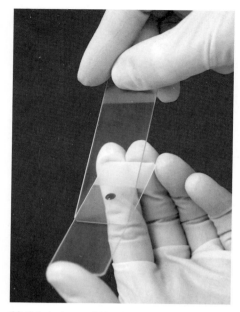

Figure 10-14 A drop of blood on a slide with pusher slide placed in front.

Exerting more pressure will only distort the smear. Increasing the angle of the spreader slide or using a smaller drop will make an even shorter smear.
REVIEW: Yes ☐   No ☐

69. **Answer: a**

WHY: Dirt or fingerprints on the slide and fat globules or lipids in the specimen can result in holes in a blood smear. Blood with a low hemoglobin level may be thin and require a smaller drop or adjustment of the pusher slide to create a proper smear, but it would not normally cause holes in a blood smear.
REVIEW: Yes ☐   No ☐

70. **Answer: c**

WHY: Malaria can be caused by any of four different species of microorganisms called plasmodia. It is diagnosed by detecting the presence of plasmodia organisms in a peripheral blood smear. Diagnosis typically requires the evaluation of both regular and thick blood smears. Presence of the organism is observed most frequently in a thick smear; however, identification of the species requires evaluation of a regular blood smear.
REVIEW: Yes ☐   No ☐

71. **Answer: b**

WHY: The total blood volume of infants, especially premature infants, is a very important consideration when ordering tests. The amount needed

for the test and amount the infant can safely lose should be calculated by the physician and also the person doing the phlebotomy. Table 10-1 in TEXTBOOK shows the percentage that a 10-mL sample is of the total blood volume when drawn from an infant. A 10-mL sample is considered an acceptable amount to draw from an adult, but if this amount is drawn frequently from an infant, it could result in anemia and the need for a transfusion.
REVIEW: Yes ☐   No ☐

72. **Answer: b**

WHY: Capillary blood gases (CBGs) are less dangerous to collect than arterial blood gases (ABGs). However, CBG results are *not* as accurate as ABG results because of the partial arterial composition of capillary blood and because the open system of collection temporarily exposes the specimen to air, which can affect test results.
REVIEW: Yes ☐   No ☐

73. **Answer: a**

WHY: Bilirubin can cross the blood–brain barrier in infants, accumulating to toxic levels that can cause permanent brain damage or even death. A transfusion may be needed if levels increase at a rate equal to or greater than 5 mg/dL per hour or when levels exceed 18 mg/dL.
REVIEW: Yes ☐   No ☐

74. **Answer: c**

WHY: Phenylketonuria (PKU) is a hereditary disorder caused by an inability to metabolize the amino acid phenylalanine. Patients with PKU lack the enzyme necessary to convert phenylalanine to tyrosine. Phenylalanine accumulates in the blood and can rise to toxic levels. PKU cannot be cured, but it can normally be treated with a diet low in phenylalanine. If left untreated or if not treated early on, PKU can lead to brain damage and mental deficiencies.
REVIEW: Yes ☐   No ☐

75. **Answer: b**

WHY: Newborn screening is the term used to describe testing of newborns for the presence of genetic, or inherited, diseases such as galactosemia (GALT). Bilirubin, hemoglobin, and hematocrit (H & H), and white blood cell (WBC) counts may be performed on newborns but are not screening tests.
REVIEW: Yes ☐   No ☐

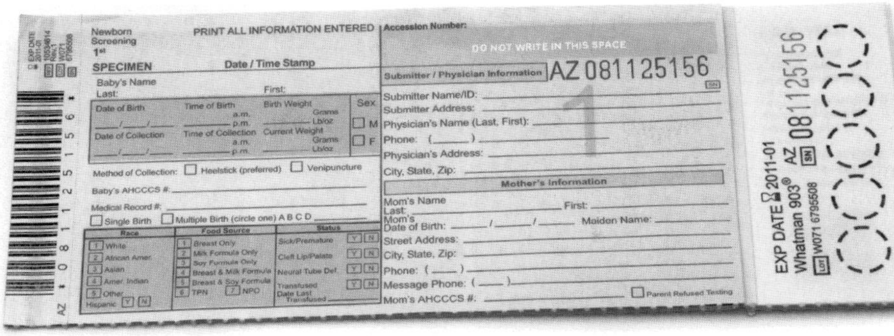

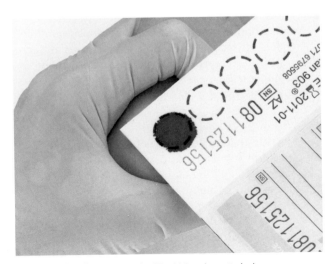

Figure 10-15 A newborn screening form with collection circles displayed.

76. Answer: b

WHY: Bilirubin is broken down in the presence of light. Collecting the specimen too slowly or failing to protect the specimen from light after collection allows the specimen to be exposed to light for longer than necessary and leads to falsely decreased results.

REVIEW: Yes ☐ No ☐

77. Answer: d

WHY: Isopropyl alcohol is the recommended antiseptic for cleaning prior to capillary puncture, including heel punctures performed to collect PKU specimens. If proper technique is used (i.e., the alcohol is allowed to dry before puncture and the first drop of blood is wiped away) alcohol contamination is unlikely to be an issue. PKU specimens are collected by placing large drops of blood within circles on special filter paper that is typically part of the test requisition (Fig. 10-15). Using the first drop of blood can contaminate an entire blood spot with tissue fluid and lead to erroneous results. Blood spots can also be contaminated by touching the circles with hands (with or without gloves) before, during, or after specimen collection. Stacking filter paper requisitions together after collection can lead to cross-contamination between different patient specimens.

REVIEW: Yes ☐ No ☐

78. Answer: d

WHY: Newborn screening blood spots must be collected properly to prevent erroneous results. Applying blood to both sides of the filter paper or layering successive drops in the same circle increase the amount of blood in the test area and can lead to erroneously increased results. Hanging specimens to dry can cause the blood to migrate and concentrate toward the lower end of the filter paper. This leaves the upper areas of the circle with less blood and the lower areas with more

blood than required for testing. In this case, the results will be erroneous on any area that is used for testing. Letting one large drop of blood entirely fill a circle (Fig. 10-16) is correct procedure.

REVIEW: Yes ☐ No ☐

79. Answer: d

WHY: Newborn screening to detect PKU, galactosemia (GALT), and hypothyroidism is required by law in all 50 states in the United States.

REVIEW: Yes ☐ No ☐

80. Answer: a

WHY: High levels of bilirubin in the blood result in jaundice, a condition characterized by yellow color of the skin, whites of the eyes, mucous membranes, and body fluids.

REVIEW: Yes ☐ No ☐

81. Answer: d

WHY: Adhesive bandages can irritate the tender skin of infants, come off and become a choking hazard, or tear the skin when removed. Consequently, they

Figure 10-16 A correctly filled blood spot circle.

should not be used on infants or children younger than 2 years.

REVIEW: Yes ☐ No ☐

82. **Answer: c**

WHY: Heel puncture includes the following steps: (1) *warm* the site; (2) *clean* the site; (3) *puncture* the site; (4) *wipe* away the first blood drop; and (5) *collect* the specimen.

REVIEW: Yes ☐ No ☐

83. **Answer: a**

WHY: Capillary specimens should be handled gently, just like venous blood specimens. After capping, gentle inversions are required to adequately mix an anticoagulant microtube without hemolyzing red blood cells. Tapping the tube gently on a hard surface can be used to settle blood to the bottom of the tube during collection but is not adequate to mix the specimen. Tapping sharply can hemolyze the specimen. Rolling the specimen in the hands may not mix the specimen adequately.

REVIEW: Yes ☐ No ☐

84. **Answer: b**

WHY: Strong repetitive pressure such as squeezing or milking the site can contaminate a capillary specimen with excess tissue fluid, hemolyze the red blood cells, and compromise test results. If adequate blood flow cannot be obtained without such action, a new puncture should be made at a different site. Venous blood flows out of the area, not into it.

REVIEW: Yes ☐ No ☐

85. **Answer: c**

WHY: Hematocrit tubes fill automatically when they come in contact with a drop of blood (Fig. 10-17) by a force called capillary action or attraction. Blood drops must be dripped onto filter paper circles for newborn screening tests and into microtubes or bullets regardless of the type or stopper color.

REVIEW: Yes ☐ No ☐

86. **Answer: d**

WHY: Capillary puncture is preferred for infants because a venipuncture can cause damage to their tiny veins and the tissue around the vein. This is especially true if the vein is difficult to access or is punctured too frequently. Tests performed in the laboratory for infants are the same as for adults and the results from capillary collection are often not as accurate as venous specimens.

REVIEW: Yes ☐ No ☐

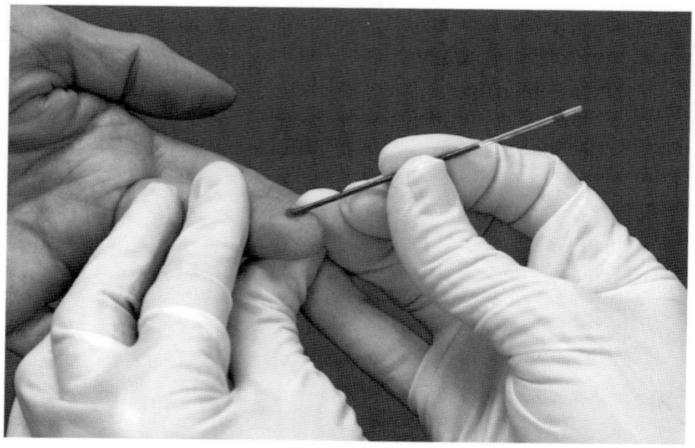

Figure 10-17 Filling an hematocrit tube by capillary action.

87. **Answer: c**

WHY: Used lancets must be disposed of in a sharps container even though the blades are permanently retractable.

REVIEW: Yes ☐ No ☐

88. **Answer: b**

WHY: Capillary puncture is generally not appropriate for patients who are dehydrated because specimens may be hard to obtain and results may not be representative of blood elsewhere in the body.

REVIEW: Yes ☐ No ☐

89. **Answer: a**

WHY: A bandage should not be applied to an infant or child younger than 2 years because it can pose a choking hazard. In addition, bandage adhesive can stick to the paper thin skin of newborns and tear it when removed.

REVIEW: Yes ☐ No ☐

90. **Answer: b**

WHY: A blood smear must be allowed to air dry naturally. Blowing on it or waving it dries it too quickly, which can distort red blood cells and also introduce contaminants. A blood smear should not be placed in alcohol before it is stained.

REVIEW: Yes ☐ No ☐

91. **Answer: a**

WHY: Blood cultures cannot be collected by capillary puncture because the volume of blood required for the tests is too large and the open collection method increases the possibility of contamination. Electrolytes, hemoglobin, and lithium levels can all be collected by capillary puncture.

REVIEW: Yes ☐ No ☐

92. **Answer: c**

    WHY: Newborn screening is the routine testing of newborns (neonates) for the presence of certain genetic (inherited), metabolic, hormonal, and functional disorders that can cause severe mental handicaps or other serious abnormalities if not detected and treated early. The disorders are not contagious and do not normally show symptoms at birth.

    REVIEW: Yes ☐ No ☐

93. **Answer: b**

    WHY: Most microhematocrit tubes are either plain, meaning they have no additive, or are coated with ammonium heparin. Color-coding does not correspond to ETS tubes or microtubes. Nonadditive microhematocrit tubes have a blue band on one end; those containing heparin have a red band on one end.

    REVIEW: Yes ☐ No ☐

94. **Answer: a**

    WHY: The area of an infant's heel that is richest in capillary loop is located in the dermis between 0.35 and 0.82 mm deep (Fig. 10-9). Pain fibers increase in abundance below 2.4 mm.

    REVIEW: Yes ☐ No ☐

95. **Answer: c**

    WHY: Use only enough pressure to keep the lancet firmly against the skin. Pressing down hard on the lancet compresses the skin and can result in a deeper puncture than intended.

    REVIEW: Yes ☐ No ☐

96. **Answer: d**

    WHY: The cross-section of full-term infant's heel (Fig. 10-8) shows that the pain fibers begin to appear in the subcutaneous layer just below the dermis, and below 2.4 mm, the pain fibers increase in abundance.

    REVIEW: Yes ☐ No ☐

97. **Answer: d**

    WHY: Newborn/neonatal screening is the state mandated testing of newborns for the presence of certain genetic (inherited), metabolic, hormonal, and functional disorders that can cause severe abnormalities if not detected and treated early. Screening for phenylketonuria (PKU), galactosemia, and hypothyroidism is required by law in all 50 states and U.S. territories.

    REVIEW: Yes ☐ No ☐

98. **Answer: b**

    WHY: The ability of a liquid to be automatically drawn into a narrow space or tube is called capillary action. If a microhematocrit tube is held in a vertical position above or in a horizontal position beside a blood drop and one end touched to the blood drop, blood will be automatically drawn into it by capillary action.

    REVIEW: Yes ☐ No ☐

99. **Answer: c**

    WHY: Maple syrup urine disease (MSUD) is an inherited amino acid metabolism disorder. GALT (classic galactosemia) is a rare genetic disease that involves the inability to metabolize the sugar galactose. Hb SS (sickle cell anemia) is a hemoglobinopathy, an inherited disease that involves abnormal hemoglobin structure.

    REVIEW: Yes ☐ No ☐

100. **Answer: b**

    WHY: Gentle pressure is correct procedure and is usually needed to keep the blood flowing during a capillary puncture. Gentle pressure should not hemolyze red blood cells, but strong pressure or squeezing the site could. Alcohol residue is removed by wiping away the first drop of blood.

    REVIEW: Yes ☐ No ☐

Chapter 11

Special Collections and Point-of-Care Testing

Study Tips

- Study the key points in the corresponding chapter of the TEXTBOOK.

- Make a list of six items that are typically required on labels for blood bank specimens.

- Find a special ID bracelet and compare it to the regular ID band.

- Make a table with three columns. In the first column list the drug categories that are subject to therapeutic drug monitoring. In the second column, list two examples of each drug. In the third column, tell why the drug is used.

- On a sheet of paper make two columns and label one "Forensic BACs" and the other "Clinical BACs." Under each heading, list, compare, and contrast the collection process.

- List all of the POCT glucose-testing instruments that are found in the chapter.

- List five POCT coagulation-testing instruments found in the chapter and tell which coagulation test they can perform.

- Using the formula found in the chapter, calculate an INR if the patient's results are 15 seconds and the PT normal is 12 seconds.

- Complete the activities in Chapter 11 of the companion WORKBOOK.

Overview   This chapter describes special tests and point-of-care testing (POCT). Collecting specimens for these tests requires additional knowledge and may involve different preparation for collection and handling. POCT specimens are collected using capillary puncture or venipuncture, and the small, portable, and often handheld testing devices that process the specimens bring laboratory testing to the location of the patient. Some of the most commonly encountered special blood test and POCT procedures are described in this chapter. Procedures in this chapter conform to CLSI standards.

Review Questions

Choose the BEST answer.

1. Forensic toxicology is concerned with
   a. deliberate, not accidental, toxin contact.
   b. legal consequences of toxin exposure.
   c. toxin contamination in water resources.
   d. treatment for the effects of toxins.

2. TB test administration involves
   a. applying pressure right after injection.
   b. checking for a reaction in 12 to 24 hours.
   c. cleaning the site with povidone–iodine.
   d. injecting the antigen just under the skin.

3. All of the following are included in the DOT's 10 Steps to Collection Site Security and Integrity EXCEPT
   a. ensure that video monitoring equipment is working during specimen collection.
   b. inspect the site to ensure that no foreign or unauthorized substances are present.
   c. secure any water sources or otherwise make them unavailable to employees.
   d. tape or otherwise secure shut any movable toilet tank top, or put bluing in the tank.

4. The correct order in collecting a blood culture is
   a. cleanse bottle tops, select equipment, perform friction scrub, and perform venipuncture.
   b. perform friction scrub, select equipment, perform venipuncture, and cleanse bottle tops.
   c. select equipment, cleanse bottle tops, perform friction scrub, and perform venipuncture.
   d. select equipment, perform friction scrub, cleanse bottle tops, and perform venipuncture.

5. False-positive results of lactose tolerance tests have been found in all of the following conditions EXCEPT
   a. congenital cystic fibrosis.
   b. male multiple myeloma.
   c. patients with flat GTTs.
   d. slow gastric emptying.

6. The preferred sample for parentage testing is
   a. amniotic fluid.
   b. blood sample.
   c. buccal swab.
   d. chorionic villi.

7. Which one of the following should be deleted from the list of those allowed to order paternity testing?
   a. Child support agent
   b. Child who is a minor
   c. Defense attorney
   d. Family physician

8. What is the recommended disinfectant for blood culture sites in infants 2 months and older?
   a. Isopropyl alcohol swab
   b. Chlorhexidine gluconate
   c. Benzalkonium chloride
   d. Povidone–iodine swab

9. Which one of the following statements about autologous donations is untrue?
   a. Blood can be collected up to 72 hours before surgery
   b. Patients must have a written order from their physician
   c. Unused autologous units may be used by other patients
   d. Using the patient's own blood eliminates many risks

10. The CPD additive in a donor unit of blood is least likely to
    a. control bacterial contamination.
    b. prevent the blood from clotting.
    c. provide nutrition for the cells.
    d. stabilize the pH of the plasma.

11. A transfusion of incompatible blood is often fatal because it causes
    a. a major allergic reaction, releasing too much histamine.
    b. lysis, or rupturing, of RBCs, within the vascular system.
    c. the patient's lungs to fill with nonfunctioning RBCs.
    d. hemochromatosis in the patient's circulatory system.

12. In using a cell-salvaging procedure during surgery, before the patient's blood can be reinfused it must be evaluated for
    a. chemical toxin.
    b. free hemoglobin.
    c. plasma glucose.
    d. white cell count.

13. Which one of the donor unit collection principles below is untrue? The collection bag
    a. contains the two additives, EDTA and sodium fluoride.
    b. employs a closed system connected to a 16- to 18-gauge needle.
    c. fills by weight and when full, normally corresponds to 450 mL.
    d. is placed on a continuous mixing unit while the blood is drawn.

14. Which of the following are coagulation tests that can be monitored using a POC instrument?
    a. BNP and Hct
    b. BUN and UA
    c. HCO3⁻ and TnI
    d. INR and PTT

15. Some individuals lack the necessary mucosal enzyme to convert which of the following sugars so that it can be digested?
    a. Glucose
    b. Glucagon
    c. Lactose
    d. Pentose

16. Blood gases can be monitored using the
    a. AVOXimeter.
    b. Cholestech.
    c. Stratus CS.
    d. Triage Cardiac.

17. This point-of-care testing instrument has recently been recognized as an accurate predictor of developing diabetic complications.
    a. Accu-Chek
    b. DCA Vantage
    c. HB 201
    d. XceedPro

18. Potassium is least likely to play a major role in
    a. muscle function.
    b. nerve conduction.
    c. osmotic pressure.
    d. transporting Hgb.

19. All POC glucose analyzers approved for hospital use have which of the following in common?
    a. The ability to use capillary, venous, or arterial blood samples
    b. Data can be downloaded to a data management program
    c. They require the use of an authorized operator ID number
    d. All of the above

20. ARD or FAN blood culture bottles
    a. detect problems in carbohydrate metabolism.
    b. eliminate vital interference from blood cells.
    c. remove any antibiotics that are in the blood.
    d. treat blood-borne pathogens in the circulation.

21. Septicemia is
    a. a positive test for transmissible disease.
    b. bacteria measurement in whole blood.
    c. fever in which the cause is not known.
    d. presence of microorganisms in the blood.

22. The Siemens Patient Identification Check system is a
    a. complete management system for IV chemotherapy.
    b. plasma/low hemoglobin point-of-care analyzer system.
    c. portable bar-code scanning system for positive patient ID.
    d. special ID bracelet having a self-carbon adhesive label.

23. Eligibility requirements for donating blood include
    a. age 17 to 66 years, 110 lb or more.
    b. age 18 to 75 years, 110 lb or more.
    c. age 21 to 65 years, at least 100 lb.
    d. minimum of 21 years old, 100 lb.

24. Identify the condition in which a unit of blood is withdrawn from a patient as a treatment.
    a. ABO incompatibility
    b. Autologous donation
    c. Hemochromatosis
    d. Hemolytic anemia

25. Which test requires especially strict identification and specimen labeling procedures?
    a. Aldosterone
    b. Cross-match
    c. Plasminogen
    d. Valproic acid

26. Which of the following should be removed from a list of drugs of abuse?
    a. Amphetamines
    b. Cannabinoids
    c. "Crack" and "ice"
    d. Phenobarbital

27. Donor units of blood are typically collected using needles that are
    a. 16 to 18 gauge.
    b. 18 to 28 gauge.
    c. 20 to 22 gauge.
    d. 23 to 25 gauge.

28. A typical unit of donated blood contains approximately
    a. 250 mL.
    b. 450 mL.
    c. 750 mL.
    d. 1 L.

29. Which of the following tests is collected from patients with FUO to rule out septicemia?
    a. Blood cultures times two
    b. Nasopharyngeal culture
    c. Urine culture and sensitivity
    d. Wound and skin culture

30. Of the following tubes, which should be eliminated for use in collecting blood bank specimens?
    a. Large gel-barrier tube
    b. Lavender-top tube
    c. Nonadditive red-top tube
    d. Pink-stopper EDTA tube

31. Which of the following tests is collected using special skin decontamination procedures?
    a. Blood urea nitrogen
    b. Complete blood count
    c. Set of blood cultures
    d. Type and cross-match

32. Under which area of clinical testing does paternity testing fall?
    a. Chemistry
    b. Coagulation
    c. Molecular genetics
    d. Hematology

33. Why would blood cultures be collected with an antimicrobial adsorbing resin?
    a. The patient has fever spikes for more than a week
    b. The patient is taking a broad-spectrum antibiotic
    c. To eliminate contaminating normal skin flora
    d. To absorb and remove bacteria-caused contamination

34. Which specimen tubes must contain a 9-to-1 ratio of blood to anticoagulant to be accepted for testing?
    a. Blood bank
    b. Chemistry
    c. Coagulation
    d. Hematology

35. What type of additive is best for collecting an ethanol specimen?
    a. CPD + adenine
    b. Potassium EDTA
    c. Sodium citrate
    d. Sodium fluoride

36. Which BC is inoculated first when the specimen has been collected by needle and syringe?
    a. Aerobic media
    b. Anaerobic vial
    c. ARD container
    d. It does not matter

37. The most critical aspect of blood culture collection is
    a. media inoculation.
    b. needle gauge.
    c. skin antisepsis.
    d. specimen handling.

38. A site for blood culture collection can typically be cleaned with which of the following?
    a. Chlorhexidine gluconate
    b. Hydrogen peroxide
    c. Sodium hypochlorite
    d. All of the above

39. Which of the following additives is sometimes used to collect blood culture specimens?
    a. ACD
    b. CPD
    c. EDTA
    d. SPS

40. Which type of specimen may require collection of a discard tube before the test specimen is collected?
    a. Blood culture
    b. Coagulation
    c. Drug testing
    d. Paternity

41. The oral glucose challenge test
    a. detects high blood glucose levels.
    b. is a 1-hour glucose screening test.
    c. screens for gestational diabetes.
    d. All of the above.

42. Which test is used as a screening test for glucose metabolism problems?
    a. 2-hour PP
    b. GTT
    c. Lactose
    d. WBC

43. Which of the following activities is acceptable during a glucose tolerance test (GTT)?
    a. Chewing sugarless gum
    b. Drinking tea without sugar
    c. Lying down during the test
    d. Smoking low-tar cigarettes

44. When does the timing of specimen collection begin during a GTT?
    a. After the fasting blood specimen has been collected
    b. As soon as the patient begins to drink the beverage
    c. Before the fasting blood specimen is to be collected
    d. When the patient has finished the glucose beverage

45. A phlebotomist arrives to collect a 2-hour post-prandial glucose specimen on an inpatient and discovers that 2 hours have not elapsed since the patient's last meal. What should the phlebotomist do?
    a. Ask the patient's nurse to verify the correct collection time
    b. Come back later at the time the patient tells you is correct
    c. Draw the specimen and write the time collected on the label
    d. Fill out an incident report form and return to the laboratory

46. A patient undergoing a GTT vomits within 30 minutes of drinking the glucose beverage. What action should the phlebotomist take?
    a. Continue the test and note on the laboratory slip that the patient vomited and at what time
    b. Discontinue the test and write on the requisition that the patient vomited the drink
    c. Give the patient another dose of the glucose beverage and continue with the test
    d. Notify the nurse or physician immediately to see if the test should be rescheduled

47. Increased blood glucose is called
    a. hyperglycemia.
    b. hyperinsulinism.
    c. hyperkalemia.
    d. hypernatremia.

48. When does a blood glucose level in normal individuals typically peak after glucose ingestion?
    a. In 15 to 20 minutes
    b. In ½ hour to 1 hour
    c. In 1 to 1½ hours
    d. In roughly 2 hours

49. Which of the following must remain consistent throughout an oral glucose challenge test?
    a. Arm used for the draw
    b. Blood specimen source
    c. Position of the patient
    d. Size of ETS tubes used

50. Patient preparation before a GTT involves
    a. eating meals with a measured amount of carbohydrate 3 days prior.
    b. exercising for 3 hours a day for a week before having the test.
    c. fasting for at least 2 hours before having the fasting specimen drawn.
    d. no chewing gum before or during the test unless it is sugarless.

51. Which of the following can be used to clean a site before a blood alcohol specimen is collected?
    a. Diluted methanol
    b. Isopropyl alcohol
    c. Tincture of iodine
    d. Zephiran chloride

52. Which of the following specimens may require chain-of-custody documentation when it is collected?
    a. Blood culture
    b. Cross-match
    c. Drug screen
    d. Trace elements

53. The purpose of TDM is to
    a. determine and maintain a beneficial drug dosage.
    b. maintain peak levels of drug in a patient's system.
    c. prevent trough levels of drug in a patient's system.
    d. screen for illegal drug use using multiple samples.

54. Which of the following tests would not be subject to therapeutic drug monitoring?
    a. Digitoxin
    b. Gentamicin
    c. Phenylalanine
    d. Theophylline

55. A peak drug level has been ordered for 0900 hours. You draw the specimen 10 minutes late because of unavoidable circumstances. What additional action does this necessitate?
    a. Draw two tubes for duplicate drug screening.
    b. Establish the last dosage time from the chart.
    c. Fill out a delay slip and leave at the desk.
    d. Record the actual time of specimen collection.

56. A trough drug level is collected
    a. 30 minutes after administration of the drug intravenously.
    b. immediately before the next scheduled drug dose is given.
    c. immediately after administration of the drug by the nurse.
    d. when the highest serum concentration of drug is expected.

57. Which test requires the collection of multiple specimens?
    a. ACT
    b. GTT
    c. HCT
    d. PTT

58. Timing of collection is most critical for drugs with short half-lives, such as
    a. digitoxin.
    b. gentamicin.
    c. methotrexate.
    d. phenobarbital.

59. Molecular tests can be used to
    a. classify the genetic makeup of an individual.
    b. determine increased risk of a certain disease.
    c. identify genetic changes that cause a disease.
    d. All of the above.

60. The most common reason for glucose monitoring through POCT is to
    a. check for sporadic glucose in the urine.
    b. diagnose glucose metabolism problems.
    c. monitor glucose levels for diabetic care.
    d. control medication-induced mood swings.

61. Which one of the following tests could be collected using a tube other than a trace element–free tube?
    a. Copper
    b. Lead
    c. Sodium
    d. Zinc

62. The definition of toxicology is
    a. a protocol for drug trafficking.
    b. the scientific study of poisons.
    c. the study of drug therapy levels.
    d. the tracking of illicit drug trade.

63. Which test typically has the shortest TAT if performed by POCT?
    a. BUN
    b. DNA
    c. GTT
    d. PSA

64. Which of the following is not a POCT analyzer?
    a. ABL80
    b. CoaguChek
    c. GEM 4000
    d. BacT/ALERT

65. To prevent introducing a contaminating substance into a trace-element collection tube, it is suggested that you
    a. collect the royal-blue tube last in the order of draw.
    b. draw it by itself using a syringe or evacuated tube system.
    c. use a syringe and transfer blood into the royal-blue tube last.
    d. use only a royal-blue short-draw tube with heparin or EDTA.

66. Which of the following is one of the most common bedside or POCT tests?
    a. Bilirubin
    b. Cholesterol
    c. Glucose
    d. Troponin

67. Which of the following tests is used to monitor heparin therapy?
    a. ACT
    b. BNP
    c. BT
    d. PT

68. Tan top tubes containing K_2ETDA can be used to collect specimens for this test.
    a. Blood alcohol
    b. Glucose screen
    c. Lead analysis
    d. Protime/INR

69. The CAP requires QC for many waived tests to be performed
    a. before each patient test performed.
    b. daily and when a new kit is opened.
    c. on a weekly basis as a minimum.
    d. when test manufacturer specifies.

70. A noninvasive transcutaneous method can now be used to measure
    a. C-reactive protein.
    b. glycosylated Hgb.
    c. infant lead levels.
    d. neonatal bilirubin.

71. The accumulation of this substance in the blood can cause metabolic acidosis.

    a. Copper
    b. Lactate
    c. Mercury
    d. Troponin

72. This test can determine if an individual has developed antibodies to a particular antigen.

    a. Hematocrit
    b. Skin test
    c. Strep test
    d. Troponin T

73. Ionized calcium plays a critical role in all of the following but this.

    a. Blood clotting
    b. Cardiac function
    c. Glycosylation
    d. Nerve impulses

74. Below-normal blood pH is referred to as

    a. blood acidosis.
    b. blood alkalosis.
    c. hypokalemia.
    d. hyponatremia.

75. Which of the following is a protein that is specific to heart muscle?

    a. ALT
    b. BNP
    c. LDL
    d. TnT

76. B-type natriuretic peptide is a cardiac

    a. antibody.
    b. enzyme.
    c. hormone.
    d. protein.

77. This test is used to evaluate long-term effectiveness of diabetes therapy.

    a. 2-hour postprandial
    b. Glucose tolerance
    c. Hemoglobin A1c
    d. Random glucose

78. This test is also referred to as packed cell volume.

    a. ESR
    b. HCT
    c. Hgb
    d. HMT

79. This test detects occult blood.

    a. BAC
    b. Guaiac
    c. Lactose
    d. Skin test

80. Which of the following is a skin test for tuberculosis exposure?

    a. BNP
    b. GTT
    c. PPD
    d. PSA

81. The hormone detected in urine pregnancy testing is

    a. ACT.
    b. hCG.
    c. PPD.
    d. TSH.

82. Which point-of-care blood analyzer uses a microcuvette instead of a test strip?

    a. Cascade POC
    b. HemoCue HB201+
    c. I-STAT system
    d. Precision XceedPro

83. An uncorrected imbalance of this analyte in a patient can quickly lead to death.

    a. Hemoglobin
    b. Potassium
    c. Prothrombin
    d. Troponin T

84. The POC instrument VerifyNow does platelet testing to

    a. continuously check the glycemic index.
    b. determine response to aspirin therapy.
    c. evaluate the warfarin or heparin therapy.
    d. measure abnormal increase in thrombocytes.

85. How much diluted antigen is injected when a PPD test is performed?

    a. 0.01 mL
    b. 0.1 mL
    c. 0.5 mL
    d. 1.0 mL

86. *Erythema* means

    a. hardness.
    b. inflamed.
    c. redness.
    d. swollen.

87. In reading a patient's tuberculin (TB) test, there is an area of induration and erythema that measures 7 mm in diameter. The result of the test is

    a. doubtful.
    b. negative.
    c. positive.
    d. unreadable.

88. Point-of-care detection of group A strep normally requires a
    a. blood sample.
    b. nasal collection.
    c. throat swab.
    d. urine specimen.

89. Which one of the following analytes is undetectable in urine when a urine dipstick is used?
    a. Bilirubin
    b. Glucose
    c. Leukocytes
    d. Thrombin

90. Which point-of-care test helps a physician detect low-grade inflammation even in asymptomatic individuals?
    a. ALT
    b. BNP
    c. CRP
    d. TnT

91. A chain-of-custody is
    a. a special protocol used when collecting forensic specimens.
    b. necessary in patient management for therapeutic phlebotomy.
    c. required for the POC quality assurance program for nursing.
    d. part of the type and cross-match procedure for blood bank.

92. Drug screening in major companies is
    a. part of their annual healthcare screening.
    b. performed in three consecutive days.
    c. required after extended leave of absence.
    d. standard for all preemployment assessment.

93. An illicit drug is a
    a. any drug that is abused and becomes addictive.
    b. one that is not manufactured in this country.
    c. prescription drug used without authorization.
    d. synthetic type of a barbiturate or an opiate.

94. The mission to lead the nation in bringing the power of science to bear on drug abuse and addiction is that of
    a. CDC.
    b. DOT.
    c. NIDA.
    d. OSHA.

95. The NPSG Goal to improve the accuracy of patient identification is set by the
    a. American Hospital Association.
    b. Clinical Laboratory Standards Institute.
    c. Occupational Safety & Health Assoc.
    d. Joint Commission organization.

Answers and Explanations

1. **Answer: b**

    WHY: Toxicology is the scientific study of toxins (poisons). Forensic toxicology is concerned with the legal consequences of toxin exposure, both intentional and accidental. Clinical toxicology is concerned with the detection of toxins and treatment for the effects they produce. Toxicology tests examine blood, hair, urine, and other body substances for the presence of toxins, often present in very small amounts.
    REVIEW: Yes ☐   No ☐

2. **Answer: d**

    WHY: When one is administering a tuberculin (TB) skin test, the antigen must be injected just beneath the skin for accurate interpretation of the results. Appearance of the bleb, or wheal, is a sign that the antigen has been injected properly (Fig. 11-1). Applying pressure after injection of the antigen

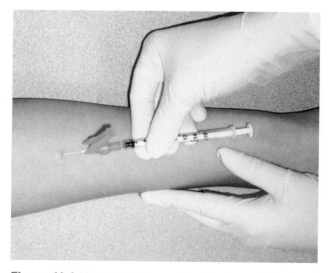

Figure 11-1 Wheal (bleb) formed by intradermal injection of antigen during skin test procedure.

could force it out of the site. The injection site should be cleaned with alcohol and allowed to dry before injection. The site should be checked for a reaction in 48 to 72 hours.

REVIEW: Yes ☐ No ☐

3. **Answer: a**

WHY: DOT does not require video monitoring during specimen collection.

REVIEW: Yes ☐ No ☐

4. **Answer: d**

WHY: Blood culture procedure steps in correct order are as follows: aseptically select and assemble the equipment, perform the friction scrub for 30 to 60 seconds, and allow the site to dry because antisepsis does not occur instantly. Next cleanse the culture bottle stopper while the site is drying and then perform the venipuncture without touching or repalpating the site.

REVIEW: Yes ☐ No ☐

📖 *Do Skills Drill Exercise 11-3 in the WORKBOOK to reinforce your understanding of blood culture procedure.*

5. **Answer: b**

WHY: False-positive results for the lactose tolerance test have been demonstrated in patients with disorders such as slow gastric emptying and cystic fibrosis but not multiple myeloma. If the patient is lactose intolerant, the glucose curve will be flat. Some individuals normally have a flat GTT curve; it is suggested that they have a 2-hour GTT performed the day before the lactose tolerance so results can be evaluated adequately.

REVIEW: Yes ☐ No ☐

6. **Answer: b**

WHY: Blood is the preferred sample for parentage testing, however the use of buccal samples is increasing. Obtaining amniotic fluid or a sample of chorionic villus tissue can only be done before the child is born.

REVIEW: Yes ☐ No ☐

7. **Answer: b**

WHY: Paternity testing is performed to determine the probability that a specific individual fathered a particular child. Unlike routine clinical tests, which require an order from a physician, paternity testing can be requested by lawyers, child support enforcement bureaus, physicians, and individuals with the exception of minor children.

REVIEW: Yes ☐ No ☐

8. **Answer: b**

WHY: According to the Clinical and Laboratory Standards Institute (CLSI), chlorhexidine gluconate is the recommended disinfectant for blood culture sites in infants 2 months of age and older.

REVIEW: Yes ☐ No ☐

9. **Answer: c**

WHY: An autologous donation is the process by which a person donates blood for his or her own use. This is done for elective surgeries when it is anticipated that a transfusion will be needed, because using one's own blood eliminates many risks associated with transfusions. Although blood is normally collected several weeks prior to the scheduled surgery, the minimum time between donation and surgery can be as little as 72 hours. To be eligible to make an autologous donation, a person must have a written order from a physician. If autologous units of blood are not used by the person who donated them, they must be discarded.

REVIEW: Yes ☐ No ☐

10. **Answer: a**

WHY: Citrate phosphate dextrose (CPD) is an anticoagulant and preservative that is typically used in collecting units of blood for transfusion purposes. The citrate prevents clotting by chelating (removing) calcium. A phosphate compound stabilizes the pH, and the dextrose provides energy to the cells and helps keep them alive. There is nothing in CPD that serves to control bacterial contamination.

REVIEW: Yes ☐ No ☐

11. **Answer: b**

WHY: A transfusion of donor blood that is not compatible with the patient's blood can be fatal because it causes agglutination (clumping) and lysis (rupturing) of the red blood cells within the patient's circulatory system. This massive destruction of red blood cells can overwhelm the patient's liver and kidneys causing death.

REVIEW: Yes ☐ No ☐

12. **Answer: b**

WHY: When patients request reinfusion of their own blood to replace blood lost during surgery, the blood must be salvaged and washed before being reinfused. Prior to reinfusion, it is recommended that the salvaged blood be tested for residual free hemoglobin. A high free hemoglobin level indicates that too many red cells were destroyed during the salvage process, and renal dysfunction could result if the blood were reinfused. Free hemoglobin can be detected using point-of-care instruments such as

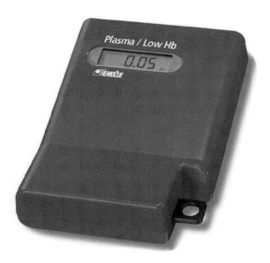

Figure 11-2 HemoCue Plasma/Low Hb. (HemoCue, Inc., Lake Forest, CA.)

the HemoCue Plasma/Low Hemoglobin Analyzer, as seen in Figure 11-2.

REVIEW: Yes ☐ No ☐

13. **Answer: a**

WHY: The additive in a unit of blood is CPD (citrate phosphate dextrose) or CPD plus adenine (CPDA). The collection unit is a sterile, closed system consisting of a blood bag connected by a length of tubing to a sterile 16- to 18-gauge needle. The collection bag contains an anticoagulant and preservative solution and is placed on a mixing unit while the blood is being drawn to keep the blood from clotting. The unit is normally filled by weight but typically contains around 450 mL of blood when full.

REVIEW: Yes ☐ No ☐

14. **Answer: d**

WHY: The prothrombin time (PT) or international normalized ratio (INR) and the partial thromboplastin time (PTT) are coagulation tests that are monitored through point-of-care testing by analyzers such as the CoaguChek (Roche Diagnostics) (Fig. 11-3). The INR is a system established by international committees for reporting standardized results for all PT testing. Because the results are so critical to the therapy given, the standardization using the international sensitivity index for PT calculation permits a person on warfarin to obtain comparable results wherever he or she may be tested.

REVIEW: Yes ☐ No ☐

15. **Answer: c**

WHY: The milk sugar lactose is converted by the body into glucose and galactose by the action of an

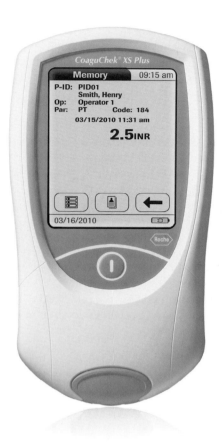

Figure 11-3 CoaguChek XS Plus for PT/INR testing (Courtesy of Roche Diagnostics Corporation, Indianapolis, IN.)

enzyme called mucosal lactase. A person lacking this enzyme has gastrointestinal distress and diarrhea when milk and other lactose-containing foods are consumed. Symptoms are relieved by eliminating milk from the diet.

REVIEW: Yes ☐ No ☐

16. **Answer: a**

WHY: The AVOXimeter 4000 (ITC) (Fig. 11-4) is designed to provide quick blood gas results owing to POC availability. It offers comprehensive evaluation of blood gases in approximately 10 seconds, enabling the physician to make critical decisions concerning care and treatment without delay. The other choices are POCT instruments designed to test C-reactive protein, lipids, and troponin, respectively.

REVIEW: Yes ☐ No ☐

17. **Answer: b**

WHY: The DCA Vantage (Siemens Health Care Diagnostics) (Fig. 11-5) measures glycosylated hemoglobin and is reported as a percentage of the total hemoglobin within an erythrocyte. Glycosylated hemoglobin is a diagnostic tool for monitoring

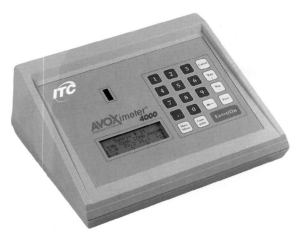

Figure 11-4 AVOXimeter for blood gases. (Courtesy of ITC, Edison, NJ.)

diabetes therapy. It was recently accepted as a more accurate predictor of complications in patients with diabetes than has been achieved with earlier techniques.

REVIEW: Yes ☐   No ☐

18. **Answer: d**

WHY: Potassium plays a major role in nerve conduction, muscle function, acid–base balance, and osmotic pressure. It has no role in transporting hemoglobin (Hgb).

REVIEW: Yes ☐   No ☐

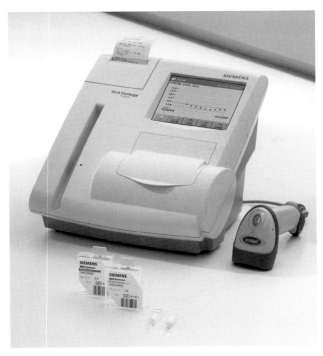

Figure 11-5 DCA Vantage and two different A1c test cartridges. (Courtesy of Siemens Healthcare Diagnostics, Deerfield, IL.)

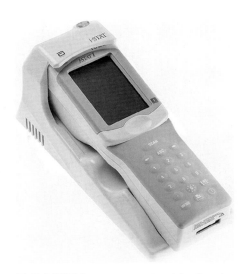

Figure 11-6 i-STAT instrument seated in the downloader/recharger. (Courtesy of Abbott Diagnostics, Abbott Park, IL.)

19. **Answer: d**

WHY: All glucose analyzers approved for use in healthcare facilities are made with the capability to download data to a data management system for the purposes of quality assurance, as shown in the photo of the iSTAT seated in the downloader/recharger (Fig. 11-6). To use one of these glucose analyzers, a person must be an authorized operator with an ID number. All instruments can use whole blood, and that blood can come from the capillary, venous, or arterial system.

REVIEW: Yes ☐   No ☐

20. **Answer: c**

WHY: It is not unusual for patients to be on antimicrobial (antibiotic) therapy at the time blood culture specimens are collected. The presence of the antimicrobial agent in the patient's blood can inhibit any growth of microorganisms in the blood culture bottle. Antimicrobial removal device (ARD) or fastidious antimicrobial neutralization (FAN) blood culture bottles (Fig. 11-7) contain, respectively, resins or activated charcoal that will neutralize antibiotics.

REVIEW: Yes ☐   No ☐

21. **Answer: d**

WHY: Septicemia is defined as microorganisms or their toxins in the blood. Bacteremia is a type of septicemia, but it is more specific to bacteria in the bloodstream.

REVIEW: Yes ☐   No ☐

📖 *Do Matching Exercise 11-1 in the WORKBOOK to reinforce your understanding of terminology in this chapter.*

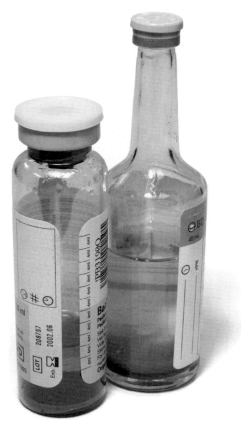

Figure 11-7 FAN and ARD blood culture bottles.

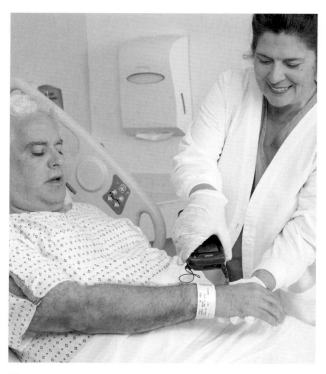

Figure 11-8 Siemens Patient Identification Check. (Courtesy of Siemens Medical Solutions, Malvern, PA.)

22. **Answer: c**

    WHY: The Siemens Patient Identification Check-Blood Administration system, as seen in Figure 11-8, is an example of an electronic blood bank ID system. It is a portable bedside bar code scanning system that provides electronic verification and tracing of the blood transfusion process. The bar-coded data are used throughout the transfusion process and appear on the unit of blood prepared for transfusion.

    REVIEW: Yes ☐ No ☐

23. **Answer: a**

    WHY: To donate blood, an individual must normally be between the ages of 17 and 66 and weigh at least 110 lb.

    REVIEW: Yes ☐ No ☐

24. **Answer: c**

    WHY: Hemochromatosis is a disease characterized by excess iron deposits in the tissues. Periodic removal of single units of blood gradually depletes excess iron stores, because the body then uses iron to make new red blood cells to replace those removed.

    REVIEW: Yes ☐ No ☐

25. **Answer: b**

    WHY: Specimens for cross-match testing require especially strict identification and labeling procedures. Misidentification of a specimen for a cross-match can cause a patient to receive an incompatible unit of blood and have a serious and possibly fatal transfusion reaction. Special blood bank specimen identification systems intended to reduce errors are available. Figure 11-9 shows a phlebotomist comparing information on a blood bank tube containing a label peeled from a special blood bank ID bracelet, with the carbon copy of the label on the bracelet attached to the patient's arm.

    REVIEW: Yes ☐ No ☐

26. **Answer: d**

    WHY: Amphetamines ("ice") and cocaine ("crack") are classified as drugs of abuse, as are cannabinoids (marijuana compounds). Phenobarbital is a drug that is prescribed for epilepsy, seizure prevention, and mood stabilization; it typically requires therapeutic monitoring.

    REVIEW: Yes ☐ No ☐

27. **Answer: a**

    WHY: Large-bore (16- to 18-gauge) needles are used to collect donor units. The large bore helps

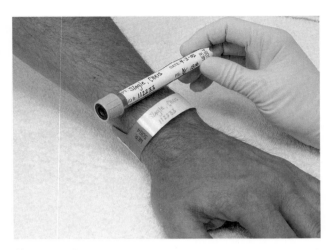

Figure 11-9 A phlebotomist compares a labeled blood bank tube with a blood bank ID bracelet.

keep the blood flowing freely and minimizes the hemolysis of red blood cells during collection.
REVIEW: Yes ☐   No ☐

28. **Answer: b**

WHY: A donor unit is filled by weight but typically contains around 450-mL blood.
REVIEW: Yes ☐   No ☐

29. **Answer: a**

WHY: The body's response to septicemia is to raise body temperature to kill the microorganisms. When a patient experiences fever with no known cause (referred to as fever of unknown origin, or FUO), a physician may suspect septicemia and order blood cultures. Figure 11-10 shows the equipment necessary for collecting a blood culture. Blood cultures are typically ordered immediately before or after anticipated fever spikes, when bacteria are most likely to be present. Recent studies have shown that the best chance of detecting bacteremia exists between 30 minutes and 2½ hours prior to the fever peak, before the body can eliminate some of the microorganisms. Therefore timely collection is essential.
REVIEW: Yes ☐   No ☐

30. **Answer: a**

WHY: A type and screen can be performed on a specimen collected in a nonadditive red-top, a lavender-top EDTA, or a special pink-top EDTA tube, depending on laboratory preference. Blood bank specimens are never collected in gel-barrier tubes because the gel and clot activator could affect antigen and antibody testing and cause erroneous results.
REVIEW: Yes ☐   No ☐

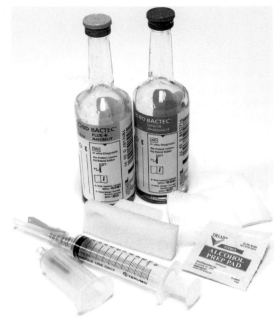

Figure 11-10 Blood culture equipment.

31. **Answer: c**

WHY: Skin antisepsis is a critical part of blood culture collection. A special skin decontamination procedure must be used when collecting blood cultures because the culture can become contaminated by normal microbial flora on the skin if these flora are not removed. This causes a major difficulty in interpreting the results.
REVIEW: Yes ☐   No ☐

32. **Answer: c**

WHY: A paternity test can determine the probability that a specific individual was the father of a particular child. Results of paternity tests can exclude an individual as the father rather than prove that he is the father.
REVIEW: Yes ☐   No ☐

33. **Answer: b**

WHY: It is not unusual for patients to be on antibiotics when a blood culture specimen is collected. Antibiotic present in the specimen can inhibit the growth of microorganisms and lead to a false-negative result. The special resin removes or neutralizes antibiotics. The blood is then cultured by conventional techniques.
REVIEW: Yes ☐   No ☐

34. **Answer: c**

WHY: Coagulation specimens must have a 9-to-1 ratio of blood to anticoagulant, or test results on the specimen will not be accurate. If a coagulation tube is not filled completely, this ratio is altered and the laboratory will not accept the specimen for testing.
REVIEW: Yes ☐   No ☐

35. **Answer: d**

    WHY: The recommended additive for collecting blood alcohol (ETOH) specimens is the antiglycolytic agent sodium fluoride. This agent prevents the breakdown of ETOH and stops the growth of bacteria; consequently, inhibiting possible bacterial fermentation that could increase the ETOH.

    REVIEW: Yes ☐   No ☐

36. **Answer: b**

    WHY: If both aerobic and anaerobic cultures are collected at one time, the anaerobic bottle is inoculated first when filled from a syringe. If a butterfly with tubing is used and blood is collected directly into the bottles, the aerobic bottle is filled first because air from the tubing will be drawn into the bottle ahead of the blood. The antimicrobial removal device (ARD) is a resin that is typically found in the bottles of aerobic and anaerobic media. Therefore inoculation into a separate container would not be required.

    REVIEW: Yes ☐   No ☐

37. **Answer: c**

    WHY: Skin antisepsis or asepsis, the destruction of microorganisms on the skin, is a critical part of the blood culture collection procedure, as seen in Figure 11-11. Failure to follow proper antiseptic technique can result in contamination of the blood culture by skin-surface bacteria or other microorganisms and interfere with the interpretation of results. The laboratory must report all microorganisms detected, so it is up to the patient's physician to determine whether the organism is clinically significant or merely a contaminant.

    REVIEW: Yes ☐   No ☐

38. **Answer: a**

    WHY: Antiseptic or sterile technique for blood culture collection varies slightly from one laboratory to another. Tincture of iodine, chlorhexidine gluconate, and a povidone/70% ethyl alcohol

    combination have all been shown to be effective in cleaning the collection site.

    REVIEW: Yes ☐   No ☐

39. **Answer: d**

    WHY: Blood is sometimes collected in an intermediate collection tube rather than blood culture bottles. A yellow-top sodium polyanethol sulfonate (SPS) tube is acceptable for this purpose. Other anticoagulants are toxic to bacteria and are not recommended.

    REVIEW: Yes ☐   No ☐

40. **Answer: b**

    WHY: If a coagulation specimen in a light blue-top tube is the first or only tube collected with a winged blood collection needle (butterfly) a discard tube must be collected first to prime the tubing. Otherwise, air in the tubing will take the place of blood in the specimen tube and the critical 9-to-1 ratio of blood to anticoagulant will be adversely affected.

    REVIEW: Yes ☐   No ☐

41. **Answer: d**

    WHY: Some pregnant women develop high blood glucose levels during pregnancy, a condition called gestational diabetes. The oral glucose challenge test (OGCT) is a modified version of the OGTT that screens for gestational diabetes. It is also called a 1-hour glucose screening test or gestational glucose screening test

    REVIEW: Yes ☐   No ☐

42. **Answer: a**

    WHY: *Postprandial* (PP) means "after a meal." Glucose levels in blood specimens obtained 2 hours after a meal are rarely elevated in normal individuals but may be significantly increased in diabetic patients. Therefore a glucose test on a specimen collected 2 hours after a meal (2-hour PP) is an excellent screening test for diabetes and other metabolic problems.

    REVIEW: Yes ☐   No ☐

43. **Answer: c**

    WHY: Chewing sugarless gum, drinking sugarless tea, and smoking cigarettes all stimulate the digestive process and therefore can affect GTT results. A person may feel nauseated during the testing and need to lie down, which is perfectly acceptable and does not affect the test results.

    REVIEW: Yes ☐   No ☐

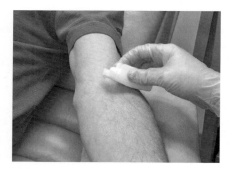

Figure 11-11 Performing a friction scrub.

44. **Answer: d**

WHY: The timing of specimen collection during a GTT begins as soon as the patient finishes the glucose beverage. For example, if a patient finishes the glucose beverage at 0805 hours, the ½-hour specimen is collected at 0835 hours, the 1-hour specimen is collected at 0905 hours, and so on. Timing of specimen collection is critical for computation of the GTT curve and correct interpretation of results.

REVIEW: Yes ☐ No ☐

45. **Answer: a**

WHY: If there is a discrepancy concerning the timing of a 2-hour postprandial specimen, the patient's nurse should be consulted to establish the correct time to draw the specimen. It is not a good idea to ask the patient because he or she may not know the correct time or understand the importance of exact timing. The specimen should not be collected early because glucose levels may still be elevated, leading to the misinterpretation of results. Filling out an incident report and returning to the laboratory may cause the correct collection time to be missed.

REVIEW: Yes ☐ No ☐

46. **Answer: d**

WHY: If a patient undergoing a GTT vomits within 30 minutes of drinking the glucose beverage, his or her nurse or physician should be notified immediately to determine if the test should be continued or rescheduled.

REVIEW: Yes ☐ No ☐

47. **Answer: a**

WHY: Increased blood glucose (sugar) is called hyperglycemia. Hyperinsulinism is excessive blood insulin levels, hyperkalemia is excessive blood potassium levels, and hypernatremia is excess sodium in the blood.

REVIEW: Yes ☐ No ☐

48. **Answer: b**

WHY: Blood glucose levels in normal individuals typically peak within 30 minutes to 1 hour of glucose ingestion and return to normal fasting levels within 2 hours. GTT specimen results are plotted on a graph to create what is referred to as a GTT curve. Figure 11-12 shows a graph with examples of normal and abnormal GTT curves.

REVIEW: Yes ☐ No ☐

49. **Answer: b**

WHY: OGTT is another name for a glucose tolerance test. Blood glucose levels vary according to the source of the specimen. It is important that the specimen source be consistent for the duration of the test for proper interpretation of results. Consequently, GTT blood specimens can be collected by capillary puncture or venipuncture but not by a combination of the two methods if at all possible.

REVIEW: Yes ☐ No ☐

50. **Answer: a**

WHY: Proper patient preparation before a GTT involves eating balanced meals containing 150 g of carbohydrate for 3 days prior to the test, fasting for at least 12 hours before the test, and avoiding smoking or chewing gum before or during the test. There is no exercise requirement.

REVIEW: Yes ☐ No ☐

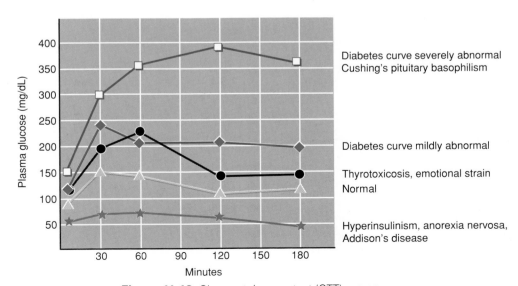

Figure 11-12 Glucose tolerance test (GTT) curves.

51. Answer: d

WHY: Zephiran chloride (benzalkonium chloride) and povidone–iodine are the preferred antiseptics for blood alcohol collection. Isopropyl alcohol (isopropanol) and methanol are types of alcohol. Alcohol solutions or alcohol-based antiseptics can cause problems in blood alcohol testing and should not be used to clean a site prior to the collection of a specimen for blood alcohol testing. Tincture of iodine cannot be used because tinctures contain alcohol.

REVIEW: Yes ☐   No ☐

52. Answer: c

WHY: Chain-of-custody documentation is required for legal or forensic specimens. Whether it is performed for legal reasons or not, drug screening

ORDERING PHYSICIAN/COMPANY OR FACILITY	SPECIMEN ID NO.	0000000	VARIABLE BARCODE
		Sonora Quest Laboratories	1255 West Washington Street
		A Subsidiary of Laboratory Sciences of Arizona	Tempe, Arizona 85281
			602.685.5000 • 800.766.6721
	LAB ACCESSION NO.		

CHAIN OF CUSTODY REQUISITION FORM

STEP 1: COMPLETED BY COLLECTOR OR EMPLOYER REPRESENTATIVE

Donor SSN or Employee I.D. No.

Donor Name: Last: First:

Donor ID Verified: ☐ Photo ID   ☐ Emp. Rep. _____

Reason for Test: ☐ Pre-employment   ☐ Random   ☐ Reasonable Suspicion/Cause   ☐ Post-Accident   ☐ Promotion
                    ☐ Return to Duty   ☐ Follow-up   ☐ Other (specify) _____

Drug Tests to be Performed:

STEP 2: COMPLETED BY COLLECTOR (Collector Instructions)

| Read specimen temperature within 4 minutes. Is temperature between 90° and 100° F? ☐ Yes ☐ No, Enter Remark | Specimen Collection: ☐ Split   ☐ Single   ☐ None Provided (Enter Remark)   ☐ Observed (Enter Remark) |
| REMARKS | |

Collection Site Address/Site Code:

Collector Phone No. _____

Collector Fax No. _____

STEP 3: Collector affixes bottle seal(s) to bottle(s). Collector dates seal(s). Donor initials seal(s). Donor completes STEP 5
STEP 4: CHAIN OF CUSTODY - INITIATED BY COLLECTOR AND COMPLETED BY LABORATORY

I certify that the specimen given to me by the donor identified in step 1 of this form was collected, labeled, sealed and released to the Delivery Service noted.

X _____
Signature of Collector   Time of Collection   AM/PM   ► **SPECIMEN BOTTLE(S) RELEASED TO:**

_____   _____
(PRINT) Collector's Name (First, MI, Last)   Date (Mo./Day/Yr.)   ►   Name of Delivery Service Transferring Specimen to Lab

RECEIVED AT LAB: | **Primary Specimen Bottle Seal Intact** | **SPECIMEN BOTTLE(S) RELEASED TO:** |
X _____ | | |
Signature of Accessioner | | |
_____ | ☐ Yes | |
(PRINT) Accessioner's Name (First, MI, Last)   Date (Mo./Day/Yr.) | ☐ No, Enter Remark Below | |

STEP 5: COMPLETED BY DONOR

I certify that I provided my urine specimen to the collector; that I have not adulterated it in any manner; each specimen bottle used was sealed with a tamper-evident seal in my presence; and that the information numbers provided on this form and on the label affixed to each specimen bottle is correct.

X _____
Signature of Donor   (PRINT) Donor's Name (First, MI, Last)   Date (Mo./Day/Yr.)

Daytime Phone No. (   )   Evening Phone No. (   )   Date of Birth   __/__/__   Mo. Day Yr.

Sonora Quest Laboratories
Q7230 (Rev. 9/07)

COPY 1 - LABORATORY   COPY 2 - COLLECTOR COPY   COPY 3 - COMPANY/MRO COPY   COPY 4 - LABORATORY-CONFIDENTIAL DONOR

Figure 11-13 Chain-of-custody requisition form. (Courtesy of Sonora Quest Laboratories, Tempe, AZ.)

has legal implications that require the use of a chain-of-custody protocol. Figure 11-13 shows an example of a chain-of-custody requisition form.

REVIEW: Yes ☐ No ☐

53. Answer: a

WHY: Therapeutic drug monitoring (TDM) is performed to determine and maintain a beneficial drug dosage for a patient. Peak drug levels represent the highest serum concentrations of a drug and are collected during TDM to screen for drug toxicity. Trough drug levels are monitored during TDM to ensure that drug levels stay within the therapeutic or effective range. TDM has nothing to do with screening for illegal drug use.

REVIEW: Yes ☐ No ☐

📖 ***Try Knowledge Drill 11-5 in the WORKBOOK if you would like to review the therapeutic drugs and the conditions associated with them.***

54. Answer: c

WHY: Digitoxin, gentamicin, and theophylline are drugs. Phenylalanine is an amino acid, not a drug.

REVIEW: Yes ☐ No ☐

55. Answer: d

WHY: Timing of TDM specimens is extremely important. A pharmacist calculates drug dosages based on blood levels of the drug at specific times. If a specimen is collected late, it is important that the actual time of collection be recorded so that the pharmacist will be aware of the time change and can calculate values accordingly. It is not the phlebotomist's responsibility to establish the collection time. Not collecting the specimen and leaving a notification with the desk clerk or at the nursing station could cause an unnecessary and expensive delay.

REVIEW: Yes ☐ No ☐

56. Answer: b

WHY: A trough, or minimum drug level, is collected when the lowest serum concentration of the drug is expected. A trough drug level is easiest to obtain because it is collected immediately before administration of the next scheduled drug dose.

REVIEW: Yes ☐ No ☐

57. Answer: b

WHY: A GTT involves the collection of multiple blood specimens. Blood specimens are serially collected at specific times throughout the duration of the test. Urine specimens are sometimes collected at the same time as the blood specimens.

REVIEW: Yes ☐ No ☐

58. Answer: b

WHY: A half-life is the time required for the body to metabolize half the amount of the drug. Timing of collection is most critical for aminoglycoside drugs with short half-lives, such as gentamicin, amikacin, and tobramycin. Timing is less critical for drugs such as phenobarbital, methotrexate, and digitoxin, which have longer half-lives.

REVIEW: Yes ☐ No ☐

59. Answer: d

WHY: Clinical molecular genetic testing provides for detection of genetic variations that can (1) identify whether an individual has a certain genetic disease, (2) determine whether an individual has an increased risk for a particular disease, (3) classify an individual's genetic makeup to determine whether a drug and dosage is suitable for a particular patient, and (4) examine the whole genome to discover genetic alterations that may cause disease.

REVIEW: Yes ☐ No ☐

60. Answer: c

WHY: Glucose monitoring in patients with diabetes mellitus is the most common reason for performing glucose testing through point-of-care testing (POCT) for glucose. An example of a POCT glucose analyzer is seen in Figure 11-14, Accu-Chek Inform II System kit.

REVIEW: Yes ☐ No ☐

61. Answer: c

WHY: Traces of elements or minerals such as copper, lead, and zinc can be contaminants in glass

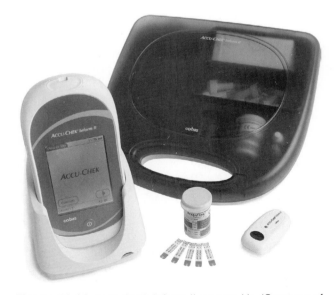

Figure 11-14 Accu-Chek Inform II system kit. (Courtesy of Roche Diagnostics, Indianapolis, IN.)

and other materials used to make blood collection tubes and stoppers and can leach from the tube into the specimen. Trace element–free tubes have the lowest possible contaminating amounts of these elements. Iron, lead, and zinc are all elements or minerals measured in such small quantities that it is best if they are collected in trace element–free tubes. Sodium is not considered a trace element.

REVIEW: Yes ☐ No ☐

62. **Answer: b**

WHY: *Toxicology* is defined as the scientific study of poisons or toxins. There are two types: clinical toxicology and forensic toxicology. Clinical toxicology comprises the detection of toxins and treatment of their effects. Forensic toxicology is concerned with the legal consequences of both intentional and accidental exposure to toxins.

REVIEW: Yes ☐ No ☐

63. **Answer: a**

WHY: Turnaround time (TAT) in laboratory testing is the amount of time that elapses between when a test is ordered and when the results are returned. BUN results are part of a panel that can be performed on small, portable handheld instruments, such as the I-STAT. Once the instrument's cartridge is injected with blood, the BUN test results are available in approximately 2 minutes. Calibration of the instrument, which is done internally by the instrument every 8 hours, does not add any appreciable time. A GTT is a timed test involving the collection of serial specimens over a period of 1 to 6 hours, depending on how the test is ordered by the physician. A DNA profile can be performed on buccal samples, which are collected by rubbing a swab against the inside of the cheek to collect loose cells. DNA results are not immediate; TAT may be several days. PSA is not a POC test and must be collected by venipuncture, processed in the laboratory, and delivered for testing, which makes for a TAT of several hours at least.

REVIEW: Yes ☐ No ☐

64. **Answer: d**

WHY: ABL80, CoaguChek, and GEM Premier 4000 are all POCT analyzers. BacT/ALERT, as shown in Figure 11-15, is a blood culture media bottle with collection adapter.

REVIEW: Yes ☐ No ☐

📖 *Try to match the POCT analyzer with the name in Labeling Exercise 11-1 in the WORKBOOK.*

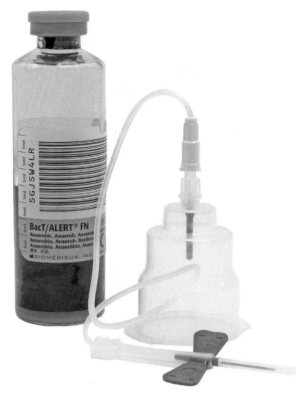

Figure 11-15 BacT/ALERT FN anaerobic blood culture bottle including a specially designed holder for a butterfly needle. (bioMerieux Inc., Durham, NC.)

65. **Answer: b**

WHY: In collecting trace elements, it is important to prevent introducing even the smallest amount of the contaminating substance into the tube, since the amounts being tested are in the range of micro- or nanograms. Contaminants in the stoppers accumulate in the needle each time a different tube is pierced in a multiple-tube collection. That accumulation can then carry over to the royal blue–stoppered tube, thus changing the results. When a trace-element test is ordered, it is best to draw it by itself if you are using a needle/tube assembly or to use a syringe. For best results, change the syringe transfer device before filling the royal-blue tube.

REVIEW: Yes ☐ No ☐

66. **Answer: c**

WHY: Whole-blood glucose or bedside glucose monitoring is one of the most common point-of-care tests. Troponin and cholesterol are point-of-care tests but are not performed nearly as often. Bilirubin testing is not commonly performed at the bedside.

REVIEW: Yes ☐ No ☐

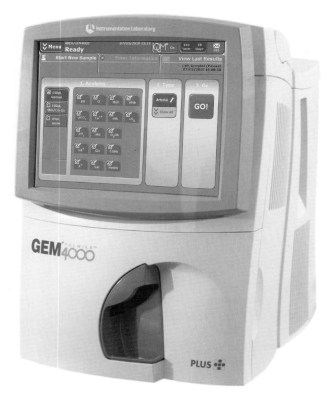

Figure 11-16 GEM Premier 4000 used for ACT determinations. (Courtesy of Instrumentation Laboratory, Lexington, MA.)

67. **Answer: a**

    WHY: The activated clotting time (ACT) test is used to monitor heparin therapy. The GEM Premier 4000 (Fig. 11-16) analyzer is an example of a POCT instrument used to perform ACT tests. The prothrombin time (PT) is used to monitor warfarin (Coumadin) therapy. The bleeding-time test (BT) evaluates platelet function. B-type natriuretic peptide (BNP) is a cardiac hormone produced by the heart; it helps physicians differentiate chronic obstructive pulmonary disease (COPD) from congestive heart failure (CHF).

    REVIEW: Yes ☐   No ☐

68. **Answer: c**

    WHY: Lead is a trace element that can be collected in a royal-blue trace element–free tube that contains K_2ETDA, or a special tan-top tube that contains K_2ETDA.

    REVIEW: Yes ☐   No ☐

69. **Answer: d**

    WHY: At one time all POCT required external quality control (QC) to be performed daily if any patient testing was to be done that day. Today the College of American Pathologists (CAP) requires that external liquid control be performed only as specified

by the manufacturer's instructions on many of the waived tests.

    REVIEW: Yes ☐   No ☐

70. **Answer: d**

    WHY: The new Bilichek meter (Philips Healthcare) allows for a noninvasive, transcutaneous bilirubin measurement system for newborns. Using light from the meter on the baby's head or sternum, the meter can measure bilirubin levels across the depth of the skin and can be done wherever the newborn is, even in the mother's room. Instruments such as this take optical density readings that show a linear correlation with the serum total bilirubin concentration.

    REVIEW: Yes ☐   No ☐

71. **Answer: b**

    WHY: A type of metabolic acidosis called lactic acidosis is due to hyperlactatemia (increased lactate in the blood). Hyperlactatemia is usually present in patients with severe sepsis or septic shock.

    REVIEW: Yes ☐   No ☐

72. **Answer: b**

    WHY: Skin tests involve intradermal injection of an antigenic substance that causes an allergic response if the patient has an antibody directed against it, but testing does not cause the disease. For example, to perform a tuberculin (TB) skin test, a modified TB antigen is injected just under the skin on a patient's forearm. (Properly injected antigen forms a temporary wheal or bleb.) If the patient has TB antibodies, they will combine with the antigen to cause a visible reaction on the surface of the skin within 48 to 72 hours.

    REVIEW: Yes ☐   No ☐

73. **Answer: c**

    WHY: Ionized calcium makes up approximately 45% of the calcium in the blood. The rest is bound to protein and other substances. Only ionized calcium can be used for critical functions such as blood clotting, cardiac function, and nerve impulses. Glycosylation is the forming of links between glucose and hemoglobin. Ionized calcium does not play a critical role in this process.

    REVIEW: Yes ☐   No ☐

74. **Answer: a**

    WHY: Normal arterial blood pH is 7.35 to 7.45. Below-normal blood pH is called acidosis.

Above-normal pH is called alkalosis. Hyponatremia is reduced sodium in the blood. Hypokalemia is reduced potassium in the blood.

REVIEW: Yes ☐ No ☐

75. **Answer: d**

WHY: Troponin T (TnT) is a protein that is specific to heart muscle. It is measured in the diagnosis of acute myocardial infarction (MI), or heart attack.

REVIEW: Yes ☐ No ☐

📖 *Test your knowledge of abbreviations and terminology in this chapter with the crossword puzzle found in the WORKBOOK.*

76. **Answer: c**

WHY: B-type natriuretic peptide (BNP) is a cardiac hormone produced by the heart in response to ventricular volume expansion and pressure overload. It is the first objective measurement for congestive heart failure (CHF). This test allows the physician to differentiate between CHF and chronic obstructive pulmonary disease (COPD).

REVIEW: Yes ☐ No ☐

77. **Answer: c**

WHY: Hemoglobin A1c is a type of hemoglobin formed by glycosylation (the reaction of glucose with hemoglobin). Figure 11-5 shows a POCT meter used for hemoglobin A1c measurement. Glycosylated Hgb levels reflect the average blood glucose level during the preceding 4 to 6 weeks and therefore can be used to evaluate the long-term effectiveness of diabetes therapy.

REVIEW: Yes ☐ No ☐

78. **Answer: b**

WHY: The hematocrit (HCT) test is a measure of the volume of RBCs in a patient's blood. It is also called packed cell volume (PCV) because it can be calculated by centrifuging a specific volume of anticoagulated blood to separate the cells from the plasma, thus determining the proportion of red blood cells to plasma. The StatSpin CritSpin (Fig. 11-17) is a microhematocrit centrifuge that is small and portable enough to be used in a "point-of-care" setting.

REVIEW: Yes ☐ No ☐

79. **Answer: b**

WHY: Occult blood is hidden or present in such small amounts that it is not apparent on visual examination. The guaiac test detects hidden blood in feces by using an alcoholic solution of a tree resin called guaiac. Detection of occult blood in stool (feces) is an important tool in diagnosing gastric ulcers and screening for colon cancer.

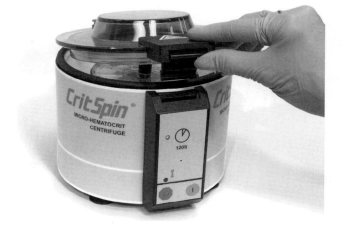

Figure 11-17 StatSpin CritSpin MicroHematocrit centrifuge. (IRIS International, Inc., Chatsworth, CA.)

Several different companies make occult blood kits containing special cards like the ones shown in Figure 11-18, on which fecal samples are collected and tested.

REVIEW: Yes ☐ No ☐

80. **Answer: c**

WHY: The test for tuberculosis exposure, the tuberculin (TB) test, is also called a PPD test because of the purified protein derivative (PPD) used in testing. The Cocci test is for an infectious fungus disease caused by *Coccidioides immitis*; the Histo test detects present or past infection with the fungus *Histoplasma capsulatum*; and the Schick test is for susceptibility to diphtheria.

REVIEW: Yes ☐ No ☐

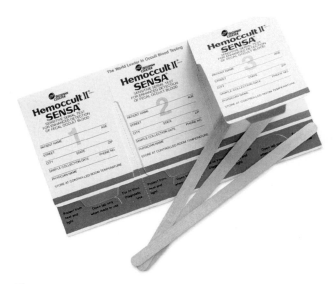

Figure 11-18 Hemoccult II Sensa occult blood collection cards. (Beckman Coulter, Fullerton, CA.)

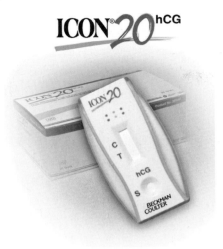

Figure 11-19 Icon 20 HCG urine assay. (Beckman Coulter, Inc., San Diego, CA.)

81. **Answer: b**

    WHY: Most rapid urine pregnancy tests detect human chorionic gonadotropin (hCG), a hormone produced by the placenta that appears in both urine and serum beginning approximately 10 days after conception. Peak urine levels of hCG occur at approximately 10 weeks of gestation. An example of a urine pregnancy testing kit is the Beckman Coulter Icon hCG urine assay (Fig. 11-19).

    REVIEW: Yes ☐   No ☐

82. **Answer: b**

    WHY: HemoCue HB 201+ blood analyzer (Fig. 11-20) uses a microcuvette instead of a test strip. The Cascade POC uses assay reagent cards, and the Precision Xceed uses a reagent strip for testing. The i-STAT uses a special cartridge for testing.

    REVIEW: Yes ☐   No ☐

83. **Answer: b**

    WHY: Potassium is an electrolyte. The body maintains electrolytes in specific proportions within narrow ranges, and any uncorrected imbalance can lead to death. Potassium plays a major role in nerve conduction, muscle function, acid–base balance, and osmotic pressure. It influences cardiac output by helping to control the rate and force of heart contraction.

    REVIEW: Yes ☐   No ☐

84. **Answer: b**

    WHY: Platelet function testing allows the clinician to determine a patient's response to medication before open heart surgery or cardiac catheterization. This can help prevent excessive bleeding or blood clots. The testing can be done with an automated

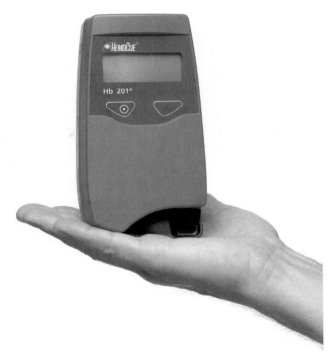

Figure 11-20 HB 201+ blood analyzer for measuring hemoglobin in arterial, venous, or capillary blood. (Courtesy of HemoCue, Inc., Lake Forest, CA.)

analyzer and single-use, disposable assays; it is called the VerifyNow System (Fig. 11-21). This system uses whole-blood samples and gives measurements that correlate with laboratory testing. The VerifyNow System Aspirin Assay, which is CLIA-waived, provides a measurement to determine whether or not a patient is responding to aspirin therapy.

REVIEW: Yes ☐   No ☐

85. **Answer: b**

    WHY: When one is performing a PPD or tuberculin (TB) test, 0.1 mL of diluted antigen is injected under the skin. The antigen injected is purified protein derivative, or PPD.

    REVIEW: Yes ☐   No ☐

86. **Answer: c**

    WHY: *Erythema* means redness.

    REVIEW: Yes ☐   No ☐

87. **Answer: a**

    WHY: Skin-test reactions often produce erythema (redness), induration (hardness), or both around the injection site. Interpretation of a TB skin test is based on the presence or absence of induration, or a firm raised area of swelling around the injection site. A positive test results when the area of induration measures 10 mm or greater in diameter. An

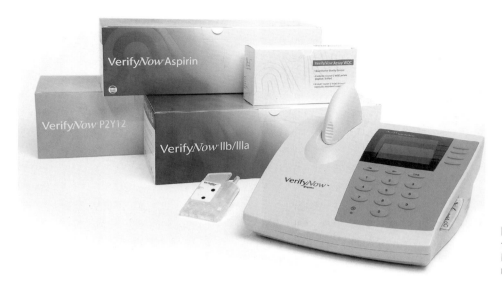

Figure 11-21 VerifyNow System is used to measure platelet function. (Courtesy of Accumetrics, San Diego, CA.)

area between 5 and 9 mm is considered doubtful. An area of less than 5 mm is considered negative.
REVIEW: Yes ☐ No ☐

88. **Answer: c**

WHY: Point-of-care detection of group A strep normally requires a throat-swab specimen. Secretions from the swab are tested for the presence of strep A antigen. Several different companies make special test kits (Fig. 11-22) for the rapid detection of strep A.
REVIEW: Yes ☐ No ☐

89. **Answer: d**

WHY: Bilirubin, glucose, and leukocytes are all commonly detected in urine by reagent-strip methods. Reagent strips also typically detect bacteria, blood, pH, protein, specific gravity, and urobilinogen. A

chemical reaction resulting in color changes to the strip takes place when the strip is dipped in a urine specimen. Results are determined by visually comparing color changes on the strip with a chart of color codes on the reagent-strip container (Fig. 11-23). Thrombin is a clot activator found in the RST tube.
REVIEW: Yes ☐ No ☐

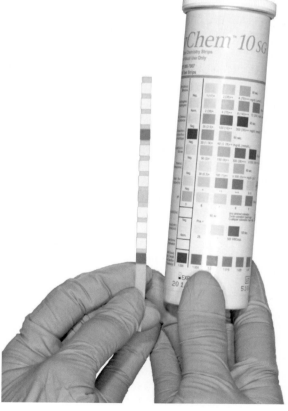

Figure 11-23 Technician comparing a urine reagent strip with the chart on a reagent-strip container.

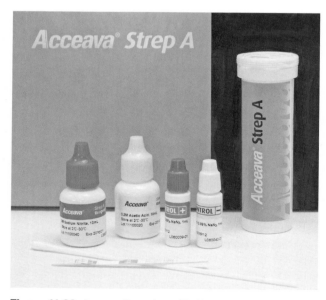

Figure 11-22 Acceava Strep A test kit. (Alere Inc., Waltham, MA.)

90. **Answer: c**

WHY: C-reactive protein (CRP) is a β-globulin found in the blood that responds to inflammation and can be used as a nonspecific marker of systemic inflammation. Alanine transferase (ALT) is a liver enzyme that is monitored when a patient is on lipid-lowering medication. B-type natriuretic peptide (BNP) is a cardiac hormone and a measurement for congestive heart failure (CHF). TnT is a protein specific to heart muscle and is measured to assist in the diagnosis of acute myocardial infarction.

REVIEW: Yes ☐ No ☐

91. **Answer: a**

WHY: The term "chain-of-custody" refers to the paper trail associated with detailed documentation of forensic specimen collection from the time of collection to the reporting of results. The specimen must be accounted for at all times. This special protocol must be strictly followed so that any legal action is not compromised.

REVIEW: Yes ☐ No ☐

92. **Answer: d**

WHY: Many healthcare organizations, sports associations, and major companies require workplace drug screening for preemployment, prepromotion, postaccident or injury, random screening (without prior notice), reasonable suspicion and for any other situation that they deem important. It is not necessarily part of an annual health screening or an extended leave of absence. The normal

procedure is for a designated person or collector to oversee the complete process of urine collection on a specified day and time.

REVIEW: Yes ☐ No ☐

93. **Answer: d**

WHY: An illicit drug is one that is prohibited by law to be used. Synthetic types of illicit drugs are also prohibited.

REVIEW: Yes ☐ No ☐

94. **Answer: c**

WHY: It is the National Institute on Drug Abuse (NIDA) that is undertaking this project because there have been major advances in understanding drug use, addiction, and recovery. NIDA will support more research that has to be done and then the sharing of the results of the research quickly and effectively so that drug abuse can be prevented, treated and policies can be formed on how to handle addiction and abuse.

REVIEW: Yes ☐ No ☐

95. **Answer: d**

WHY: The Joint Commission's National Patient Safety Goals (NPSGs) program is the overall CQI requirements for accreditation. For 2015, NPSG Goal 01.01.01 is to use at least two ways to identify patients. For example, use the patient's name and date of birth. This is done to make sure that each patient gets the correct medicine and treatment.

REVIEW: Yes ☐ No ☐

Chapter 12

Computers and Specimen Handling and Processing

Study Tips

- Study the key points and cautions in the corresponding chapter of the TEXTBOOK. Describe a theme they all indicate. Place a "P" next to caution statements that address a patient safety issue. Place an "S" next to those that address specimen quality issues. Use a "P" and an "S" for statements that address both issues.

- Make a flow sheet to trace what happens to the test request once it is entered into the LIS on nursing unit. Use LIS terminology when describing the process.

- Boldly write the headers as listed in Box 12-1 on individual sticky notes, and put them on a wall or white board. Then write each source of preanalytical error on individual sticky notes. Mix them up as you stick them on a wall or board and then rearrange them under the headers.

- Find every different collection tube you have access to and describe how you would handle a specimen in that tube when received in central processing.

- Complete the activities in Chapter 12 of the companion WORKBOOK.

Overview

Today many aspects of patient care are connected through computerized networking, even in the smallest clinic or physician's office. The phlebotomist is involved in certain aspects of the laboratory computer information system as it tracks patient specimens from the time they are collected until the results are reported. This chapter covers knowledge of computer components, general computer skills, and associated terminology. The chapter also addresses proper specimen handling and processing, including how to recognize sources of preanalytical error that may have occurred previous to receiving the specimen in the laboratory. A thorough understanding of handling and processing helps the phlebotomist avoid preanalytical errors that can render the most skillfully obtained specimen useless and also helps ensure that results obtained on a specimen accurately reflect the status of the patient.

Review Questions

Choose the BEST answer.

1. A mnemonic is a
   a. memory aid.
   b. number code.
   c. program icon.
   d. secret phrase.

2. A barcode is a
   a. coded instruction needed to control computer hardware.
   b. confidential computer code that is required by the HIPAA.
   c. series of bars and spaces representing numbers or letters.
   d. unique number given to each test request for ID purposes.

3. A pneumatic tube is a
   a. pressurized air transportation system.
   b. temporary computer data storage unit.
   c. tube connection between two computers.
   d. type of collection tube for blood gases.

4. This is permanent computer memory that instructs the computer to carry out user-requested operations.
   a. CPU
   b. LIS
   c. RAM
   d. ROM

5. Computerized analyzers in the laboratory can read barcodes and ID patients if the
   a. barcode is anywhere on the specimen.
   b. label is placed horizontally on the tube.
   c. label is placed correctly on the tube.
   d. specimen is in the right evacuated tube.

6. Which one of the following methods should be used to prevent exposure to aerosols generated when transferring plasma or serum to the aliquot tube?
   a. Pipetting liquid into the secondary tube held behind a shield
   b. Pouring the serum from primary tube into an aliquot tube
   c. Withdrawing the specimen through the stopper by syringe
   d. All of the above

7. Which one of the following describes proper aliquot preparation?
   a. Immediately covering aliquot tubes after transferring the specimen
   b. Labeling tubes after pipetting the sample into the aliquot tube
   c. Pouring plasma from different additive tubes into one aliquot tube
   d. Pouring samples into aliquot tubes instead of using transfer pipettes

8. This organization develops standards for specimen handling and processing.
   a. CDC
   b. CLIA
   c. CLSI
   d. FDA

9. Interface means
   a. checking quality control results on instrumentation.
   b. entering data into a laboratory information system.
   c. interacting through the connection of computers.
   d. standardizing all laboratory ordering and testing.

10. ESR determinations on specimens held at room temperature must be made within
    a. 1 hour.
    b. 4 hours.
    c. 12 hours.
    d. 24 hours.

11. Which of the following is the best way to prepare routine blood specimen tubes for transportation to an off-site lab?
    a. Place the tubes in ice slurry.
    b. Seal the tubes in plastic bags.
    c. Wipe each tube with alcohol.
    d. Wrap the tubes in the requisitions.

12. Which of the following specimens is least likely to require special handling?
    a. Bilirubin
    b. Cholesterol
    c. Gastrin
    d. Homocysteine

13. This is an example of a preanalytical error made at the time of collection.
    a. Delay in transporting
    b. Failing to mix tubes
    c. Incomplete requisition
    d. Waiting to centrifuge

14. Transferring specimens into aliquot tubes has inherent risks. Which of the following involves the least risk?
    a. Aerosols created during transfer
    b. Aliquot tubes that are prelabeled
    c. Serum and plasma's similar color
    d. Specimens that are biohazardous

15. This is a source of preanalytical error that occurs before specimen collection.
    a. Dehydrated patient
    b. Incorrect needle size
    c. Mislabeled ETS tube
    d. Wrong collection time

16. HIPAA was enacted to
    a. examine all patient healthcare records.
    b. protect HCW from malpractice issues.
    c. provide guidelines for sharing of PHI.
    d. standardize patient electronic records.

17. Special handheld computer systems used in laboratory medicine are capable of
    a. displaying what tubes to collect.
    b. generating labels for specimens.
    c. reading barcodes on ID bracelets.
    d. all of the above.

18. Critical values (test values that are considered life-threatening) are also called
    a. alarm values.
    b. at-risk values.
    c. panic values.
    d. unstable values.

19. Which of the following would be a preanalytical error related to specimen storage?
    a. Exposure to light
    b. Faulty technique
    c. Inadequate fast
    d. Underfilled tube

20. Which of the following would be a preanalytical error related to specimen transport?
    a. Agitation-induced hemolysis
    b. Contamination caused by dust
    c. Incorrect collection tube
    d. Strenuous, recent exercise

21. A USB drive is a
    a. network connection device.
    b. secondary storage device.
    c. terminal linking device.
    d. word processing device.

22. Cellular metabolism in specimens that have not been separated from the cells will affect which of the following analytes?
    a. Amylase
    b. Calcitonin
    c. Hemoglobin
    d. Triglycerides

23. Glycolysis by the cells in blood specimens can falsely lower glucose values at a rate of
    a. 1% to 3% per hour.
    b. 3% to 5% per hour.
    c. 4% to 6% per hour.
    d. 5% to 7% per hour.

24. Which of the following samples are time-sensitive?
    a. ESR determinations in EDTA tubes
    b. PTT samples that have been opened
    c. RNA samples collected in PPT tubes
    d. All of the above

25. Which of the following temperatures is acceptable for a specimen that requires transportation and handling at room temperature?
    a. −20°C
    b. 8°C
    c. 25°C
    d. 37°C

26. Some blood specimens require cooling to
    a. avoid hemolysis of RBCs.
    b. prevent premature clotting.
    c. promote serum separation.
    d. slow metabolic processes.

27. Which one of the following activities is least likely to take place in central processing or triage?
    a. Accessioning or logging
    b. Analysis and reporting
    c. Evaluation for suitability
    d. Sorting by department

28. It is unlikely that removing the stopper from a specimen will cause
    a. contamination.
    b. evaporation.
    c. increase in pH.
    d. loss of iCa^{2+}.

29. If a specimen has inadequate identification, the specimen processor may
    a. add the missing information to the label.
    b. ask the phlebotomist to get a new sample.
    c. contact the patient for correct information.
    d. refer the tube to the laboratory supervisor.

30. RFID, as used in health care, is a/an
    a. abbreviation for a new disinfectant.
    b. LIS mnemonic for a chemistry test.
    c. method of specimen identification.
    d. a new fire extinguisher safety code.

31. An example of a preanalytical error happening during specimen processing is
    a. faulty collection technique.
    b. inadequate centrifugation.
    c. insufficient specimen.
    d. patient stress and anxiety.

32. To be considered computer literate, an individual must be able to
    a. explain how POCT instruments are connected to the LIS.
    b. design programs for job-specific problems in your area.
    c. perform daily QA documentation in database software.
    d. understand the computer and the functions it performs.

33. This is a term for a group of computers linked together for the purpose of sharing information.
    a. Junction
    b. Network
    c. Node unit
    d. Terminal

34. Data can be entered or input into a computer from
    a. applications.
    b. modems.
    c. printers.
    d. scanners.

35. Which of the following tests requires only 3 to 4 inversions of the collection tube?
    a. CBC
    b. HbA1c
    c. PTT
    d. RBC

36. Which of the following is a function of a computer monitor?
    a. Instructs the computer to carry out user-requested operations
    b. Manages the processing and completion of user-required tasks
    c. Performs mathematical processes and comparisons of data
    d. Provides visible display of all the information being processed

37. Random access memory (RAM)
    a. can be lost when the computer program is closed.
    b. includes data, software, hardware, and peripherals.
    c. instructs the computer to carry out user operations.
    d. is permanent memory installed by manufacturers.

38. According to CLSI, which tubes should be placed upright as soon as they are mixed?
    a. Gel tubes with anticoagulant
    b. Light green gel barrier tubes
    c. Light blue coagulation tubes
    d. Nonanticoagulant gel tubes

39. Systems software includes
    a. coded instructions that control processing of data.
    b. programs from software companies sold as a unit.
    c. the central processing unit and all hardware additions.
    d. word processing, spreadsheet, and graphic programs.

40. The laboratory has a computerized laboratory information system (LIS). Once an inpatient specimen has been collected by a phlebotomist and returned to the laboratory, what occurs next?
    a. A collection list is generated.
    b. All lab test orders are retrieved.
    c. Collection labels are printed.
    d. Specimen collection is verified.

41. A computer terminal is a
    a. keyboard and computer screen workstation.
    b. last computer in a series of matching terminals.
    c. printer where information can be displayed.
    d. screen that visually displays data to the user.

42. A test sample that is not recommended to be sent in a pneumatic tube is
    a. alkaline phosphatase.
    b. blood creatinine.
    c. serum potassium.
    d. total bilirubin.

43. Which of the following would be described as logging on?
    a. Accessing the Internet from a computer
    b. Entering a password to access the LIS
    c. Turning the computer terminal to "on"
    d. Using menus to navigate the program

44. To process input data, a computer user must
    a. log off of the Web.
    b. move the cursor.
    c. press the enter key.
    d. select an LIS icon.

45. Computer verification of test orders is *best* described as a process that allows a user to
    a. access the system to view the patient's diagnosis.
    b. confirm that the test was ordered by a physician.
    c. establish that the appropriate test was ordered.
    d. modify, delete, or accept test orders after review of data.

46. The "order inquiry" function allows the user to
    a. check the physician's diagnosis.
    b. edit or delete duplicate test orders.
    c. find errors in patient identification.
    d. retrieve all test orders on a patient.

47. Which of the following is confidential and unique to a single computer user?
    a. Entry icon
    b. ID code
    c. LIS menu
    d. Password

48. Central processors who send out specimens to another location must be certified by
    a. ASCP.
    b. CLIA.
    c. CLSI.
    d. DOT.

49. What does the laboratory use to identify a specimen throughout the testing process?
    a. Accession number
    b. Hospital number
    c. LIS image/icon
    d. Mnemonic code

50. Using the information from the computer requisition in Figure 12-1, identify the number that points to the time the specimen is to be collected.
    a. 1
    b. 6
    c. 7
    d. 9

51. Using the information from the computer requisition in Figure 12-1, identify the number that points to the color of tube required.
    a. 4
    b. 5
    c. 7
    d. 10

52. Using the information from the computer requisition in Figure 12-1, identify the number that points to the specimen accession number.
    a. 1
    b. 3
    c. 6
    d. 9

53. When using computer-generated specimen labels, what information must typically be added to the label after a specimen is collected?
    a. Medical record number
    b. Patient's complete name
    c. Patient's date of birth
    d. Phlebotomist's initials

54. A bidirectional computer interface allows
    a. computer RAM storage capacity to double in size.
    b. data to upload or download between two systems.
    c. information to go from two analyzers to the LIS.
    d. two persons to use a computer at the same time.

55. According to CLSI, there is a 2-hour time limit for separating serum and plasma from the cells for which of the following tests?
    a. Lactic acid
    b. Creatinine
    c. Total bilirubin
    d. Troponin T

56. In computer language, "hard copy" is
    a. data stored on disks or USB drives.
    b. information displayed on the CRT.
    c. lab results stored on the hard drive.
    d. processed data printed on paper.

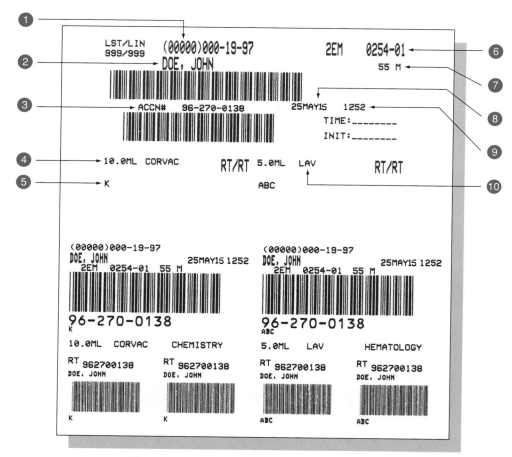

Figure 12-1 Computer requisition with bar code.

57. The Cobas, an automated chemistry instrument, is temporarily inoperable because of a serum sample. What could be the cause?
    a. Fibrin clot in the SST
    b. Hemolysis in a PST
    c. Lipemia in the SST
    d. Microclots in an EDTA

58. In specimen handling it is very important to appreciate that
    a. effects of mishandling the specimen are not always obvious.
    b. centrifuging specimens are considered to be error-free.
    c. most laboratory errors occur in the postanalytical phase.
    d. quality of results is not affected by collection procedure.

59. Proper specimen handling begins
    a. as soon as the specimen is collected.
    b. during specimen collection procedures.
    c. in the course of patient identification.
    d. when the physician orders the test.

60. You are the only phlebotomist in an outpatient drawing station. A physician orders a test with which you are not familiar. What is the appropriate action to take?
    a. Call the physician's office for assistance.
    b. Draw both a serum and a plasma specimen.
    c. Refer to the user manual for instructions.
    d. Send the patient to another drawing station.

61. The number of tube inversions required during specimen collection depends on
    a. how difficult it is to collect the blood.
    b. manufacturer-recommended inversions.
    c. the amount of blood in the evacuated tube.
    d. which needle gauge is used in collection.

62. Inadequate mixing of an anticoagulant tube can lead to
    a. hemolysis of the specimen.
    b. lipemia of the specimen.
    c. microclots in the specimen.
    d. the sample clotting too fast.

63. Which tube does not require mixing?
    a. Clot activator
    b. Gel separator
    c. Liquid EDTA
    d. Red/light gray

64. Transporting blood specimens with the stopper up has nothing to do with
    a. encouraging complete clot formation.
    b. maintaining the sterility of the sample.
    c. minimizing stopper-caused aerosols.
    d. reducing agitation-caused hemolysis.

65. Clinical and Laboratory Standards Institute (CLSI) and Occupational Safety and Health Administration (OSHA) guidelines do *not* require specimen transport bags to have
    a. a visible biohazard logo.
    b. liquid-tight closure top.
    c. shock-resistant features.
    d. slip pockets for paperwork.

66. Which one of the following agencies sets guidelines for specimens transported by courier and other air or ground mail systems?
    a. CLIA
    b. CMS
    c. FDA
    d. IATA

67. Which of the following specimens is unlikely to be rejected for analysis? A specimen for
    a. electrolytes that are hemolyzed.
    b. fasting glucose that is lipemic.
    c. platelet count with microclots.
    d. total bilirubin that is icteric.

68. It is unnecessary to protect this specimen from light.
    a. Ammonia
    b. Bilirubin
    c. Vitamin B$_2$
    d. Vitamin C

69. Rough handling during transport is bad for specimens, but it will not
    a. activate the platelets.
    b. affect coagulation tests.
    c. elevate WBC counts.
    d. hemolyze red blood cells.

70. Which specimen needs to be transported on ice?
    a. Ammonia
    b. Bilirubin
    c. Carotene
    d. Potassium

71. The *best* way to chill a specimen is to
    a. cool the tube before the venipuncture.
    b. place it in a chilled canister of water.
    c. put it in a small container of ice cubes.
    d. transport in a commercial cooling tray.

72. Chilling can cause erroneous results for this analyte.
    a. Ammonia
    b. Glucagon
    c. Lactic acid
    d. Potassium

73. How should a cryofibrinogen specimen be transported?
    a. At room temperature
    b. Immersed in ice slurry
    c. In a 37°C heat block
    d. Protected from light

74. The most probable reason a phlebotomist would wrap a specimen in aluminum foil (Fig. 12-2) would be to
    a. cool down the specimen.
    b. cover a contaminated tube.
    c. maintain 37°C temperature.
    d. protect it from room light.

75. A specimen must be transported at or near normal body temperature. Which of the following temperatures meets this requirement?
    a. 25°C
    b. 37°C
    c. 50°C
    d. 98°C

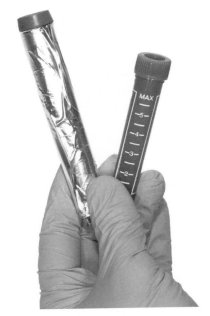

Figure 12-2 Specimen wrapped in aluminum foil.

76. According to CLSI, when an uncentrifuged blood specimen is sent to the lab from a drawing station, the blood must
    a. arrive in a time limit that protects analyte stability.
    b. be kept at body temperature until it is centrifuged.
    c. have a clot activator added prior to transportation.
    d. remain refrigerated until arrival at the laboratory.

77. A separator gel prevents glycolysis
    a. after the specimen has been centrifuged.
    b. as soon as the specimen is collected.
    c. in tubes used for serum samples only.
    d. when the specimen is thoroughly mixed.

78. A glucose specimen collected in a sodium fluoride tube is generally stable at room temperature for
    a. 6 hours.
    b. 12 hours.
    c. 24 hours.
    d. 48 hours.

79. Which specimen has priority over all other specimens during processing and testing?
    a. ASAP
    b. Fasting
    c. STAT
    d. Timed

80. Which of the following specimens does not need to be centrifuged?
    a. BUN in a red/gray SST
    b. CBC in a lavender tube
    c. Potassium in a green tube
    d. PTT in a light blue tube

81. Which of the following is not a valid reason for why blood slides made from EDTA specimens must be prepared within 1 hour of specimen collection? To
    a. ensure they are made before clots appear.
    b. minimize RBC distortion on the smear.
    c. preserve the integrity of the blood cells.
    d. prevent artifact formation from additive.

82. Processing specimens requires various types of protection, but this PPE is unnecessary.
    a. Covers for footwear
    b. Disposable gloves
    c. Fluid-resistant apron
    d. Protective goggles

83. This specimen would most likely be accepted for testing despite this problem.
    a. Expired evacuated tube
    b. Incomplete identification
    c. Not initialed by collector
    d. Quantity is not sufficient

84. Which of the following actions will compromise the quality of the specimen?
    a. Drawing a BUN in an amber serum tube
    b. Mixing an SST by inverting it five times
    c. Only partially filling a liquid EDTA tube
    d. Transporting a cryofibrinogen at 37°C

85. Results for this test should be normal despite a delay in processing longer than 2 hours.
    a. Carbon dioxide
    b. Fasting glucose
    c. Ionized calcium
    d. Pregnancy test

86. An aliquot is a
    a. filter for separating serum from cells.
    b. portion of a specimen being tested.
    c. specimen being prepared for testing.
    d. tube used to balance the centrifuge.

87. Which specimen is most likely to be rejected if the tube is not filled until the normal vacuum is exhausted?
    a. Complete blood count
    b. Plasma electrolytes
    c. Postprandial glucose
    d. Prothrombin time

88. Which of the following tests is unaffected by hemolysis?
    a. Amylase
    b. Hemoglobin
    c. Magnesium
    d. Potassium

89. Tests performed on plasma samples are
    a. collected in red/gray top tubes.
    b. drawn in anticoagulant tubes.
    c. hematology or serology tests.
    d. obtained from clotted blood.

90. Chemistry tests are often collected in heparin tubes to
    a. ensure adequate coagulation.
    b. maximize diagnosis potential.
    c. minimize effects of hemolysis.
    d. reduce the turnaround time.

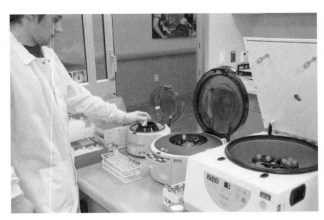

Figure 12-3 Specimen processor loading a centrifuge.

91. It is important to note the type of heparin in a collection tube because
    a. a few types of heparin do not require tube inversions.
    b. not all types of heparin prevent complete coagulation.
    c. some types of heparin can affect results of certain tests.
    d. some types of heparin make centrifugation unnecessary.

92. To avoid airborne infection while processing specimens
    a. apply the brake when stopping the centrifuge.
    b. "pop" tube stoppers when opening serum tubes.
    c. pour spun specimens into labeled aliquot tubes.
    d. remove tube stoppers behind a splash shield.

93. When a nonadditive specimen is spun in a centrifuge (Fig. 12-3), the substance that comes to the top is
    a. buffy coat.
    b. plasma.
    c. red cells.
    d. serum.

94. If a serum specimen is not completely clotted before it is centrifuged, the
    a. buffy coat may not form properly.
    b. red blood cells in it may hemolyze.

c. separator gel may come to the top.
d. serum may have a fibrin clot in it.

95. Which of the following collection circumstances is least likely to delay clotting in a serum gel tube?
    a. Collection was difficult, hemolyzing red cells
    b. Patient has an elevated white blood cell count
    c. Patient is taking an anticoagulant medication
    d. Specimen is chilled soon after being collected

96. Types of intrafacility specimen transport systems include
    a. pneumatic tube
    b. robot couriers
    c. vertical track
    d. all of the above

97. Stoppers should be left on tubes awaiting centrifugation to prevent
    a. analyte dilution.
    b. contamination.
    c. decrease in pH.
    d. all of the above.

98. Minimum precentrifugation time for specimens drawn in serum separator tubes is
    a. 10 minutes.
    b. 15 minutes.
    c. 20 minutes.
    d. 30 minutes.

99. Repeated centrifugation of a specimen can
    a. alter the test results.
    b. deteriorate analytes.
    c. result in hemolysis.
    d. all of the above.

100. Which statement describes proper centrifuge operation?
    a. Balance specimens by placing tubes of equal volume and size opposite one another.
    b. Centrifuge serum specimens before they start to form clots on the sides of the tubes.
    c. Never centrifuge serum specimens and plasma specimens in the same centrifuge.
    d. Remove the stoppers from evacuated tubes before placing them in the centrifuge.

Answers and Explanations

1. **Answer: a**

   WHY: A mnemonic is a memory-aiding code or abbreviation, such as 5.0 mL LAV, which tells the phlebotomist the tube type to choose (lavender) and the amount of blood to draw (5 mL).

   REVIEW: Yes ☐   No ☐

2. **Answer: c**

   WHY: A barcode is a parallel array of alternately spaced black bars and white spaces representing a code. The code may represent numbers or letters.

   REVIEW: Yes ☐   No ☐

3. **Answer: a**

   WHY: Pneumatic tube systems (often referred to simply as pneumatic tubes) use pressurized air to transport cylinders that contain items such as patient records, medications, test results, and all types of laboratory specimens to and from various locations in a facility.

   REVIEW: Yes ☐   No ☐

4. **Answer: d**

   WHY: Read-only memory (ROM) is a computer memory installed by the manufacturer. It is permanently stored inside the computer and instructs the computer to carry out operations requested by the user.

   REVIEW: Yes ☐   No ☐

5. **Answer: c**

   WHY: One of the benefits of computerization of laboratory instrumentation has meant that analyzers can read/scan the bar code labels on a patient's primary tube for identification, but only if the labels are properly placed on the tube after drawing so that the scanner can read it correctly. See Figure 12-4.

   REVIEW: Yes ☐   No ☐

6. **Answer: a**

   WHY: To prevent exposure to aerosol formation when one is opening a tube, the stopper should be removed while the specimen is held behind a safety shield or removed using a safety stopper removal device. If the tube has a conventional stopper, the stopper should be covered with a 4 × 4-in gauze square during removal. Pouring the serum from the primary tube to a secondary or aliquot tube has been shown to create aerosols.

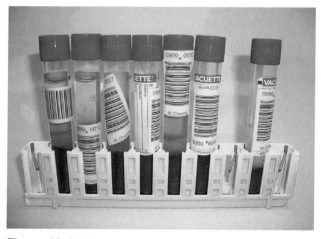

Figure 12-4 Gel tubes with examples of applied labels.

   Never withdraw a sample from a tube using a syringe because it is against Occupational Safety and Health Administration (OSHA) regulations and can hemolyze the specimen.

   REVIEW: Yes ☐   No ☐

7. **Answer: a**

   WHY: Proper aliquot preparation involves capping or covering tubes as soon as they are filled. Disposable transfer pipettes (Fig. 12-5) should be used instead of pouring specimens into aliquot tubes. Never put serum or plasma specimens from different additive tubes into one aliquot tube. Always place the aliquot in a prelabeled tube that matches the original tube.

   REVIEW: Yes ☐   No ☐

8. **Answer: c**

   WHY: The Clinical and Laboratory Standards Institute (CLSI) develops and publishes standards for handling and processing blood specimens and many other laboratory procedures. The U.S. Food and Drug Administration (FDA), Centers for Disease Control and Prevention (CDC), and the Clinical Laboratory Improvement Amendments (CLIA) have regulations that affect laboratories, but they do not develop standards for handling or processing blood specimens.

   REVIEW: Yes ☐   No ☐

9. **Answer: c**

   WHY: Many laboratory analyzers have sophisticated computer systems that manage patient data

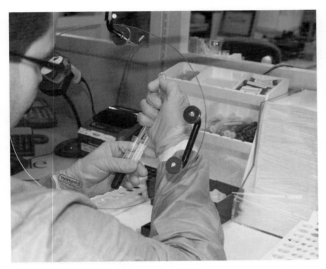

Figure 12-5 A sample being transferred from the collection tube to an aliquot tube behind a splash screen.

and interface (connect for the purpose of interaction) with the main hospital information system and many other software system in the healthcare facility.

REVIEW: Yes ☐   No ☐

10. **Answer: b**

WHY: When an erythrocyte sedimentation rate (ESR) is ordered on an EDTA specimen that is held at room temperature, the test must be performed within 4 hours. If the specimen is refrigerated, the time to perform the test is extended up to 12 hours.

REVIEW: Yes ☐   No ☐

11. **Answer: b**

WHY: Blood specimen tubes being transported from one facility to another must be placed in leakproof plastic bags with a biohazard logo, a liquid-tight closure, and a slip pocket for paperwork (Fig. 12-6). Several organizations have regulations for transporting biohazardous materials, such as blood specimens. DOT, IATA, and OSHA impose penalties if the regulations are violated.

REVIEW: Yes ☐   No ☐

12. **Answer: b**

WHY: Bilirubin and serum folate specimens must be protected from light. Gastrin, lactic acid, homocysteine, and renin specimens should be chilled in crushed ice slurry. Cholesterol and uric acid specimens do not require special handling.

REVIEW: Yes ☐   No ☐

📖 *WORKBOOK Labeling Exercise 12-3 will help you distinguish between preanalytical collection errors and other specimen issues.*

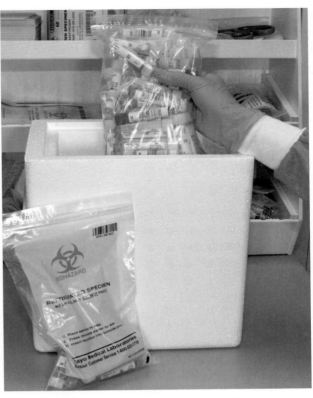

Figure 12-6 Processing tech packages specimens for send out.

13. **Answer: b**

WHY: Failure to mix tubes using the required number of inversions at the time of collection is a preanalytical error that can lead to microclot formation or insufficient clotting.

REVIEW: Yes ☐   No ☐

14. **Answer: b**

WHY: Aliquot tubes are supposed to be prelabeled to help avoid transfer errors. Great care must still be taken to match each specimen with the corresponding labeled aliquot tube to avoid the risk of misidentified samples. Different types of specimens, such as serum and plasma, are virtually indistinguishable once they have been transferred into aliquot tubes, so to avoid errors it is important to match the specimen with the aliquot tube of the requested test as well as the patient. In addition, there is risk of exposure to biohazardous material from spills, splashes, and aerosols if specimens are not handled and transferred carefully.

REVIEW: Yes ☐   No ☐

15. **Answer: a**

WHY: Dehydration of a patient can affect test results and is a source of error that occurs before specimen collection. A misidentified patient, mislabeled tube, and wrong collection time are also sources of preanalytical error; however, they occur at the time of collection.

REVIEW: Yes ☐ No ☐

16. **Answer: c**

    WHY: Computer technology makes sharing of information so simple that patient confidentiality can be easily violated. The Health Insurance Portability and Accountability Act (HIPAA) is designed to protect the privacy and security of patient information by standardizing the electronic transfer of data and providing guidelines for sharing protected health information (PHI). It was not enacted to have patient healthcare records examined, protect healthcare workers (HCWs) from malpractice issues, or standardize patient electronic records.

    REVIEW: Yes ☐ No ☐

17. **Answer: d**

    WHY: Handheld computer systems (HPCs) used in laboratory medicine are ideal for patient identification using barcode systems and paperless collection of data because they can go anywhere the patient may be. Today they are being used to read barcodes on patient ID bands (Fig. 12-7) and generate the labels used for specimen collection at the patient's bedside, display the required collection tubes and the order of draw, and identify the person who is performing the phlebotomy.

    REVIEW: Yes ☐ No ☐

18. **Answer: c**

    WHY: A critical laboratory value, also called a panic value, is a test result that represents such a variance from normal values as to be a threat to the patient's life and requires the immediate attention of the physician. The Clinical and Laboratory Standards Institute requires critical values to be reported to the physician as soon as possible.

    REVIEW: Yes ☐ No ☐

19. **Answer: a**

    WHY: Proper handling from the time a specimen is collected until the test is performed helps ensure that results obtained on the specimen accurately reflect the status of the patient. Exposure to light during the time a specimen is being stored while awaiting testing can affect test results on several specimens, including bilirubin, carotene, and serum folate.

    REVIEW: Yes ☐ No ☐

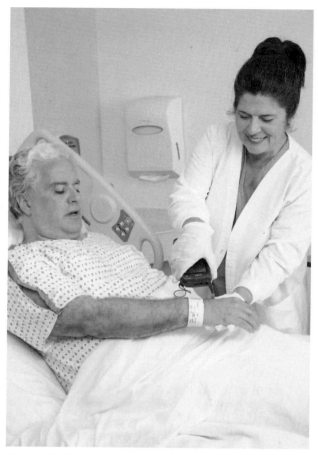

Figure 12-7 A phlebotomist scans an ID band. Siemens Patient Identification Check being used to scan a wristband. (Courtesy Siemens Healthcare, Malvern, PA.)

20. **Answer: a**

    WHY: It is important to handle and transport blood specimens carefully. Rough handling and agitation can hemolyze specimens.

    REVIEW: Yes ☐ No ☐

21. **Answer: b**

    WHY: Secondary storage is storage outside of a computer central processing unit (CPU). A Universal Serial Bus (USB) drive (Fig. 12-8) is one type of permanent secondary storage device. Other types include external hard drives, CDs, and the cloud.

    REVIEW: Yes ☐ No ☐

22. **Answer: b**

    WHY: Prompt delivery and separation minimize the effects of metabolic processes such as glycolysis. Cellular metabolism is known to affect calcitonin and other analytes, such as aldosterone, enzymes, and phosphorus.

    REVIEW: Yes ☐ No ☐

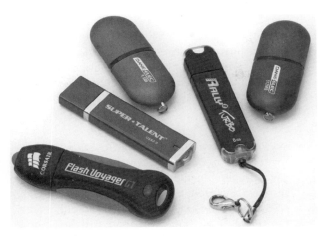

Figure 12-8 Assortment of USB drives.

23. **Answer: d**

WHY: Glycolysis, breaking down of glucose, by erythrocytes and leukocytes in blood specimens can falsely lower glucose values by 5% to 7% per hour. For this reason, glucose specimens must be separated from the cells within 2 hours of collection or collected in tubes containing an antiglycolytic agent, such as sodium fluoride. Glucose specimens collected in sodium fluoride tubes are generally stable for 24 hours at room temperature and up to 48 hours when refrigerated at 2° to 8°C.

REVIEW: Yes ☐   No ☐

24. **Answer: d**

WHY: Specimens for erythrocyte sedimentation rate (ESR) determinations must be tested within 4 hours at room temperature or within 12 hours if refrigerated. Partial thromboplastin time (PTT) test specimens require analysis within 4 hours of collection regardless of storage conditions. Specimens for molecular determinations, such as RNA, must be tested as soon as possible because these substances are extremely unstable.

REVIEW: Yes ☐   No ☐

25. **Answer: c**

WHY: A temperature of 25°C is considered normal room temperature and would not hurt the specimen. A temperature of −20°C is below freezing and could damage the specimen. A temperature of 8°C, which is around 45°F, is above freezing but well below room temperature. A temperature of 37°C is body temperature and well above the required temperature.

REVIEW: Yes ☐   No ☐

26. **Answer: d**

WHY: Metabolic processes can continue in a blood specimen after collection and negatively affect

some analytes. Cooling slows down metabolic processes. Some analytes are more affected by metabolic processes than others and must be cooled immediately after collection and during transportation. Cooling can delay clotting but is not a desired effect. Cooling does not promote serum separation, nor does it help to avoid hemolysis.

REVIEW: Yes ☐   No ☐

27. **Answer: b**

WHY: Most large laboratories have a specific area, called central processing, where specimens are triaged or screened and prioritized in preparation for testing. Here the specimens are identified, logged/accessioned, sorted by department, and evaluated for suitability for testing. Analysis of specimens and reporting of test results are performed in respective test areas by technicians or technologists after the specimen has been properly processed.

REVIEW: Yes ☐   No ☐

28. **Answer: d**

WHY: Stoppers should remain on tubes awaiting centrifugation. Removing the stopper from a specimen can cause loss of CO_2 and increase the pH, leading to inaccurate results for tests such as pH, CO_2, and acid phosphatase. In addition, leaving the stopper off exposes the specimen to evaporation and contamination, but should not result in loss of ionized calcium.

REVIEW: Yes ☐   No ☐

29. **Answer: b**

WHY: Suitable specimens are required for accurate laboratory results. Unsuitable specimens must be rejected for testing and new specimens obtained. A properly identified specimen is essential because it links the test results to the patient. Consequently, inadequate patient information on a specimen is a reason for rejection by the specimen processor and a request for a new specimen.

REVIEW: Yes ☐   No ☐

30. **Answer: c**

WHY: Radio frequency identification (RFID) is a form of identification using computer technology that is rapidly emerging in health care for identifying and tracking records, equipment and supplies, specimens, and patients. RFID tags are tiny silicon chips that transmit data to a wireless receiver. With this technique, it is possible to identify or track many items simultaneously.

REVIEW: Yes ☐   No ☐

31. **Answer: b**

    WHY: A preanalytical error that could happen during specimen processing is inadequate centrifugation. Not centrifuging long enough or fast enough would cause incomplete separation of the sample and contamination of the serum with cells and fibrin.

    REVIEW: Yes ☐ No ☐

32. **Answer: d**

    WHY: Computer literacy involves the ability to understand a computer and how it functions, perform basic computer operations, and be able to adapt to changes that computers are creating in our lives. One does *not* have to be able to explain how POCT instruments connect to the LIS, design job-specific programs, or perform advanced computer operations, such as to QA documentation, to be considered computer literate.

    REVIEW: Yes ☐ No ☐

    📖 *WORKBOOK Matching Exercise 12-3 is a good way to review parts of a computer and familiarize yourself with the terminology.*

33. **Answer: b**

    WHY: When a number of computers are linked together for the purpose of sharing information, it is called a computer network. The computers can be linked because of the software called middleware that connects two applications and passes data between them.

    REVIEW: Yes ☐ No ☐

34. **Answer: d**

    WHY: "Input" is the term for data entered into a computer. Data can be entered in several different ways, such as by using keyboards, scanners, and light pens. Applications are software programs prepared by software companies or in-house programmers to perform specific tasks required by users. Printers are output devices.

    REVIEW: Yes ☐ No ☐

35. **Answer: c**

    WHY: All additives except sodium citrate require from 5 to 10 inversions depending on manufacturer instructions. Sodium citrate tubes are used to collect PT and PTT tests and they require only 3 to 4 inversions.

    REVIEW: Yes ☐ No ☐

36. **Answer: d**

    WHY: Visible display of data is a function of the computer monitor or display screen. The

central processing unit (CPU) is the thinking part of the computer that instructs the computer to carry out user requests, manages tasks, and performs mathematical processes and data comparisons.

REVIEW: Yes ☐ No ☐

37. **Answer: a**

    WHY: Random access memory (RAM) is temporary storage of data that can be lost if it is not saved to permanent storage before the computer program is closed. Storage can be on CDs, DVDs, USB drives, and external drives. Read-only memory (ROM) is permanent memory installed by the manufacturer that instructs the computer to carry out user-requested operations.

    REVIEW: Yes ☐ No ☐

38. **Answer: d**

    WHY: Nonanticoagulant gel tubes should be placed in an upright position as soon as they are mixed. This upright position aids clot formation and prevents the clot from attaching to the stopper.

    REVIEW: Yes ☐ No ☐

39. **Answer: a**

    WHY: Software is the programming, or coded instructions that control computer hardware in the processing of data. There are two types of software, systems software and applications software. Systems software controls the normal operation of the computer. Applications software refers to programs developed by software companies or computer programmers to perform specific tasks and includes graphics, spreadsheet, and word processing programs. The central processing unit is hardware.

    REVIEW: Yes ☐ No ☐

40. **Answer: d**

    WHY: On returning to the lab with a specimen, the first thing a phlebotomist must do is to verify collection so that nursing personnel will know the specimen has been collected and no one else will attempt to collect it. Before the specimen is collected, patient information is entered into the system and labels and collection lists are generated. Verification of a specimen does not involve retrieval of all test orders.

    REVIEW: Yes ☐ No ☐

    📖 *WORKBOOK Labeling Exercise 12-1 will give you an opportunity to review the work flow when a specimen is brought to the lab.*

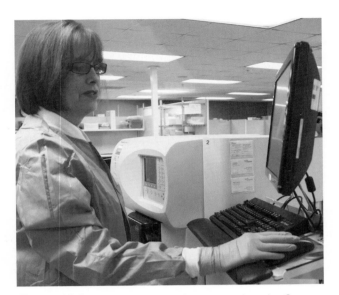

Figure 12-9 Computer terminal connected to the Sysmex hematology instrument.

41. **Answer: a**

    WHY: As a minimum, a computer terminal (Fig. 12-9) consists of a monitor or computer screen and a keyboard.

    REVIEW: Yes ☐ No ☐

42. **Answer: c**

    WHY: According to CLSI, abnormalities have been recorded in serum potassium, acid phosphatase, lactic dehydrogenase, and plasma hemoglobin after having been sent to the laboratory in a pneumatic tube system.

    REVIEW: Yes ☐ No ☐

43. **Answer: b**

    WHY: Entering a password to gain access to a computer or computer system is called logging on.

    REVIEW: Yes ☐ No ☐

44. **Answer: c**

    WHY: After necessary information has been input into the computer, the "enter" key must be pressed for information to be processed. When entering patient information in a laboratory information system (LIS), the cursor will automatically reset itself at the correct point for data input after the "enter" key is pressed.

    REVIEW: Yes ☐ No ☐

45. **Answer: d**

    WHY: The process of verifying an order allows the user to review the information and choose at that point to modify, delete, or accept it before

entering. It is not a phlebotomist's duty to determine the appropriateness of a physician's order. Confirmation of the test order takes place before the specimen is collected.

REVIEW: Yes ☐ No ☐

46. **Answer: d**

    WHY: Selecting the "order inquiry" function allows the user to retrieve any or all test orders associated with a particular patient.

    REVIEW: Yes ☐ No ☐

47. **Answer: d**

    WHY: A password uniquely identifies a person and allows that person to gain entrance into a computer system as a user. ID codes are not always confidential. An icon is an image that represents a document or software program. The LIS menu is a listing of icons or mnemonic codes for selecting a computer function or program to use to enter data into the computer system.

    REVIEW: Yes ☐ No ☐

48. **Answer: d**

    WHY: Hazardous biological samples can pose a danger if someone should come in contact with the contents of the shipping container; consequently, it is critical to follow DOT and IATA regulations. Any person who packages such materials must show proof of training and certification by DOT or IATA.

    REVIEW: Yes ☐ No ☐

49. **Answer: a**

    WHY: An accession number is a unique number given to a test order. The number is used throughout the collection, handling, processing, and testing process to identify the specimen with its test order. Each new test order will have a different accession number. A hospital or medical record number is unique to the patient and remains the same throughout the patient's hospital stay. A mnemonic code is a memory-aiding code or abbreviation. The LIS image/icon is used to select the appropriate program from the LIS so that patient information can be entered.

    REVIEW: Yes ☐ No ☐

50. **Answer: d**

    WHY: Military, or 24-hour time, is used on computer-generated labels to eliminate confusion between AM and PM. The specimen in the requisition example (Fig. 12-1) should be collected at 1252, which is 12:52 PM.

    REVIEW: Yes ☐ No ☐

51. **Answer: d**

    WHY: The code on the requisition (Fig. 12-1) indicated by number 10 is LAV, which indicates that a lavender top tube should be collected. The size of the lavender tube is indicated as 5.0 mL.
    REVIEW: Yes ☐ No ☐

52. **Answer: b**

    WHY: An accession number is a unique number generated when the test request is entered. The accession number on the requisition example (Fig. 12-1) is 96-270-0138, and is easily spotted because of the preceding abbreviation "ACCN#."
    REVIEW: Yes ☐ No ☐

53. **Answer: d**

    WHY: A computer-generated label typically contains the patient's name, medical record number, and date of birth or age. The actual time collected and the phlebotomist's initials are added to the label that is placed on the collection tube immediately after the specimen is collected.
    REVIEW: Yes ☐ No ☐

54. **Answer: b**

    WHY: A bidirectional computer interface allows data to upload (transfer from analyzer to LIS) or download (transfer from LIS to analyzer) between two systems.
    REVIEW: Yes ☐ No ☐

55. **Answer: a**

    WHY: Ideally, specimens that require separation of the serum or plasma from the cells should be centrifuged upon arrival in the lab, and the liquid portion removed from contact with the cells as soon as possible. CLSI sets 2 hours as the maximum time for separating serum and plasma from cells for the lactic acid, glucose, catecholamines, homocysteine, LD, ionized calcium, and potassium.
    REVIEW: Yes ☐ No ☐

    📖 *The crossword in Chapter 12 of the WORKBOOK is a fun way to review many words associated with computers.*

56. **Answer: d**

    WHY: In computer language, "hard copy" is data printed on paper.
    REVIEW: Yes ☐ No ☐

57. **Answer: a**

    WHY: It is very important to allow complete clotting of gel barrier tubes before centrifugation.

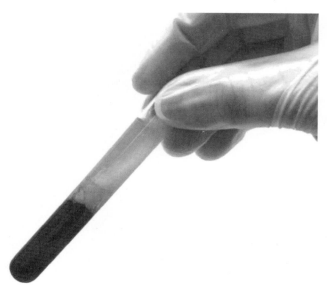

Figure 12-10 Clotted serum.

Any automated chemistry instrument that samples serum from gel barrier tubes for analysis can be greatly affected by latent fibrin formation. A clotted serum (Fig. 12-10) will interfere with performance of the test by not allowing any of the sample to be aspirated from the primary tube OR by plugging the sampler completely.
REVIEW: Yes ☐ No ☐

58. **Answer: a**

    WHY: Proper collection procedures, including specimen handling, are important for quality test results. Testing personnel may not be aware that the integrity of a specimen is compromised because effects of mishandling are not always obvious. Most effects of mishandling *cannot* be corrected. It has been estimated that 50% to 70% of all lab errors occur in the preanalytical phase.
    REVIEW: Yes ☐ No ☐

59. **Answer: d**

    WHY: Proper specimen handling begins when a test is ordered and continues throughout the testing process, and until the results are reported out.
    REVIEW: Yes ☐ No ☐

60. **Answer: c**

    WHY: Procedures and policies concerning specimen collection can be found in the laboratory user manual. A phlebotomist who is unfamiliar with a requested test should consult the user manual for instructions.
    REVIEW: Yes ☐ No ☐

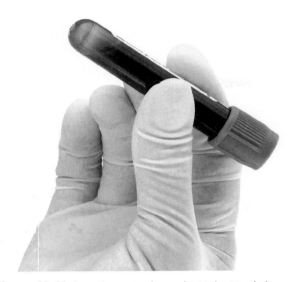

Figure 12-11 Inverting an anticoagulant tube to mix it.

61. Answer: b

WHY: The number of times a specimen tube should be inverted (Fig. 12-11) depends on whether or not the tube contains an additive and on the manufacturer's instructions. Nonadditive tubes do not require inverting. Additive tubes typically require from 3 to 10 inversions, depending on manufacturer instructions, to mix the additive adequately with the blood in the tube. The difficulty of the draw, the amount of blood in the tube, and the gauge of the needle used have no relationship to the number of tube inversions required.

REVIEW: Yes ☐ No ☐

62. Answer: c

WHY: Inadequate mixing of an anticoagulant tube can lead to microclots in the specimen. Hemolysis can occur if the specimen is mixed too vigorously. Lipemia is a patient condition that is unrelated to mixing the specimen. An anticoagulant specimen is not supposed to clot.

REVIEW: Yes ☐ No ☐

63. Answer: d

WHY: Additive tubes require tube inversions to mix the additive adequately with the blood; nonadditive tubes do not. BD's red/light gray top does not contain an additive such as a clot activator. Consequently, it does not require mixing. A serum separator tube (SST), also called a gel separator, requires mixing because it contains a clot activator. An EDTA tube needs to be mixed regardless of whether or not the anticoagulant EDTA is in liquid or dry form.

REVIEW: Yes ☐ No ☐

64. Answer: b

WHY: Transporting tubes with the stopper up aids clotting of serum tubes, allows fluids to drain away from the stopper to minimize aerosol generation when the stopper is removed, and reduces the chance of hemolysis caused by agitation of the tube contents during transportation. If the tube contents are sterile, they will remain that way until the tube is opened, regardless of tube position during transport.

REVIEW: Yes ☐ No ☐

65. Answer: c

WHY: CLSI and OSHA guidelines require a specimen transport bag to have a biohazard logo, a liquid-tight closure, and a slip pocket for paperwork. Pneumatic tube system specimen carriers, as in Figure 12-12, need to have shock-resistant features to prevent breakage of specimens, but regular transport bags do not need this feature.

REVIEW: Yes ☐ No ☐

66. Answer: d

WHY: Specimens transported by courier or other air or ground mail systems must follow guidelines defined by the Department of Transportation (DOT), the International Air Transport Association (IATA).

REVIEW: Yes ☐ No ☐

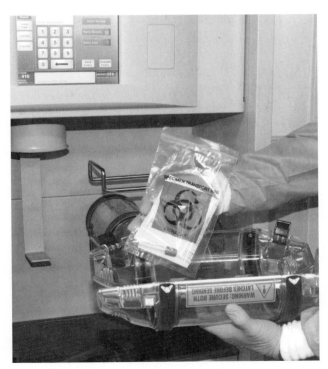

Figure 12-12 Specimen prepared for transport through pneumatic tube system.

67. **Answer: d**

WHY: Specimens with high bilirubin levels typically have an abnormal yellow color described as icterus, and the specimen is said to be icteric. Icterus can be expected in some bilirubin specimens and would not be a reason to reject them for testing. A specimen for a platelet count with clots in it would be rejected because clots cause false low results for cell counts, platelet counts in particular. Hemolysis invalidates electrolyte results, potassium results in particular. A lipemic specimen is a clue that the patient may not have been fasting. A nonfasting specimen might be rejected if a fasting specimen was specifically requested.

REVIEW: Yes ☐ No ☐

68. **Answer: a**

WHY: Bilirubin and vitamins C and B_2 are all analytes that can be broken down in the presence of light. Ammonia requires ASAP transportation in ice slurry, but is not affected by light exposure.

REVIEW: Yes ☐ No ☐

📖 *Box 12-1, Possible Sources of Preanalytical Error, in the TEXTBOOK will give you an overview of many other error possibilities throughout the analytical process.*

69. **Answer: c**

WHY: It is important to handle and transport blood specimens carefully. Rough handling and agitation can activate platelets and affect coagulation tests, hemolyze specimens, and even crack or break tubes. Rough handling does not elevate white blood cell (WBC) counts, however.

REVIEW: Yes ☐ No ☐

70. **Answer: a**

WHY: Ammonia specimens are extremely volatile and must be transported ASAP on ice. The expression "on ice" means in an ice slurry (Fig. 12-13) or cooling rack. Bilirubin and carotene specimens require protection from light. A potassium specimen should be collected and transported at room temperature.

REVIEW: Yes ☐ No ☐

71. **Answer: d**

WHY: The best way to chill a specimen is to immerse it in an ice and water slurry or put it in a commercial cooling tray. Ice cubes without added water may prevent adequate cooling of the specimen. Specimens in contact with a solid piece of ice may freeze in the area touched by the ice, resulting in hemolysis and possible breakdown of the analyte. A chilled canister of water is

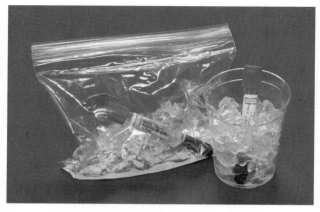

Figure 12-13 Specimen immersed in crushed ice and water slurry.

inadequately cooled to protect the analyte being measured.

REVIEW: Yes ☐ No ☐

72. **Answer: d**

WHY: The energy needed to pump potassium into the cells is provided by glycolysis. Cold inhibits glycolysis, causing potassium to leak from the cells, falsely elevating test results. Cooling can also cause hemolysis, which also elevates test results. If a potassium test is ordered along with other tests that require cooling, it must be collected in a separate tube that is not cooled. Ammonia, glucagon, and lactic acid all require cooling for accurate test results.

REVIEW: Yes ☐ No ☐

73. **Answer: c**

WHY: A cryofibrinogen specimen should be transported at body temperature, which is normally 37°C. Small portable heat blocks that hold a 37°C temperature for approximately 15 minutes are available.

REVIEW: Yes ☐ No ☐

74. **Answer: d**

WHY: Wrapping a specimen in aluminum foil (Fig. 12-2) is an easy way to protect it from light. A specimen that needs to be cooled quickly should be placed in ice slurry or cooling tray (Fig. 12-14). Heat blocks or special warmers are used to keep specimens warm. A contaminated tube should be wiped with disinfectant and placed in a secondary bag or container.

REVIEW: Yes ☐ No ☐

75. **Answer: b**

WHY: Normal body temperature is approximately 37°C (98.6°F).

REVIEW: Yes ☐ No ☐

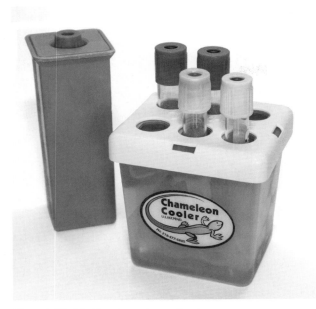

Figure 12-14 Specimen in cooling tray.

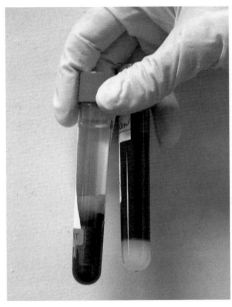

Figure 12-15 Serum gel tubes. *Right,* before being centrifuged. *Left,* after being centrifuged.

76. **Answer: a**

    WHY: All specimens should be transported to the laboratory promptly. According to Clinical and Laboratory Standards Institute (CLSI) guidelines, unless conclusive evidence indicates that longer times do not affect the accuracy of test results, specimens should be separated from the cells as soon as possible, with a maximum time limit of 2 hours.
    REVIEW: Yes ☐ No ☐

77. **Answer: a**

    WHY: Separator gel has a density between that of serum or plasma and cells. During centrifugation, it undergoes a change in viscosity and ends up between the liquid portion of the specimen and the cells becoming a physical barrier between the serum or plasma and the cells, which prevents glycolysis. Figure 12-15 shows two serum gel separator tubes, one before centrifugation and the other after.
    REVIEW: Yes ☐ No ☐

78. **Answer: c**

    WHY: Sodium fluoride can prevent changes in glucose concentration for up to 24 hours at room temperature and up to 48 hours if the tube is refrigerated.
    REVIEW: Yes ☐ No ☐

79. **Answer: c**

    WHY: STAT, or medical emergency specimens, require immediate collection, processing, and testing and have priority over all other specimens.
    REVIEW: Yes ☐ No ☐

80. **Answer: b**

    WHY: A complete blood count (CBC) is performed on whole blood, and the specimen should never be centrifuged.
    REVIEW: Yes ☐ No ☐

81. **Answer: a**

    WHY: A well-mixed EDTA specimen should never form a clot. Prolonged contact with EDTA can distort blood cells, change their staining characteristics, and result in artifact formation. To preserve the integrity of the blood cells and prevent artifact formation, slides made from EDTA specimens must be prepared within 1 hour of specimen collection. If microclots appear on a slide made from an EDTA specimen, it is usually because the specimen was not properly mixed after collection.
    REVIEW: Yes ☐ No ☐

82. **Answer: a**

    WHY: Occupational Safety and Health Administration (OSHA) regulations require the wearing of protective equipment when processing specimens. Protective equipment includes gloves, fully closed, fluid-resistant lab coats or aprons, and protective face gear, such as masks and goggles with side shields or chin-length face shields. Shoe covering is not required.
    REVIEW: Yes ☐ No ☐

83. **Answer: c**

    WHY: Reasons for rejecting a specimen for analysis include missing or incomplete identification, collection in an expired tube, and an insufficient quantity of specimen (referred to as QNS, or quantity not sufficient) to perform the test. If the collector's initials do not appear on the specimen, the specimen is still analyzed even though the collector is unknown.

REVIEW: Yes ☐ No ☐

84. **Answer: c**

WHY: The additive in a tube is designed to work most effectively with an amount of blood that fills the tube until the normal vacuum is exhausted. Results on a specimen from a partially filled liquid EDTA tube may be compromised. Although a blood urea nitrogen (BUN) level does not need to be protected from light, it would not hurt to draw it in an amber serum tube. Serum separator tubes *should* be mixed five times. A cryofibrinogen specimen *should* be transported at 37°C.

REVIEW: Yes ☐ No ☐

85. **Answer: d**

WHY: A delay in processing beyond 2 hours can lead to erroneously decreased results for carbon dioxide, glucose, and calcium. A pregnancy testing specimen is not affected by a delay in processing.

REVIEW: Yes ☐ No ☐

86. **Answer: b**

WHY: An aliquot is a portion of a specimen being tested. When several tests are to be performed on the same specimen, portions of the specimen are transferred into separate tubes so that each test has its own tube of specimen. Each portion is called an aliquot, and the tubes containing each portion are called aliquot tubes. Each aliquot tube is labeled with the same identifying information as the original tube.

REVIEW: Yes ☐ No ☐

87. **Answer: d**

WHY: A prothrombin time (PT) is a coagulation test collected in a light blue sodium citrate tube. Coagulation tests require a critical 9-to-1 ratio of blood to anticoagulant for test results to be valid. Therefore, an underfilled light blue top for a PT test would not be accepted for testing (Fig. 12-16). All anticoagulant tubes should be filled until the vacuum is exhausted for best results; however, with the exception of sodium citrate tubes, slightly underfilled anticoagulant tubes are usually accepted for testing. Underfilled serum tubes are almost always accepted

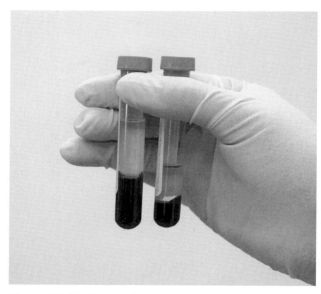

Figure 12-16 Coagulation tubes. *Right,* correctly filled. *Left,* not filled enough.

for testing provided there is sufficient specimen to perform the test.

REVIEW: Yes ☐ No ☐

88. **Answer: b**

WHY: Hemolysis, regardless of the cause, affects amylase, magnesium, and potassium levels. Hemolysis should not affect hemoglobin levels because the cells are lysed in the testing process in order to measure hemoglobin. Other hematology tests, however, are affected by hemolysis and should not be performed on a hemolyzed specimen.

REVIEW: Yes ☐ No ☐

89. **Answer: b**

WHY: Plasma samples are obtained from blood collected in anticoagulant tubes. A tube containing an anticoagulant must be spun in a centrifuge to obtain plasma for testing. Most coagulation tests, for example, are performed on plasma obtained from light-blue–top sodium citrate tubes. Hematology specimens are collected in lavender top tubes containing the anticoagulant EDTA, but the tests are performed on whole blood, not plasma. Serology tests are usually performed on serum. Blood collected in red/light gray–top tubes will clot. Clotted blood yields serum, not plasma.

REVIEW: Yes ☐ No ☐

📖 **WORKBOOK** Matching Exercise 12-4 will remind you of the role that specimen processing plays in analysis preparation.

90. **Answer: d**

    WHY: The preferred specimen for many chemistry tests is serum. However, to obtain serum, the blood must first be allowed to clot completely before it can be centrifuged and separated. Complete clotting takes anywhere from 30 to 60 minutes at room temperature and even longer if the patient is on a blood thinner or has a high WBC count. Heparin is an anticoagulant. Anticoagulant specimens do not clot and can be spun in a centrifuge immediately to obtain plasma for testing. Collecting chemistry specimens in heparin reduces turnaround time (TAT), which is especially important for STAT tests.

    REVIEW: Yes ☐ No ☐

91. **Answer: c**

    WHY: There are three types of heparin: ammonium, lithium, and sodium heparin. Ammonium heparin is primarily found in capillary tubes for hematocrit determinations; however, sodium heparin and lithium heparin are commonly found in evacuated tubes. It is important to note the type of heparin in a collection tube to prevent interference in test results. For example, sodium heparin must not be used for electrolytes, because sodium is one of the electrolytes measured. Lithium heparin must not be used for lithium levels. All heparin tubes prevent coagulation regardless of the type of heparin they contain provided they are mixed properly, and all heparin tubes require mixing. All types of heparin require centrifugation if plasma is needed for testing.

    REVIEW: Yes ☐ No ☐

92. **Answer: d**

    WHY: Tube stoppers should be removed using commercially available stopper removal devices, by use of robotics, or after covering conventional stoppers (Fig. 12-17) with a 4 × 4-in gauze or tissue to catch any aerosol that may be released. In addition, the tube should be held behind a "splash shield" while the stopper is removed. Applying the brake to stop a centrifuge, "popping" stoppers when opening tubes, and pouring specimens directly into aliquot tubes instead of using transfer pipettes are all activities that should be avoided because they can generate infectious aerosols.

    REVIEW: Yes ☐ No ☐

93. **Answer: d**

    WHY: Blood in a nonadditive tube will eventually clot. When a clotted specimen is centrifuged, the clear liquid that separates from the cells and

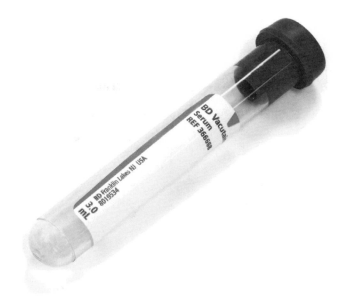

Figure 12-17 Evacuated collection tube with conventional stopper.

comes to the top of the specimen is called serum. Blood in an anticoagulant tube does not clot. When an anticoagulant tube is centrifuged or allowed to settle, the clear liquid that separates from the cells is called plasma. The red blood cells (RBCs) are heaviest and are at the bottom. The white blood cells and platelets are lighter and form a thin layer on top of the red blood cells called the buffy coat.

REVIEW: Yes ☐ No ☐

94. **Answer: d**

    WHY: If a serum specimen is not completely clotted before it is centrifuged, latent fibrin formation may cause the serum to clot. Incomplete clotting does not affect the action of the separator gel or cause hemolysis of the red blood cells. Buffy coat forms when a whole blood specimen is centrifuged. Clotted specimens do not form a buffy coat.

    REVIEW: Yes ☐ No ☐

95. **Answer: a**

    WHY: A serum specimen may take longer than normal to clot completely if the patient has a high white blood cell count or is on anticoagulant medication. Chilling also delays clot formation. A difficult collection or hemolysis does not normally delay clotting.

    REVIEW: Yes ☐ No ☐

96. **Answer: d**

    WHY: If the laboratory is on site, specimens are either hand delivered by the phlebotomist or

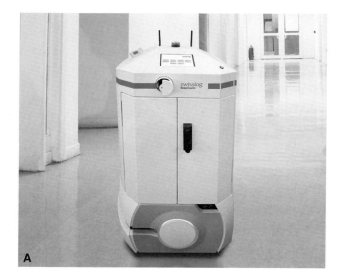

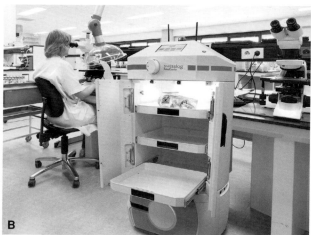

Figure 12-18 Robot system delivers specimens in the laboratory. (Courtesy Swisslog Healthcare Solutions North America, Denver, CO.)

other healthcare workers who have collected them or sent to the lab by means of an automated internal transportation system such as vertical track, pneumatic tube, or robot system (Fig. 12-18).

REVIEW: Yes ☐ No ☐

97. **Answer: b**

WHY: Stoppers should be left on tubes awaiting centrifugation to prevent contamination, evaporation (which *concentrates* analytes), loss of CO_2, and *increase* in PH.

REVIEW: Yes ☐ No ☐

98. **Answer: d**

WHY: Specimens drawn in gel barrier tubes generally clot within 30 minutes. Consequently, to prevent latent fibrin formation in the serum, the minimum precentrifugation time for this tube is 30 minutes.

REVIEW: Yes ☐ No ☐

99. **Answer: d**

WHY: A specimen should be centrifuged only once. Repeated centrifugation can cause hemolysis or otherwise deteriorate analytes and lead to erroneous test results.

REVIEW: Yes ☐ No ☐

100. **Answer: a**

WHY: Proper centrifuge operation involves balancing the centrifuge by placing tubes of equal volume and size opposite one another. Specimens should never be centrifuged before they are completely clotted. Specimens should always be centrifuged with the stoppers on to prevent evaporation of the specimen and generation of aerosols. Plasma and serum specimens can be centrifuged at the same time in the same centrifuge.

REVIEW: Yes ☐ No ☐

Chapter 13

Nonblood Specimens and Tests

Study Tips

- Complete the activities in Chapter 13 of the companion WORKBOOK.

- Draw an outline of the body. Make a numbered list of nonblood specimens and mark the location of the source of the specimen with an "x" and the number from the list.

- Make a table listing nonblood specimens, their sources, reasons for collecting them, and examples of tests performed on them.

- Make flash cards for the various nonblood specimens with the name of the fluid on one side and the source and reasons for collecting it on the other.

- See how many nonblood body fluids you can list in 1 minute.

- Study the steps and rationales for the various specimen collection procedures in Chapter 13 of the TEXTBOOK.

- Describe the various specimen collection procedures to one of your friends and have them repeat what they heard.

Overview

Although blood is the specimen of choice for many laboratory tests, various other body substances are also analyzed. The phlebotomist may be involved in obtaining the specimens (e.g., throat swab collection), test administration (e.g., sweat chloride collection), instruction (e.g., urine collection), processing (accessioning and preparing the specimen for testing), or simply verifying labeling and transporting the specimens to the laboratory. As with other laboratory specimens, standard precautions must be followed when handling nonblood specimens. This chapter addresses routine and special nonblood specimens and procedures, including the collection and handling of urine specimens and other nonblood body fluids and substances. A phlebotomist with a thorough understanding of all aspects of nonblood specimen collection helps ensure the quality of the specimens and the accuracy of test results.

Review Questions

Choose the BEST answer.

1. An antibiotic susceptibility test determines which antibiotics
   a. are effective against a particular microbe.
   b. cause an allergic reaction in the patient.
   c. cause the fewest side effects in the patient.
   d. reduce a patient's susceptibility to infection.

2. This microbe is often the causative agent of hospital-acquired diarrhea.
   a. *Clostridium difficile*
   b. *Helicobacter pylori*
   c. *Neisseria meningitidis*
   d. *Staphylococcus aureus*

3. A catheterized urine specimen is collected
   a. after stimulating urine production with intravenous histamine.
   b. by aspirating it with a sterile syringe inserted into the bladder.
   c. following midstream, clean-catch urine collection procedures.
   d. from a sterile tube passed through the urethra into the bladder.

4. CSF is the abbreviation for fluid that comes from the
   a. joint cavities.
   b. lung cavity.
   c. pelvic cavity.
   d. spinal cavity.

5. *Clean catch* refers to the collection of urine
   a. after cleaning the genital area.
   b. from a catheter in the bladder.
   c. in a container that is sterile.
   d. first thing in the morning.

6. A test that identifies bacteria and the antibiotics that can be used against them is the
   a. AFP test.
   b. C&S test.
   c. guaiac test.
   d. O&P test.

7. Which of the following types of infections would be classified as a UTI?
   a. Bladder
   b. Lung
   c. Nasal
   d. Throat

8. Fluid aspirated from the sac that surrounds the heart is called
   a. amniotic fluid.
   b. pericardial fluid.
   c. peritoneal fluid.
   d. synovial fluid.

9. This test includes a physical, chemical, and microscopic analysis of the specimen.
   a. AFP
   b. C&S
   c. GTT
   d. UA

10. A technician is aspirating a specimen from flexible tube coming out of a patient's nose. What type of test was most likely ordered?
    a. Gastric analysis
    b. *H. pylori* culture
    c. Sputum culture
    d. Stomach biopsy

11. This type of specimen is obtained by inserting a flexible swab through the nose.
    a. AFP
    b. Buccal
    c. Gastric
    d. NP

12. This test can be used to evaluate stomach acid production.
    a. C-urea breath
    b. Gastric analysis
    c. Hydrogen breath
    d. Sweat chloride

13. A technician collects a specimen from a child's mouth by rubbing a swab on the inside of the cheek. What type of specimen is most likely being collected?
    a. Breath
    b. Buccal
    c. Sputum
    d. Throat

14. A type of bacterium that can damage the stomach lining is
    a. *Bordetella pertussis*.
    b. *Helicobacter pylori*.
    c. *Neisseria meningitidis*.
    d. *Staphylococcus aureus*.

15. An exocrine gland disorder that primarily affects the lungs, upper respiratory tract, liver, and pancreas is
    a. cystic fibrosis.
    b. emphysema.
    c. herpes zoster.
    d. tuberculosis.

16. A term used to describe blood that cannot be seen with the naked eye is
    a. guaiac.
    b. micro.
    c. occult.
    d. serous.

17. What special information in addition to routine identification information is required in labeling a nonblood specimen?
    a. Any special handling needs
    b. Biohazard warning sticker
    c. Ordering physician's name
    d. Type and source of specimen

18. Which type of specimen must be handled and analyzed STAT?
    a. Buccal swab
    b. Gastric fluid
    c. Spinal fluid
    d. Throat swab

19. The most frequently analyzed nonblood specimen is
    a. feces.
    b. saliva.
    c. CSF.
    d. urine.

20. Which of the following can occur in urine specimens that are not processed in a timely fashion?
    a. Breakdown of bilirubin
    b. Decomposition of cells
    c. Overgrowth of bacteria
    d. All of the above

21. Which specimen is ideal for most urine tests?
    a. 8-hour
    b. 24-hour
    c. Fasting
    d. Random

22. A buccal swab can now be used for the diagnosis of
    a. bladder cancer
    b. herpes simplex
    c. tuberculosis
    d. whooping cough

23. Which of the following is typically included in a routine UA?
    a. Chemical analysis
    b. C&S
    c. Cytological analysis
    d. Drug screening

24. A urine C&S is typically ordered to
    a. check for glucose in the urine.
    b. diagnose urinary tract infection.
    c. evaluate the function of the kidneys.
    d. monitor urinary protein levels.

25. Urine cytology studies look for the presence of
    a. abnormal cells.
    b. heavy metals.
    c. illegal drugs.
    d. microbe toxins.

26. Urine drug screening is unable to
    a. detect prescription drug abuse.
    b. detect the use of illegal drugs.
    c. identify a deliberate overdose.
    d. monitor therapeutic drug use.

27. Suspected pregnancy is typically confirmed by testing urine for the presence of
    a. ADH.
    b. FSH.
    c. HCG.
    d. TSH.

28. Which type of urine specimen is best for pregnancy testing?
    a. 24-hour
    b. Clean-catch
    c. First-voided
    d. Random

29. Which type of specimen is typically used for routine urinalysis?
    a. 24-hour
    b. Double-voided
    c. First morning
    d. Random

30. Which urine specimen is normally the most concentrated?
    a. 24-hour
    b. First morning
    c. Random
    d. Timed

31. The patient must follow strict dietary restrictions for 72 hours before and during collection of this timed urine specimen.
    a. 2-hour postprandial glucose
    b. 5-hydroxyindolacetic acid
    c. Creatinine clearance
    d. Quantitative porphyrins

32. What is the recommended procedure for collecting a 24-hour urine specimen?
    a. Collect the first morning specimen and all other urine for 24 hours except the first specimen the following morning.
    b. Collect the first morning specimen and all urine for 24 hours including the first specimen the following morning.
    c. Discard the first morning specimen, start timing, and collect all urine for 24 hours including the next morning specimen.
    d. Start the timing and collect and preserve every urine specimen that is voided in any consecutive 24-hour period.

33. Which of the following statements is true of a urine creatinine clearance test?
    a. A 24-hour urine specimen is required.
    b. A fasting blood creatinine is required
    c. All of the urine is to be double voided.
    d. The urine is kept at body temperature.

34. This type of specimen is sometimes used to compare urine concentrations of glucose and ketones to blood concentrations.
    a. 8-hour
    b. 24-hour
    c. Double-voided
    d. Pooled time

35. Which urine test requires a midstream clean-catch specimen?
    a. Creatinine clearance
    b. Culture and sensitivity
    c. Glucose tolerance test
    d. Routine urinalysis

36. Which of the following midstream urine collection steps are in the proper order?
    a. Void into container; void into second container; void last urine into toilet
    b. Void into container; void into toilet; void remaining urine into container
    c. Void into toilet; void into container; void any remaining urine into toilet
    d. Void into toilet; void into container; void into toilet; void into container

37. Midstream clean-catch urine specimens require
    a. a preservative in the container.
    b. collection in a sterile container.
    c. timing of specimen collection.
    d. transportation at 37°C.

38. Which urine specimen is obtained by inserting a sterile needle directly into the urinary bladder and aspirating a sample of urine?
    a. Catheterized
    b. Double-voided
    c. Pediatric
    d. Suprapubic

39. Which of the following tests is sometimes performed on amniotic fluid?
    a. Alkaline phosphatase
    b. Alpha-fetoprotein
    c. Lactic dehydrogenase
    d. Reticulocyte count

40. Amniotic fluid comes from the
    a. cavity surrounding the spinal cord.
    b. membranes that enclose the lungs.
    c. sac containing a fetus in the womb.
    d. spaces within the moveable joints.

41. CSF analysis is used in the diagnosis of
    a. meningitis.
    b. osteoporosis.
    c. pneumonia.
    d. renal failure.

42. Tests commonly performed on CSF include
    a. cell counts.
    b. glucose.
    c. total protein.
    d. all of the above.

43. This test requires intravenous administration of histamine or pentagastrin.
    a. Alpha-fetoprotein
    b. Gastric analysis
    c. Sweat chloride
    d. Urine porphyrins

44. An NP culture swab is sometimes collected to detect the presence of organisms that cause
    a. inflamed throats.
    b. stomach ulcers.
    c. urinary infection.
    d. whooping cough.

45. Saliva tests can identify
    a. arthritis antibodies.
    b. chronic drug abuse.
    c. heavy metal intake.
    d. recent use of drugs.

46. Semen analysis can be performed to
    a. detect bladder infection.
    b. evaluate fertility status.
    c. identify cancerous cells.
    d. monitor prostate growth.

47. A semen specimen is unlikely to be accepted for testing if it is
    a. collected in a condom.
    b. collected on site.
    c. in a sterile container.
    d. kept at 37°C.

48. Which of the following fluids is obtained through lumbar puncture?
    a. Amniotic
    b. Gastric
    c. Pleural
    d. Spinal

49. Which of the following is a type of serous fluid?
    a. Gastric
    b. Pleural
    c. Seminal
    d. Synovial

50. Peritoneal fluid comes from the
    a. abdominal cavity.
    b. lung cavities.
    c. pericardial sac.
    d. spinal cavity.

51. Fluid from joint cavities is called
    a. pericardial fluid.
    b. peritoneal fluid.
    c. pleural fluid.
    d. synovial fluid.

52. Pleural fluid is aspirated from the
    a. lungs.
    b. joints.
    c. spine.
    d. stomach.

53. Accumulation of excess fluid in the peritoneal cavity is called
    a. ascites.
    b. edema.
    c. peritonitis.
    d. septicemia.

54. What is sputum?
    a. Gastric fluid
    b. Nasal fluid
    c. Phlegm
    d. Saliva

55. Sputum specimens are collected in the diagnosis of
    a. genetic defects.
    b. lung maturity.
    c. strep throat.
    d. tuberculosis.

56. This test is used to diagnose cystic fibrosis.
    a. C-urea breath
    b. CSF analysis
    c. Gastric studies
    d. Sweat chloride

57. Which of the following types of ETS tubes are used for synovial fluid specimens?
    a. ACD, CPD, and serum separator
    b. Citrate, EDTA, and gel separator
    c. EDTA, heparin, and nonadditive
    d. Sodium fluoride, CPD, and heparin

58. Synovial fluid can be tested to identify
    a. arthritis and gout.
    b. *H. pylori* and TB.
    c. hemolytic anemia.
    d. lactose intolerance.

59. A process called iontophoresis is used to collect
    a. breath.
    b. semen.
    c. sweat.
    d. tears.

60. Bone marrow is typically aspirated from the
    a. iliac crest.
    b. left femur.
    c. vertebrae.
    d. wrist bone.

61. Bone marrow is studied to identify
    a. arthritic disease.
    b. blood disorders.
    c. diabetes mellitus.
    d. osteochondritis.

62. A breath specimen can be used to detect
    a. bacterial meningitis.
    b. *H. pylori.*
    c. pertussis microbes.
    d. whooping cough.

63. Which of the following tests may require a 72-hour stool specimen?
    a. Fecal fat analysis
    b. Fecal occult blood
    c. O&P
    d. Stool culture

64. The sweat of a child can be up to five times saltier than normal if they have
    a. cystic fibrosis
    b. strep throat
    c. tuberculosis
    d. whooping cough

65. The guaiac test detects
    a. cystic fibrosis.
    b. lung maturity.
    c. occult blood.
    d. tuberculosis.

66. Which type of sample can be tested to detect chronic drug abuse?
    a. Blood
    b. Hair
    c. Saliva
    d. Urine

67. What type of specimen is required for a "rapid strep" test?
    a. Buccal swab
    b. Stool sample
    c. Throat swab
    d. Urine sample

68. What type of specimen is collected during a biopsy?
    a. Blood
    b. Stool
    c. Sweat
    d. Tissue

69. Which site is typically used when performing a sweat chloride test on a toddler?
    a. Arm
    b. Hand
    c. Thigh
    d. Wrist

70. The first tube of cerebrospinal fluid (CSF) collected is typically used for
    a. chemistry studies.
    b. counting the cells.
    c. immunology tests.
    d. microbiology tests.

71. A minimally invasive way of obtaining cells for DNA analysis is to collect a
    a. breath sample.
    b. buccal swab.
    c. stool sample.
    d. throat swab.

72. This fluid comes from the male reproductive system.
    a. Pleural
    b. Seminal
    c. Serous
    d. Synovial

73. This type of sample is sometimes collected for drug testing because it is not easily tampered with or altered.
    a. Bone marrow
    b. Buccal swab
    c. Hair sample
    d. Urine sample

74. This test detects parasites and their eggs in feces.
    a. C&S
    b. FOBT
    c. HCG
    d. O&P

75. The hydrogen breath test detects
    a. *H. pylori* bacteria.
    b. lactose intolerance.
    c. respiratory disease.
    d. whooping cough.

76. Why is a first morning urine specimen undesirable for cytology studies?
    a. Abnormal concentration of protein causes false positive
    b. Cells may have disintegrated in the bladder overnight
    c. Microorganisms could masks the cells being studied
    d. pH of first morning specimen interferes with test results

77. Why is the morning specimen at the end of a 24-hour collection so important?
    a. It is diluted because the kidneys work while the body is at rest.
    b. It is less in volume, but more ketones and glucose are present.
    c. It is normally the largest by volume and the most concentrated.
    d. It has a higher pH and protein than other day-time specimens.

78. From which of the following substances is an AFB smear made?
    a. Saliva
    b. Semen
    c. Sputum
    d. Sweat

79. Which of the following is a test that can be performed on hair, but the sample must be plucked rather than cut?
    a. Alcohol
    b. DNA
    c. FOBT
    d. Lead

80. VRE is sometimes detected using a/an
    a. AFP smear
    b. buccal smear
    c. NP swab
    d. rectal swab

Answers and Explanations

1. **Answer: a**

   WHY: An antibiotic susceptibility test is the sensitivity part of a culture and sensitivity (C&S) test. If a microorganism is identified by culture, a sensitivity test is performed to determine which antibiotics will be effective against the microorganism—in other words, which antibiotics the microorganism is susceptible to and thus, can be used to treat the patient.
   REVIEW: Yes ☐ No ☐

2. **Answer: a**

   WHY: *Clostridium difficile* (*C. difficile*) is a bacterium that can inhabit the intestinal tract and proliferate at the expense of normal bacteria in patients on antibiotic therapy. Although it is not commonly found in healthy adults, it is frequently found in hospitalized patients and is implicated as a causative agent of hospital-acquired diarrhea. Although cases are usually mild and subside when the antibiotic is discontinued, symptoms can persist and may become severe in some individuals, especially those who are immunocompromised.
   REVIEW: Yes ☐ No ☐

3. **Answer: d**

   WHY: A urine catheter is a narrow flexible tube inserted through the urethra directly into the bladder. A catheterized urine specimen is collected when a patient is having trouble urinating or is already catheterized for other reasons. Catheterized specimens are sometimes collected on infants to obtain C&S specimens, on female patients to prevent vaginal contamination of the specimen, and

on bedridden patients when serial urine specimens are needed.
REVIEW: Yes ☐ No ☐

4. **Answer: d**

   WHY: Cerebrospinal fluid (CSF) is the normally clear, colorless fluid that surrounds the brain and spinal cord.
   REVIEW: Yes ☐ No ☐

5. **Answer: a**

   WHY: *Clean catch* refers to a urine specimen collected after following a special cleaning procedure used to ensure that the specimen is free of contaminating material from the external genital area. A catheterized specimen is collected from a catheter inserted into the bladder. A urine specimen collected in a sterile container is not necessarily a clean-catch specimen, although a clean-catch specimen *is* supposed to be collected in a sterile container. Urine collected first thing in the morning is called an 8-hour or first-voided specimen and is not necessarily collected by clean-catch procedures.
   REVIEW: Yes ☐ No ☐

   📖 *Test your knowledge of the entire clean-catch procedure with WORKBOOK Knowledge Drill 13-4.*

6. **Answer: b**

   WHY: A urine C&S is a test that is sometimes ordered on patients with symptoms of urinary tract infection (UTI). In the culture portion of the test, urine is placed on a nutrient medium that encourages the growth of bacteria. Any bacteria that grow are identified and a sensitivity test is performed.

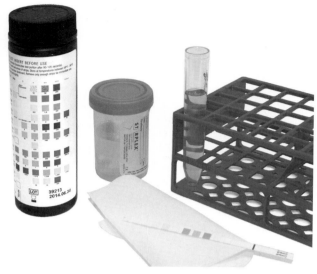

Figure 13-1 Urinalysis specimen, reagent strip for chemical testing and urine in a conical tube ready to centrifuge for microscopic examination.

A sensitivity test identifies antibiotics that will be effective against the bacteria.

REVIEW: Yes ☐ No ☐

7. **Answer: a**

WHY: A urinary tract infection (UTI) is an infection anywhere in the urinary system. The bladder is part of the urinary tract.

REVIEW: Yes ☐ No ☐

8. **Answer: b**

WHY: The sac that surrounds the heart is called the pericardium. Fluid found in this sac is called pericardial fluid.

REVIEW: Yes ☐ No ☐

9. **Answer: d**

WHY: A urinalysis (UA) test typically includes the physical, chemical, and microscopic analysis of a urine specimen (Fig. 13-1). The physical analysis includes macroscopic observations of color, clarity, and odor and measurements of volume and specific gravity. Chemical analysis detects the presence of substances such as bacteria, blood, white blood cells, protein, and glucose. The microscopic analysis identifies components in the urine such as cells, crystals, and microorganisms.

REVIEW: Yes ☐ No ☐

10. **Answer: a**

WHY: A gastric analysis test examines stomach contents for abnormal substances and measures gastric acid concentration to evaluate stomach acid production. A gastric analysis specimen is aspirated through a tube passed through the mouth and throat or nose and throat into the stomach.

REVIEW: Yes ☐ No ☐

11. **Answer: d**

WHY: A nasopharyngeal (NP) specimen is collected using a special flexible swab inserted gently through the nose into the nasopharynx (Fig. 13-2). Alpha-fetoprotein (AFP) is a type of test that can be performed on amniotic fluid to assess fetal development. Buccal (cheek) specimens for DNA analysis are collected by swabbing the inside of the cheek. Gastric specimens are collected by passing flexible tubing through the mouth and throat (oropharynx) or nose and throat (nasopharynx) into the stomach and aspirating stomach (gastric) fluid through the tubing.

REVIEW: Yes ☐ No ☐

1. Use a cotton-tipped aluminum wire swab.
2. Grasp the shaft, using the thumb and forefinger, about 3" from the tip.
3. Gently insert the swab into one nostril stopping when the swab contacts the mid-inferior portion of the inferior tubinate (1/3 to 1/2 way up the shaft).
4. Gently rotate the swab tip several times to loosen and collect material.
5. Gently withdrawal the swab and place in VTM. Refrigerate and send to lab.

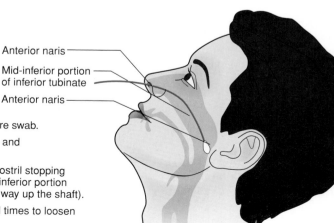

Anterior naris
Mid-inferior portion of inferior tubinate
Anterior naris

70°

Patient's head should be inclined from vertical as shown for proper specimen recovery.

Figure 13-2 Nasopharyngeal (NP) swab collection procedure.

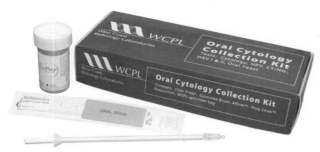

Figure 13-3 Buccal swab collection kit.

12. **Answer: b**

    WHY: *Gastric* means "of the stomach." A gastric analysis test examines fluid material from the stomach for abnormal substances and measures the acid concentration in it to evaluate stomach acid production. The C-urea breath test detects *Helicobacter pylori* (*H. pylori*) bacteria. A hydrogen breath test detects lactose intolerance. A sweat chloride test is used in the diagnosis of cystic fibrosis.

    REVIEW: Yes ☐   No ☐

13. **Answer: b**

    WHY: The specimen being collected is most likely a buccal (cheek) specimen for DNA analysis. (A buccal swab collection kit is shown in Fig. 13-3.) Such a specimen is collected by swabbing the inside of the cheek. DNA is later extracted from cells on the swab.

    REVIEW: Yes ☐   No ☐

14. **Answer: b**

    WHY: *Helicobacter pylori* (*H. pylori*) is a bacteria normally found in the stomach of some people; this bacteria secretes substances that damage the lining of the stomach, causing chronic gastritis that can lead to peptic ulcer disease.

    REVIEW: Yes ☐   No ☐

15. **Answer: a**

    WHY: Cystic fibrosis is a disorder of the exocrine glands that affects many body systems but primarily the lungs, upper respiratory tract, liver, and pancreas. Emphysema and tuberculosis affect the respiratory system but are not exocrine gland disorders. Herpes zoster (shingles) is an infection caused by varicella zoster virus; it results in a painful eruption of blisters along the course of a nerve.

    REVIEW: Yes ☐   No ☐

16. **Answer: c**

    WHY: *Occult* means "hidden or concealed." Occult blood is blood in feces that is present in such tiny amounts that it cannot be seen with the naked eye. Guaiac is a type of tree resin containing a chemical that can detect blood. Tests for occult blood that use this chemical are called guaiac tests.

    REVIEW: Yes ☐   No ☐

17. **Answer: d**

    WHY: As a minimum, nonblood specimens should be labeled with the same identification information as blood specimens. However, because many nonblood specimens are similar in appearance, it is very important to include information on the type and source of the specimen.

    REVIEW: Yes ☐   No ☐

18. **Answer: c**

    WHY: Spinal fluid (cerebrospinal fluid or CSF) is obtained by a physician through lumbar puncture. It should be delivered to the laboratory stat and analysis started immediately. CSF specimens are not easily recollected and the procedure can be uncomfortable and costly. It also involves greater risk and often produces a higher level of patient anxiety than the collection of most other types of laboratory specimens. If immediate testing is not possible chemistry and serology tubes are typically frozen, microbiology tubes can remain at room temperature, and hematology tubes are refrigerated. Specimens that are over 24 hours old when delivered to the laboratory are normally considered unacceptable for testing and will most likely be rejected by the laboratory.

    REVIEW: Yes ☐   No ☐

19. **Answer: d**

    WHY: Urine is fairly easy to obtain and provides valuable information in a number of circumstances including monitoring wellness, diagnosing and treating urinary tract infections, detecting and monitoring metabolic disease, and drug screening. Consequently it is the most frequently analyzed nonblood specimen.

    REVIEW: Yes ☐   No ☐

20. **Answer: d**

    WHY: Some components in a urine sample are not stable. If a urine specimen is not processed in a timely fashion, any bilirubin in the sample can break down to biliverdin, cellular elements can decompose, and bacteria can multiply.

    REVIEW: Yes ☐   No ☐

21. **Answer: a**

    WHY: Although not always required, a first morning (also called first-voided or 8-hour) specimen is

the ideal specimen for most urine studies because
it is the most concentrated.

REVIEW: Yes ☐ No ☐

22. **Answer: b**

WHY: A buccal swab (Fig. 13-3) allows the laboratory to collect DNA from the cells on the inside
of a person's cheek for testing. This method of
collecting a sample offers a rapid and sensitive way
to test for specific DNA using polymerase chain
reaction (PCR) testing. PCR is a type of testing
that can detect pieces of DNA from viruses such as
Herpes simplex.

REVIEW: Yes ☐ No ☐

23. **Answer: a**

WHY: A routine urinalysis typically includes a
physical, chemical, and microscopic analysis
(Fig. 13-1). Physical analysis notes the color, odor,
transparency, and specific gravity of the specimen.
Chemical analysis typically involves dipping a
reagent strip into the specimen to detect the presence of bacteria, blood, white blood cells, protein,
glucose, and other substances. A microscopic
analysis of urine sediment identifies urine components such as casts, cells, and crystals. Cytological
analysis of urine is performed to detect cancer,
cytomegalovirus, and other viral and inflammatory
diseases of the bladder, as well as other structures
of the urinary system, but it is not part of a routine
urinalysis. Culture and sensitivity (C&S) testing
and drug screening can be performed on urine but
are not part of a routine UA.

REVIEW: Yes ☐ No ☐

24. **Answer: b**

WHY: The most common reason for ordering a
culture and sensitivity (C&S) on a urine specimen
is to diagnose urinary tract infection (UTI). Urine
C&S testing can detect the presence of UTI through
culturing (growing) and identifying microorganisms present in the urine. When microorganisms
are identified an antibiotic susceptibility test is
performed to determine which antibiotics are
effective against the microorganism.

REVIEW: Yes ☐ No ☐

25. **Answer: a**

WHY: Urine cytology studies look for the presence
of abnormal cells that have been shed from the
urinary tract into the urine. Cytological analysis of
urine can detect cancer, cytomegalovirus, and other
viral and inflammatory diseases of the bladder and
other structures of the urinary system.

REVIEW: Yes ☐ No ☐

26. **Answer: c**

WHY: Urine drug screening can be used to detect
illegal drug use or abuse, unwarranted use of pre-
scription drugs, and use of performance-enhancing
steroids as well as to monitor therapeutic drug use
to minimize withdrawal symptoms or confirm drug
overdose. Drug screening identifies drugs in urine
but cannot prove whether or not a drug overdose
was intentional.

REVIEW: Yes ☐ No ☐

27. **Answer: c**

WHY: Pregnancy can be confirmed by testing urine
for the presence of human chorionic gonadotropin
(HCG), a hormone produced by cells within a developing placenta. This hormone appears in serum
and urine approximately 8 to 10 days after concep-
tion or fertilization.

REVIEW: Yes ☐ No ☐

28. **Answer: c**

WHY: Although a random urine specimen can be
used for testing, the first morning (also called
first-voided or 8-hour) specimen is preferred
because it is normally the most concentrated and
therefore would have the highest HCG concentration if the patient is pregnant.

REVIEW: Yes ☐ No ☐

29. **Answer: d**

WHY: Random urine specimens are typically used
for routine urinalysis. *Random* refers only to the
timing of the specimen and not the method of
collection.

REVIEW: Yes ☐ No ☐

30. **Answer: b**

WHY: The first morning specimen is usually the
most concentrated.

REVIEW: Yes ☐ No ☐

31. **Answer: b**

WHY: 5-hydroxyindolacetic acid (HIAA), is a metab-
olite of serotonin that is measured in the diagnosis
of and monitoring of a particular type of tumor
that produces serotonin. Consequently the patient
must not eat certain foods that have high serotonin
content (including avocados, bananas, kiwi fruit,
specific kinds of nuts, and tomato products) for a
72-hour period prior to and during collection.

REVIEW: Yes ☐ No ☐

32. **Answer: c**

WHY: A 24-hour urine specimen is collected to
allow quantitative analysis of a urine analyte.

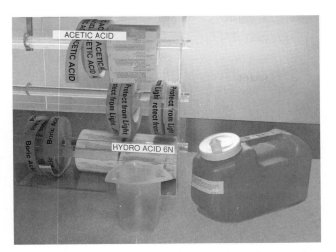

Figure 13-4 A 24-hour urine specimen collection container with collection cup and an assortment of labeling tapes and instructions to be placed on collection containers.

Collection of all urine voided in the 24-hour period is critical. A special large collection container (Fig. 13-4) is required. The best time to begin a 24-hour collection is when the patient wakes in the morning, typically between 6 and 8 AM. The first morning specimen is from the previous 24 hours and must be voided and discarded before timing is started. All urine voided over the next 24 hours is collected, including the next morning's specimen.

REVIEW: Yes ☐ No ☐

33. **Answer: a**

WHY: A urine creatinine clearance requires collection of a 24-hour urine, which is kept refrigerated throughout the collection period. A blood creatinine specimen is also required, but it is ideally collected 12 hours into the urine collection and is not a fasting specimen. All urine voided in the 24-hour period is carefully collected in a special container (Fig. 13-4). A double-voided urine is a type of specimen collected to compare the urine concentrations of an analyte to its concentration in the blood and is not part of creatinine clearance test.

REVIEW: Yes ☐ No ☐

34. **Answer: c**

WHY: A double-voided specimen is collected to compare the urine concentration of an analyte to its concentration in the blood. It is most commonly used to test urine for glucose and ketones. A fresh double-voided specimen is thought to more accurately reflect the blood concentration of an analyte than a specimen that has been held in the bladder for some time.

REVIEW: Yes ☐ No ☐

35. **Answer: b**

WHY: A urine culture and sensitivity test is most often ordered to detect urinary tract infection. It calls for the collection of a midstream clean-catch specimen in a sterile container. Midstream clean-catch procedures are necessary to ensure that the specimen is free of contamination by microorganisms from the external genital area. A creatinine clearance test requires a 24-hour urine specimen. At one time urine specimens were collected during a glucose tolerance test (GTT) but they are rarely required anymore. A routine urinalysis requires a regular-voided random urine specimen.

REVIEW: Yes ☐ No ☐

36. **Answer: c**

WHY: A midstream urine collection is performed to obtain a specimen that is free of genital secretions, pubic hair, and bacteria from the area around the urinary opening. To collect a midstream urine specimen, the patient voids initial urine into the toilet and then brings the container into the urine stream until a sufficient amount of urine is collected. Any excess urine is voided into the toilet.

REVIEW: Yes ☐ No ☐

📖 *See how well you understand the rationale for the clean-catch urine collection procedure with WORKBOOK Knowledge Drill 13-4.*

37. **Answer: b**

WHY: A midstream clean-catch urine collection is typically performed to obtain a specimen for culture and sensitivity testing to detect urinary tract infection. It is important that the specimen be free of genital secretions, pubic hair, and bacteria that surround the urinary opening. This requires cleaning of the genital area before collecting a midstream specimen into a sterile container (Fig. 13-5) and prompt processing

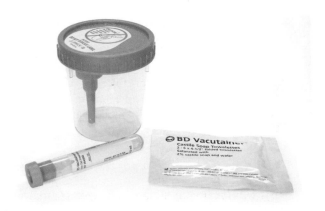

Figure 13-5 Sterile kit for urine culture and sensitivity (C & S) testing (Sterile Cup, preservative, urine tube, and castile soap towelettes).

to prevent overgrowth of any microorganisms present, decomposition of the specimen, and misinterpretation of results. A preservative is not normally required. No special timing is normally involved and the specimen is transported at room temperature, not 37°C.

REVIEW: Yes ☐ No ☐

38. **Answer: d**

WHY: A suprapubic urine specimen is collected in a sterile syringe by inserting the needle directly into the urinary bladder and aspirating urine directly from the bladder. Suprapubic collection is used to obtain samples for microbial analysis or cytology studies.

REVIEW: Yes ☐ No ☐

39. **Answer: b**

WHY: Alpha-fetoprotein (AFP) is an antigen normally present in the human fetus; it is also found in amniotic fluid and maternal serum. Abnormal AFP levels may indicate problems in fetal development, such as neural tube defects. AFP testing is initially performed on maternal serum and abnormal results are confirmed by AFP testing on amniotic fluid.

REVIEW: Yes ☐ No ☐

40. **Answer: c**

WHY: Amniotic fluid is the clear, almost colorless to pale-yellow fluid filling the membrane (amnion or amniotic sac) containing the fetus within the uterus. It is obtained by transabdominal amniocentesis, a procedure that involves inserting a needle through the mother's abdominal wall into the uterus and aspirating approximately 10 mL of fluid from the amniotic sac.

REVIEW: Yes ☐ No ☐

📖 *Test your knowledge of the source of non-blood specimens with WORKBOOK Labeling Exercise 13-2.*

41. **Answer: a**

WHY: The primary reason for collecting cerebrospinal fluid (CSF) is to diagnose meningitis. An increased white blood cell count in spinal fluid is most often associated with bacterial or viral meningitis.

REVIEW: Yes ☐ No ☐

42. **Answer: d**

WHY: Routine tests performed on cerebrospinal fluid include cell counts, glucose, chloride, and total protein. Other tests (e.g., cytology tests) are performed if indicated.

REVIEW: Yes ☐ No ☐

43. **Answer: b**

WHY: A typical gastric analysis, called a basal gastric analysis, involves aspirating a sample of gastric secretions by means of a tube passed through the mouth and throat (oropharynx) or nose and throat (nasopharynx) into the stomach following a period of fasting. This sample is tested to determine acidity. After the basal sample has been collected, a gastric stimulant, most commonly histamine or pentagastrin, is administered intravenously and several more samples are collected at timed intervals. Serum gastrin levels may also be collected.

REVIEW: Yes ☐ No ☐

44. **Answer: d**

WHY: Nasopharyngeal (NP) secretions can be collected on a special swab and cultured to detect the presence of microorganisms that cause diphtheria, meningitis, pneumonia, and whooping cough (pertussis).

REVIEW: Yes ☐ No ☐

45. **Answer: d**

WHY: Saliva specimens are increasingly being used to detect or confirm alcohol and drug abuse and monitor hormone levels because they can be collected quickly and easily in a noninvasive manner. Detection of drugs in saliva is a sign of recent drug use.

REVIEW: Yes ☐ No ☐

46. **Answer: b**

WHY: Semen is the sperm-containing thick fluid discharged during male ejaculation. Analysis of semen is primarily ordered to assess fertility or determine the effectiveness of sterilization after vasectomy.

REVIEW: Yes ☐ No ☐

47. **Answer: a**

WHY: Semen specimens should be collected in sterile containers, kept warm at or near body temperature of 37°C, and delivered to the laboratory immediately, which means that an on-site collection is ideal. Semen specimens should *never* be collected in a condom unless the condom was specifically designed for semen collection. Condoms often contain spermicides (substances that kill sperm), which invalidate test results.

REVIEW: Yes ☐ No ☐

📖 *WORKBOOK Labeling Exercise 13-2 will help you practice identifying the types of fluid that come from the different areas of the body.*

48. **Answer: d**

WHY: Cerebrospinal fluid (CSF) is obtained from the spinal cavity by lumbar puncture, also called a spinal tap. The spinal cord ends near the first or second lumbar vertebrae. To avoid injury to the spinal cord, the needle used to withdraw the CSF is inserted between the third and fourth or the fourth and fifth lumbar vertebrate, well below where the spinal cord ends. Amniotic fluid is aspirated from the sac that surrounds a fetus in the womb. Gastric fluid is aspirated from the stomach via a tube passed through the mouth and throat or nose and throat into the stomach. Pleural fluid is aspirated from the pleural (lung) cavity.

REVIEW: Yes ☐ No ☐

49. **Answer: b**

WHY: Serous fluid is a pale-yellow watery fluid resembling serum that is found between the double-layered membranes enclosing the pleural, pericardial, and peritoneal cavities; it is identified according to the cavity of origin. Gastric fluid is liquid material from the stomach. Seminal fluid (semen) is a thick yellowish-white fluid. Synovial fluid is a clear, viscous, pale-yellow fluid that comes from movable joints.

REVIEW: Yes ☐ No ☐

50. **Answer: a**

WHY: Peritoneal fluid is aspirated from within the membranes lining the abdominal cavity. Fluid from the lung cavity is called pleural fluid. Fluid from the pericardial sac surrounding the heart is called pericardial fluid. Fluid from the cavities surrounding the brain and spinal cord is called cerebrospinal fluid (CSF) or spinal fluid for short.

REVIEW: Yes ☐ No ☐

51. **Answer: d**

WHY: The clear, pale-yellow, viscous fluid found in movable joint cavities is called synovial fluid. This fluid lubricates the joints and decreases friction in them. It is normally present in small amounts but increases when inflammation is present. The aspirated fluid can be tested to identify or differentiate arthritis, gout, and other inflammatory conditions. Pleural fluid comes from the lungs. Pericardial fluid comes from the pericardial sac surrounding the heart. Peritoneal fluid comes from within the membranes that line the abdominal cavity.

REVIEW: Yes ☐ No ☐

52. **Answer: a**

WHY: Pleural fluid is aspirated from within the pleural membranes in the lungs. Peritoneal fluid is aspirated from within the membranes that line the abdominal cavity. Synovial fluid is aspirated from joint cavities. Fluid from the spinal cavity is

called cerebrospinal fluid (CSF), or simply spinal fluid.

REVIEW: Yes ☐ No ☐

53. **Answer: a**

WHY: Ascites (a-si'-tez) is the accumulation of excess serous fluid in the peritoneal cavity. Edema is the accumulation of excess fluid in the tissues. Peritonitis is inflammation of the peritoneum, the membranes lining the abdominal cavity. Septicemia is the presence of pathogenic microbes or their toxins in the bloodstream.

REVIEW: Yes ☐ No ☐

54. **Answer: c**

WHY: Sputum is mucus or phlegm that is ejected from the trachea, bronchi, and lungs by deep coughing.

REVIEW: Yes ☐ No ☐

📖 *See if you can identify a sputum collection container and other nonblood specimen containers in WORKBOOK Labeling Exercise 13-1.*

55. **Answer: d**

WHY: Sputum specimens are sometimes collected and cultured to detect the presence of microorganisms in the diagnosis or monitoring of lower respiratory tract infections such as tuberculosis (TB). The sputum test for TB is called an acid-fast bacillus (AFB) culture. A sputum collection container is shown in Figure 13-6.

REVIEW: Yes ☐ No ☐

56. **Answer: d**

WHY: A sweat chloride test analyzes a sweat specimen for chloride content in the diagnosis of cystic fibrosis in children and adolescents. Patients with cystic fibrosis have abnormally high (two to five times normal) levels of chloride in their sweat.

REVIEW: Yes ☐ No ☐

57. **Answer: c**

WHY: Synovial fluid is typically collected in an EDTA or heparin tube for cell counts, identification of crystals, and smear preparations; in a nonadditive tube for macroscopic appearance, chemistry, and immunology tests and to observe clot formation; and in a sterile tube or container for culture and sensitivity testing.

REVIEW: Yes ☐ No ☐

58. **Answer: a**

WHY: Synovial fluid is normally present in small amounts, but levels increase when inflammation is present. Synovial fluid specimens can be

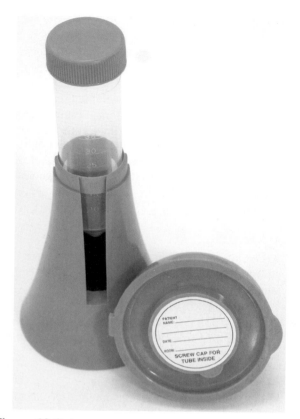

Figure 13-6 A sputum collection container.

aspirated from joints and tested to identify or differentiate arthritis, gout, and other inflammatory conditions.

REVIEW: Yes ☐ No ☐

59. **Answer: c**

WHY: A sweat chloride test involves producing measurable quantities of sweat by transporting pilocarpine (a sweat-stimulating drug) into the skin by means of electrical stimulation (iontophoresis) from electrodes placed on the skin. Sweat is then collected, weighed to determine the volume, and analyzed for chloride content.

REVIEW: Yes ☐ No ☐

60. **Answer: a**

WHY: A physician obtains a bone marrow specimen by inserting a special large-gauge needle into the iliac crest (hip bone) or sternum (breast bone) and aspirating some of the marrow into a syringe.

REVIEW: Yes ☐ No ☐

61. **Answer: b**

WHY: Because it is the site of blood cell production, bone marrow may be obtained and examined to detect and identify blood disorders.

REVIEW: Yes ☐ No ☐

62. **Answer: b**

WHY: Breath specimens are collected and analyzed in the detection of *H. pylori*, a type of bacterium that secretes substances that damage the lining of the stomach, causing chronic gastritis and leading to peptic ulcer disease.

REVIEW: Yes ☐ No ☐

63. **Answer: a**

WHY: A fecal fat analysis sometimes requires a 72-hour refrigerated stool specimen. Fecal occult blood testing (FOBT) typically requires small amounts of feces collected on special test cards on three separate days. Ova and parasite (O&P) testing typically requires small amounts of feces from a fresh stool specimen that are placed in special vials containing preservative (Fig. 13-7). A stool culture requires a single fresh specimen.

REVIEW: Yes ☐ No ☐

64. **Answer: a**

WHY: Cystic fibrosis is a disorder of the exocrine glands that affects many body systems but primarily the lungs, upper respiratory tract, liver, and pancreas. The sweat of patients with CF can be up to five times saltier than normal because their sweat contains two to five times the normal amount of chloride.

REVIEW: Yes ☐ No ☐

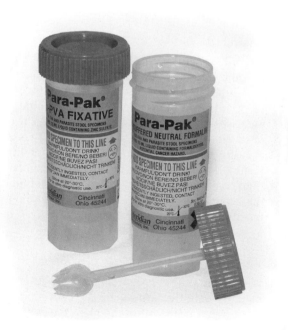

Figure 13-7 Ova and parasite transfer containers.

65. Answer: c

WHY: Occult blood is blood present in such tiny amounts that it is invisible to the naked eye. Guaiac is a type of tree resin containing a chemical that can detect small amounts of blood. Tests that use this chemical to detect blood in feces are called guaiac tests.

REVIEW: Yes ☐   No ☐

66. Answer: b

WHY: Samples of hair are sometimes analyzed to detect drugs of abuse. Hair can show evidence of chronic drug use rather than recent use. Use of hair samples for drug testing is advantageous because hair cannot easily be altered.

REVIEW: Yes ☐   No ☐

67. Answer: c

WHY: Throat swab specimens (Fig. 13-8) are most often collected to aid in the diagnosis of streptococcal (strep) infections. A throat culture is typically collected using a special kit containing a sterile polyester-tipped swab in a covered transport tube containing transport medium. A throat swab is used for a "rapid strep" test because the test is used to diagnose strep throat. Results are typically ready in minutes.

REVIEW: Yes ☐   No ☐

68. Answer: d

WHY: A biopsy involves collection of a tissue sample from the area in question and its subsequent examination.

REVIEW: Yes ☐   No ☐

69. Answer: c

WHY: The forearm is the preferred site for sweat chloride testing in adults, but the leg or thigh is often used in infants or toddlers.

REVIEW: Yes ☐   No ☐

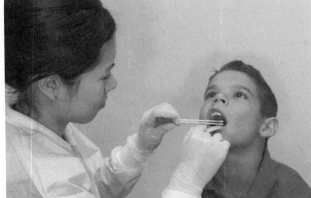

Figure 13-8 Throat swab being collected from a child for rapid strep test.

70. Answer: a

WHY: CSF is generally collected in three or four special sterile tubes numbered in order of collection. Laboratory protocol dictates which tests are to be performed on each particular tube unless indicated otherwise by the physician. Normally, the first tube is used for chemistry and immunology tests, the second tube for microbiology studies, and the third tube for cell count and differential. If a fourth tube is collected, it is typically used for cytology or other special tests, or as an extra tube.

REVIEW: Yes ☐   No ☐

📖 *Match other nonblood tests with equipment, procedure, or specimen requirements with WORKBOOK Matching Exercise 13-3.*

71. Answer: b

WHY: Collection of a buccal (cheek) swab is a less invasive and painless alternative to blood collection to obtain cells for DNA analysis. The phlebotomist collects the sample by gently massaging the mouth on the inside of the cheek with a special swab (Fig. 13-3). DNA is later extracted from cells on the swab.

REVIEW: Yes ☐   No ☐

72. Answer: b

WHY: Semen (seminal fluid) is the sperm-containing thick, yellowish-white fluid discharged during male ejaculation. It is analyzed to assess fertility or to determine the effectiveness of sterilization following vasectomy.

REVIEW: Yes ☐   No ☐

73. Answer: c

WHY: Use of hair samples is advantageous for drug testing because hair is easy to obtain and cannot be as easily tampered with as a urine sample. In addition, hair can show evidence of chronic drug abuse. Hair samples can also be used for trace and heavy metal analysis. Bone marrow is not easily obtained, requires a physician to collect, and is typically used to identify blood disorders, not drug abuse. Buccal swabs are most commonly used for DNA analysis.

REVIEW: Yes ☐   No ☐

74. Answer: d

WHY: An ova and parasite (O&P) test is typically performed on a stool (feces) specimen to detect intestinal parasites and their eggs (ova). Ova and parasite testing typically requires small amounts of feces from a fresh stool specimen that are placed in special vials containing preservative (Fig. 13-7). A culture and sensitivity test detects the presence of microorganisms and determines appropriate antibiotics to use against them. A fecal occult blood test (FOBT) detects hidden, tiny amounts of blood in feces. An HCG test detects human chorionic gonadotropin (HCG) in urine to confirm pregnancy.

REVIEW: Yes ☐ No ☐

75. **Answer: b**

WHY: The hydrogen breath test is used to evaluate lactose tolerance and is thought to be the most accurate lactose tolerance test.

REVIEW: Yes ☐ No ☐

76. **Answer: b**

WHY: Cytology studies are performed to detect cancer, cytomegalovirus, and other viral and inflammatory diseases of the bladder and other structures of the urinary system. Cells from the lining of the urinary tract are readily shed into the urine, and a smear containing them can easily be prepared from urinary sediment or filtrate. A fresh clean-catch specimen is required for the test. It should not be a first morning specimen because the cells may have disintegrated in the bladder overnight.

REVIEW: Yes ☐ No ☐

77. **Answer: c**

Why: Collection and pooling of all urine voided during the designated 24-hour period is critical. The last specimen will be collected at the same time the following morning. This last sample is normally the largest by volume and the most concentrated after having been in the bladder overnight.

REVIEW: Yes ☐ No ☐

78. **Answer: c**

Why: The diagnosis of TB is made from a sputum test that is often called an acid-fast bacillus (AFB) culture, and the slide made from sputum is called an AFB smear. First morning specimens are preferred, as secretions tend to collect in the lungs overnight and a larger volume of specimen can be produced. The patient must cough up material from deep in the respiratory tract and not simply spit into the container.

REVIEW: Yes ☐ No ☐

79. **Answer: b**

Why: The typical hair sample requirement is a lock of hair the width of a pencil and at least three inches in length. Hair samples are typically collected close to the scalp. For DNA analysis, the hair must include the root so samples must be plucked, not cut. Head hair is the preferred specimen, but beard, chest, mustache, or pubic hair can sometimes be used. Specimens can normally be submitted at room temperature.

REVIEW: Yes ☐ No ☐

80. **Answer: d**

Why: Microbiological tests on feces (stool) samples include culture to detect the presence of pathogenic bacteria, such as a type of bacteria called enterococci that have developed resistance to many antibiotics, especially vancomycin. Rectal swabs can be used to detect vancomycin-resistant enterococcus (VRE).

REVIEW: Yes ☐ No ☐

Chapter 14
Arterial Puncture Procedures

Study Tips

- Locate the brachial artery on a partner or yourself, noting how close it is to the pulse of the brachial artery.

- Locate the radial and ulnar arteries on a partner, perform the modified Allen test, and be able to describe a positive result and what it means.

- List the advantages of various arterial puncture sites on the front of a sheet of paper and disadvantages on the back. Quiz yourself over both.

- Study the ABG analytes in Table 14-1 and radial ABG Procedure 14-3 in the TEXTBOOK.

- The cautions in Chapter 14 of the TEXTBOOK describe things that you should not do when you are collecting ABGs. Be able to explain the reason or the proper procedure that is given for each caution.

- Make a table of arterial puncture complications, sampling errors, and specimen rejection criteria. Include descriptions of how to prevent or identify and handle them.

Overview Arterial puncture is technically difficult and potentially more painful and hazardous than venipuncture. Consequently, arterial specimens are *not* normally used for routine blood tests, even though arterial blood composition is more consistent throughout the body than venous, which varies relative to the metabolic needs of the area it serves. The primary reason for arterial puncture is to obtain blood for **arterial blood gas (ABG)** tests. **ABGs** evaluate respiratory function. Arterial blood is the best specimen for evaluating respiratory function because of its normally high oxygen content and consistency of composition. Capillary blood, which is similar to arterial blood in composition provided that the puncture site is warmed prior to specimen collection, is sometimes used to test blood gases in infants (see Chapter 10).

Those who collect ABG specimens must have a thorough understanding of all aspects of collection in order to ensure accurate results and the safety of the patient. This chapter addresses advantages and disadvantages of using various arterial puncture sites, radial ABG procedures, ABG analytes, and arterial puncture hazards, complications, sampling errors, and specimen rejection criteria.

Review Questions

Choose the BEST answer.

1. Arteriospasm is defined as
   a. artery contraction due to pain, irritation by a needle, or anxiety.
   b. fainting related to hypotension caused by a nervous response.
   c. pain that shoots up the side of the arm after needle penetration.
   d. tingling felt in the fingertips when the needle enters the artery.

2. Formation of a thrombus during arterial puncture can result from an
   a. extremely tight tourniquet.
   b. impaired collateral artery.
   c. injury to the arterial wall.
   d. unaddressed arteriospasm.

3. Significantly inaccurate ABG values can result from
   a. collection from a femoral artery.
   b. improperly applied antiseptic.
   c. microclots that are undetected.
   d. testing with a POCT instrument.

4. The integrity of a blood gas specimen can be affected by
   a. increased vagus nerve activity.
   b. ratio of blood to anticoagulant.
   c. use of a syringe instead of ETS.
   d. use of the anticoagulant heparin.

5. The thumb should not be used to feel for an artery because it
   a. has a pulse.
   b. is insensitive.
   c. is too large.
   d. is too strong.

6. A patient complication associated with arterial puncture is
   a. hemolysis.
   b. numbness.
   c. phlebitis.
   d. venostasis.

7. The radial artery is located in the
   a. antecubital fossa.
   b. crease of the groin.
   c. pinky side of the wrist.
   d. thumb side of the wrist.

8. Why is arterial blood better for blood gas determination than venous blood?
   a. Analytes in venous specimens are not very stable.
   b. Arterial puncture is technically easier to perform.
   c. Composition of arterial blood is more consistent.
   d. Venous blood is subject to more collection error.

9. The blood gas parameter HCO_3 measures the amount of
   a. bicarbonate circulating in the blood.
   b. carbon dioxide dissolved in the blood.
   c. oxygen dissolved in the bloodstream.
   d. oxygen that is bound to hemoglobin.

10. Which of the following tests requires an arterial specimen?
    a. Blood culture
    b. Blood gases
    c. Blood glucose
    d. Blood typing

11. Which of the following analytes is routinely part of a blood gas analysis?
    a. CO
    b. NH_3
    c. PaO_2
    d. PO_4

12. Arterial blood gas evaluation would *most* likely be performed on a patient with
    a. chronic hepatitis.
    b. hypothyroidism.
    c. osteochondritis.
    d. pulmonary disease.

13. Arterial puncture instruction typically includes
    a. bedside patient diagnosis.
    b. minimal theory training.
    c. observation of procedures.
    d. practice on other students.

14. Arterial puncture site selection is based on the
    a. absence of underlying ligaments.
    b. available equipment in the room.
    c. existence of collateral circulation.
    d. presence of a strong rapid pulse.

15. One reason to favor a site as a choice for arterial puncture is
    a. a recent puncture can provide a landmark.
    b. an active fistula can be used for the draw.
    c. that an IV in the arm is placed distal to the site.
    d. that it has very little tissue covering the artery.

16. The preferred and most common site for arterial puncture is the
    a. brachial artery.
    b. femoral artery.
    c. radial artery.
    d. ulnar artery.

17. Which artery is generally easiest to access during low cardiac output?
    a. Brachial
    b. Femoral
    c. Radial
    d. Ulnar

18. The *biggest* advantage of choosing the radial artery for ABG collection is that
    a. it can be felt during low blood pressure.
    b. it is easy to compress it to stop bleeding.
    c. it is superficial and very easy to palpate.
    d. it usually has good collateral circulation.

19. Which of the following is a disadvantage of using the radial artery for ABG collection?
    a. It has a high risk of hematoma.
    b. It has no collateral circulation.
    c. It is not easy to compress fully.
    d. It is small and difficult to feel.

20. Which of the following is an advantage of using the brachial artery for arterial blood collection?
    a. It is large and fairly easy to palpate.
    b. It is not as deep as the radial artery.
    c. Risk of hematoma formation is low.
    d. The artery is very easy to compress.

21. One disadvantage of puncturing the brachial artery is that it
    a. has irregular blood pressure.
    b. has ligaments underlying it.
    c. is superficial and rolls easily.
    d. lies near the median nerve.

22. Which arterial site poses the greatest risk of infection?
    a. Brachial
    b. Femoral
    c. Radial
    d. Ulnar

23. Of the following arteries, the best choice for arterial specimen collection would be the
    a. brachial artery of an infant or child.
    b. common carotid artery in the neck.
    c. dorsalis pedis artery of most adults.
    d. ulnar artery of a nondominant arm.

24. Supplemental information on an arterial blood gas requisition typically includes
    a. age at onset of respiratory disease.
    b. patient activity and body position.
    c. previous arterial blood gas values.
    d. the required blood collection system.

25. Which of the following is required for ABG collection?
    a. A 1- to 5-mL self-filling syringe
    b. A container full of crushed ice
    c. A disposable tourniquet strap
    d. A povidone–iodine prep pad

26. Arterial blood gas specimens are collected in syringes rather than tubes because
    a. a syringe holds the right amount of blood.
    b. anaerobic conditions are easier to maintain.
    c. evacuated tube pressure can change results.
    d. the sterility of the specimen is guaranteed.

27. PPE used when collecting arterial specimens includes
    a. gloves and hair cover.
    b. lab coat and gloves.
    c. N95-type respirator.
    d. mask and shoe covers.

28. Commercially prepared arterial sampling kits rarely contain a
    a. 1% lidocaine-filled syringe.
    b. cover for the syringe hub.
    c. needle with safety device.
    d. special heparinized syringe.

29. Heparin is used in arterial sample collection to
    a. increase blood flow in the area.
    b. numb the area around the site.
    c. prevent clotting of the specimen.
    d. stabilize the oxygen content.

30. Lidocaine is sometimes used during arterial puncture to
    a. anesthetize the site prior to the puncture.
    b. help dissolve air bubbles in the specimen.
    c. keep clots from forming in the specimen.
    d. maintain the specimen in an anaerobic state.

31. Prior to ABG collection, a patient should have been in a steady state for at least
    a. 5 to 10 minutes.
    b. 10 to 15 minutes.
    c. 15 to 20 minutes.
    d. 20 to 30 minutes.

32. A patient in a steady state for ABG collection has
    a. been fasting for at least 8 hours.
    b. been sleeping for at least an hour.
    c. had no oxygen therapy for 12 hours.
    d. had no suction changes in 20 minutes.

33. The purpose of performing the modified Allen test prior to arterial specimen collection is to
    a. assess patient ventilation status.
    b. determine collateral circulation.
    c. locate the pulse in the ulnar artery.
    d. measure the radial artery pressure.

34. When performing the modified Allen test, which artery is released first?
    a. Brachial
    b. Femoral
    c. Radial
    d. Ulnar

35. What constitutes a positive modified Allen test?
    a. The blood pressure increases in the radial artery.
    b. The color drains from the hand within 30 seconds.
    c. The hand color returns to normal in 15 seconds.
    d. The pulse in the ulnar artery becomes irregular.

36. Which of the following is proper procedure if the Allen test is negative?
    a. Check collateral circulation in the other arm.
    b. Collect the specimen from the femoral artery.
    c. Perform arterial puncture on the radial artery.
    d. Perform arterial puncture on the ulnar artery.

37. A patient who has collateral circulation
    a. does not need respiratory therapy or assessment.
    b. does not need to undergo radial artery puncture.
    c. has multiple arteries supplying blood to an area.
    d. has normal arterial pressure in both wrist areas.

38. Which of the following actions associated with the radial ABG procedure are in the correct order?
    a. Assess, position, clean, puncture, fill, expel, label
    b. Clean, position, assess, puncture, fill, label, expel

c. Label, clean, position, puncture, fill, assess, expel
d. Position, clean, assess, puncture, fill, expel, label

39. Which one of the following radial ABG specimen collection steps is optional?
    a. Administration of local anesthetic
    b. Assessment of collateral circulation
    c. Determination of current steady state
    d. Verification of required conditions

40. Positioning of the arm for radial ABG specimen collection includes
    a. placing the arm higher than the heart.
    b. having the dorsal side of the hand face up.
    c. having the patient's hand support the arm.
    d. extending the wrist approximately 30 degrees.

41. Which of the following would be a reason to terminate an arterial puncture?
    a. Bright red blood spurting into the syringe
    b. Missing the artery so that needle redirection is required
    c. The patient's complaints of extreme pain and discomfort
    d. A dark reddish blue color of the specimen

42. An example of improper antisepsis prior to arterial specimen collection would be
    a. allowing the site to air-dry before puncturing.
    b. cleaning the phlebotomist's nondominant finger.
    c. maintaining antisepsis at the puncture site.
    d. scrubbing the site with alcohol for 2 minutes.

43. In performing arterial puncture, the needle must be directed
    a. away from the hand, facing the blood flow.
    b. bevel-down to prevent reflux of the blood.
    c. perpendicular to the wrist and lower arm.
    d. toward the hand, against the blood flow.

44. Which of the following is an acceptable angle of needle insertion for drawing radial arterial blood gases?
    a. 15 degrees
    b. 20 degrees
    c. 45 degrees
    d. 90 degrees

45. The proper angle of needle insertion for drawing femoral arterial blood gas is
    a. 15 degrees
    b. 30 degrees
    c. 45 degrees
    d. 90 degrees

46. The typical needle used to collect blood from a radial artery is
    a. 18-gauge, 1 in.
    b. 22-gauge, 1 in.
    c. 23-gauge, 1½ in.
    d. 25-gauge, 1½ in.

47. How do you know when you have "hit" an artery during arterial blood gas collection?
    a. A flash of blood appears in the syringe hub.
    b. Blood immediately seeps around the needle.
    c. The pulse in the artery becomes very erratic.
    d. The syringe needle bends owing to resistance.

48. Which of the following is the best way to tell if a specimen is arterial? As the specimen is collected, the blood will
    a. appear bright red in color.
    b. contain small air bubbles.
    c. look darker than venous blood.
    d. pump or pulse into the syringe.

49. As soon as the needle is withdrawn following ABG specimen collection, the
    a. nurse should apply a special arterial puncture bandage.
    b. patient should apply pressure to the site for 3 to 5 minutes.
    c. phlebotomist should apply a pressure bandage to the site.
    d. phlebotomist should apply site pressure for 3 to 5 minutes.

50. Proper specimen handling immediately following collection involves
    a. mixing the specimen to prevent clotting.
    b. placing the specimen in a green-top tube.
    c. removing only excess air bubbles from it.
    d. using the safety needle to cap the syringe.

51. After performing arterial puncture, the phlebotomist should check the pulse
    a. distal to the puncture site.
    b. in the ulnar artery in the wrist.
    c. medial to the puncture site.
    d. proximal to the puncture site.

52. What should the phlebotomist do if the pulse is absent or faint following ABG collection?
    a. Apply a pressure bandage as soon as possible.
    b. Gently massage the patient's wrist and hand.
    c. Nothing, because an arteriospasm is expected.
    d. Notify the patient's nurse or the lab supervisor.

53. An arterial specimen collected in an appropriate plastic syringe is typically transported
    a. at room temperature.
    b. in a small heat block.
    c. in a cup of ice slurry.
    d. vertically in a syringe.

54. Specimens for electrolyte testing in addition to arterial blood gas analysis should be
    a. kept in a heat block during delivery.
    b. placed in a cup of ice slurry ASAP.
    c. transferred to a red-top test tube.
    d. transported at room temperature.

55. If the patient has an elevated white blood cell count, the ABG specimen should be
    a. analyzed ASAP.
    b. collected in EDTA.
    c. kept in a heat block.
    d. mixed continually.

56. Which of the following is a common arterial puncture complication even when proper procedure is used?
    a. Arteriospasm
    b. Bacteremia
    c. Clot formation
    d. Hematoma

57. Blood gas specimen rejection criteria include
    a. improper labeling or missing label.
    b. inadequate volume of the specimen.
    c. visible hemolysis of the specimen.
    d. all of the above.

58. Sudden fainting during arterial puncture is
    a. called vasovagal syncope.
    b. caused by anesthetic use.
    c. related to hypoglycemia.
    d. triggered by hypertension.

59. Which of the following is most likely to cause erroneous ABG results?
    a. An arteriospasm during the draw
    b. Failure to place the syringe on ice
    c. Microclots present in the specimen
    d. Testing 25 minutes after collection

60. Which ABG specimen is most likely to be rejected for testing?
    a. A specimen drawn in a heparinized syringe
    b. A specimen maintained at 37°C until tested
    c. A specimen that is dark bluish-red in color
    d. A specimen that was capped before mixing

Answers and Explanations

1. **Answer: a**

   WHY: Pain or irritation caused by needle penetration of the artery muscle and even patient anxiety can cause a reflex (involuntary) contraction of the artery referred to as an arteriospasm. This condition is transitory but can make it difficult to obtain a specimen.

   REVIEW: Yes ☐ No ☐

   Have some fun by finding this term in the scrambled words activity in the WORKBOOK. Take a look at Matching Exercise 14-1 in the WORKBOOK to see if you can define other key terms.

2. **Answer: c**

   WHY: Injury to the intima, or inner wall of the artery, can lead to thrombus, or clot formation. A tourniquet is not used during arterial puncture. An arteriospasm does not damage the intima. A thrombus can impair the artery drawn, not the one providing collateral circulation. An arterial puncture should not be performed if the artery that provides collateral circulation is already impaired.

   REVIEW: Yes ☐ No ☐

3. **Answer: c**

   WHY: Undetected microclots can lead to erroneous results. Applying the antiseptic improperly could result in infection at the site but should not affect testing. Blood cells continue to metabolize at room temperature, so testing the specimen as soon as possible using a point of care testing analyzer would help ensure accurate results. All acceptable sites for arterial puncture will result in accurate values if the procedure is performed correctly.

   REVIEW: Yes ☐ No ☐

4. **Answer: b**

   WHY: The integrity of a blood gas specimen can be affected if the blood-to-anticoagulant ratio is not correct. Vasovagal syncope (faintness or fainting due to increased vagus nerve activity on the artery) can occur during arterial puncture but will not affect the integrity of the sample. The ETS system should not be used to collect an ABG specimen because the tube's vacuum can affect test results. Heparin is the anticoagulant of choice for collecting an ABG specimen.

   REVIEW: Yes ☐ No ☐

5. **Answer: a**

   WHY: The thumb should never be used to feel for an artery because it has a pulse, which could be misleading in locating an artery.

   REVIEW: Yes ☐ No ☐

6. **Answer: b**

   WHY: Numbness is a complication associated with arterial puncture. Hemolysis, the breaking of red cells, is not a complication for the patient but an issue with the blood sample. Phlebitis is inflammation of a vein and not a consideration in arterial puncture. Venostasis is defined as trapping of blood in an extremity by compression of the veins and is usually the result of tying the tourniquet too tight and leaving it in place for too long. A tourniquet is not used for arterial punctures.

   REVIEW: Yes ☐ No ☐

7. **Answer: d**

   WHY: The radial artery is located in the thumb side of the wrist. The brachial artery is located in the antecubital area. The femoral artery is located in the groin. The ulnar artery is located in the little finger (pinky) side of the wrist.

   REVIEW: Yes ☐ No ☐

8. **Answer: c**

   WHY: Arterial blood is the ideal specimen for many blood tests because its composition is fairly consistent throughout the body, whereas the composition of venous blood varies relative to the metabolic needs of the area it serves. Analytes in venous specimens are relatively stable with proper handling. Arterial puncture is technically *more difficult* to perform. Both arterial and venous blood specimens are subject to collection error.

   REVIEW: Yes ☐ No ☐

9. **Answer: a**

   WHY: HCO_3 is bicarbonate. This ABG component is a measure of the amount of bicarbonate in the blood and is used to evaluate the bicarbonate buffer system of the kidneys. Metabolic disturbances alter HCO_3 levels.

   REVIEW: Yes ☐ No ☐

10. **Answer: b**

    WHY: The primary reason for performing arterial puncture is to obtain blood for evaluation of arterial blood gases (ABGs). Blood cultures, blood glucose, and blood typing are typically performed on venous specimens.

REVIEW: Yes ☐   No ☐

11. **Answer: c**

WHY: Arterial blood gas components commonly measured include $paCO_2$, pH, and PaO_2. PO_4 is the designation for phosphate and is not a blood gas component. NH_3 is the designation for ammonia, which is not a blood gas component. CO stands for carbon monoxide, which is not part of a routine blood gas analysis.

REVIEW: Yes ☐   No ☐

📖 *More routine ABG analytes can be found in Table 14-1 of the TEXTBOOK.*

12. **Answer: d**

WHY: Arterial blood gas evaluation is used in the diagnosis and management of respiratory or pulmonary disease to provide information about a patient's oxygenation, ventilation, and acid–base balance.

REVIEW: Yes ☐   No ☐

13. **Answer: c**

WHY: Personnel who perform ABG procedures are normally certified by their healthcare institutions after successfully completing extensive training involving theory, demonstration of technique, observation of the actual procedure, and performance of arterial puncture under the supervision of qualified personnel. Diagnosis is not part of the phlebotomist's training or duties. Due to the hazardous nature of arterial puncture, practice on other students is not normally part of arterial puncture instruction.

REVIEW: Yes ☐   No ☐

14. **Answer: c**

WHY: One of the main criteria for arterial puncture site selection is the presence of collateral circulation. The presence—not the absence—of underlying ligaments to support compression is a reason to choose a site. Several different sites can be used for arterial puncture, and the choice of site is never based on what equipment is available in the room or on the phlebotomist's tray. A strong pulse may make it easier to palpate an artery, but a rapid pulse has no bearing on site selection.

REVIEW: Yes ☐   No ☐

15. **Answer: d**

WHY: An artery that has very little tissue covering it is relatively close to the surface. This is a reason to favor the site because it should make it easier

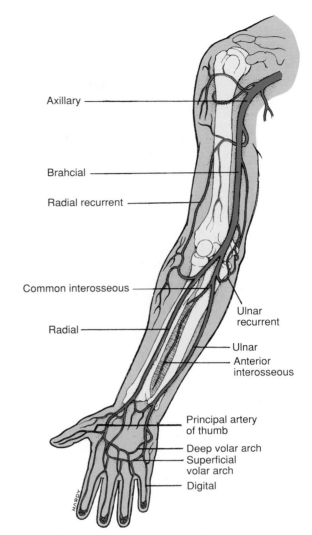

Figure 14-1 Arteries of the arm and hand.

Axillary

Brahcial

Radial recurrent

Common interosseous

Radial

Ulnar recurrent

Ulnar

Anterior interosseous

Principal artery of thumb

Deep volar arch

Superficial volar arch

Digital

to locate and puncture the artery. The presence of an IV, fistula, or recent arterial puncture at the site are reasons to avoid a site as a choice for arterial puncture.

REVIEW: Yes ☐   No ☐

16. **Answer: c**

WHY: The radial artery (Fig. 14-1) located on the thumb side of the wrist is the preferred and therefore the first choice and most common site used for arterial puncture. The brachial artery is the second choice. Puncture of the femoral artery (Fig. 14-2) is typically performed only in emergency situations by physicians and specially trained emergency room personnel. The ulnar artery is reserved to provide collateral circulation to the hand if the radial artery is damaged; it is never used for arterial puncture.

REVIEW: Yes ☐   No ☐

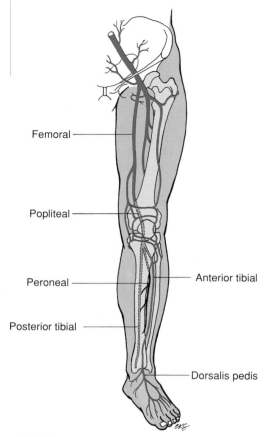

Figure 14-2 Arteries of the leg.

17. Answer: b

WHY: The femoral artery is large and easily located and punctured. It is sometimes the only site where arterial sampling is possible on patients with low cardiac output.

REVIEW: Yes ☐ No ☐

18. Answer: d

WHY: The biggest advantage of choosing the radial artery for ABG collection is that it normally has good collateral circulation. Collateral circulation means that more than one artery supplies blood to the area. If the radial artery were to be inadvertently damaged, the ulnar artery would still supply blood to the hand.

REVIEW: Yes ☐ No ☐

📖 *Do WORKBOOK activity Matching 14-2 to test your knowledge of the advantages and disadvantages of all the arteries commonly used to collect ABGs. Review advantages and disadvantages of all three main arteries used for ABG collection in Chapter 14 of the TEXTBOOK.*

19. Answer: d

WHY: One disadvantage of collecting ABGs from the radial artery is that it takes considerable skill to

puncture successfully since it is so small. The presence of ligaments and bone in the area makes it easy to compress and *decreases* the risk of hematoma formation, which are advantages. The presence of collateral circulation via the ulnar artery is also an advantage.

REVIEW: Yes ☐ No ☐

20. Answer: a

WHY: One advantage of using the brachial artery is that it is normally large and fairly easily palpated. However, it is located deeper than the radial artery, rather than not as deep, which is a disadvantage. In addition, there is increased risk of hematoma formation, not less, because the lack of underlying ligaments or bones to support compression makes it harder to compress.

REVIEW: Yes ☐ No ☐

21. Answer: d

WHY: Disadvantages of puncturing the brachial artery are that it is deeper and harder to palpate than the radial artery; it lies close to the basilic vein and the median nerve, both of which could be inadvertently punctured, and the area lacks bone and ligaments to support compression of the artery after puncture. Blood pressure in the brachial artery should be consistent with the arterial system throughout the body and would not be significantly different than that of the radial artery.

REVIEW: Yes ☐ No ☐

22. Answer: b

WHY: The femoral artery (Fig. 14-2) is located superficially in the groin lateral to the pubic bone. This area poses the greatest risk of infection because the presence of pubic hair makes it difficult to achieve an aseptic site.

REVIEW: Yes ☐ No ☐

23. Answer: c

WHY: In addition to the radial, brachial, and femoral arteries, arterial specimens may be obtained from the dorsalis pedis (foot) arteries of adults, scalp and umbilical arteries in infants, and indwelling lines. The brachial artery of a child is not a good choice and is not normally used because it has no collateral circulation. Arterial specimens should *not* be collected from the carotid artery, or the ulnar artery.

REVIEW: Yes ☐ No ☐

24. Answer: b

WHY: An ABG requisition typically includes the patient's body temperature, respiratory rate,

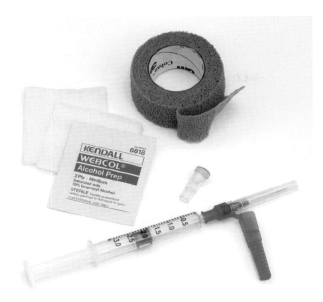

Figure 14-3 ABG equipment.

method of ventilation or delivery, and patient activity and body position in addition to normal patient identification information. The patient's age at onset of respiratory disease, previous blood gas values, or information on the type of equipment to use is not found on the requisition.

REVIEW: Yes ☐ No ☐

25. **Answer: a**

WHY: An ABG specimen is typically collected in a 1- to 5-mL syringe. Ice is no longer required for ABG specimen transportation except under special circumstances. A tourniquet is not needed to find an artery and is not used when collecting an arterial specimen. Povidone–iodine is no longer the recommended antiseptic for arterial puncture. The current recommended antiseptic for ABG collection is isopropyl alcohol. Arterial blood gas equipment is shown in Figure 14-3.

REVIEW: Yes ☐ No ☐

📖 *See the list of ABG equipment in Box 14-2 in the TEXTBOOK.*

26. **Answer: c**

WHY: Arterial blood gas specimens are not collected in evacuated tubes because the tube pressure or vacuum would alter test results.

REVIEW: Yes ☐ No ☐

27. **Answer: b**

WHY: Personal protective equipment (PPE) required in collecting arterial specimens includes a fluid-resistant lab coat, gown, or apron, gloves, and face protection. An N-95 respirator is not required

unless the patient is in airborne isolation. Hair covering, or shoe covering is not normally required.

REVIEW: Yes ☐ No ☐

28. **Answer: a**

WHY: Commercially prepared arterial sampling kits are available from several manufacturers. A kit typically contains a safety needle, a heparinized syringe with a filter that removes residual air, and a cap or other device to plug or cover the syringe hub after specimen collection so as to maintain anaerobic conditions. Use of local anesthetic is optional; consequently equipment to administer local anesthetic (e.g., a lidocaine-filled syringe) is *not* normally part of a prepared ABG kit.

REVIEW: Yes ☐ No ☐

29. **Answer: c**

WHY: Arterial blood gas tests are performed on whole-blood specimens. Therefore an anticoagulant is needed to keep the specimen from clotting. The anticoagulant of choice is heparin.

REVIEW: Yes ☐ No ☐

30. **Answer: a**

WHY: Lidocaine is sometimes used to numb the site before arterial puncture. Although once part of standard arterial puncture procedure, use of a local anesthetic is now optional. The advent of improved thin-wall needles that make arterial puncture less painful has made the routine administration of anesthetic prior to arterial puncture unnecessary.

REVIEW: Yes ☐ No ☐

31. **Answer: d**

WHY: Current body temperature, breathing pattern, and the concentration of oxygen inhaled all affect arterial blood gas results. Consequently it is best if a patient has been in a steady state (i.e., no exercise, suctioning, or respirator changes) for 20 to 30 minutes before blood gases are obtained.

REVIEW: Yes ☐ No ☐

32. **Answer: d**

WHY: Steady state, which is required prior to ABG collection, means that the patient has had no exercise, suctioning, or respiratory changes during the 20 to 30 minutes immediately preceding specimen collection.

REVIEW: Yes ☐ No ☐

33. **Answer: b**

WHY: The modified Allen test, as shown in Figures 14-4 and 14-5, is performed to determine the presence of collateral circulation. Collateral circulation means that the area of the body receives blood

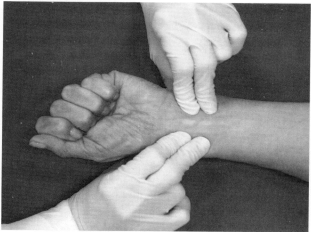

Figure 14-4 Obstruction of radial and ulnar arteries during the Allen test.

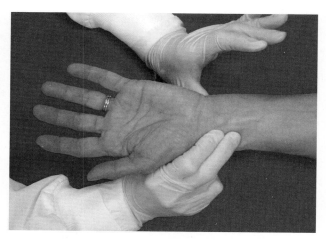

Figure 14-5 Ulnar artery released to allow return of blood to the hand.

from more than one artery. Collateral circulation is necessary in the event that damage to the artery occurs during arterial puncture. If the patient has circulation through an alternate artery, the area of the body that is normally fed by the damaged artery will receive blood from the alternate artery.

REVIEW: Yes ☐ No ☐

📖 *Test your grasp of the Allen test procedure by doing Skills Drill 14-3 in the WORKBOOK.*

34. **Answer: d**

WHY: The modified Allen test checks for the presence of collateral circulation to the hand via the ulnar artery. Circulation via the ulnar artery is important in the event that the radial artery is damaged during arterial puncture. Consequently, when one is performing the modified Allen test, the ulnar artery is released first (Fig. 14-5).

REVIEW: Yes ☐ No ☐

📖 *Review all the steps of this important test in Procedure 14-1 in the TEXTBOOK.*

35. **Answer: c**

WHY: When one is performing the modified Allen test, both the ulnar and radial arteries are compressed to stop arterial flow to the hand. With both arteries compressed, the hand should appear blanched, or drained of color. If the patient has collateral circulation, the hand will flush pink or normal color when the ulnar artery is released even though the radial artery is still compressed. The presence of collateral circulation constitutes a positive modified Allen test.

REVIEW: Yes ☐ No ☐

36. **Answer: a**

WHY: If the modified Allen test result is negative, the patient does not have collateral circulation and

arterial puncture cannot be performed on the radial artery of that arm. At this point, the phlebotomist should check for collateral circulation in the other arm. Phlebotomists are not normally trained to perform femoral punctures. Arterial puncture should never be performed on the ulnar artery.

REVIEW: Yes ☐ No ☐

37. **Answer: c**

WHY: A patient who has collateral circulation has more than one artery supplying blood to that area of the body.

REVIEW: Yes ☐ No ☐

38. **Answer: a**

WHY: Radial ABG procedure includes the following steps: (1) *assess* steady state, (2) *position* arm, (3) *clean* the site, (4) *puncture* at a 30- to 45-degree angle, (5) *fill* the syringe to a proper level, (6) *expel* air bubbles, and (7) *label* the specimen.

REVIEW: Yes ☐ No ☐

📖 *If your knowledge of radial ABG procedure needs firming up, go over Procedure 14-3 in the TEXTBOOK and Skills Drill 14-4 in the WORKBOOK to assess your knowledge of this procedure.*

39. **Answer: a**

WHY: Administration of local anesthetic to numb the site before arterial puncture is optional. Verification of required conditions, assessment of steady state, and determination of the presence of collateral circulation are mandatory steps of the procedure.

REVIEW: Yes ☐ No ☐

40. **Answer: d**

WHY: Proper arm positioning before puncture of the radial artery includes having the patient's arm

abducted (out to the side), with the palm up and the wrist extended at approximately 30 degrees and supported (e.g., by a rolled towel placed under it).
REVIEW: Yes ☐   No ☐

41. **Answer: c**

WHY: Arterial puncture is typically more painful than venipuncture but should not cause the patient extreme pain. Extreme or significant pain indicates nerve involvement and requires immediate termination of the procedure. It is not unusual for arterial blood to spurt into the syringe during collection. Arterial blood from a patient with pulmonary function problems may be dark reddish blue (because of reduced oxygen content) rather than the typical bright red of normal arterial blood. Slight redirection of the needle to successfully access the artery is acceptable.
REVIEW: Yes ☐   No ☐

42. **Answer: d**

WHY: Proper antisepsis before collecting an arterial specimen is important. The site must be cleaned using a suitable antiseptic such as isopropanol and allowed to air-dry. The phlebotomist's nondominant index finger should be prepped in the same manner because it will be used to relocate the artery. Antisepsis of the site must be maintained. Scrubbing the site with alcohol for 2 minutes is unnecessary and may irritate the skin at the site.
REVIEW: Yes ☐   No ☐

43. **Answer: a**

WHY: During puncture of the radial artery, the needle with the bevel up is directed away from the hand, facing the arterial blood flow.
REVIEW: Yes ☐   No ☐

44. **Answer: c**

WHY: An acceptable angle of needle insertion during radial arterial blood gas collection is between 30 and 45 degrees (Fig. 14-6).
REVIEW: Yes ☐   No ☐

45. **Answer: d**

WHY: The proper angle of needle insertion in collecting femoral arterial blood gases is 90 degrees, owing to the deep location of the femoral artery.
REVIEW: Yes ☐   No ☐

46. **Answer: b**

WHY: 20- to 23-gauge and 25-gauge needles can be used for arterial puncture, depending on the collection site. However, a 22-gauge 1-in needle is most commonly used for radial artery puncture. Needles

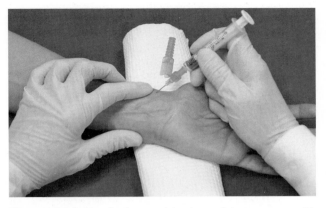

Figure 14-6 Needle inserted in the radial artery at a 45-degree angle.

1½ in long are generally reserved for brachial and femoral punctures.
REVIEW: Yes ☐   No ☐

47. **Answer: a**

WHY: Under normal circumstances, a flash of blood appears in the hub of the syringe when an artery is entered, and blood continues to pump into the syringe under its own power.
REVIEW: Yes ☐   No ☐

48. **Answer: d**

WHY: Blood pumping into the syringe under its own power is the best way to be certain that a specimen is arterial. Color is not a reliable indicator of successful arterial puncture. Although normal arterial blood is bright red, arterial blood of patients with abnormal pulmonary function may appear almost as dark as venous blood. Arterial specimens do not normally contain air bubbles. Introduction of air into the specimen causes erroneous results and should be avoided.
REVIEW: Yes ☐   No ☐

49. **Answer: d**

WHY: The phlebotomist should apply manual pressure (Fig. 14-7) to the site for 3 to 5 minutes as soon as the needle is withdrawn following arterial puncture. The patient should never be allowed to hold pressure because he or she may not apply it firmly enough. A pressure bandage should never be used in place of manual pressure over the site. A pressure bandage can be applied after manual pressure has been held for the appropriate amount of time and bleeding has stopped.
REVIEW: Yes ☐   No ☐

50. **Answer: a**

WHY: As soon as the arterial blood gas needle is removed from the arm, the needle safety feature

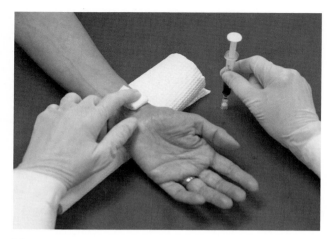

Figure 14-7 Clean folded gauze held firmly over the site after needle removal.

is activated. The needle is then removed from the syringe, air bubbles are ejected from the specimen, and the syringe is capped with a device that prevents exposure of the specimen to air. The specimen is mixed as soon as possible to prevent clotting and transported to the lab in the syringe. An arterial blood gas specimen must be maintained in anaerobic conditions and consequently cannot be transferred to an evacuated tube at any time. In addition, if the blood is drawn into an evacuated tube from the syringe, evacuated tube pressure can affect ABG results negatively.

REVIEW: Yes ☐ No ☐

51. **Answer: a**

WHY: After performing arterial puncture, the pulse is checked distal to or below the puncture site to ensure that blood flow is normal and no damage has occurred during the draw. If the pulse is faint or absent, a blood clot, or thrombus, may be obstructing blood flow, and the patient's nurse or physician must be notified immediately so that steps can be taken to restore proper circulation.

REVIEW: Yes ☐ No ☐

52. **Answer: d**

WHY: An absent or faint pulse following arterial puncture is not normal and indicates that blood flow may be partially or completely blocked by a blood clot, or thrombus. The patient's nurse or physician must be notified immediately so that steps can be taken to restore proper circulation. An arteriospasm does not cause a faint or absent pulse.

REVIEW: Yes ☐ No ☐

📖 *An absent pulse is serious; if you aren't sure what to do, see Procedure 14-3 in the TEXTBOOK.*

53. **Answer: a**

WHY: An arterial specimen should be transported ASAP according to laboratory protocol. At one time it was standard procedure to transport arterial blood gas (ABG) specimens on ice. The Clinical and Laboratory Standards Institute (CLSI) guidelines now call for transporting ABG specimens at room temperature provided that they are to be analyzed within 30 minutes of collection. If the patient has an elevated white blood cell or platelet count, the specimen should be analyzed within 5 minutes of collection. If a delay is expected, the specimen should be collected in a glass syringe and placed in ice slurry.

REVIEW: Yes ☐ No ☐

54. **Answer: d**

WHY: Specimens for electrolyte testing in addition to arterial blood gas (ABG) analysis should be transported at room temperature. They should never be placed on ice because cooling affects potassium levels. Placing the specimen in a heat block would adversely affect both ABG and electrolyte results. The vacuum draw of a test tube can negatively affect ABG results.

REVIEW: Yes ☐ No ☐

55. **Answer: a**

WHY: If the patient has an elevated white blood cell count, an ABG specimen should be transported at room temperature and analyzed within 5 minutes of collection. If analysis cannot occur within 5 minutes, the specimen should be collected in a glass syringe and transported in ice slurry. ABG specimens should never be placed in a heat block or collected in EDTA. An ABG specimen should not be mixed continually because hemolysis may result.

REVIEW: Yes ☐ No ☐

56. **Answer: a**

WHY: Arteriospasm is a reflex constriction of the artery, which can occur even when proper technique is used. It can be caused by patient anxiety, pain during the procedure, or irritation caused by needle penetration of the artery muscle. Although this common complication is transitory, it may make it difficult to obtain a specimen. Hematoma, thrombus (clot) formation, and infection are less common complications that are often the result of improper technique.

REVIEW: Yes ☐ No ☐

57. **Answer: d**

    WHY: Blood gas rejection criteria include improper or missing labeling, inadequate volume of specimen, and visible hemolysis of the specimen.

    REVIEW: Yes ☐   No ☐

    📖 *Look up other ABG specimen rejection criteria in Box 14-3 in the TEXTBOOK.*

58. **Answer: a**

    WHY: Vasovagal syncope is sudden fainting related to hypotension caused by a nervous system response to abrupt pain or trauma. It is not triggered by hypertension or related to hypoglycemia. Use of an anesthetic can result in an allergic reaction but not sudden fainting. Hypoglycemia can make a person feel faint but is associated with a low glucose level and would not come on as suddenly.

    REVIEW: Yes ☐   No ☐

59. **Answer: c**

    WHY: Microclots in the specimen can cause erroneous ABG results and also machine malfunction.

An arteriospasm can make it difficult to collect a specimen but should not affect test results. CLSI guidelines no longer recommend transporting ABG specimens on ice provided that they are processed within 30 minutes of collection.

REVIEW: Yes ☐   No ☐

📖 *Explore other causes of erroneous ABG results in Chapter 14 of the TEXTBOOK.*

60. **Answer: b**

    WHY: An ABG specimen would be automatically rejected if the syringe were brought to the testing site in a 37-degree heat block or warmer. An ABG specimen *should* be drawn in a heparinized syringe; it should be capped and mixed immediately after collection in order to avoid microclots and air exposure. A dark bluish-red color to the ABG specimen may cause suspicion that it is a venous specimen but is not an automatic cause for rejection. Low oxygen content causes some arterial specimens to appear dark bluish-red, or wine-colored, rather than bright red.

    REVIEW: Yes ☐   No ☐

Appendix A

Laboratory Tests

Review Questions

Choose the *BEST* answer.

1. The abbreviation for another name for alanine aminotransferase (ALT) is:
   a. ALP.
   b. ANA.
   c. SGOT.
   d. SGPT.

2. A chemistry test that may require the patient to be in an upright position for a minimum of 30 minutes before specimen collection is:
   a. aldosterone.
   b. catecholamine.
   c. plasma renin
   d. Stypven time.

3. Which test should be collected in a royal blue-top tube?
   a. Aluminum
   b. Calcitonin
   c. Lipoprotein
   d. Magnesium

4. A specimen for hemoglobin A1c goes to:
   a. chemistry.
   b. coagulation.
   c. hematology.
   d. microbiology.

5. This is the abbreviation for a chemistry test that is typically collected in a lavender-top tube.
   a. BUN
   b. CO
   c. ESR
   d. GC

6. Which of the following is an abbreviation for a type of antibody?
   a. AFB
   b. CEA
   c. IgM
   d. PSA

7. Most coagulation tests require a plasma specimen collected in a:
   a. gray-top tube.
   b. lavender-top tube.
   c. light blue-top tube.
   d. plasma separator tube.

8. Which of the following is a drug used in the treatment of epilepsy?
   a. Carbamazepine
   b. Lithium
   c. Phenytoin
   d. Theophylline

9. Which of the following is a hematology test?
   a. A/G ratio
   b. Acid-p'tase
   c. Differential
   d. HbA1c

10. Which test requires a minimum 12-hour fast before specimen collection?
    a. ADH
    b. CK-MB
    c. HDL/LDL
    d. uric acid

11. Which of the following tests is collected in a red-top tube or serum gel-barrier?
    a. Ammonia
    b. DIC panel
    c. ETOH
    d. SPEP

12. A tube without gel barrier should be used to collect a specimen for this test.
    a. Acid phosphatase
    b. Alpha-fetoprotein
    c. Salicylate level
    d. Thyroid profile

13. Which test is used in the detection of allergies?
    a. CEA
    b. D-dimer
    c. Ferritin
    d. RAST

14. Which of the following is a chemistry test performed on whole blood?
    a. AFB
    b. ANA
    c. Cyclosporine
    d. Plasminogen

15. Which test requires a whole blood specimen?
    a. CBC
    b. CMV
    c. CRP
    d. EBV

16. Immunology tests are most often performed on:
    a. plasma.
    b. serum.
    c. urine.
    d. whole blood.

17. Using this tube to collect blood bank specimens is unacceptable.
    a. Lavender top
    b. Nonadditive red top
    c. Pink top EDTA
    d. Serum separator tube

18. This test is used as a tumor marker.
    a. AT-III
    b. BMP
    c. CA 125
    d. HLA

19. Which tests are used in the diagnosis of pancreatitis?
    a. Amylase, lipase
    b. BUN, creatinine
    c. HCT, indices
    d. RPR, FTA

20. Name the type of specimen required and the department that performs the CMV test.
    a. Plasma, chemistry
    b. Serum, immunology
    c. Urine, microbiology
    d. Whole blood, hematology

21. This test requires whole blood collected from a stasis-free vein.
    a. Calcitonin
    b. Fibrinogen
    c. Lactic acid
    d. Zinc RBC

22. Identify the type of tube required and the department that performs the plasminogen test.
    a. Green top or PST, chemistry
    b. Light blue top, coagulation
    c. Red top or SST, chemistry
    d. Yellow top, microbiology

23. Microbiology tests on can be performed on:
    a. blood.
    b. sputum.
    c. urine.
    d. all of the above.

24. Which of the following tubes is usually required for hematology tests?
    a. Green top
    b. Lavender top
    c. Light blue top
    d. White top

25. Which of the following is actually a panel of several tests?
    a. BMP
    b. ESR
    c. PTT
    d. TSH

26. An HLA specimen is collected in a tube containing:
    a. ACD.
    b. EDTA.
    c. silica.
    d. thrombin.

27. Which department performs ETOH tests?
    a. Chemistry
    b. Coagulation
    c. Immunology
    d. Microbiology

28. Carbamazepine levels are determined in this department.
    a. Blood bank
    b. Chemistry
    c. Hematology
    d. Immunology

29. Specimens to be tested for glucose-6-phosphate dehydrogenase deficiency are typically collected in tubes containing:
    a. citrate.
    b. EDTA.
    c. heparin.
    d. oxalate.

30. Which of the following is a blood bank test?
    a. AFP
    b. DAT
    c. NH4
    d. Retic

Answers and Explanations

1. **Answer: d**

   WHY: An older name and abbreviation for alanine transferase (ALT) is serum glutamic-pyruvic transaminase (SGPT). ALP is the abbreviation for alkaline phosphatase. ANA is the abbreviation for antinuclear antibody. Serum glutamic-oxaloacetic transaminase (SGOT) is an older name for aspartate aminotransferase (AST).

   REVIEW: Yes ☐   No ☐

2. **Answer: a**

   WHY: Aldosterone is an adrenal hormone that plays a role in the absorption of sodium and water in the renal distal tubules. The test is performed in the chemistry department and typically requires the patient to be in an upright position and ambulatory for a minimum of 30 minutes before specimen collection. Catecholamines are a group of organic compounds that include dopamine, epinephrine, and norepinephrine. Catecholamine plasma specimens are ideally collected after the patient has rested quietly in a recumbent (lying down) position for 30 minutes following insertion of a venous catheter. Renin is an enzyme that plays a role in hypertension. Renin levels are best collected after the patient has been resting quietly in a supine position for 2 hours. The specimen is typically collected in EDTA and chilled during transportation and centrifugation. The Stypven time test is a coagulation test collected in a light blue-top sodium citrate tube. It is also called a Russell viper venom time (RVVT) or lupus anticoagulant test.

   REVIEW: Yes ☐   No ☐

3. **Answer: a**

   WHY: Aluminum is a metal that can be toxic to humans in elevated amounts. It requires collection in a trace-element–free royal blue-top tube. Calcitonin is collected in a red-top tube. Lipoprotein can be collected in a red-top, serum gel-barrier tube, or green-top plasma gel-barrier tube. A magnesium (Mg) can be collected in a gel-barrier tube such as a serum separator tube (SST) or a plasma gel-barrier tube (PST).

   REVIEW: Yes ☐   No ☐

4. **Answer: a**

   WHY: Hemoglobin A1c (HbA1c) is also called glycohemoglobin, glycosylated hemoglobin, and glycated hemoglobin. Glycation is a process in which glucose is bound to hemoglobin. Formation of glycated hemoglobin is irreversible, and the rate of formation is directly proportional to the concentration of glucose in the blood. HbA1c concentration therefore reflects the blood glucose concentration over the preceding 6 to 8 weeks. The test is performed in the chemistry department and is ordered to assess long-term glucose control in diabetic patients.

   REVIEW: Yes ☐   No ☐

5. **Answer: b**

   WHY: Carbon monoxide (CO) is a chemistry test that is typically collected in a lavender-top tube. CO more readily binds to hemoglobin than oxygen and can lead to CO poisoning, which can be fatal. CO bound to hemoglobin is called carboxyhemoglobin (HbCO). Blood urea nitrogen (BUN) is a chemistry test typically performed on serum. The erythrocyte sedimentation rate (ESR) is collected in a lavender-top tube, but it is a hematology test. GC stands for gonococcus, a microorganism from the species *Neisseria gonorrhoeae* that causes gonorrhea. A test that screens for GC is performed in microbiology.

REVIEW: Yes ☐ No ☐

6. **Answer: c**

WHY: An antibody is a type of protein molecule called an immunoglobulin (Ig). There are five classes of immunoglobulins: IgA, IgD, IgM, IgG, and IgE. AFB is the abbreviation for acid-fast bacillus, a type of bacteria. CEA and PSA are antigens; carcinoembryonic antigen and prostate-specific antigen, respectively.

REVIEW: Yes ☐ No ☐

7. **Answer: c**

WHY: Most coagulation tests require plasma specimens collected in light blue-top tubes containing the anticoagulant sodium citrate.

REVIEW: Yes ☐ No ☐

8. **Answer: c**

WHY: Phenytoin (Dilantin) is a drug used in the treatment of epilepsy. Lithium is a drug used to treat manic depression. Carbamazepine (Tegretol) is a drug used to treat bipolar affective disorder. Theophylline is an asthma drug.

REVIEW: Yes ☐ No ☐

9. **Answer: c**

WHY: A differential (diff) is a hematology test that classifies types of leukocytes, describes erythrocyte morphology, and estimates the platelet count. It can be performed automatically by machine or manually by looking at a stained blood smear under a microscope. Albumin/globulin (A/G) ratio, acid phosphatase (acid-p'tase) and glycosylated hemoglobin (also called hemoglobin A1c [HbA1c]) are chemistry tests.

REVIEW: Yes ☐ No ☐

10. **Answer: c**

WHY: Lipids are fats such as cholesterol. Cholesterol is transported throughout the body in complexes with protein called lipoprotein. High-density lipoprotein (HDL) is referred to as *good* cholesterol because it plays a role in removing cholesterol from the arteries and transporting it to the liver, where it is removed from the body. Low-density lipoprotein (LDL) is called *bad* cholesterol because it moves cholesterol into the arteries. Accurate measurement of HDL and LDL levels require a 12-hour fast. Antidiuretic hormone (ADH), creatine kinase MB (CK-MB), and uric acid tests do not require fasting specimens.

REVIEW: Yes ☐ No ☐

11. **Answer: d**

WHY: Serum protein electrophoresis (SPEP or PEP) requires a serum specimen collected in a red-top or serum separator tube (SST). An ammonia test requires a plasma specimen collected in a lavender-top (EDTA) tube or a green-top heparin tube. A disseminated intravascular coagulation (DIC) panel consists of several coagulation tests performed on plasma collected in a light blue-top sodium citrate tube. Ethanol (ETOH) or blood alcohol is best collected in a gray-top sodium fluoride tube.

REVIEW: Yes ☐ No ☐

12. **Answer: c**

WHY: It is recommended that salicylate (aspirin) levels be collected in tubes without gel-barrier. It is acceptable to collect acid phosphatase, alpha-fetoprotein, and thyroid profile specimens in gel-barrier tubes.

REVIEW: Yes ☐ No ☐

13. **Answer: d**

WHY: The radioallergosorbent test (RAST) is used in the detection of allergies. Carcinoembryonic antigen (CEA) is used in diagnosing and monitoring malignancies. D-dimer is a coagulation test. D-dimers are fragments produced by the action of plasmin on fibrin. Ferritin is a reliable indicator of iron stores and is measured in the diagnosis of iron-deficiency anemia and hemochromatosis.

REVIEW: Yes ☐ No ☐

14. **Answer: c**

WHY: Cyclosporine is an immunosuppressive drug used to suppress organ rejection in transplant recipients. The test can be performed on whole blood. An acid-fast bacillus (AFB) culture is a microbiology test used to diagnose tuberculosis. The antinuclear antibody (ANA) test is a serology/immunology test used in the diagnosis of systemic lupus erythematosus (SLE) and other autoimmune disorders. Plasminogen is a coagulation test performed on patients with disseminated intravascular coagulation (DIC) or thrombosis.

REVIEW: Yes ☐ No ☐

15. **Answer: a**

WHY: A complete blood count (CBC) is a hematology test performed on a whole blood specimen. Cytomegalovirus (CMV) is a herpesvirus that can cause devastating effects in a congenitally infected infant and fatal pneumonia in immunocompromised individuals. C-reactive protein (CRP) is an abnormal protein that appears in the blood during inflammatory illnesses, such as rheumatic fever, rheumatoid arthritis, and acute bacterial or viral infections, and as a response to injurious stimuli, such as myocardial infarction and malignancy. Epstein-Barr virus (EBV) is a herpesvirus that is the most common cause of infectious mononucleosis (IM). CMV, CRP, and EBV are serology/immunology tests most commonly performed on serum.

REVIEW: Yes ☐   No ☐

16. **Answer: b**

WHY: Immunology tests are most often performed on serum specimens.

REVIEW: Yes ☐   No ☐

17. **Answer: d**

WHY: Although most blood bank tests have been traditionally performed on serum and cells from clotted blood specimens, they are now more commonly performed on plasma and cells from EDTA anticoagulated specimens obtained in lavender-top tubes or special pink-top tubes. Gel-barrier tubes such as serum separator tubes (SSTs) cannot be used for blood bank tests.

REVIEW: Yes ☐   No ☐

18. **Answer: c**

WHY: A tumor marker is a substance found in blood, other body fluids, and tissues that may indicate the existence of malignancy or cancer. Cancer antigen 125 (CA 125) is an antigen that appears in the blood in increased amounts in the presence of ovarian and endometrial tumors. It is detected using an antibody called OC 125. Antithrombin III (AT-III) is the main physiologic inhibitor of thrombin and is measured in the identification of clotting factor deficiencies. A basic metabolic panel (BMP) is a designated number of tests covering a certain body system. Antigens that can be detected on white blood cells are called human leukocyte antigens (HLAs). HLA typing is used in tissue typing for parentage determination and transplant compatibility between donor and recipient.

REVIEW: Yes ☐   No ☐

19. **Answer: a**

WHY: Amylase and lipase are enzymes found in greatest concentrations in the pancreas. They are measured in the diagnosis and treatment of pancreatic disease as well as in differentiating pancreatitis from other abdominal disorders. Urea is an end-product of protein metabolism. In the past it was indirectly measured as blood urea nitrogen (BUN). Most analyzers now measure urea directly, but the term "BUN" may still be used. Creatinine is a product of creatine metabolism in the muscles. Its formation is related to muscle mass, and values vary according to age and gender. BUN and creatinine are excreted by the kidneys and measured in the assessment of kidney function. Hematocrit (HCT) and red blood cell indices are hematology tests used to detect abnormal bleeding and anemia. Rapid plasma reagin (RPR) is a nonspecific test used to screen for syphilis antibodies. The fluorescent treponemal antibody (FTA) test specifically detects antibodies to *Treponema pallidum*, the microorganism that causes syphilis, and is used to confirm positive RPR results.

REVIEW: Yes ☐   No ☐

20. **Answer: b**

WHY: Cytomegalovirus (CMV) is a herpesvirus that can cause devastating effects in a congenitally infected infant and fatal pneumonia in immunocompromised individuals. It is a serology/immunology test most commonly performed on serum.

REVIEW: Yes ☐   No ☐

21. **Answer: c**

WHY: Lactic acid is a product of carbohydrate metabolism. Excess amounts are produced during hypoxic (oxygen deficiency) states such as shock, hypovolemia (diminished blood volume), and left ventricular failure, and certain metabolic disease states such as diabetes mellitus and drug toxicity. Excess lactic acid in the blood is called lactic acidosis. Strict patient preparation and sample collection and handling procedures must be followed to ensure accurate testing. Patients should be fasting and at rest for 2 hours before testing. Patients should be instructed not to make a fist before or during specimen collection, and specimens should be obtained without the use of a tourniquet because blood levels are affected by stasis (stoppage of blood flow) and hemoconcentration.

REVIEW: Yes ☐   No ☐

22. **Answer: b**

WHY: Plasminogen is a coagulation test collected in a light blue-top tube. Plasminogen is a precursor of plasmin, an enzyme that dissolves fibrin and fibrinogen. It circulates in the blood until activated and is converted to plasmin during fibrin clot formation. Its normal function is to dissolve the fibrin clot when healing has occurred and the clot is no longer needed. Substances called antiplasmins destroy any plasmin released into the blood. When pathologic processes such as thrombosis or disseminated intravascular coagulation (DIC) occur, excess amounts of plasmin are released into the blood and begin destroying other coagulation factors, including fibrinogen.

REVIEW: Yes ☐   No ☐

23. **Answer: d**

WHY: The most common type of testing performed in microbiology is culture and sensitivity (C & S) testing of blood and other body fluids and substances such as urine and sputum.

REVIEW: Yes ☐   No ☐

24. **Answer: b**

WHY: Most hematology tests are performed on whole blood specimens collected in lavender or purple-top tubes containing the anticoagulant ethylenediaminetetraacetate (EDTA). The most common use of heparin-containing green-top tubes is to provide plasma for chemistry tests. Light blue-top tubes containing sodium citrate are used for coagulation tests. A white- (or pearl-)-top tube is a plasma preparation tube (PPT) and is used to provide EDTA plasma for molecular diagnostic tests.

REVIEW: Yes ☐   No ☐

25. **Answer: a**

WHY: A basic metabolic panel (BMP) includes a designated number of body system chemistry tests. Erythrocyte sedimentation rate (ESR), partial thromboplastin time (PTT), and thyroid-stimulating hormone (TSH) are individual tests.

REVIEW: Yes ☐   No ☐

26. **Answer: a**

WHY: Human leukocyte antigen (HLA) specimens are typically collected in tubes containing acid citrate dextrose (ACD), although they are sometimes collected in heparin tubes.

REVIEW: Yes ☐   No ☐

27. **Answer: a**

WHY: Blood alcohol (ethanol or ETOH) tests are performed in the toxicology area of the chemistry department. The test can be performed on serum, plasma, or whole blood, but plasma obtained from specimens collected in gray-top tubes containing sodium fluoride is typically preferred when a specimen is collected for legal reasons, especially if it is sent off site to a reference laboratory for testing. The test can be performed on serum, plasma, or whole blood, but plasma obtained from specimens collected in gray-top tubes containing sodium fluoride is Alcohol is volatile, and specimens must be kept capped during handling and processing to prevent evaporation of the analyte.

REVIEW: Yes ☐   No ☐

28. **Answer: b**

WHY: Carbamazepine (trade name, Tegretol) is a drug used to treat seizure disorders. Drug levels are measured in the toxicology area of the chemistry department.

REVIEW: Yes ☐   No ☐

29. **Answer: b**

WHY: Glucose-6-phosphate dehydrogenase (G-6-PD) is an enzyme that plays a role in glucose metabolism and ultimately in protecting hemoglobin from oxidation. A deficiency of G-6-PD is an inherited sex-linked disorder that can lead to hemolytic anemia. The test for G-6-PD deficiency is commonly performed on a solution of hemolyzed red blood cells obtained from an EDTA specimen. Testing for elevated levels of G-6-PD is performed on serum.

REVIEW: Yes ☐   No ☐

30. **Answer: b**

WHY: The direct antiglobulin test (DAT) is a blood bank or immunohematology test that detects antigen-antibody complexes on the red blood cells, and red blood cell sensitization. It is useful in evaluating hemolytic disease of the newborn (HDN), acquired hemolytic anemias, transfusion reactions, and drug-induced red blood cell sensitization. The alpha-fetoprotein test (AFP) and the ammonia test (NH_4) are chemistry tests. A reticulocyte (retic) count is a hematology test.

REVIEW: Yes ☐   No ☐

Appendix B

Laboratory Mathematics

Review Questions

1. 10 cc of blood equals approximately:
   a. 1.0 mL of blood.
   b. 5.0 mL of blood.
   c. 10 mL of blood.
   d. 20 mL of blood.

2. 200 µL is equal to:
   a. 2 mL.
   b. 0.2 mL.
   c. 0.02 mL.
   d. 0.002 mL.

3. Your requisition says that a specimen is to be drawn at 1530. What time would that be in 12-hour time?
   a. 1:30 AM
   b. 3:30 PM
   c. 5:30 AM
   d. 7:30 PM

4. 1:00 PM in 24-hour time is:
   a. 100.
   b. 0100.
   c. 1300.
   d. 01300.

5. Body temperature in centigrade degrees is:
   a. 98.6.
   b. 37.0.
   c. 25.0.
   d. 32.0.

6. If room temperature is 77°F, what is the temperature in centigrade?
   a. 20
   b. 25
   c. 32
   d. 37

7. A specimen must be transported at body temperature, plus or minus 5° Fahrenheit. Which of the following temperature readings is within that range?
   a. 25°C
   b. 35°C
   c. 37°F
   d. 90°F

8. Your text says that factor VIII is the antihemophilic factor. What common Arabic number is this factor?
   a. 4
   b. 8
   c. 13
   d. 23

9. How is the number 12 written in Roman numerals?
   a. IIV
   b. VII
   c. IIX
   d. XII

10. Your paper says that you got 45 of 50 questions correct. What is your grade expressed as a percentage?
    a. 45%
    b. 75%
    c. 90%
    d. 95%

11. If a red blood cell is 8 µm in diameter, what is its size in millimeters?
    a. 0.8
    b. 0.08
    c. 0.008
    d. 0.0008

12. One teaspoon is approximately:
    a. 1 mL.
    b. 5 mL.
    c. 10 mL.
    d. 15 mL.

13. A blood culture bottle containing 45 mL of media requires a 1:10 dilution of specimen. How much blood should be added?
    a. 4 mL
    b. 5 mL
    c. 8 mL
    d. 10 mL

14. Normal infant blood volume is approximately 100 mL/kg. Calculate the approximate blood volume of a baby who weighs 6 lb.
    a. 1.2 L
    b. 2.7 L
    c. 270 mL
    d. 600 mL

15. Normal adult blood volume is approximately 70 mL per kilogram. A patient weighs 130 lb. What is the patient's blood volume?
    a. 1300 mL
    b. 1.3 L
    c. 59 kg
    d. 4.1 L

16. To prepare 100 mL of a 1:10 dilution of bleach, add:
    a. 1 mL water to 100 mL bleach.
    b. 1 mL bleach to 99 mL water.
    c. 10 mL bleach to 90 mL water.
    d. 10 mL water to 100 mL bleach.

17. The basic unit of volume in the metric system is the:
    a. gram.
    b. liter.
    c. meter.
    d. ounce.

18. In the metric system, a millimeter (mm) is:
    a. 1/10 meter.
    b. 1/100 meter.
    c. 1/1000 meter.
    d. 1/10,000 meter.

19. 1.2 kg is equal to how many grams?
    a. 12
    b. 120
    c. 1200
    d. 12,000

20. What does 2.2 pounds (lb) equal in the metric system?
    a. 1 kg
    b. 44 g
    c. 100 g
    d. 454 kg

21. The basic unit of weight in the metric system is the:
    a. gram.
    b. liter.
    c. meter.
    d. ounce.

22. In the metric system the prefix for 1000 is:
    a. centi-.
    b. deci-.
    c. kilo-.
    d. milli-.

23. In the metric system a meter is a measure of:
    a. mass.
    b. density.
    c. distance.
    d. volume.

24. A patient voids 1200 mL of urine for a creatinine clearance test. How much urine is this?
    a. less than a liter
    b. less than a quart
    c. more than a liter
    d. more than 2 liters

25. A test requires 3 mL serum. The laboratory requires that the amount of blood collected be 250% of the volume of specimen required to perform the test. Which size tube should you use to collect the specimen?
    a. 4 mL
    b. 5 mL
    c. 10 mL
    d. 15 mL

Answers and Explanations

1. **Answer: c**

   WHY: For practical purposes, *mL* and *cc* are equivalent and the terms are often used interchangeably in a laboratory setting. Both are approximately equal to one-thousandth of a liter. The term *milliliter* (ml) is used when referring to liquid volume; *cubic centimeter* (cc) is used when referring to volume of gas. However, syringes that are used to extract liquid volume are often calibrated in cc rather than in mL.
   REVIEW: Yes ☐   No ☐

2. **Answer: b**

   WHY: When converting small units to larger units, the decimal point moves to the left the number of spaces determined by subtracting the exponent of the smaller unit from the exponent of the larger unit. A milliliter (mL) is one-thousandth of a liter (L), or 10^{-3} liters. A microliter (μL) is one-millionth of a liter, or 10^{-6} liters. Microliters are smaller than milliliters. Therefore, subtract –6 (μL exponent) from –3 (mL exponent). The result is 3, which means the decimal point moves three places to the left.
   Solution: $-3 - (-6) = -3 + 6 = 3$
   $200.0 = 0.2$ mL
   REVIEW: Yes ☐   No ☐

3. **Answer: b**

   WHY: To change 24-hour time to 12-hour time, subtract 1200 from any time after 1300. 1530 in 24-hour time less 1200 is 330, which written in 12-hour time format with the colon is 3:30 PM. A clock showing standard and 24-hour (military) time is shown in Fig. AppB-1.
   REVIEW: Yes ☐   No ☐

4. **Answer: c**

   WHY: To convert 12-hour time to 24-hour time, add 1200 to the time (minus the colon) from 1 PM on. 1:00 without the colon is 100. 100 plus 1200 becomes 1300 (see Fig. AppB-1).
   REVIEW: Yes ☐   No ☐

5. **Answer: b**

   WHY: Body temperature in centigrade is 37°. To calculate body temperature in centigrade when given a Fahrenheit reading, subtract 32 from the Fahrenheit temperature and multiply by 5/9.
   Note: A healthcare worker should memorize the centigrade body temperature value along with a few other centigrade temperatures that are common when working in healthcare (Fig. AppB-2).
   REVIEW: Yes ☐   No ☐

6. **Answer: b**

   WHY: Centigrade and Celsius are equal. To convert 77° Fahrenheit (F) temperature to centigrade (C) or Celsius (C), subtract 32 from the Fahrenheit value and multiply the result by 5/9.
   Formula: $C = 5/9 (F - 32)$
   Solution: $F - 32 = 77 - 32 = 45$
   $5/9 (45) = 5/9 \times 45/1$
   $5/9 \times 45/1 = 225/9$
   $225/9 = 25°C$
   Room temperature in Celsius or centigrade is 25°C. Healthcare workers should memorize this commonly referenced centigrade temperature (Fig. AppB-2).
   REVIEW: Yes ☐   No ☐

7. **Answer: b**

   WHY: Fahrenheit body temperature is 98.6° (Fig. AppB-2). Once we add and subtract 5, we know that we are looking for a temperature that is between 93.6°F and 103.6°F. This eliminates 37°F and 90°F. 25°C (Celsius or centigrade) is the same as 77°F. (See answer 6.) The remaining choice

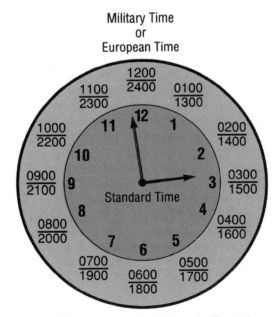

Figure AppB-1 Clock showing 24-hour (military) time.

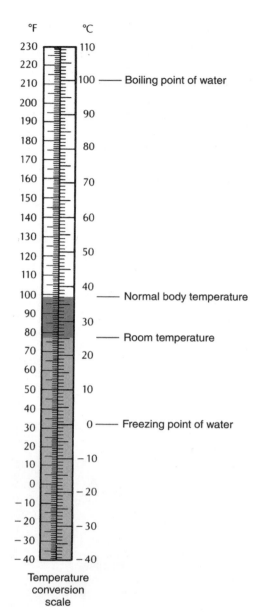

°F   °C

230 — 110
220
210 — 100 —— Boiling point of water
200
190 — 90
180 — 80
170
160 — 70
150
140 — 60
130
120 — 50
110
100 — 40 —— Normal body temperature
90
80 — 30
70 —— Room temperature
60 — 20
50 — 10
40
30 — 0 —— Freezing point of water
20
10 — -10
0
-10 — -20
-20 — -30
-30
-40 — -40

Temperature
conversion
scale

Figure AppB-2 Thermometer showing both Fahrenheit and Celsius degrees. (Memmler RL, Cohen BJ, Wood DL.)

is 35°C. To verify that this is the correct answer, convert 35°C to Fahrenheit temperature:

Formula: F = 9/5 C + 32

Solution: (9/5 × 35) + 32 = 63 + 32 = 95°F

35°C is the correct answer because it is same as 95°F, which meets the transportation temperature requirement.

REVIEW: Yes ☐   No ☐

8. **Answer: b**

WHY: Coagulation factors such as the antihemophilic factor are written in Roman numerals. In Roman numerals, letters equal numbers.

The Roman numeral V equals 5, and the Roman numeral I equals 1. When numerals of the same value follow in sequence, their values are added. When a numeral is followed by one or more numerals of a lower value, the values are added. Therefore:

VIII = 5 + 1 + 1 + 1 = 5 + 3 = 8

REVIEW: Yes ☐   No ☐

9. **Answer: d**

WHY: Roman numerals are written from left to right in decreasing value (except for numerals that are to be subtracted from subsequent numerals). In addition, there can never be more than three of the same numeral in a sequence. To write a number, you should start with the closest base number and add or subtract other numbers until you reach the desired value. The closest base number to 12 is X, which equals 10. Then add one I for every number 1. Therefore:

12 = X + I + I = XII

REVIEW: Yes ☐   No ☐

10. **Answer: c**

WHY: To calculate a percentage, a number must be converted to parts per 100. First, make the number a fraction. Then multiply the numerator of the fraction by 100, divide by the denominator, and add a percent sign.

Solution: 45 of 50 = 45/50

45/50 × 100 = 4500/50

4500 ÷ 50 = 90

Or reduce the fractions first as follows:

45/50 × 100/1 = 45/1 × 2/1 = 45 × 2 = 90%

REVIEW: Yes ☐   No ☐

11. **Answer: c**

WHY: A micrometer (μm), or micron is equal to one-millionth (10^{-6}) of a meter and a millimeter (mm) is equal to one-thousandth (10^{-3}) of a meter, which means you are converting smaller units to larger units (Table AppB-1). When converting small units to larger units the decimal point moves to the left the number of spaces determined by subtracting the exponent of the smaller unit from the exponent of the larger unit. Therefore, subtract −6 (mL exponent) from −3 (mm exponent). The result is 3, which means the decimal point moves three places to the left.

Solution: −3 − (−6) = −3 + 6 = 3

008.0 μm = 0.008 mm

REVIEW: Yes ☐   No ☐

Table AppB-1: Commonly Used Metric Measurement Prefixes

Prefix	Multiple	Unit of Measure		
		Meter	**Gram**	**Liter**
Kilo- (k)	1000 (10^3)	km	kg	kL
Deci- (d)	1/10 (10^{-1})	dm	dg	dL
Centi- (c)	1/100 (10^{-2})	cm	cg	cL
Milli- (m)	1/1000 (10^{-3})	mm	mg	mL
Micro- (μ)	1/1,000,000 (10^{-6})	μm	μg	μL

12. Answer: b

WHY: By using an English-Metric conversion chart (Table AppB-2), you can find the right answer, or you may choose to memorize certain common conversions, such as 1 tsp = 5 mL.

REVIEW: Yes ☐   No ☐

13. Answer: b

WHY: A blood culture dilution of 1:10 means there is 1 mL of blood and 9 mL of media for every 10 mL of blood culture specimen. Forty-five milliliters of media is five times the original proportion of nine milliliters. To maintain the same 1:10 dilution, you must also have five times the original 1 mL proportion of blood. That means you will need to add 5 mL blood to the 45 mL media.

REVIEW: Yes ☐   No ☐

14. Answer: c

WHY: Normal infant blood volume is approximately 100 mL/kg. If a baby's weight is given in pounds, it must be converted to kilograms by multiplying the pounds by the conversion factor 0.454. Once the weight is established in kilograms, multiply that number by 100, because for every kilogram there are 100 mL of blood.

Table AppB-2: English Metric Equivalents

	English	= Metric
Distance	Yard (yd)	= 0.9 meters (m)
	Inch (in)	= 2.54 centimeters (cm)
Weight	Pound (lb)	= 0.454 kilograms (kg) or 454 grams (g)
	Ounce (oz)	= 28 grams (g)
Volume	Quart (qt)	= 0.95 liters (L)
	Fluid ounce (fl oz)	= 30 milliliters (mL)
	Tablespoon (tbsp)	= 15 milliliters (mL)
	Teaspoon (tsp)	= 5 milliliters (mL)

Example:

6 lb × 0.454 = 2.7 kg
(rounded to nearest tenth)

2.7 kg × 100 mL/kg = 270 mL

270 mL/1000 = 0.27 L

REVIEW: Yes ☐   No ☐

15. Answer: d

WHY: Normal adult blood volume is approximately 70 mL per kilogram of weight. If the weight is given in pounds, it must be converted to kilograms by multiplying by the conversion factor 0.454 (Table AppB-1). The weight in kilograms is multiplied by 70 because we know that for every kilogram of weight in an adult there is approximately 70 mL of blood. Divide the result by 1000 because adult blood volume is reported in liters and 1 L equals 1000 mL.

Example:

130 lb × 0.454 = 59.02 kg

59 kg × 70 mL/kg = 4130 mL

4130/1000 = 4.13 L

REVIEW: Yes ☐   No ☐

16. Answer: c

WHY: A 1:10 dilution of bleach means there is 1 mL of bleach and 9 mL of water for every 10 mL of solution. One hundred milliliters of a 1:10 dilution is 10 times the original 10-mL proportion. That means you will also need 10 times the original amount of bleach and water, or 10 mL bleach and 90 mL water.

REVIEW: Yes ☐   No ☐

17. Answer: b

WHY: The basic unit of volume in the metric system is the liter (L), as shown in Table AppB-3 (Metric-English Equivalents). It is easier to remember that the liter is the basic metric unit of volume than to remember other

Table AppB-3: Metric-English Equivalents

	Metric	English
Distance	Meter (m)	= 3.3 fee/39.37 inches
	Centimeter (cm)	= 0.4 inches
	Millimeter (mm)	= 0.04 inches
Weight	Gram (g)	= 0.0022 pounds
	Kilogram (kg)	= 2.2 pounds
Volume	Liter (L)	= 1.06 quarts
	Milliliter (mL)^a	= 0.03 fluid
ounces	Milliliter (mL)^a	= 0.20 or 1/5 tsp

^{a}A milliliter (mL) is approximately equal to a cubic centimeter (cc) and the two terms are often used interchangeably.

metric measurements, because the soft drink industry in the United States has converted much of their packaging to metric measurements, and we see advertisements for liters of soft drinks all the time.

REVIEW: Yes ☐   No ☐

18. **Answer: c**

WHY: A millimeter (mm) is 1/1000 meter, or 10^{-3} m (Table AppB-2).

REVIEW: Yes ☐   No ☐

19. **Answer: c**

WHY: When converting large units to smaller units, the decimal point moves to the right. To convert large units to basic units, move the decimal point to the right the value of the exponent of the larger unit. A kilogram (k) is 1000 or 10^3 grams (Table AppB-2). The exponent is 3, so the decimal point moves three places to the right.

Solution: 1.200 kg = 1200 g.

REVIEW: Yes ☐   No ☐

20. **Answer: a**

WHY: One kilogram equals 2.2 lb (Table AppB-3). This is a conversion factor that should be memorized. A helpful hint might be to remember that weight in kilograms is approximately half (divide

by 2) the number given in pounds. However, it is important to remember that this number will always be slightly higher than an actual calculation.

REVIEW: Yes ☐   No ☐

21. **Answer: a**

WHY: The basic unit of weight in the metric system is the gram (Table AppB-3).

REVIEW: Yes ☐   No ☐

22. **Answer: c**

WHY: Kilo-, abbreviated "k," means 1000 (Table AppB-1). It can be used with each of the three basic units of measure in the metric system.

Example:

kilogram (kg) = 1000 grams (g)

kiloliter (kL) = 1000 liters (L)

kilometer (km) = 1000 meters (m)

REVIEW: Yes ☐   No ☐

23. **Answer: c**

WHY: Metric-English conversion equivalent for distance (or length) is the meter (m), as shown in Table AppB-3.

REVIEW: Yes ☐   No ☐

24. **Answer: c**

WHY: A liter is equal to 1000 mL and a quart is equal to 950 mL; therefore, 1200 mL is 200 mL more than a liter, 250 mL more than a quart, and 800 mL less than 2 liters (Table AppB-1 and AppB-2).

REVIEW: Yes ☐   No ☐

25. **Answer: c**

WHY: The laboratory needs 250%, or two and one-half times, the 3 mL required for the test. Two times 3 mL is 6 mL. One-half of 3 mL is 1½ mL (or you can multiply 3 times 2.5). Therefore, you need 7½ mL to do the test. The closest tube choice is 10 mL.

REVIEW: Yes ☐   No ☐

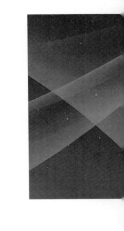

Part 3

Pretest and Written Comprehensive Mock Exam

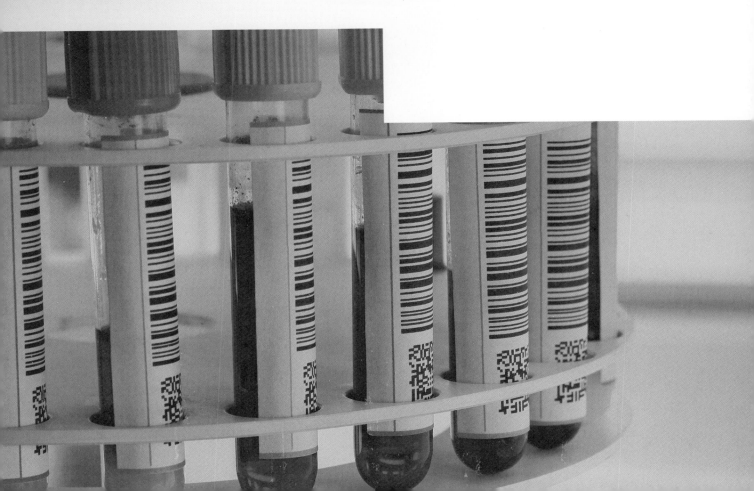

Pretest

1. Which of the following was developed by AMA to provide a terminology and coding system for physician billing:
   a. APC
   b. CPT.
   c. DRG.
   d. Medicare.

2. The patient is very emotional and cannot understand what the phlebotomist is asking him to do. This is an example of:
   a. a communication barrier.
   b. invasion of the intimate zone.
   c. lack of professionalism.
   d. all of the above.

3. Which of the following is an example of negative kinesics?
   a. eye contact
   b. frowning
   c. good grooming
   d. smiling

4. Part of the phlebotomist's role is to promote good public relations because:
   a. close personal relationships with the patients are essential.
   b. laboratorians are not recognized as part of the healthcare team.
   c. patients equate this interaction with the overall caliber of care.
   d. skilled public relations overcomes inexperience and insecurity.

5. Which manual describes the chemical, electrical, and radiation safety for the laboratory?
   a. Infection control manual
   b. Lab Test Catalog
   c. Procedure manual
   d. Safety manual

6. An individual who has little resistance to an infectious microbe is referred to as a susceptible:
   a. agent.
   b. host.
   c. pathway.
   d. reservoir.

7. SDS information includes:
   a. general and emergency information.
   b. highly technical chemical formulas.
   c. information on competitor products.
   d. product manufacturing conditions.

8. A person who has recovered from a particular virus and has developed antibodies against that virus is said to be:
   a. a carrier.
   b. immune.
   c. infectious.
   d. susceptible.

9. All pathogens are:
   a. communicable microorganisms.
   b. microbes that can cause disease.
   c. microorganisms that live in soil.
   d. normal flora found on the skin.

10. These are the initials of the two organizations responsible for the latest *Guideline for Isolation Precautions in Hospitals.*
    a. CDC and HICPAC
    b. CLSI and OSHA
    c. HICPAC and NIOSH
    d. NIOSH and OSHA

11. Informed consent means that:
    a. a patient's medical records are available for review by all healthcare workers.
    b. all consequences of a medical procedure have been given to the patient.
    c. the patient received a book outlining all procedures and their consequences.
    d. the patient's confidentiality has been breached during the assessment process.

12. This equipment is required when collecting a specimen from a patient in airborne isolation.
    a. eye protection
    b. full face shield
    c. mask and goggles
    d. N95 respirator

13. Which of the following is an example of a *work practice* control that reduces risk of exposure to bloodborne pathogens?
    a. ordering self-sheathing needles
    b. reading the exposure control plan
    c. receiving an HBV vaccination
    d. wearing gloves to draw blood

14. Which of the following statements complies with electrical safety guidelines?
    a. Electrical equipment should be unplugged while being serviced.
    b. Extension cords should be used to conveniently place equipment.
    c. It is safe to use an electrical cord if it is only slightly frayed.
    d. Use electrical equipment carefully if it is starting to malfunction.

15. The "Right to Know" law primarily deals with:
    a. electrical safety issues.
    b. exposure to pathogens.
    c. hazard communication.
    d. labeling of specimens.

16. A phlebotomist using an armband for patient ID must also:
    a. check the room number for additional verification.
    b. have the patient state additional ID information.
    c. make certain requisition matches wristband.
    d. write down location of the patient on the requisition.

17. A laboratory technician asked a phlebotomist to recollect a specimen on a patient. When the phlebotomist asked what was wrong with the specimen, the technician replied, "The specimen was OK, but the results were inconsistent." How would the laboratory technician have decided that the results were questionable? The results did not:
    a. compare with previous results after delta check.
    b. match results of patients with the same diagnosis.
    c. measure up to the results on the control specimens.
    d. relate well to other patients tested at the same time.

18. Which of the following would violate a patient's right to confidentiality?
    a. Discussing the nature of a patient's test results with the family.
    b. Giving the patient a physician's name that you know and trust.

    c. Sharing information on a "difficult draw" with a coworker
    d. Showing a patient his or her lab results when requested.

19. In performing a glucose tolerance test, the fasting specimen is drawn at 6:15 A.M. and the patient finishes the glucose beverage at 6:30 A.M. When should the 2-hour specimen be collected?
    a. 8:15
    b. 8:30
    c. 9:15
    d. 9:30

20. Which one of the following can be eliminated from a list of antecubital veins?
    a. accessory cephalic.
    b. median.
    c. median basilic.
    d. subclavian.

21. In collecting blood cultures, one of the most frequent errors made is
    a. failure to inoculate two media bottles.
    b. improper cleansing of the collection site.
    c. incorrect labeling of the media bottles.
    d. not noting the venipuncture location.

22. This ion is essential to the coagulation process.
    a. calcium.
    b. chloride.
    c. potassium.
    d. sodium.

23. Which of the following tests does not require special chain-of-custody documentation when collected?
    a. BAC
    b. Drug screen
    c. Paternity testing
    d. TDM

24. QC protocols prohibit use of outdated evacuated tubes because:
    a. additives that speed up clotting become crystallized in the tube.
    b. bacteria begin to grow in these tubes, yielding erroneous results.
    c. stoppers may shrink, allowing specimen leakage if the tube is inverted.
    d. tubes may not fill completely, changing additive-to-sample ratios.

25. What word is used to describe the breakdown of red blood cells?
    a. erythema
    b. erythrocytosis
    c. hemolysis
    d. hemostasis

26. Which of the following word parts are prefixes?
    a. al, lysis, pnea
    b. gastr, lip, onc
    c. ices, ina, nges
    d. iso, neo, tachy

27. A patient who is NPO:
    a. cannot have any food or drink.
    b. cannot have anything but water.
    c. is in critical, but stable condition.
    d. is recovering from minor surgery.

28. There is a sign above the patient's bed that reads, "No blood pressures or venipuncture, right arm". The patient has an IV in the left forearm. You have a request to collect a complete blood count on the patient. How should you proceed?
    a. Ask the patient's nurse to collect the specimen from the IV.
    b. Ask the patient's nurse what to do when the sign is posted.
    c. Collect a CBC from the right arm without using tourniquet.
    d. Collect the specimen from the left hand by finger puncture.

29. Molecular genetic testing requires:
    a. chain of custody protocol to be followed
    b. freezing of the spun sample immediately
    c. RNA tubes to be incubated at 37°C
    d. specimens to be collected in sterile EDTA

30. It is incorrect to say that this tube stopper color indicates the presence of a certain additive in the tube.
    a. green.
    b. lavender.
    c. light blue.
    d. royal blue.

31. What is the purpose of an antiglycolytic agent?
    a. enhance the clotting process
    b. inhibit electrolyte breakdown
    c. preserve glucose
    d. prevent clotting

32. Which one of the following tubes is filled first when multiple tubes are filled using an evacuated tube system?
    a. blood culture (SPS) tube
    b. complete blood count tube
    c. nonadditive discard tube
    d. STAT potassium tube

33. The purpose of a tourniquet in the venipuncture procedure is to:
    a. block the flow of arterial blood into the area.
    b. enlarge veins so they are easier to find and enter.
    c. obstruct blood flow to concentrate the analyte.
    d. redirect more blood flow to the venipuncture site.

34. Which type of test is most affected by tissue thromboplastin contamination?
    a. chemistry
    b. coagulation
    c. microbiology
    d. serology

35. Which of the following tests would be most affected by carryover of K_2EDTA?
    a. blood urea nitrogen
    b. glucose
    c. potassium
    d. sodium

36. Which one of the following can be deleted from a list of symptoms of needle phobia?
    a. arrhythmia.
    b. fainting.
    c. lightheadedness.
    d. muscle cramps.

37. Steps taken to unmistakably connect a specimen and the accompanying paperwork to a specific individual are called:
    a. accessioning the specimen.
    b. barcoding specimen labels.
    c. collection verification.
    d. patient identification.

38. What is the recommended disinfectant for blood culture sites in infants 2 months and older?
    a. Isopropyl alcohol swab
    b. Chlorhexidine gluconate
    c. Benzalkonium chloride
    d. Povidone–iodine swab

39. Which BC is inoculated first when the specimen has been collected by needle and syringe?
    a. Aerobic media
    b. Anaerobic vial
    c. ARD container
    d. It does not matter

40. Latent fibrin formation in serum can result from:
    a. a centrifuge speed that is set too high.
    b. a long delay before centrifugation.
    c. gross hemolysis of the specimen.
    d. incomplete clotting when centrifuged.

41. You must collect a light blue top for a special coagulation test from a patient who has an IV in the left wrist area and dermatitis all over the right arm and hand. The veins on the right arm and hand are not readily visible. What is the best way to proceed?
    a. Apply a tourniquet on the right arm over a towel & do the draw.
    b. Ask the patient's nurse to collect the specimen from the IV line.
    c. Collect from the left antecubital area without using a tourniquet.
    d. Collect the specimen by capillary puncture from the left hand.

42. What is the *best* thing to do if the vein can be felt but not seen, even with the tourniquet on?
    a. Insert the needle where you think it is and probe until you find it.
    b. Keep the tourniquet on while cleaning the site and during the draw.
    c. Look for visual clues on the skin to remind you where the vein is.
    d. Mark the spot using a felt tip pen and clean it off when finished.

43. When is the best time to release the tourniquet during venipuncture?
    a. After the last tube has been filled completely.
    b. After the needle is withdrawn and covered.
    c. As soon as blood begins to flow into the tube.
    d. As soon as the needle penetrates the skin.

44. All of the following are proper techniques for collecting specimen tubes when using the evacuated tube method EXCEPT:
    a. collect sterile specimens before all other specimens.
    b. draw a "clear" tube before special coagulation tests.
    c. fill each tube until the normal vacuum is exhausted.
    d. position the arm so tubes fill from stopper end up.

45. It is important to fill anticoagulant tubes to the proper level to ensure that:
    a. the specimen yields enough serum for the required tests.
    b. there is a proper ratio of blood to anticoagulant additive.
    c. there is an adequate amount of blood to perform the test.
    d. tissue fluid contamination of the specimen is minimized.

46. You have just made two unsuccessful attempts to collect a fasting blood specimen from an outpatient. The patient rotates his arm, and you notice a large vein that you had not seen before. How do you proceed?
    a. Ask another phlebotomist to collect the fasting specimen.
    b. Ask the patient to come back later so that you can try again.
    c. Call the supervisor for permission to make a third attempt.
    d. Make a third attempt on the newly discovered large vein.

47. When drawing blood from an older child the most important consideration is:
    a. assuring the child that it won't be painful.
    b. explaining all of the tests being collected.
    c. explaining the importance of holding still.
    d. offering the child a reward for not crying.

48. According to CLSI this test is negatively affected by tube system transportation.
    a. albumin
    b. creatinine
    c. potassium
    d. uric acid

49. It is untrue that capillary specimens contain:
    a. arterial blood
    b. serous fluids
    c. tissue fluids
    d. venous blood

50. Which two federal agencies work together to regulate the transporting of biological specimens off site?
    a. CAP & CLSI
    b. CLIA & IATA
    c. DOT & IATA
    d. FDA & OSHA

51. It is necessary to control the depth of lancet insertion during heel puncture to avoid:
    a. damage to the tendons.
    b. injuring the calcaneus.
    c. puncturing an artery.
    d. unnecessary bleeding.

52. In which of the following areas does capillary specimen collection differ from routine venipuncture when collecting a BUN and CBC?
    a. additives used
    b. antiseptic used
    c. ID procedures
    d. order of draw

53. A blood smear prepared from an EDTA specimen should be made:
    a. after the blood cells settle in the tube.
    b. at the time the specimen is collected.
    c. before the specimen has been mixed.
    d. within 1 hour of specimen collection.

54. An infant may require a blood transfusion if blood levels of this substance exceed 18 mg/dL.
    a. bilirubin
    b. carnitine
    c. galactose
    d. thyroxine

55. Phenylketonuria is a:
    a. contagious condition caused by lack of phenylalanine.
    b. disorder caused by excessive phenylalanine ingestion.
    c. genetic disorder involving phenylalanine metabolism.
    d. temporary condition caused by lack of phenylalanine.

56. Arteriospasm is defined as:
    a. artery contraction due to pain, irritation by a needle, or anxiety.
    b. fainting related to hypotension caused by a nervous response.
    c. pain that shoots up the side of the arm after needle penetration.
    d. tingling feeling in the fingertips when a needle enters an artery.

57. When thawing a frozen sample, the procedure is to:
    a. heat it in a warm waterbath; invert it occasionally.
    b. thaw it in the refrigerator; mix only when thawed.
    c. warm it at 25 deg C; invert 10-20 times after thawing.
    d. warm it at 37 deg C; mixing it when ready for testing.

58. Computerized analyzers in the laboratory can read barcodes and ID patients if the:
    a. barcode is anywhere on the specimen
    b. label is placed horizontally on the tube
    c. label is placed correctly on the tube
    d. specimen is in the right evacuated tube

59. This is an example of a preanalytical error made at the time of collection.
    a. delay in transporting
    b. failing to mix tubes
    c. incomplete requisition
    d. waiting to centrifuge

60. What constitutes a positive modified Allen test? The
    a. blood pressure increases in the radial artery.
    b. color drains from hand at least 30 seconds.
    c. hand color returns to normal in 15 seconds.
    d. pulse in the ulnar artery becomes irregular.

61. Some blood specimens require cooling to:
    a. avoid hemolysis of RBCs.
    b. prevent premature clotting.
    c. promote serum separation.
    d. slow metabolic processes.

62. All of the following are correct in stating the importance of specimen handling EXCEPT:
    a. Effects of mishandling are not always obvious.
    b. Improper handling can affect quality of results.
    c. Many lab errors occur in the preanalytical phase.
    d. Mishandling effects can be corrected if identified.

63. Which of the following actions will compromise the quality of the specimen?
    a. drawing a BUN in an amber serum tube
    b. mixing an SST by inverting it five times
    c. only partially filling a liquid EDTA tube
    d. transporting a cryofibrinogen at 37°C

64. Which of the following analytes does not require protection from light?
    a. ammonia.
    b. bilirubin.
    c. vitamin B_{12}.
    d. vitamin C.

65. Chilling can cause erroneous results for this analyte.
    a. ammonia
    b. glucagon
    c. lactic acid
    d. potassium

66. An example of a QA indicator is:
    a. all phlebotomists will follow universal precautions.
    b. blood culture contamination rates will not exceed 3 percent.
    c. laboratory personnel will not wear lab coats when on break.
    d. no eating, drinking, or smoking is allowed in lab work areas.

67. According to CLSI, which tubes should be placed upright as soon as they are mixed?
    a. gel tubes with anticoagulant
    b. light green gel barrier tubes
    c. light blue coagulation tubes
    d. nonanticoagulant gel tubes

68. Reference values for this test are higher for capillary specimens.
    a. calcium
    b. glucose
    c. phosphorous
    d. total protein

69. If a specimen has inadequate identification, the specimen processor may:
    a. add the missing information to the label.
    b. ask the phlebotomist to get a new sample.
    c. contact the patient for correct information.
    d. refer the tube to the laboratory supervisor.

70. According to CLSI, the maximum time limit for separating serum or plasma from cells is:
    a. 15 minutes from the time of collection.
    b. 30 minutes from the time of collection.
    c. 1.0 hour from the time of collection.
    d. 2.0 hours from the time of collection.

71. An aliquot is a:
    a. filter for separating serum from cells.
    b. portion of a specimen being tested.
    c. specimen being prepared for testing.
    d. tube used to balance the centrifuge.

72. Which of the following is the best way to prepare routine blood specimen tubes for transportation to the lab?
    a. Place the tubes in ice slurry.
    b. Seal the tubes in plastic bags.
    c. Wipe each tube with alcohol.
    d. Wrap them in the requisitions.

73. All of the following are a reason for transporting tubes with the stoppers up EXCEPT:
    a. encourages complete clot formation.
    b. maintains the sterility of the sample.
    c. minimizes stopper caused aerosols.
    d. reduces agitation caused hemolysis.

74. It is incorrect to say that specimen transported by courier or other transport systems must follow guidelines defined by:
    a. DOT.
    b. FAA.
    c. FDA.
    d. OSHA.

75. Which specimen may need to be transported on ice?
    a. ammonia
    b. bilirubin
    c. carotene
    d. potassium

76. A specimen must be transported at or near normal body temperature. Which of the following temperatures meets this requirement?
    a. 25°C
    b. 37°C
    c. 50°C
    d. 98°C

77. The liquid portion of a clotted specimen is called:
    a. fibrinogen.
    b. plasma.
    c. saline.
    d. serum.

78. A less invasive way than venipuncture to collect a specimen for DNA analysis is by:
    a. buccal swab
    b. NP swab
    c. sweat swab
    d. throat swab

79. The specimen for this test requires STAT handling and is typically collected by a physician in three or four sterile tubes.
    a. CSF analysis
    b. Gastric analysis
    c. Nasopharyngeal culture
    d. Suprapubic urine specimen

80. *Clean-catch* refers to the collection of urine:
    a. after cleaning the genital area.
    b. from a catheter in the bladder.
    c. in a container that is sterile.
    d. the first thing in the morning.

81. The patient has an IV in the left forearm and a large hematoma in the antecubital area of the right arm. The *best* place to collect a specimen by venipuncture is the:
    a. left arm above the IV entry point.
    b. left arm below the IV entry point.
    c. right arm distal to the hematoma.
    d. right arm in the antecubital area.

82. When a blood specimen is collected from a saline lock, it is important to draw:
    a. a 5-mL discard tube before the specimen tubes.
    b. coagulation specimens before other specimens.
    c. extra tubes in case other tests are ordered later.
    d. two tubes per test in case one is contaminated.

83. The most common reason for glucose monitoring through POCT is to:
    a. check for sporadic glucose in the urine.
    b. control medication induced mood swings.
    c. diagnose glucose metabolism problems.
    d. monitor glucose levels for diabetic care.

84. It is *not* a good idea to collect a CBC from a screaming infant because the:
    a. chance of hemolysis is increased.
    b. platelets are more likely to clump.
    c. specimen may be hemoconcentrated.
    d. WBCs may be temporarily elevated.

85. Point-of-care detection of Group A strep normally requires a:
    a. blood sample.
    b. nasal collection.
    c. throat swab.
    d. urine specimen.

86. Which of the following *cannot* be detected in urine on a special reagent strip that is dipped in the urine specimen and then compared visually against color codes on the reagent strip container?
    a. bilirubin
    b. glucose
    c. leukocytes
    d. thrombin

87. The AMT, ACA, and ASCP are agencies that:
    a. accredit phlebotomy programs
    b. certify laboratory professionals
    c. license allied health professionals
    d. monitor communicable diseases

88. Which of the following is the name or abbreviation for the federal law that established standards for the electronic exchange of patient information?
    a. CLIA
    b. HIPAA
    c. Medicare
    d. OSHA

89. A quadriplegic patient:
    a. can feel pain if there is no sensory damage.
    b. cannot speak due to upper body paralysis.
    c. is paralyzed only from the waist down.
    d. must have blood drawn by a physician.

90. According to CLSI depth of heel puncture should not exceed:
    a. 1.5 mm.
    b. 2.0 mm.
    c. 2.4 mm.
    d. 4.9 mm.

91. The standard of care used in phlebotomy malpractice cases is often based on guidelines from this organization.
    a. CAP
    b. CLIA
    c. CLSI
    d. NAACLS

92. The abbreviation for the federal regulations that established quality standards to ensure the accuracy, reliability, and timeliness of patient test results, regardless of the size, type, or location of the laboratory.
    a. BBP Standard
    b. CLIA '88
    c. JCAHO
    d. OSHA

93. Which of the following is most likely to result in exposure to an aerosol generated when a specimen tube stopper is removed?
    a. Covering the stopper with a 4 × 4 gauze while removing it.
    b. Removing the stopper with the tube held behind a shield
    c. Using a specially designed safety stopper removal device
    d. Withdrawing the specimen through the stopper by syringe.

94. Drawing a patient's blood without his or her permission can result in a charge of:
    a. assault and battery.
    b. breach of confidentiality.
    c. malpractice.
    d. negligence.

95. Failure to keep privileged medical information private is:
    a. breach of confidentiality.
    b. invasion of privacy.
    c. *res ipsa loquitur.*
    d. vicarious liability.

96. Malpractice is a claim of:
    a. breach of confidentiality.
    b. improper treatment.
    c. invasion of privacy.
    d. res ipsa loquitur.

97. When selecting a venipuncture site do not use an arm with:
    a. a very strong basilic pulse.
    b. an active AV graft or fistula.
    c. evidence of a recent draw.
    d. tattoos from elbow to wrist.

98. Which of the following specimens would most likely be rejected for testing?
    a. A hemolyzed potassium specimen
    b. An icteric bilirubin specimen
    c. A nonfasting glucose specimen
    d. An underfilled serum tube

99. If you have no choice but to collect a specimen from an arm with a hematoma, collect the specimen:
    a. above the hematoma.
    b. beside the hematoma.
    c. distal to the hematoma.
    d. through the hematoma.

100. The ratio of blood to anticoagulant is *most* critical for which of the following tests?
    a. alkaline phosphatase
    b. complete blood count
    c. glycohemoglobin
    d. prothrombin time

Pretest Answers

1. **Answer: b**

   Subject: Laboratory Operations/Coding/Billing

   Why: The current procedural terminology (CPT) codes were originally developed in the 1960s by the American Medical Association to provide a terminology and coding system for physician billing. Physicians' offices have continued to use it to report their services. Now all types of HC providers use CPT.

   Reference: Chapter 1, *Phlebotomy Essentials* 6e.

2. **Answer: a**

   Subject: Laboratory Operations/Communications

   Why: Language, age and emotions can all be barriers to communication and require special communication techniques for effective exchange of information to occur. In the case of a very emotional patient who cannot understand what the phlebotomist is asking of him, it is the responsibility of the phlebotomist to recognize the problem and do whatever it takes to be easily understood by patients.

   Reference: Chapter 1, *Phlebotomy Essentials* 6e.

3. **Answer: b**

   Subject: Laboratory Operations/Communications

   Why: Kinesics is the study of nonverbal communication or body language. Frowning is an example of negative kinesics or body language. Eye contact, good grooming, and smiling are all examples of positive body language.

   Reference: Chapter 1, *Phlebotomy Essentials* 6e.

4. **Answer: c**

   Subject: Laboratory Operations/Professionalism

   Why: As the "public relations officer" everything the phlebotomist does reflects on the whole facility. The phlebotomist is often the only real contact the patient has with the laboratory. In many cases, the patient equates this encounter with the caliber of care they receive while in the hospital. Positive public relations promotes good will and harmonious relationships with employees and patients. Mastering good public relations does not ever cover up for inexperience and lack of skills.

   Reference: Chapter 1, *Phlebotomy Essentials* 6e.

5. **Answer: d**

   Subject: Laboratory Operations/Professionalism

   Why: The Safety Manual contains policies and procedures related to chemical, electrical, fire, and radiation safety: exposure control; and disaster plans as well as complete details on how to handle hazardous materials. OSHA regulations require every business to have a workplace safety manual.

   Reference: Chapter 2, *Phlebotomy Essentials* 6e.

6. **Answer: b**

   Subject: Laboratory Operations/Infection Control

   Why: In healthcare, a susceptible host is someone with decreased ability to resist infection. A microbe responsible for an infection is called the causative or infectious agent. An exit or entry pathway is the way an infectious microbe is able respectively, to leave or to enter a host. A reservoir is a place where an infectious microbe can survive and multiply, and includes humans, animals, food, water, soil, contaminated articles, and equipment.

   Reference: Chapter 3, *Phlebotomy Essentials* 6e.

7. **Answer: a**

   Subject: Laboratory Operations/Infection Control

   Why: SDS stands for safety data sheet, a document that contains general, precautionary, and emergency information for a product with a hazardous warning on the label. The OSHA Hazard Communication (HazCom) Standard requires manufacturers to supply t an SDS for every hazardous product they make. Employers are required to obtain the SDS for every hazardous chemical present in the workplace and have them readily accessible to employees.

   Reference: Chapter 3, *Phlebotomy Essentials* 6e.

8. **Answer: b**

Subject: Laboratory Operations/Infection Control

Why: Immunity to a particular virus normally exists when a person's blood has antibodies directed against that virus. A person who has recovered from infection with a virus has antibodies directed against it and is considered immune. A person who does not display symptoms of a virus such as hepatitis B, but whose blood contains the virus, is capable of transmitting it to others and is called a carrier. A person who is susceptible to a virus has no antibodies against it.

Reference: Chapter 3, *Phlebotomy Essentials* 6e.

9. **Answer: b**

Why: Microorganisms (microbes) that are capable of causing disease are called pathogens. Communicable microorganisms are pathogens that can be spread from person to person. Only some pathogenic microbes live in the soil. Normal flora (microorganisms that live on the skin) do not cause disease under normal conditions.

Reference: Chapter 3, *Phlebotomy Essentials* 6e.

10. **Answer: a**

Subject: Laboratory Operations/Infection Control

Why: The CDC and HICPAC together developed the latest *Guideline for Isolation Precautions in Hospitals.* The guideline identifies two tiers of precautions; standard precautions to be used in the care of all patients, and transmission-based precautions to be used in addition to standard precautions for patients with certain highly transmissible diseases.

Reference: Chapter 3, *Phlebotomy Essentials* 6e.

11. **Answer: b**

Subject: Laboratory Operations/Professional Ethics

Why: Informed consent implies voluntary and competent permission for a medical procedure, test or medication. It requires that the patient be given adequate information regarding the method, risks, and consequences of a procedure before consenting to it.

Reference: Chapter 2, *Phlebotomy Essentials* 6e.

12. **Answer: d**

Subject: Laboratory Operations/Infection Control

Why: Anyone entering the room of a patient with airborne precautions must wear an N95 respirator, unless the precautions are for rubeola or varicella and the individual entering the room is immune.

Reference: Chapter 3, *Phlebotomy Essentials* 6e.

13. **Answer: d**

Subject: Laboratory Operations/Infection Control

Why: Work practice controls are routines that alter the manner in which a task is performed to reduce likelihood of exposure to bloodborne pathogens (BBPs). Wearing gloves to draw blood reduces the chance of exposure to BBPs. Ordering self-sheathing needles, reading the exposure control plan, and receiving an HBV vaccination are all important in reducing the risk of exposure to BBPs, but do not in themselves alter the actual performance of a task and are not considered work practice controls.

Reference: Chapter 3, *Phlebotomy Essentials* 6e.

14. **Answer: a**

Subject: Laboratory Operations/Safety

Why: Electrical equipment should be unplugged before servicing to avoid electrical shock. The use of extension cords should be avoided because they lead to circuit overload, incomplete connections, and potential clutter in the path of workers. Frayed electrical cords are dangerous and should be replaced rather than used. Malfunctioning equipment should be unplugged and not used until fixed.

Reference: Chapter 3, *Phlebotomy Essentials* 6e.

15. **Answer: c**

Subject: Laboratory Operations/Safety

Why: The OSHA HazCom Standard, which is called the "Right to Know Law", requires manufacturers of hazardous materials to provide an SDS for every hazardous products. An SDS contains general, precautionary, and emergency information about the product.

Reference: Chapter 3, *Phlebotomy Essentials* 6e.

16. **Answer: b**

Subject: Specimen Collections/Patient Identification

Why: The process of verifying a patient's identity, is the most important step in specimen collection. The patient must be actively involved in the identification process. When identifying a patient, ask the patient to state his or her full name and date of birth. In addition, the CLSI guideline GP33-A (*Accuracy in Patient and Sample Identification*) recommends having the patient spell the last name.

Reference: Chapter 8, *Phlebotomy Essentials* 6e.

17. **Answer: A**

Subject: Laboratory Operations/Quality Control

Why: Delta checks compare current results of a test with previous results for the same test on the same patient. Although some variation is to be expected, a major difference in results could indicate error and require investigation.

Reference: Chapter 2, *Phlebotomy Essentials* 6e.

18. **Answer: a**

    Subject: Laboratory Operations/Patient Confidentiality

    Why: Patient confidentiality is seen by many as the ethical cornerstone of professional behavior in the healthcare field. It serves to protect both the patient and the practitioner. The healthcare provider must recognize that all patient information is absolutely private and confidential. Healthcare providers are bound by ethical standards and various laws to maintain the confidentiality of each person's health information. Any questions relating to patient information should be referred to the proper authority.

    Reference: Chapter 6, *Phlebotomy Essentials* 6e.

19. **Answer: b**

    Subject: Specimen Collections/Glucose Tolerance

    Why: Note the time that the patient finishes the beverage, start the timing for the test, and calculate the collection times for the rest of the specimens based on this time. It is important to remember that the timing starts from beverage completion, not from the fasting or before the drink has been consumed. GTT specimens are typically collected 30 minutes, 1 hour, 2 hours, 3 hours, and so forth, after the patient finishes the glucose beverage.

    Reference: Chapter 11, *Phlebotomy Essentials* 6e.

20. **Answer: d**

    Subject: Circulatory System

    Why: The subclavian vein begins in the shoulder area and leads into the chest. The accessory cephalic median basilic, and median veins all have portions that are in the antecubital fossa.

    Reference: Chapter 6, *Phlebotomy Essentials* 6e.

21. **Answer: b**

    Subject: Specimen Collection/Blood Cultures

    Why: **Skin antisepsis,** the destruction of microorganisms on the skin, is a critical part of the blood culture collection procedure. Failure to carefully disinfect the venipuncture site can introduce skin-surface bacteria into the blood culture bottles and interfere with interpretation of results. The laboratory must report all microorganisms detected; it is then up to the patient's physician

to determine whether the organism is clinically significant or merely a contaminant. If a contaminating organism is misinterpreted as pathogenic, it could result in inappropriate treatment.

Reference: Chapter 11, *Phlebotomy Essentials* 6e.

22. **Answer: a**

    Subject: Circulatory System

    Why: Ions are particles that carry an electrical charge. The coagulation process requires the presence of calcium ions, which have a positive charge, for proper function. An anticoagulant prevents coagulation by binding or chelating calcium and not allowing it to enter into the coagulation process for which it is essential. Chloride, sodium and potassium are also ions. They function in other body processes, however.

    Reference: Chapter 6, *Phlebotomy Essentials* 6e.

23. **Answer: d**

    Subject: Specimen Collection/Chain of Custody

    Why: When specimens are collected for blood alcohol, other drugs or paternity testing, a special protocol, referred to as the **chain of custody,** must be strictly followed. Chain of custody requires detailed documentation that tracks the specimen from the time it is collected until the results are reported. The specimen must be accounted for at all times in case there is a reason that it might be taken to court. If documentation is incomplete, legal action may be compromised.

    Reference: Chapter 11, *Phlebotomy Essentials* 6e.

24. **Answer: d**

    Subject: Specimen Collection/Equipment

    Why: Outdated tubes should never be used. The tube vacuum and the integrity of any additive that might be in the tube are guaranteed by the manufacturer, but only if the tube is used before the expiration date. After that date, the additive may break down and no longer function as intended. In addition, outdated tubes may lose some of the vacuum and no longer fill completely changing the additive to sample ratio. In either situation, the results may be incorrect or erroneous. It has not been shown that the tube stoppers actually shrink when held past the expiration date or that bacteria start to grow in outdated tubes. It is important to note that some additives can be seen on the sides of tubes before blood is added because they are made this way at the factory.

    Reference: Chapter 7, *Phlebotomy Essentials* 6e.

25. **Answer: c**

    Subject: Terminology

    Why: Hemolysis is the breakdown of red blood cells. The combining form *hemo* means blood. The suffix *lysis* means breakdown.

    Reference: Chapter 4, *Phlebotomy Essentials* 6e.

26. **Answer: d**

    Subject: Terminology

    Why: The word parts *iso-*, *neo-*, and *tachy-* are prefixes. The word parts *-al -lysis,* and *-pnea* are suffixes; *gastr, lip* and *onc* are word roots; and *ices, ina,* and *nges* are plural endings.

    Reference: Chapter 4, *Phlebotomy Essentials* 6e.

27. **Answer: a**

    Subject: Specimen Collection/Patient Considerations

    Why: NPO comes from Latin (*nil per os*) and means nothing by mouth. Patients who are NPO cannot have food or drink, not even water. Patients are typically NPO before surgery, not after.

    Reference: Chapter 8, *Phlebotomy Essentials* 6e.

28. **Answer: d**

    Subject: Tests and Disorders

    Why: Because the specimen is a complete blood count (CBC), it can easily be collected by fingerstick from the left hand. The right arm should not be used. Collecting the CBC from the IV is not worth the risk when it can easily be collected by capillary puncture. A competent phlebotomist should be able to decide what to do in this situation without having to ask the nurse.

    Reference: Chapter 1, *Phlebotomy Essentials* 6e.

29. **Answer: d**

    Subject: Specimen Collection/Special Tests

    Why: Before specimen collection for molecular genetic testing, essential information must be obtained. The patient's demographics are required and an informed consent form must be signed. Sterile whole blood specimens for molecular genetic testing are generally collected in the lavender-top EDTA tubes or tubes specially designed for this type of diagnostic study, ie, white-top gel tubes from Greiner Bio-One. When a test for RNA is ordered, the blood specimen must be sent for testing immediately or collected in a special stabilizing reagent. Blood specimens will be rejected if frozen, hemolyzed or clotted.

    Reference: Chapter 11, *Phlebotomy Essentials* 6e.

30. **Answer: d**

    Subject: Specimen Collection/Equipment

    Why: Most tube stopper colors indicate the presence (or absence) and type of additive in a tube. A green stopper indicates heparin, a lavender stopper indicates EDTA, and light blue normally indicates sodium citrate. A royal blue stopper, however, indicates that the tube and stopper are virtually trace-element–free. A royal blue top can contain no additive, potassium EDTA, or sodium heparin. Additive color-coding of a royal blue top tube is typically indicated on the label.

    Reference: Chapter 7, *Phlebotomy Essentials* 6e.

31. **Answer: c**

    Subject: Specimen Collection Equipment

    Why: An antiglycolytic agent is a substance that inhibits or prevents glycolysis (metabolism of glucose) by the cells of the blood. The most common glycolytic inhibitors are sodium fluoride and lithium iodoacetate.

    Reference: Chapter 7, *Phlebotomy Essentials* 6e.

32. **Answer: a**

    Subject: Specimen Collection Equipment

    Why: Tubes or containers for specimens such as blood cultures that must be collected in a sterile manner are always collected first in both the syringe and ETS system of venipuncture.

    Reference: Chapter 7, *Phlebotomy Essentials* 6e.

33. **Answer: b**

    Subject: Specimen Collection Equipment

    Why: The purpose of a tourniquet in the venipuncture procedure is to block the venous flow, not the arterial flow, so that blood flows freely into the area but not out. This causes the veins to enlarge, making them easier to find and penetrate with a needle. The tourniquet does not redirect blood flow, but does change the volume of the flow. The tourniquet must not be left on for longer than 1 minute because obstruction of blood flow changes the concentration of some analytes, leading to erroneous test results.

    Reference: Chapter 7, *Phlebotomy Essentials* 6e.

34. **Answer: b**

    Subject: Specimen Collection Equipment

    Why: Tissue thromboplastin affects coagulation tests the most because it is a substance found in tissue that activates the extrinsic coagulation pathway. Tissue thromboplastin is picked up by the needle as it penetrates the skin during venipuncture and is flushed into the first tube filled during ETS collection, or mixed with blood collected in a syringe. Although it is no longer considered a significant problem for prothrombin time (PT) and partial thromboplastin time (PTT) tests unless the draw is difficult or involves a lot of needle manipulation, it may compromise results of other coagulation tests. Therefore, any time a coagulation test other than PT or PTT is the first or only tube collected, a few milliliters of blood should be drawn into a "discard" tube.

Reference: Chapter 7, *Phlebotomy Essentials* 6e.

35. **Answer: c**

Subject: Specimen Collection Equipment

Why: K$_2$EDTA contains potassium. (K is the chemical symbol for potassium, and K$_2$EDTA is an abbreviation for dipotassium EDTA.) Carryover of potassium EDTA formulations into tubes for potassium testing have been known to significantly increase potassium levels in the specimen, causing erroneously elevated test results.

Reference: Chapter 7, *Phlebotomy Essentials* 6e.

36. **Answer: d**

Subject: Specimen Collection/Venipuncture

Why: Symptoms of needle phobia include pallor (paleness), profuse sweating, lightheadedness, nausea, and fainting. In severe cases, patients have been known to suffer arrhythmia and even cardiac arrest, but not muscle cramps.

Reference: Chapter 8, *Phlebotomy Essentials* 6e.

37. **Answer: a**

Subject: Specimen Collection/Venipuncture

Why: The steps taken to unmistakably connect a specimen and the accompanying paperwork to a specific individual is called accessioning the specimen. The accession number is automatically assigned when the request is entered into the computer.

Reference: Chapter 8, *Phlebotomy Essentials* 6e.

38. **Answer: b**

Subject: Specimen Collection/Blood Cultures

Why: According to the CLSI, chlorhexidine gluconate is the recommended blood culture site disinfectant for infants 2 months and older and patients with iodine sensitivity.

Reference: Chapter 11, *Phlebotomy Essentials* 6e.

39. **Answer: a**

Subject: Specimen Collection/Blood Cultures

Why: To transfer blood from the syringe to the culture bottles, activate the needle's safety device as soon as the needle is removed from the vein. Remove the needle and attach a safety transfer device to the syringe. Inoculate the aerobic bottle first and then the anaerobic.

Reference: Chapter 11, *Phlebotomy Essentials* 6e.

40. **Answer: d**

Subject: Specimen Processing and Handling

Why: If clotting is not complete when serum specimen tubes are centrifuged, latent fibrin formation may form a clot in the serum after centrifugation. Residual fibrin can also be present as invisible fibrin strands or microfibers that can directly affect some tests or cause problems with instrumentation. Consequently, serum tubes cannot be centrifuged until it is determined that clotting is complete.

Reference: Chapter 12, *Phlebotomy Essentials* 6e.

41. **Answer: a**

Subject: Specimen Collection Venipuncture

Why: When a person has dermatitis and there is no other site available, it is acceptable to apply the tourniquet over a towel or washcloth placed over the patient's arm. A coagulation test should not be collected from an IV and a coagulation tube cannot be collected by fingerstick. The area above an IV must not be used regardless of whether or not you use a tourniquet.

Reference: Chapter 8, *Phlebotomy Essentials* 6e.

42. **Answer: c**

Subject: Specimen Collection/Venipuncture

Why: If the vein can be felt, but not seen, try to mentally visualize its location. It often helps to note the position of the vein in reference to a mole, hair, or skin crease. Never insert the needle blindly or probe to find a vein as damage to nerves and tissue may result. Never leave the tourniquet on for more than 1 minute as hemoconcentration of the specimen may result. Marking the site with a felt tip pen could contaminate the specimen or transfer disease from patient to patient.

Reference: Chapter 8, *Phlebotomy Essentials* 6e.

43. **Answer: c**

Subject: Specimen Collection/Venipuncture

Why: According to CLSI guidelines, the tourniquet should be released as soon as blood flow is established. Releasing the tourniquet as well as having the patient release the fist minimizes the effects of stasis and hemoconcentration on the specimen. A tourniquet should not remain in place longer than 1 minute.

Reference: Chapter 8, *Phlebotomy Essentials* 6e.

44. **Answer: d**

    Subject: Specimen Collection/Venipuncture

    Why: The arm should be in a downward position during venipuncture so that tubes fill from the bottom up and *not* from the stopper end first. This keeps blood in the tube from coming in contact with the needle, preventing reflux of tube contents into the patient's vein, and minimizing the chance of additive carryover between tubes. Collecting sterile specimens before filling tubes for other specimens, clearing for special coagulation tests, and filling tubes until the normal vacuum is exhausted are all part of proper venipuncture technique.

    Reference: Chapter 8, *Phlebotomy Essentials* 6e.

45. **Answer: b**

    Subject: Specimen Collection/Venipuncture

    Why: It is important to fill additive tubes to the proper fill level to ensure a proper ratio of additive to blood. The proper fill level is attained by allowing the tube to fill until the normal vacuum is exhausted and blood ceases to flow into the tube. Tubes will not fill completely as there is always dead space at the top. Blood in an anticoagulant tube does not clot. A partially filled tube would likely yield enough specimen to perform the test; however, the results would be inaccurate. Tissue thromboplastin is a problem for some tests, particularly special coagulation tests collected in light blue tops. However, contamination can be minimized by first collecting a discard tube to flush the tissue thromboplastin out of the needle.

    Reference: Chapter 8, *Phlebotomy Essentials* 6e.

46. **Answer: a**

    Subject: Specimen Collection/Venipuncture

    Why: After two unsuccessful attempts at blood collection, *do not* try a third time. Ask another phlebotomist to take over. Unsuccessful venipuncture attempts are frustrating to the patient and the phlebotomist. With the exception of STAT and other priority specimens, if the second phlebotomist is also unsuccessful, it is a good idea to give the patient a rest and come back at a later time. An outpatient may be given the option of returning another day after consultation with his or her physician.

    Reference: Chapter 8, *Phlebotomy Essentials* 6e.

47. **Answer: c**

    Subject: Specimen Collection/Venipuncture

    Why: Older children appreciate honesty and will be more cooperative if you explain what you are going to do and stress the importance of holding still.

    Never tell the child it won't hurt, because chances are it will, even if just a little. It is all right to offer the child a reward for being brave, but *do not* put conditions on receiving the reward such as, "You can only have the reward if you don't cry." Some crying is to be anticipated, and it is important to let the child know that it is all right to cry.

    Reference: Chapter 8, *Phlebotomy Essentials* 6e.

48. **Answer: c**

    Subject: Specimen Processing and Handling/Transporting

    Why: Each facility's pneumatic tube system should be carefully evaluated for the effects of shock and vibration on the validity of laboratory test results. CLSI Guideline GP44-A4, states that in general, tests negatively affected by PTS transport are those influenced by red cell damage, and include potassium, plasma hemoglobin, acid phosphatase, and lactate dehydrogenase.

    Reference: Chapter 12, *Phlebotomy Essentials* 6e.

49. **Answer: b**

    Subject: Specimen Collection/Capillary

    Why: Capillary specimens are a mixture of arterial and venous blood, and tissue fluids that include interstitial fluid from the tissue spaces between the cells, and intracellular fluid from within the cells. Serous fluids are pale yellow watery fluids similar to serum that are found between double-layered membranes that line the pleural, pericardial, and peritoneal cavities.

    Reference: Chapter 10, *Phlebotomy Essentials* 6e.

50. **Answer: c**

    Subject: Specimen Processing and Handling/Agencies

    Why: Diagnostic specimens that are transported out of the area by public transportation are covered by **U.S. Department of Transportation (DOT)**, and **International Air Transport Association (IATA)** regulations for transportation of infectious substances.

    Reference: Chapter 12, *Phlebotomy Essentials* 6e.

51. **Answer: b**

    Subject: Specimen Collection/Capillary

    Why: The depth of lancet insertion must be controlled to avoid injuring the heel bone. The medical term for the heel bone is calcaneus. Puncturing an artery or damaging tendons is avoided by puncturing in a recommended area. A deep puncture does not necessarily produce more bleeding.

    Reference: Chapter 10, *Phlebotomy Essentials* 6e.

52. **Answer: d**

    Subject: Specimen Collection/Capillary

    Why: Capillary puncture releases tissue thromboplastin, which activates the coagulation process and leads to platelet clumping and microclot formation in specimens that are not collected quickly. This affects hematology specimens the most, consequently they are collected first. Serum specimens are collected last because they are supposed to clot. In the order of draw for venipuncture, which was designed to minimize problems caused by additive carryover between tubes, serum specimens are collected before hematology specimens. Carryover is not an issue with capillary collection. Isopropyl alcohol is the recommended antiseptic for capillary puncture and routine venipuncture. Patient identification is the same regardless of specimen collection method. Additives in microcollection tubes and stopper colors correspond to those of evacuated tubes.

    Reference: Chapter 10, *Phlebotomy Essentials* 6e.

53. **Answer: d**

    Subject: Specimen Collection/Capillary

    Why: A blood smear prepared from an EDTA specimen should be made within 1 hour of collection to prevent cell distortion caused by prolonged contact with the anticoagulant.

    Reference: Chapter 10, *Phlebotomy Essentials* 6e.

54. **Answer: a**

    Subject: Specimen Collection/Capillary

    Why: Bilirubin can cross the blood–brain barrier in infants, accumulating to toxic levels that can cause permanent brain damage or even death. A transfusion may be needed if levels increase at a rate equal to or greater than 5 mg/dL per hour or when levels exceed 18 mg/dL.

    Reference: Chapter 10, *Phlebotomy Essentials* 6e.

55. **Answer: c**

    Subject: Specimen Collection/Capillary

    Why: Phenylketonuria (PKU) is a hereditary (i.e., genetic) disorder caused by an inability to metabolize the amino acid phenylalanine. Patient's with PKU lack the enzyme necessary to convert phenylalanine to tyrosine. Phenylalanine accumulates in the blood and can rise to toxic levels. PKU cannot be cured but it can normally be treated with a diet low in phenylalanine. If left untreated or not treated early on, PKU can lead to brain damage and mental retardation.

    Reference: Chapter 10, *Phlebotomy Essentials* 6e.

56. **Answer: a**

    Subject: Specimen Collection/Arterial Blood Gases

    Why: Pain or irritation caused by needle penetration of the artery muscle and even patient anxiety can cause a reflex (involuntary) contraction of the artery referred to as an arteriospasm. The condition is transitory but can make it difficult to obtain a specimen.

    Reference: Chapter 14, *Phlebotomy Essentials* 6e.

57. **Answer: c**

    Subject: Specimen Processing and Handling

    Why: Some tests require the specimen to be refrigerated or frozen for analyte stability, especially if testing is to be delayed. Frozen samples should be thawed at room temperature (approximately 25 °C) and inverted 10 to 20 times after thawing before testing. It is important to consult the procedure manual for specific instructions.

    Reference: Chapter 12, *Phlebotomy Essentials* 6e.

58. **Answer: c**

    Subject: Specimen Collection/Labeling

    Why: One of the benefits of computerization of laboratory instrumentation has meant that analyzers can read/scan the bar code labels on a patient's primary tube for identification, but only if the labels are properly placed on the tube after drawing so that the scanner can read it correctly.

    Reference: Chapter 12, *Phlebotomy Essentials* 6e.

59. **Answer: b**

    Subject: Specimen Collection/Preanalytical Error

    Why: Failure to mix tubes using the required number of inversions at the time of collection is a preanalytical error that can lead to microclot formation or insufficient clotting.

    Reference: Chapter 12, *Phlebotomy Essentials* 6e.

60. **Answer: c**

    Subject: Specimen Collection/Arterial Blood Gases

    Why: When performing the modified Allen test, both the ulnar and radial arteries are compressed to stop arterial flow to the hand. With both arteries compressed the hand should appear blanched or drained of color. If the patient has collateral circulation, the hand will flush pink or normal color when the ulnar artery is released even though the radial artery is still compressed. The presence of collateral circulation constitutes a positive modified Allen test.

    Reference: Chapter 14, *Phlebotomy Essentials* 6e.

61. **Answer: d**

    Subject: Specimen Processing and Handling

    Why: Metabolic processes can continue in a blood specimen after collection and negatively affect some analytes. Cooling slows down metabolic processes. Some analytes are more affected by metabolic processes than others and must be cooled immediately after collection and during transportation. Cooling can delay clotting, but is not a desired effect. Cooling does not promote serum separation, nor does it help to avoid hemolysis.

    Reference: Chapter 12, *Phlebotomy Essentials* 6e.

62. **Answer: d**

    Subject: Specimen Processing and Handling

    Why: Proper handling of specimens is important for quality results. It has been estimated that 46 to 68% of all lab errors occur in the preanalytical phase. Proper handling is important because personnel may not be aware that the integrity of a specimen is compromised because effects of mishandling are not always obvious. Most effects of mishandling *cannot* be corrected.

    Reference: Chapter 12, *Phlebotomy Essentials* 6e.

63. **Answer: c**

    Subject: Specimen Processing and Handling

    Why: The additive in a tube is designed to work most effectively with an amount of blood that fills the tube until the normal vacuum is exhausted. Results on a specimen from a partially filled liquid EDTA tube may be compromised. Although a blood urea nitrogen (BUN) level does not need to be protected from light, it would not hurt to draw it in an amber serum tube. Serum separator tubes *should* be mixed. A cryofibrinogen specimen *should* be transported at 37°C.

    Reference: Chapter 12, *Phlebotomy Essentials* 6e.

64. **Answer: a**

    Subject: Specimen Processing and Handling

    Why: Bilirubin, and vitamins C and B_{12} are all analytes that can be broken down in the presence of light. Ammonia requires ASAP transportation in ice slurry, but is not affected by light exposure.

    Reference: Chapter 4, *Phlebotomy Essentials* 6e.

65. **Answer: d**

    Subject: Specimen Processing and Handling

    Why: The energy needed to pump potassium into the cells is provided by glycolysis. Cold inhibits glycolysis, causing potassium to leak from the cells, falsely elevating test results. Cooling can also cause hemolysis, which also elevates test results. If a potassium test is ordered along with other tests that require cooling, it must be collected in a separate tube that is not cooled. Ammonia, glucagon, and lactic acid all require cooling for accurate test results.

    Reference: Chapter 12, *Phlebotomy Essentials* 6e.

66. **Answer: b**

    Subject: Laboratory Operations/Regulatory Agencies

    Why: Following standard precautions guidelines, not wearing lab coats outside of work areas, and not eating, drinking or smoking in lab work areas are all safety rules. QA indicators are not considered rules but are statements that serve as monitors of patient care. By setting a limit or threshold value, the QA indicators serve as initiators of action plans.

    Reference: Chapter 2, *Phlebotomy Essentials* 6e.

67. **Answer: d**

    Subject: Specimen Processing and Handling/ Transporting

    Why: Nonanticoagulant gel tubes should be placed in an upright positon as soon as they are mixed. This upright position aids clot formation and prevents the clot from attaching to the stopper.

    Reference: Chapter 12, *Phlebotomy Essentials* 6e.

68. **Answer: b**

    Subject: Specimen Collection/Capillary

    Why: Because the composition of capillary blood differs from that of venous blood, reference (normal) values may also differ. Most differences are minor, however clinically significant differences in some analytes have been reported. For example, the concentration of glucose is normally higher in capillary blood specimens, whereas bilirubin, calcium (Ca^{2+}), chloride, sodium, and total protein (TP) concentrations are lower.

    Reference: Chapter 10, *Phlebotomy Essentials* 6e.

69. **Answer: b**

    Subject: Specimen Processing and Handling

    Why: Suitable specimens are required for accurate laboratory results. Unsuitable specimens must be rejected for testing and new specimens obtained. A properly identified specimen is essential because it links the test results to the patient. Consequently, inadequate patient information on a specimen is reason for rejection by the specimen processor and a request for a new specimen.

    Reference: Chapter 12, *Phlebotomy Essentials* 6e.

70. **Answer: d**

    Subject: Specimen Processing and Handling

    Why: All specimens should be transported to the laboratory promptly. According to Clinical and Laboratory Standards Institute (CLSI) guidelines, unless conclusive evidence indicates that longer times do not affect the accuracy of test results, specimens should be separated from the cells as soon as possible with a maximum time limit of two hours.

    Reference: Chapter 12, *Phlebotomy Essentials* 6e.

71. **Answer: b**

    Subject: Specimen Processing and Handling

    Why: An aliquot is a portion of a specimen being tested. When several tests are to be performed on the same specimen, portions of the specimen are transferred into separate tubes so that each test has its own tube of specimen. Each portion is called an aliquot, and the tubes containing each portion are called aliquot tubes. Each aliquot tube is labeled with the same identifying information as the original tube.

    Reference: Chapter 12, *Phlebotomy Essentials* 6e.

72. **Answer: b**

    Subject: Specimen Processing and Handling

    Why: Blood specimen tubes are typically placed in plastic bags for transportation to the laboratory. CLSI and OSHA guidelines require specimen transport bags to have a bio-hazard logo and a liquid-tight closure.

    Reference: Chapter 12, *Phlebotomy Essentials* 6e.

73. **Answer: b**

    Subject: Specimen Processing and Handling/
    Transporting

    Why: Transporting tubes with the stopper up aids clotting of serum tubes, allows fluids to drain away from the stopper to minimize aerosol generation when the stopper is removed, and reduces the chance of hemolysis caused by agitation of the tube contents during transportation. If the tube contents are sterile they will remain that way until the tube is opened regardless of tube position during transport.

    Reference: Chapter 12, *Phlebotomy Essentials* 6e.

74. **Answer: c**

    Subject: Specimen Processing and Handling/
    Transporting

    Why: The Food and Drug Administration (FDA) does not issue guidelines for transporting specimens. Specimens transported by courier or other air or ground mail systems must follow guidelines defined by the Department of Transportation (DOT), the Federal Aviation Administration (FAA), and OSHA.

    Reference: Chapter 12, *Phlebotomy Essentials* 6e.

75. **Answer: a**

    Subject: Specimen Processing and Handling/
    Transporting

    Why: Ammonia specimens are extremely volatile and must be transported ASAP on ice. The expression "on ice" means in an ice slurry. Bilirubin and carotene specimens require protection from light. A potassium specimen should be collected and transported at room temperature.

    Reference: Chapter 12, *Phlebotomy Essentials* 6e.

76. **Answer: b**

    Subject: Specimen Processing and Handling/
    Transporting

    Why: Normal body temperature is approximately 37°C (98.6 F).

    Reference: Chapter 12, *Phlebotomy Essentials* 6e.

77. **Answer: d**

    Subject: Circulatory System

    Why: A clotted blood specimen is actually made up of two parts, a clotted portion containing cells enmeshed in fibrin, and a liquid portion called serum. The liquid portion is called serum because it does not contain fibrinogen. The fibrinogen was used up in the process of clot formation.

    Reference: Chapter 6, *Phlebotomy Essentials* 6e.

78. **Answer: a**

    Subject: Specimen Processing and Handling/
    Special Tests

    Why: Collection of a **buccal** (cheek) **swab** or oral specimen is a rapid, less invasive, and painless alternative to blood collection for obtaining cells for DNA analysis. (Plus, DNA is more easily extracted from buccal swabs than from blood samples).

    Reference: Chapter 13, *Phlebotomy Essentials* 6e.

79. **Answer: a**

    Subject: Specimen Processing and Handling/
    Special Tests

    Why: **Cerebrospinal fluid (CSF)** is the fluid that surrounds and helps cushion the brain and spinal cord. It is normally a clear, colorless liquid that has many of the same constituents as blood plasma. CSF specimens are obtained by a physician; most often through lumbar puncture (spinal tap) and are considered a "stat" test. CSF is generally collected in 3 or 4 special sterile screw top tubes specifically numbered in order of collection

Reference: Chapter 13, *Phlebotomy Essentials* 6e.

80. **Answer: a**

Subject: Specimen Processing and Handling/ Special Tests

Why: Clean catch refers to a urine specimen collected after following a special cleaning procedure used to ensure that the specimen is free of contaminating material from the external genital area. A catheterized specimen is collected from a catheter inserted into the bladder. A urine specimen collected in a sterile container is not necessarily a clean-catch specimen, although a clean-catch specimen *is* supposed to be collected in a sterile container. Urine collected first thing in the morning is called an 8-hour or first voided specimen and is not necessarily collected by clean-catch procedures.

Reference: Chapter 13, *Phlebotomy Essentials* 6e.

81. **Answer: c**

Subject: Specimen Collection

Why: When one arm has an IV it is preferred that the specimen be collected from the other arm if possible. Never collect a blood specimen above an IV or a hematoma. When there is no alternative site, perform the venipuncture below or distal to the hematoma. Venipuncture through or close to a hematoma is painful to the patient and can result in collection of blood from outside the vein that is hemolyzed or contaminated by the IV, and unsuitable for testing. Going below (distal) to the hematoma ensures collection of blood that is free-flowing and unaltered by the effects of the clotting and hemolysis in the area.

Reference: Chapter 9, *Phlebotomy Essentials* 6e.

82. **Answer: a**

Subject: Specimen Collection

Why: When a blood specimen is collected from a saline lock, a 5-mL discard tube must be drawn first to eliminate residual saline or heparin used to flush the device and keep it from clotting. The only extra tube collected is the clear tube. Drawing coagulation specimens from a saline lock is not recommended. Only nurses and specially trained personnel draw from such devices.

Reference: Chapter 9, *Phlebotomy Essentials* 6e.

83. **Answer: d**

Subject: POCT

Why: Glucose monitoring in diabetics (people with diabetes mellitus) is the most common

reason for performing glucose testing through point-of-care testing (POCT).

Reference: Chapter 11, *Phlebotomy Essentials* 6e.

84. **Answer: d**

Subject: Specimen Collection/Infant

Why: Studies performed on crying infants have demonstrated significant increases in white blood cell (WBC) counts, which are a part of a complete blood count (CBC). Counts returned to normal within 1 hour after crying stopped. For this reason, it is best if CBCs or WBC specimens are obtained after the infant has been sleeping or resting quietly for at least 30 minutes. Because an infant usually cries during blood collection, the specimens should be collected as quickly as possible. If a specimen must be collected while an infant is crying, it should be noted on the report.

Reference: Chapter 9, *Phlebotomy Essentials* 6e.

85. **Answer: c**

Subject: POCT

Why: Point-of-care detection of Group A strep normally requires a throat swab specimen. Secretions from the swab are tested for the presence of strep A antigen. A number of different companies make special test kits, for rapid detection of strep A.

Reference: Chapter 11, *Phlebotomy Essentials* 6e.

86. **Answer: d**

Subject: POCT

Why: Bilirubin, glucose, and leukocytes are all commonly detected in urine by reagent strip methods. Reagent strips also typically detect bacteria, blood, pH, protein, specific gravity, and urobilinogen, but not thrombin. A chemical reaction resulting in color changes to the strip take place when the strip is dipped in a urine specimen. Results are determined visually by comparing color changes on the strip with the chart of color codes on the reagent strip container.

Reference: Chapter 11, *Phlebotomy Essentials* 6e.

87. **Answer: b**

Subject: Laboratory Operations/Regulatory Agencies

Why: American Medical Technologists (AMT), American Certification Agency (ACA) and American Society for Clinical Pathology (ASCP) are among the agencies that offer certification for all levels of laboratory professionals. These agencies do not license allied health professionals because that is the responsibility of the states that have passed licensure laws. They do not accredit phlebotomy programs because that is the role of NAACLS.

Public Health Services (PHS) at the state and local level monitor communicable diseases.

Reference: Chapter 1, *Phlebotomy Essentials* 6e.

88. **Answer: b**

    Subject: Laboratory Operations/Regulatory Agencies

    Why: To more closely secure protected health information (PHI) and regulate patient privacy, a federal law was enacted and went into effect in 2003. The law, HIPAA, established national standards for the electronic exchange of PHI. The law, CLIA '88 mandates that all laboratories must be regulated using the same standard measurement regardless of the location, type or size.

    Reference: Chapter 1, *Phlebotomy Essentials* 6e.

89. **Answer: a**

    Subject: Specimen Collection/Preanalytical Considerations

    Why: A person who is paralyzed in both arms and legs is called a quadriplegic. Paralysis is the loss of muscle function. A person who is paralyzed can feel pain if there is no sensory damage. Quadriplegics can speak if the paralysis is only from the neck down. Phlebotomists can draw quadriplegic patients although the loss of muscle function can result in stagnation of blood flow and an increased chance of vein thrombosis that is magnified by venipuncture. Consequently strict venipuncture procedures must be followed (e.g. no probing or lateral needle redirection) and firm pressure must be held over the site after the draw until it is certain that blood flow has ceased.

    Reference: Chapter 9, *Phlebotomy Essentials* 6e.

90. **Answer: b**

    Subject: Specimen Collection/Infant

    Why: Studies have shown that heel punctures deeper than 2.0 mm risk injuring the calcaneus or heel bone. For this reason, the latest CLSI capillary puncture standard states that heel puncture depth should not exceed 2.0 mm.

    Reference: Chapter 10, *Phlebotomy Essentials* 6e.

91. **Answer: c**

    Subject: Laboratory Operations/Professional Standards

    Why: Clinical and Laboratory Standards Institute (CLSI) publishes standards for phlebotomy procedures. These national standards are recognized as the legal standard of care for phlebotomy procedures. CLIA and College of American Pathologists (CAP) set standards for healthcare organizations

and laboratories, respectively, but not specifically for phlebotomy procedures. NAACLS approves phlebotomy programs.

Reference: Chapter 2, *Phlebotomy Essentials* 6e.

92. **Answer: b**

    Subject: Laboratory Operations/Regulatory Agencies

    Why: The Clinical Laboratory Improvement Amendments of 1988 (CLIA '88) are federal regulations whose aim is to ensure the accuracy, reliability, and timeliness of patient test results no matter what the type, size, or location of the laboratory. The Occupational Safety and Health Act and also the Occupational Safety and Health Administration (OSHA) were designed to protect employee safety. The Bloodborne Pathogen (BBP) Standard was instituted to protect healthcare employees from bloodborne pathogens.

    Reference: Chapter 1, *Phlebotomy Essentials* 6e.

93. **Answer: d**

    Subject: Specimen Processing

    Why: To prevent aerosol exposure it is best to use robotics or a safety stopper removal device to open a blood specimen tube. It is also acceptable to cover the stopper with a 4 × 4 gauze to catch drips and any aerosol that might be released. Regardless, the processor should be wearing a full-length face shield or the tube should be held behind a bench-top splash shield or in a safety cabinet when the stopper is removed. Never use a syringe to withdraw a sample from a blood tube because it can create an aerosol, and it violates OHSA safety regulations.

    Reference: Chapter 12, *Phlebotomy Essentials* 6e.

94. **Answer: a**

    Subject: Laboratory Operations/Ethics

    Why: Attemping to draw a person's blood without permission can be perceived as assault, the act or threat of intentionally causing a person to be in fear of harm to his or her person. If the act or threat is actually committed than it can be perceived as battery also. Battery is defined as the intentional harmful or offensive touching of a person without consent or legal justification. Breach of confidentiality involves failure to keep medical information private or confidential. Negligence requires doing something that a reasonable person would not do, or not doing something a reasonable person would do. Malpractice is negligence by a professional.

    Reference: Chapter 2, *Phlebotomy Essentials* 6e.

95. **Answer: a**

    Subject: Laboratory Operations

    Why: Breach of confidentiality is the failure to keep privileged medical information private. An example is the unauthorized release of patient information such as laboratory results. This could lead to a lawsuit for medical malpractice if it caused harm to the patient, such as the loss of his or her job. Patient confidentiality is protected under state law.

    Reference: Chapter 2, *Phlebotomy Essentials* 6e.

96. **Answer: b**

    Subject: Laboratory Operations/Professional Ethics

    Why: Malpractice can be described as improper or negligent treatment resulting in injury, loss, or damage. Breach of confidentiality involves failure to keep medical information private or confidential as opposed to invasion of privacy, a tort that involves physical intrusion or the unauthorized publishing or releasing of private information.

    Reference: Chapter 2, *Phlebotomy Essentials* 6e.

97. **Answer: b**

    Subject: Specimen Collection/Preanalytical Considerations

    Why: A shunt is a dialysis patient's lifeline. Never apply a blood pressure cuff or tourniquet, or perform venipuncture, on an arm with any type of shunt.

    Reference: Chapter 9, *Phlebotomy Essentials* 6e.

98. **Answer: a**

    Subject: Specimen Handling and Processing/Preanalytical Considerations

    Why: Hemolyzed specimens can be attributed to invivo hemolysis due to patient conditions such as hemolytic anemia, liver disease, or a transfusion reaction, but they are more commonly the result of procedural errors in specimen collection or handling that damage the RBCs. Hemolysis can erroneously elevate a number of analytes, especially potassium. (There is 23 times as much potassium in red blood cells as in plasma).

    Reference: Chapter 9, *Phlebotomy Essentials* 6e.

99. **Answer: c**

    Subject: Specimen Handling and Processing/Preanalytical Considerations

    Why: If you have no other choice, it is acceptable to collect a blood specimen distal, or below a hematoma, where blood flow is least affected by it. A venipuncture in the area of a hematoma, including above, beside, or through it, is painful to the patient, and can yield erroneous results related to the obstruction of blood flow by the hematoma. It can also result in collection of contaminated and possibly hemolyzed blood from the hematoma, instead of blood from the vein.

    Reference: Chapter 9, *Phlebotomy Essentials* 6e.

100. **Answer: d**

    Subject: Specimen Handling and Processing/Preanalytical Considerations

    Why: A prothrombin time is a coagulation test. The ratio of blood to anticoagulant is *most* critical for coagulation tests because a ratio of nine parts blood to one part anticoagulant must be maintained for accurate test results. The excess anticoagulant in a short draw dilutes the plasma portion of the specimen used for testing, causing falsely prolonged test results.

    Reference: Chapter 9, *Phlebotomy Essentials* 6e.

Exam Topics and Study Hours by Topic

Anatomy & Physiology (5–10%)	Specimen Collection (45–50%)	Specimen Handling & Processing (15–20%)	Point-of-Care Testing (3–8%)	Non-Blood Specimens (5–10%)	Lab Operations (15–20%)
Structure & Function ☐ Recommended study time ___ hr.	Review of Orders ☐ Recommended study time ___ hr.	Accessioning ☐ Recommended study time ___ hr.	Urinalysis ☐ Recommended study time ___ hr.	Physiology ☐ Recommended study time ___ hr.	Quality Control ☐ Recommended study time ___ hr.
Blood Composition & Function ☐ Recommended study time ___ hr.	Patient Communication, ID, & Assessment ☐ Recommended study time ___ hr.	Labeling ☐ Recommended study time ___ hr.	H & H ☐ Recommended study time ___ hr.	Patient Preparation ☐ Recommended study time ___ hr.	Quality Improvement ☐ Recommended study time ___ hr.
Blood Specimen Types ☐ Recommended study time ___ hr.	Patient Prep & Site Selection ☐ Recommended study time ___ hr.	Specimen Quality ☐ Recommended study time ___ hr.	Coagulation ☐ Recommended study time ___ hr.	Collection ☐ Recommended study time ___ hr.	Interpersonal Relations ☐ Recommended study time ___ hr.
Body System Tests ☐ Recommended study time ___ hr.	Equipment & Techniques ☐ Recommended study time ___ hr.	Transport & Storage ☐ Recommended study time ___ hr.	Glucose ☐ Recommended study time ___ hr.	Handling & Processing ☐ Recommended study time ___ hr.	Professional Ethics ☐ Recommended study time ___ hr.
Terminology ☐ Recommended study time ___ hr.	Additives & Order of Draw ☐ Recommended study time ___ hr.	Equipment ☐ Recommended study time ___ hr.	Test Performance ☐ Recommended study time ___ hr.	Terminology ☐ Recommended study time ___ hr.	Standards & Regs. ☐ Recommended study time ___ hr.
	Complications ☐ Recommended study time ___ hr.	Terminology ☐ Recommended study time ___ hr.	Test Operation ☐ Recommended study time ___ hr.		Terminology ☐ Recommended study time ___ hr.
	Terminology ☐ Recommended study time ___ hr.		Terminology ☐ Recommended study time ___ hr.		

Summary of Study Hours

Study Item	Hours
Pretest Suggested Study Hours	_____
Additional study hours added for Specimen Collection and Handling which is >60% of the test questions on all exams	4
Timed mock exam (computer or written) and final prep hours	4
Total suggested minimum study hours	_____

Written Comprehensive Mock Exam

Choose the *best* answer.

1. Name the tube that a CBC is collected in, and identify the additive in the tube and the department that performs the test.
   a. Green top, heparin, chemistry
   b. Blue top, citrate, coagulation
   c. Purple top, EDTA, hematology
   d. Red top, no additive, serology

2. A phlebotomist who collects a specimen from an inpatient with this disease must wear an N-95 respirator while in the patient's room.
   a. Diabetes mellitus
   b. Infectious hepatitis
   c. Pulmonary tuberculosis
   d. Respiratory syncytial virus

3. Red blood cells are also called
   a. erythrocytes.
   b. leukocytes.
   c. lymphocytes.
   d. thrombocytes.

4. Identify the tube stopper color, department, and the order of draw for a trace-element test collected with a CBC and a protime.
   a. Green, immunology, collect it after the protime.
   b. Lavender, chemistry, the first tube to be drawn.
   c. Royal blue, chemistry, collect by separate draw
   d. Tan top, immunology, collect it last of all tubes.

5. A stat H&H on a postop patient is requested. Which of the following scenarios best describes the proper response?
   a. During the next sweep, collect that specimen first, and send it down to the lab in the tube system before proceeding with the rest.
   b. Go immediately to the surgical recovery room, collect a lavender top on the patient, and deliver it immediately to the laboratory.
   c. Proceed to postop as soon as possible, collect one red top on the patient, and return it to the laboratory as soon as possible.
   d. Proceed to surgery, collect a red top and a lavender top on the patient, and call someone from the lab to come get the specimens.

6. The phlebotomist arrives to collect a specimen on a patient named John Doe in 302B. How should the phlebotomist verify the patient's identity?
   a. Ask him, "Are you John Doe?" If he says yes, collect the specimen.
   b. Ask him to state his name and DOB and match it to the requisition.
   c. Check his ID band. If it matches the requisition, draw the specimen.
   d. Check his ID band. Then ask his nurse to verify his name.

7. A delay in processing longer than 2 hours can lead to erroneously decreased results for
   a. blood glucose.
   b. cholesterol.
   c. ionized calcium.
   d. occult blood.

8. Which type of specimen is typically used for routine urinalysis?
   a. 24-hour
   b. Double-voided
   c. First-morning
   d. Random

9. A positive FIT test indicates
   a. bleeding in the colon or rectum.
   b. *C. diff* colonization of intestines.
   c. presence of intestinal parasites.
   d. sizeable fecal fat accumulation.

10. A quick, noninvasive means of paternity testing is performed on cells from a
    a. 24-hour urine.
    b. buccal swab.
    c. CSF specimen.
    d. feces sample.

11. Hematoma formation during venipuncture could be caused by
    a. firm site pressure applied after needle removal.
    b. the needle bevel centered in the lumen of the vein.
    c. the needle bevel partially inserted into the vein.
    d. the tourniquet applied for less than one minute.

12. Accessioning a specimen involves
    a. connecting it with the correct individual.
    b. giving it a unique identification number.
    c. recording it in the order it was received.
    d. all of the above.

13. Antiseptics are
    a. corrosive liquid chemical compounds.
    b. designed to kill pathogenic microbes.
    c. safe and effective to use on human skin.
    d. used to disinfect contaminated surfaces.

14. Which of the following blood specimens has a critical blood-to-additive ratio and is most likely to be rejected by specimen processing if not filled to within 90% of the stated tube volume?
    a. ASO
    b. CBC
    c. BMP
    d. PTT

15. A breath test can be used to detect organisms that cause
    a. meningitis.
    b. peptic ulcers.
    c. tuberculosis.
    d. whooping cough.

16. A blood specimen collected in nongel tube has been centrifuged. The cells at the bottom are free flowing and can be resuspended if the tube is inverted. The term used to describe the liquid portion on top of the cells is
    a. lymph
    b. plasma
    c. serum
    d. solute

17. The composition of capillary puncture blood more closely resembles
    a. arterial blood.
    b. lymph fluid.
    c. tissue fluid.
    d. venous blood.

18. An accidental splash of bleach solution into the phlebotomist's eyes occurs while preparing it for cleaning purposes. What is the first thing to do?
    a. Blot the eyes with a wet paper towel several times.
    b. Flush the eyes with water for a minimum of 15 minutes.
    c. Proceed to the emergency room as quickly as possible.
    d. Put 10 to 20 drops of saline in the eyes and repeat twice.

19. Which specimen is most likely to be rejected for testing?
    a. Bilirubin specimen that is icteric.
    b. CBC specimen collected in EDTA.
    c. Fasting glucose specimen that is lipemic.
    d. Potassium specimen collected in heparin.

20. Which point-of-care blood analyzer uses a microcuvette instead of a test strip?
    a. AccuChek
    b. CoaguChek
    c. HemoCue HB201+
    d. I-STAT System

21. What is the *best* means of preventing an HAI?
    a. Proper immunizations
    b. Hand decontamination
    c. Isolation procedures
    d. Using disposable gloves

22. The suffix of the term hepatitis means
    a. condition.
    b. deficiency.
    c. infection.
    d. inflammation.

23. Symptoms of shock include
    a. decreased breathing.
    b. expressionless face.
    c. rapid, strong pulse.
    d. warm, moist skin.

24. The phlebotomist is unfamiliar with a test that has been ordered. The specimen collection manual says it requires a serum specimen. Which of the following tubes will yield a serum specimen?
    a. Green top
    b. Lavender top
    c. Light-blue top
    d. Plain-red top

25. Midstream clean-catch urine specimens require
    a. a preservative in the container.
    b. collection in a sterile container.
    c. timing of specimen collection.
    d. transportation at 37°C.

26. When the threshold value of a QA indicator is exceeded and a problem is identified
    a. a corrective action plan is implemented.
    b. an incident report is written and filed.
    c. patient specimens must be redrawn.
    d. patient physicians must be notified.

27. A phlebotomist arrives to collect a 2-hour postprandial glucose specimen on an inpatient and discovers that 2 hours have not elapsed since the patient's meal. What should the phlebotomist do?
    a. Ask the patient's nurse to verify the correct time to draw the specimen.
    b. Come back 2 hours from the time the patient says he finished his meal.
    c. Draw the specimen and write the time collected on the specimen label.
    d. Fill out an incident report form and give it to the phlebotomy supervisor.

28. Which of the following is referred to as a delivering chamber of the heart?
    a. Aortic arch.
    b. Left ventricle.
    c. Right atrium.
    d. Vena cava.

29. The exchange of nutrients and gases in the tissues takes place in the _____ and involves these blood cells.
    a. arterioles; granulocytes
    b. capillaries; erythrocytes
    c. lymph nodes; leukocytes
    d. venae cavae; lymphocytes

30. Which of the following would violate a patient's right to confidentiality?
    a. Discussing the nature of a patient's test results with the family.
    b. Giving the patient a physician's name that you know and trust.
    c. Sharing information on a "difficult draw" with a coworker.
    d. Showing a patient his or her lab results when requested.

31. Routine handling of additive tubes includes
    a. agitating until well mixed.
    b. mixing by 180-degree inversions.
    c. shaking gently 8 to 10 times.
    d. tilting back and forth twice.

32. What should a phlebotomist do if a patient feels faint during a blood draw?
    a. Have the patient lower his head and continue drawing the blood.
    b. Immediately stop the draw and have the patient lower his head.
    c. Remove the needle quickly and shake the patient to revive him.
    d. Use one hand to hold the patient upright and continue the draw.

33. Which of the following is an example of a nosocomial infection?
    a. Catheter site of a patient in intensive care becomes infected.
    b. Child breaks out with measles a day after hospital admission.
    c. Drug addict contracts hepatitis from a contaminated needle.
    d. Patient is admitted with symptoms suggestive of Hantavirus.

34. It is normally acceptable to perform venipuncture in this area despite the following:
    a. A massive, deep-looking scar covers the area.
    b. Petechiae appear with tourniquet application.
    c. The arm is edematous from an infiltrated IV.
    d. The only palpable vein feels hard and cord-like.

35. These are the initials of the two organizations responsible for the latest *Guideline for Isolation Precautions in Hospitals.*
    a. CDC and HICPAC
    b. CLSI and OSHA
    c. HICPAC and NIOSH
    d. NIOSH and OSHA

36. According to laboratory policy, specimens collected need to yield 2.5 times the amount of sample needed to perform the test. If a chemistry test requires 0.5 mL of serum, which of the following tubes is the smallest that can be used?
    a. Plain microtube
    b. 3-mL red top
    c. 5-mL SST
    d. 7-mL PST

37. A short in the wiring of a centrifuge causes a fire. Which type of extinguisher is best for putting it out?
    a. Class A
    b. Class B
    c. Class C
    d. Class D

38. To minimize effects of hemoconcentration caused by blockage of blood flow during venipuncture, the tourniquet should never be left in place longer than
    a. 30 seconds.
    b. 60 seconds.
    c. 2 minutes.
    d. 4 minutes.

39. Which of the following is an acceptable chemical safety procedure?
    a. Familiarize oneself with the SDS for any new reagent.
    b. If mixing acid and water together, add the water to the acid.
    c. Mix bleach with other cleaners for extra disinfecting power.
    d. Store chemicals at eye level so the labels are easy to see.

40. Which of the following would be the best vein to choose for a venipuncture on a female patient?
    a. Accessory cephalic just below the crease of the elbow.
    b. Basilic vein near the attachment of the biceps muscle.
    c. Cephalic vein proximal to the crease of the left wrist.
    d. Median vein near the middle of the antecubital fossa.

41. A newly hired phlebotomist has not been vaccinated against hepatitis B. The phlebotomist is immediately assigned to phlebotomy duties. According to federal law, the employer must offer the hepatitis B vaccination free of charge
    a. after any probationary period is over.
    b. immediately upon being hired.
    c. within 1 month of employment.
    d. within 10 working days of assignment.

42. QC protocols prohibit use of outdated evacuated tubes because
    a. additives that speed up clotting become crystallized in the tube.
    b. bacteria begin to grow in these tubes, yielding erroneous results.
    c. stoppers may shrink, allowing specimen leakage if the tube is inverted.
    d. tubes may not fill completely, changing additive-to-sample ratios.

43. Latent fibrin formation in serum can result from
    a. a centrifuge speed that is set too high.
    b. a long delay before centrifugation.
    c. gross hemolysis of the specimen.
    d. incomplete clotting when centrifuged.

44. Which of the following needles has the largest diameter?
    a. 18-gauge hypodermic needle
    b. 21-gauge multisample needle
    c. 22-gauge multisample needle
    d. 23-gauge butterfly needle

45. A phlebotomist explains to a patient that a blood specimen is going to be collected. The patient extends his arm and pushes up his sleeve. This is an example of
    a. expressed consent.
    b. implied consent.
    c. informed consent.
    d. refusal of consent.

46. The main difference between serum and plasma is
    a. plasma has fibrinogen, serum does not.
    b. plasma is obtained from clotted blood.
    c. serum is usually clear, plasma is cloudy.
    d. serum is pale yellow, plasma is colorless.

47. While processing blood specimens, blood is accidentally spilled on the countertop. What is the best way to clean it up?
    a. Absorb it with a damp cloth and wash the area with soapy water.
    b. Absorb it with a paper towel and wipe the area with disinfectant.
    c. Wait for it to dry and then scrape it into a biohazard bag.
    d. Wipe it up immediately with an alcohol pad and let it dry.

48. Which statement concerning human anatomy is true?
    a. A patient who is supine is lying down on his or her back.
    b. Phalanx is the medical term for the curved heel bone.
    c. Sagittal planes divide the body into upper and lower portions.
    d. The elbow is distal to the wrist and proximal to the shoulder.

49. Identify the tubes that can be used to collect a WBC, PT, and STAT calcium by stopper color and in the proper order of collection for a multitube draw.
    a. Gold, gray, light blue
    b. Lavender, green, royal blue
    c. Light blue, green, lavender
    d. Red, yellow, light blue

50. Which of the following would be the best site for a finger puncture?
    a. Central fleshy portion of the end segment of the index finger.
    b. Distal segment of the ring finger, slightly to one side of center.
    c. Medial or lateral fleshy pad of the nondominant index finger.
    d. Very tip of the proximal segment of the middle or ring finger.

51. The silica particles in an SST
    a. enhance the process of coagulation.
    b. keep RBCs from sticking to the tube.
    c. minimize hemolysis of blood cells.
    d. stop glycolysis by enhancing clotting.

52. Which of the following would be the best choice of equipment for drawing multiple tubes from a difficult vein?
    a. Butterfly and evacuated tube holder.
    b. Lancet and microcollection container.
    c. Needle and evacuated tube holder.
    d. Small gauge needle and 5-cc syringe.

53. A blood smear made from blood collected in EDTA must be prepared within
    a. a few minutes of collection.
    b. 30 minutes of collection.
    c. 1 hour of collection.
    d. 4 hours of collection.

54. Anaerobic conditions must be maintained when collecting and handling this specimen.
    a. Bilirubin
    b. Blood gases
    c. Glucose
    d. Plasma renin

55. Some specimens require cooling to
    a. avoid cold agglutinin activation.
    b. prevent the blood from clotting.
    c. separate serum more completely.
    d. slow down metabolic processes.

56. Which of the following represents proper collection and handling of newborn screening specimens?
    a. Apply multiple drops until all circles are filled; hang the form to dry.
    b. Completely fill at least three circles; put in a stack with others to dry.
    c. Fill circles on one side, fill them from the back side; let them air-dry.
    d. Use one free-flowing drop to fill both sides; air-dry flat and elevated.

57. It is incorrect to say that HIPAA was enacted to
    a. examine all patient healthcare records.
    b. protect privacy of patient information.
    c. provide guidelines for sharing of PHI.
    d. standardize electronic transfer of data.

58. The patient asks if the test about to be drawn is for diabetes. How should the phlebotomist answer?
    a. Explain that it is best to discuss the test with the physician.
    b. If the test is for glucose say, "Yes it is" but do not elaborate.
    c. Say, "HIPAA confidentiality rules won't let me tell you."
    d. Tell the patient that it is not for a glucose test even if it is.

59. Which of the following is a safe area for infant heel puncture?
    a. Area of the arch.
    b. Central plantar area.
    c. Medial plantar surface.
    d. Posterior curvature.

60. Generally, the minimum force and time required to result in good separation of serum or plasma from the cells is
    a. 1,000 g for 10 minutes
    b. 1,200 g for 15 minutes
    c. 1,300 g for 20 minutes
    d. 1,500 g for 30 minutes

61. The major structural difference between arteries and veins is
    a. arteries are larger in diameter.
    b. arteries have more tissue layers.
    c. veins have a thicker muscle layer.
    d. veins have valves that direct flow.

62. The phlebotomist arrives to draw a fasting specimen. The patient is eating breakfast. What should the phlebotomist do?
    a. Ask the patient's nurse if it should be collected and document it as a "nonfasting" specimen if drawn.
    b. Collect the specimen anyway, since the patient had not finished eating breakfast.
    c. Do not collect the specimen; fill out an incident report, and ask the nurse to reorder the test.
    d. Draw the specimen anyway, but write "nonfasting" on the test order and the specimen label.

63. The additive and color code associated with coagulation tests is
    a. potassium EDTA, lavender.
    b. lithium heparin, green.
    c. sodium citrate, light blue.
    d. thixotropic gel, red/gray.

64. What is the CLSI recommended blood culture site disinfectant for infants 2 months and older?
    a. Isopropyl alcohol swab
    b. Chlorhexidine gluconate
    c. Benzalkonium chloride
    d. Betadine swabsticks

65. All of the following statements concerning an employee bloodborne pathogen exposure incident are true EXCEPT
    a. all exposure incidents should be reported to the immediate supervisor.
    b. an exposed employee has access to a free confidential medical evaluation.
    c. the exposure should be documented on a standard incident report form.
    d. the source patient must submit to HIV and HBV testing within 48 hours.

66. Which additive prevents coagulation by binding calcium?
    a. Lithium heparin
    b. Potassium EDTA
    c. Sodium fluoride
    d. Thixotropic gel

67. Which of the following statements complies with electrical safety guidelines?
    a. Electrical equipment should be unplugged while being serviced.
    b. Extension cords should be used to conveniently place equipment.
    c. It is generally safe to use an electrical cord that is slightly frayed.
    d. Use electrical equipment carefully if it is starting to malfunction.

68. An ETOH specimen must be collected on a patient for forensic purposes. Which of the following tubes would be the best choice to collect the specimen?
    a. Gray-top sodium fluoride tube
    b. Green-top plasma separator tube
    c. Plain red-top clot activator tube
    d. Royal blue with green-coded label

69. Only one phlebotomist is on the night shift. Orders are received for all of the following tests within minutes of one another. Which test has the greatest collection priority?
    a. ASAP electrolytes in CCU
    b. STAT CBC in labor and delivery
    c. STAT electrolytes in the ER
    d. Timed blood cultures in ICU

70. It is necessary to control the depth of lancet insertion during capillary puncture to avoid
    a. excessive bleeding.
    b. injury to the calcaneus.
    c. puncturing an artery.
    d. specimen contamination.

71. Which of the following is the best way to tell if a specimen is arterial? As the specimen is collected, the blood
    a. appears bright cherry red.
    b. exhibits some air bubbles.
    c. looks thick and dark blue.
    d. pulses into the syringe.

72. A specimen must be collected on a 6-year old. The child is a little fearful. Which of the following is the best thing to do?
    a. Explain what is going to happen in simple terms and ask the child to cooperate.
    b. Have someone restrain the child and draw the specimen without any explanation.
    c. Offer to give the child a special treat if there is no crying during the procedure.
    d. Tell the child not to worry and to remain very still because then it will not hurt.

73. A prothrombin specimen must be collected from a patient with IVs in both arms. The best place to collect the specimen is
    a. above one of the IVs.
    b. below one of the IVs.
    c. from an ankle vein.
    d. from one of the IVs.

74. Biological Substance Category B regulations must be followed when shipping laboratory specimens for diagnostic purposes by public transportation. These regulations require the specimens to be
    a. in a container that can withstand a 8 to 10 foot drop.
    b. sealed in a secondary container made out of metal.
    c. triple packaged in a watertight primary container.
    d. all of the above.

75. A patient complains of significant pain when the needle is inserted. The pain does not subside and radiates down the patient's arm. What should the phlebotomist do?
    a. Ask the patient if it is all right to continue the draw.
    b. Collect the necessary amount as quickly as possible.
    c. Remove the needle and discontinue the draw immediately.
    d. Tell the patient there will be another stick if the draw is stopped.

76. Which of the following microcollection containers should be filled first if collected by capillary puncture?
    a. Gray top
    b. Green top
    c. Lavender top
    d. Red top

77. Which one of the following should be deleted from the list below of suggested quality assurance (QA) procedures?
    a. Checking needles for blunt tips and barbs before use
    b. Following strict requirements for labeling specimens
    c. Keeping track of and logging employee absenteeism
    d. Recording results of refrigerator temperature checks

78. Which of the following specimens is negatively affected by chilling?
    a. Ammonia
    b. Glucose
    c. Lactic acid
    d. Potassium

79. The CAP requires QC for many waived tests to be performed
    a. before each patient test performed.
    b. daily and when a new kit is opened.
    c. on a weekly basis as a minimum.
    d. when test manufacturer specifies.

80. Continuous quality improvement means
    a. accepting unionization by the hourly employees.
    b. being committed to ongoing process monitoring.
    c. overseeing employees' investments and retirement.
    d. providing annual salary increases and bonuses.

81. The most common reason for glucose monitoring through POCT is to
    a. check for sporadic glucose in the urine.
    b. control medication-induced mood swings.
    c. diagnose glucose metabolism problems.
    d. monitor glucose levels for diabetic care.

82. Which one of the following is found in a procedure manual?
    a. Description of QC checks for equipment used
    b. Instruction for reporting errors in specimen handling
    c. Listing of all revision dates for the procedure
    d. References to the applicable CLIA regulations

83. Which of the following pieces of information is typically required to be on an inpatient specimen label?
    a. Diagnosis
    b. CPT code
    c. Medications
    d. MR number

84. Which additional identification information is typically required on a nonblood specimen label?
    a. Accession number
    b. Patient diagnosis
    c. Physician's name
    d. Specimen source

85. Which of the following analytes requires protection from light?
    a. Ammonia
    b. Bilirubin
    c. Cryoglobulins
    d. Homocysteine

86. A technologist asks the phlebotomist to collect 5 cc of whole blood for a special test. What volume tube should be used?

    a. 3 mL
    b. 5 mL
    c. 10 mL
    d. 15 mL

87. A hospital uses computer-generated specimen labels. What information is typically added to the labels manually after the specimens are collected?

    a. Date, time, and collector initials
    b. MR number and admission date
    c. Patient's name and date of birth
    d. Test name and site of collection

88. Only one phlebotomist is in an outpatient drawing station. A physician orders a test that is unfamiliar to the phlebotomist. What is the appropriate action to take?

    a. Call the physician's office for assistance.
    b. Draw both a serum and a plasma specimen.
    c. Refer to the specimen collection manual.
    d. Send the patient to another drawing station.

89. CPT codes were developed by the AMA

    a. as a part of an ongoing process for monitoring CQI.
    b. so that patient information could be put into the HIS.
    c. to avoid confidentiality issues with patient information.
    d. to provide a classification system for physician billing.

90. Transporting tubes with the stopper up has nothing to do with

    a. encouraging complete clot formation.
    b. maintaining the sterility of the sample.
    c. minimizing stopper caused aerosols.
    d. reducing agitation caused hemolysis.

91. The first tube of cerebrospinal fluid (CSF) collected is typically used for

    a. chemistry studies.
    b. counting the cells.
    c. immunology tests.
    d. microbiology tests

92. Which one of the following can be deleted from a list of agencies that define guidelines for specimens transported by courier or other air and ground mail systems?

    a. DOT
    b. FAA
    c. FDA
    d. OSHA

93. Which of the following is *not* a required characteristic of a sharps container?

    a. Leak-proof
    b. Lid that locks
    c. Puncture-resistant
    d. Red in color

94. Which statement describes proper centrifuge operation?

    a. Avoid centrifuging serum specimens in the same centrifuge as plasma specimens.
    b. Balance specimens by placing tubes of equal volume and size opposite one another.
    c. Centrifuge serum specimens as soon as possible to stimulate the clotting process.
    d. Remove stoppers from the tubes before balancing specimen tubes in the centrifuge.

95. The manufacturer must supply an SDS for

    a. certain prescribed medications.
    b. fluid-resistant laboratory coats.
    c. isopropyl and methyl alcohol.
    d. isotonic sodium chloride solution.

96. Which type of specimen has processing and testing priority over all other specimens?

    a. ASAP
    b. Fasting
    c. STAT
    d. Timed

97. What is the recommended procedure for collecting a 24-hour urine specimen?

    a. Collect the first morning specimen and all other urine for 24 hours except the first specimen the following morning.
    b. Collect the first morning specimen and all other urine for 24 hours including the first specimen the next morning.
    c. Discard the first morning specimen; collect all the following specimens including the next morning's specimen.
    d. Drink 500 cc of water before starting the timing; collect all urine for a 24-hour period including the first and last.

98. The abbreviation for the federal agency that instituted and enforces regulations requiring the labeling of hazardous materials is
    a. CDC.
    b. CLSI.
    c. NFPA.
    d. OSHA.

99. A phlebotomist using an armband for patient ID must also
    a. check the room number for additional verification.
    b. have the patient state additional ID information.
    c. make certain requisition matches wristband.
    d. write down location of the patient on the requisition.

100. Point-of-care detection of group A strep normally requires a
    a. blood sample.
    b. nasal collection.
    c. throat swab.
    d. urine specimen.

Answers to the Written Comprehensive Mock Exam

Answers to the Written Comprehensive Mock Exam Topics and chapters from Phlebotomy Essentials 6th edition.

1. **Answer: c**

    COGNITIVE LEVEL: Recall & Application
    TOPIC: Specimen Collection (Venipuncture, Skin Puncture, Arterial Puncture)
    CHAPTER: 7

2. **Answer: c**

    COGNITIVE LEVEL: Application
    TOPIC: Laboratory Operations Related to Phlebotomy
    CHAPTER: 3

3. **Answer: a**

    COGNITIVE LEVEL: Recall
    TOPIC: Circulatory System
    CHAPTER: 6

4. **Answer: c**

    COGNITIVE LEVEL: Application
    TOPIC: Specimen Collection (Venipuncture, Skin Puncture, Arterial Puncture)
    CHAPTER: 7

5. **Answer: b**

    COGNITIVE LEVEL: Application
    TOPIC: Specimen Collection (Venipuncture, Skin Puncture, Arterial Puncture)
    CHAPTER: 8

6. **Answer: b**

    COGNITIVE LEVEL: Application
    TOPIC: Specimen Collection (Venipuncture, Skin Puncture, Arterial Puncture)
    CHAPTER: 8

7. **Answer: a**

    COGNITIVE LEVEL: Recall
    TOPIC: Specimen Processing and Handling
    CHAPTER: 12

8. **Answer: d**

    COGNITIVE LEVEL: Recall
    TOPIC: Nonblood Specimens (Urine, Stool, Other)
    CHAPTER: 13

9. **Answer: a**

    COGNITIVE LEVEL: Recall
    TOPIC: Nonblood Specimens (Urine, Stool, Other)
    CHAPTER: 13

10. **Answer: b**

    COGNITIVE LEVEL: Recall
    TOPIC: Nonblood Specimens (Urine, Stool, Other)
    CHAPTER: 13

11. **Answer: c**

    COGNITIVE LEVEL: Analysis
    TOPIC: Specimen Collection (Venipuncture, Skin Puncture, Arterial Puncture)
    CHAPTER: 9

12. **Answer: d**

    COGNITIVE LEVEL: Recall
    TOPIC: Specimen Collection (Venipuncture, Skin Puncture, Arterial Puncture)
    CHAPTER: 8

13. **Answer: c**

    COGNITIVE LEVEL: Application
    TOPIC: Specimen Collection (Venipuncture, Skin Puncture, Arterial Puncture)
    CHAPTER: 7

14. **Answer: d**

    COGNITIVE LEVEL: Application
    TOPIC: Specimen Collection (Venipuncture, Skin Puncture, Arterial Puncture)
    CHAPTER: 7

15. Answer: b

    COGNITIVE LEVEL: Recall
    TOPIC: Nonblood Specimens (Urine, Stool, Other)
    CHAPTER: 13

16. Answer: b

    COGNITIVE LEVEL: Analysis
    TOPIC: Circulatory System
    CHAPTER: 6

17. Answer: a

    COGNITIVE LEVEL: Recall
    TOPIC: Specimen Collection (Venipuncture, Skin Puncture, Arterial Puncture)
    CHAPTER: 10

18. Answer: b

    COGNITIVE LEVEL: Application
    TOPIC: Laboratory Operations Related to Phlebotomy
    CHAPTER: 3

19. Answer: c

    COGNITIVE LEVEL: Analysis
    TOPIC: Specimen Processing and Handling
    CHAPTER: 12

20. Answer: c

    COGNITIVE LEVEL: Recall
    TOPIC: Point-of-Care Testing (POCT)
    CHAPTER: 11

21. Answer: b

    COGNITIVE LEVEL: Recall
    TOPIC: Laboratory Operations Related to Phlebotomy
    CHAPTER: 3

22. Answer: d

    COGNITIVE LEVEL: Recall
    TOPIC: Medical Terminology
    CHAPTER: 4

23. Answer: b

    COGNITIVE LEVEL: Analysis
    TOPIC: Laboratory Operations Related to Phlebotomy
    CHAPTER: 3

24. Answer: d

    COGNITIVE LEVEL: Application
    TOPIC: Circulatory System
    CHAPTER: 6

25. Answer: b

    COGNITIVE LEVEL: Analysis
    TOPIC: Nonblood Specimens (Urine, Stool, Other)
    CHAPTER: 13

26. Answer: a

    COGNITIVE LEVEL: Application
    TOPIC: Laboratory Operations Related to Phlebotomy
    CHAPTER: 2

27. Answer: a

    COGNITIVE LEVEL: Application
    TOPIC: Specimen Collection (Venipuncture, Skin Puncture, Arterial Puncture)
    CHAPTER: 11

28. Answer: b

    COGNITIVE LEVEL: Recall
    TOPIC: Circulatory System
    CHAPTER: 6

29. Answer: b

    COGNITIVE LEVEL: Recall
    TOPIC: Circulatory System
    CHAPTER: 6

30. Answer: a

    COGNITIVE LEVEL: Analysis
    TOPIC: Laboratory Operations Related to Phlebotomy
    CHAPTER: 1

31. Answer: b

    COGNITIVE LEVEL: Analysis
    TOPIC: Specimen Collection (Venipuncture, Skin Puncture, Arterial Puncture)
    CHAPTER: 7

32. Answer: b

    COGNITIVE LEVEL: Application
    TOPIC: Specimen Collection (Venipuncture, Skin Puncture, Arterial Puncture)
    CHAPTER: 9

33. Answer: a

    COGNITIVE LEVEL: Analysis
    TOPIC: Laboratory Operations Related to Phlebotomy
    CHAPTER: 3

34. Answer: b

    COGNITIVE LEVEL: Application
    Topic 1: Problem Sites
    Topic 2: Specimen Collection (Venipuncture, Skin Puncture, Arterial Puncture)
    CHAPTER: 8

35. **Answer: a**
    COGNITIVE LEVEL: Recall
    TOPIC: Point-of-Care Testing (POCT)
    CHAPTER: 3

36. **Answer: b**
    COGNITIVE LEVEL: Analysis & Application
    TOPIC: Circulatory System
    CHAPTER: 6

37. **Answer: c**
    COGNITIVE LEVEL: Application
    TOPIC: Laboratory Operations Related to
    Phlebotomy
    CHAPTER: 3

38. **Answer: b**
    COGNITIVE LEVEL: Recall
    Topic 1: Specimen Collection (Venipuncture, Skin
    Puncture, Arterial Puncture)
    Topic 2: Specimen Quality Concerns
    Chapters: 8, 9

39. **Answer: a**
    COGNITIVE LEVEL: Analysis
    TOPIC: Laboratory Operations Related to
    Phlebotomy
    CHAPTER: 3

40. **Answer: d**
    COGNITIVE LEVEL: Analysis
    TOPIC: Specimen Collection (Venipuncture, Skin
    Puncture, Arterial Puncture)
    CHAPTER: 8

41. **Answer: d**
    COGNITIVE LEVEL: Recall
    TOPIC: Point-of-Care Testing (POCT)
    CHAPTER: 3

42. **Answer: d**
    COGNITIVE LEVEL: Analysis
    TOPIC: Laboratory Operations Related to
    Phlebotomy
    CHAPTER: 2

43. **Answer: d**
    COGNITIVE LEVEL: Analysis
    TOPIC: Specimen Processing and Handling
    CHAPTER: 12

44. **Answer: a**
    COGNITIVE LEVEL: Recall
    TOPIC: Specimen Collection (Venipuncture, Skin
    Puncture, Arterial Puncture)
    CHAPTER: 7

45. **Answer: b**
    COGNITIVE LEVEL: Application
    TOPIC: Laboratory Operations Related to
    Phlebotomy
    CHAPTER: 2

46. **Answer: a**
    COGNITIVE LEVEL: Analysis
    TOPIC: Circulatory System
    CHAPTER: 6

47. **Answer: b**
    COGNITIVE LEVEL: Application
    TOPIC: Laboratory Operations Related to
    Phlebotomy
    CHAPTER: 12

48. **Answer: a**
    COGNITIVE LEVEL: Analysis
    TOPIC: Anatomy and Physiology
    CHAPTER: 5

49. **Answer: c**
    COGNITIVE LEVEL: Application
    Topic 1: Specimen Collection (Venipuncture, Skin
    Puncture, Arterial Puncture)
    Topic 2: Order of Draw
    CHAPTER: 7

50. **Answer: b**
    COGNITIVE LEVEL: Recall
    TOPIC: Specimen Collection (Venipuncture, Skin
    Puncture, Arterial Puncture)
    CHAPTER: 10

51. **Answer: a**
    COGNITIVE LEVEL: Recall
    TOPIC: Specimen Collection (Venipuncture, Skin
    Puncture, Arterial Puncture)
    CHAPTER: 7

52. **Answer: a**
    COGNITIVE LEVEL: Application
    Topic 1: Specimen Collection (Venipuncture, Skin
    Puncture, Arterial Puncture)
    Topic 2: Butterfly Procedures
    CHAPTER: 7, 8

53. **Answer: c**
    COGNITIVE LEVEL: Recall
    TOPIC: Specimen Collection (Venipuncture, Skin
    Puncture, Arterial Puncture)
    CHAPTER: 10

54. **Answer: b**

    COGNITIVE LEVEL: Recall
    TOPIC: Specimen Processing and Handling
    CHAPTER: 12

55. **Answer: d**

    COGNITIVE LEVEL: Recall
    TOPIC: Specimen Processing and Handling
    CHAPTER: 11

56. **Answer: d**

    COGNITIVE LEVEL: Analysis & Application
    TOPIC: Specimen Collection (Venipuncture, Skin
    Puncture, Arterial Puncture)
    CHAPTER: 7

57. **Answer: a**

    COGNITIVE LEVEL: Recall
    TOPIC: Laboratory Operations Related to
    Phlebotomy
    CHAPTER: 1

58. **Answer: a**

    COGNITIVE LEVEL: Application
    TOPIC: Specimen Collection (Venipuncture, Skin
    Puncture, Arterial Puncture)
    CHAPTER: 8

59. **Answer: c**

    COGNITIVE LEVEL: Recall
    TOPIC: Specimen Collection (Venipuncture, Skin
    Puncture, Arterial Puncture)
    CHAPTER: 10

60. **Answer: a**

    COGNITIVE LEVEL: Recall
    TOPIC: Specimen Processing and Handling
    CHAPTER: 12

61. **Answer: d**

    COGNITIVE LEVEL: Application
    TOPIC: Circulatory System
    CHAPTER: 6

62. **Answer: a**

    COGNITIVE LEVEL: Analysis
    TOPIC: Specimen Collection (Venipuncture, Skin
    Puncture, Arterial Puncture)
    CHAPTER: 9

63. **Answer: c**

    COGNITIVE LEVEL: Recall
    TOPIC: Specimen Collection (Venipuncture, Skin
    Puncture, Arterial Puncture)
    CHAPTER: 7

64. **Answer: b**

    COGNITIVE LEVEL: Recall
    TOPIC: Specimen Collection (Venipuncture, Skin
    Puncture, Arterial Puncture)
    CHAPTER: 11

65. **Answer: d**

    COGNITIVE LEVEL: Analysis
    TOPIC: Laboratory Operations Related to
    Phlebotomy
    CHAPTER: 3

66. **Answer: b**

    COGNITIVE LEVEL: Recall
    TOPIC: Specimen Collection (Venipuncture, Skin
    Puncture, Arterial Puncture)
    CHAPTER: 7

67. **Answer: a**

    COGNITIVE LEVEL: Application
    TOPIC: Laboratory Operations Related to
    Phlebotomy
    CHAPTER: 3

68. **Answer: a**

    COGNITIVE LEVEL: Recall
    Topic 1: Specimen Collection (Venipuncture, Skin
    Puncture, Arterial Puncture)
    Topic 2: Toxicology Specimens
    Chapters: 7, 11

69. **Answer: c**

    COGNITIVE LEVEL: Analysis
    TOPIC: Specimen Collection (Venipuncture, Skin
    Puncture, Arterial Puncture)
    CHAPTER: 8

70. **Answer: b**

    COGNITIVE LEVEL: Recall
    TOPIC: Specimen Collection (Venipuncture, Skin
    Puncture, Arterial Puncture)
    CHAPTER: 10

71. **Answer: d**

    COGNITIVE LEVEL: Recall
    TOPIC: Specimen Collection (Venipuncture, Skin
    Puncture, Arterial Puncture)
    CHAPTER: 9

72. **Answer: a**

    COGNITIVE LEVEL: Analysis
    TOPIC: Specimen Collection (Venipuncture, Skin
    Puncture, Arterial Puncture)
    CHAPTER: 10

73. **Answer: b**
    COGNITIVE LEVEL: Application
    TOPIC: Specimen Collection (Venipuncture, Skin Puncture, Arterial Puncture)
    CHAPTER: 9

74. **Answer: c**
    COGNITIVE LEVEL: Application
    TOPIC: Specimen Processing and Handling
    CHAPTER: 12

75. **Answer: c**
    COGNITIVE LEVEL: Application
    Topic 1: Specimen Collection (Venipuncture, Skin Puncture, Arterial Puncture)
    Topic 2: Procedural Error risks
    CHAPTER: 9

76. **Answer: c**
    COGNITIVE LEVEL: Recall
    TOPIC: Specimen Collection (Venipuncture, Skin Puncture, Arterial Puncture)
    CHAPTER: 10

77. **Answer: c**
    COGNITIVE LEVEL: Application
    TOPIC: Laboratory Operations Related to Phlebotomy
    CHAPTER: 2

78. **Answer: d**
    COGNITIVE LEVEL: Recall
    TOPIC: Specimen Processing and Handling
    CHAPTER: 12

79. **Answer: d**
    COGNITIVE LEVEL: Analysis
    TOPIC: Laboratory Operations Related to Phlebotomy
    CHAPTER: 11

80. **Answer: b**
    COGNITIVE LEVEL: Recall
    TOPIC: Laboratory Operations Related to Phlebotomy
    CHAPTER: 2

81. **Answer: d**
    COGNITIVE LEVEL: Application
    TOPIC: Point-of-Care Testing
    CHAPTER: 11

82. **Answer: c**
    COGNITIVE LEVEL: Analysis
    TOPIC: Laboratory Operations Related to Phlebotomy
    CHAPTER: 2

83. **Answer: d**
    COGNITIVE LEVEL: Recall
    TOPIC: Specimen Collection (Venipuncture, Skin Puncture, Arterial Puncture)
    CHAPTER: 8

84. **Answer: d**
    COGNITIVE LEVEL: Recall
    TOPIC: Nonblood Specimens (Urine, Stool, Other)
    CHAPTER: 13

85. **Answer: b**
    COGNITIVE LEVEL: Recall
    TOPIC: Specimen Processing and Handling
    CHAPTER: 12

86. **Answer: b**
    COGNITIVE LEVEL: Application
    TOPIC: Specimen Processing and Handling
    CHAPTER: 12

87. **Answer: a**
    COGNITIVE LEVEL: Recall
    TOPIC: Specimen Collection (Venipuncture, Skin Puncture, Arterial Puncture)
    CHAPTER: 8

88. **Answer: c**
    COGNITIVE LEVEL: Application
    TOPIC: Laboratory Operations Related to Phlebotomy
    CHAPTER: 2

89. **Answer: d**
    COGNITIVE LEVEL: Application
    TOPIC: Laboratory Operations Related to Phlebotomy
    CHAPTER: 1

90. **Answer: b**
    COGNITIVE LEVEL: Application
    TOPIC: Specimen Processing and Handling
    CHAPTER: 12

91. **Answer: a**
    COGNITIVE LEVEL: Application
    TOPIC: Nonblood Specimens (Urine, Stool, Other)
    CHAPTER: 13

92. **Answer: c**
    COGNITIVE LEVEL: Recall
    TOPIC: Specimen Processing and Handling
    CHAPTER: 12

93. **Answer: d**
    COGNITIVE LEVEL: Recall
    TOPIC: Specimen Collection (Venipuncture, Skin Puncture, Arterial Puncture)
    CHAPTER: 7

94. **Answer: b**
    COGNITIVE LEVEL: Application
    TOPIC: Specimen Processing and Handling
    CHAPTER: 12

95. **Answer: c**
    COGNITIVE LEVEL: Application
    TOPIC: Laboratory Operations Related to Phlebotomy
    CHAPTER: 3

96. **Answer: c**
    COGNITIVE LEVEL: Recall
    TOPIC: Specimen Collection (Venipuncture, Skin Puncture, Arterial Puncture)
    CHAPTER: 12

97. **Answer: c**
    COGNITIVE LEVEL: Application
    TOPIC: Nonblood Specimens (Urine, Stool, Other)
    CHAPTER: 13

98. **Answer: d**
    COGNITIVE LEVEL: Recall
    TOPIC: Laboratory Operations Related to Phlebotomy
    CHAPTER: 3, 12

99. **Answer: b**
    COGNITIVE LEVEL: Recall
    TOPIC: Specimen Collection (Venipuncture, Skin Puncture, Arterial Puncture)
    CHAPTER: 8

100. **Answer: c**
     COGNITIVE LEVEL: Recall
     TOPIC: Point-of-Care Testing (POCT)
     CHAPTER: 11

Index

Note: Page number followed by f and t denotes figure and table respectively.